Patholo[gy]

Parakrama Chandrasoma, MD
Clive R. Taylor, MD

First Edition

Parakrama T. Chandrasoma, MD
Associate Professor of Pathology
University of Southern California
Director of Anatomic Pathology
Los Angeles County - University of
Southern California Medical Center

Clive R. Taylor, MD, PhD
Professor and Chairman of Pathology
University of Southern California
Director of Laboratories and Pathology
Los Angeles County - University of
Southern California Medical Center

APPLETON & LANGE
Norwalk, Connecticut/San Mateo, California

0-8385-5164-5

92 93 94 95 96 / 10 9 8 7 6 5 4 3 2 1

Prentice Hall International (UK) Limited, *London*
Prentice Hall of Australia Pty. Limited, *Sydney*
Prentice Hall Canada, Inc., *Toronto*
Prentice Hall Hispanoamericana, S.A., *Mexico*
Prentice Hall of India Private Limited, *New Delhi*
Prentice Hall of Japan, Inc., *Tokyo*
Simon & Schuster Asia Pte. Ltd., *Singapore*
Editora Prentice Hall do Brasil Ltda., *Rio de Janeiro*
Prentice Hall, *Englewood Cliffs, New Jersey*

Library of Congress Cataloging-in-Publication Data

Chandrasoma, Para.
  Pathology notes / authors, Parakrama T. Chandrasoma, Clive R. Taylor.
    p.   cm.
  Outline format of: Concise pathology.
  Rev. ed. of: Key facts in pathology. 1986.
  Includes index.
  ISBN 0-8385-5164-5
  1. Pathology—Outlines, syllabi, etc.   I. Taylor, C. R. (Clive Roy)   II. Chandrasoma, Para. Key
facts in pathology.   III. Concise pathology.   IV. Title.
  [DNLM: 1. Pathology—outlines.   QZ 18 C456p]
  RB32.C49   1991
  616.07—dc20
  DNLM/DLC
  for Library of Congress   91-22267
                                                                                CIP

PRINTED IN THE UNITED STATES OF AMERICA

CONTENTS

PREFACE

It is our experience that seconed year medical students frequently feel the need to have key facts in a review format during preparation for Part I of their National Board Examination. We have attempted to satisfy this need. *Pathology Notes* is presented in a terse, outline format with use of different levels of headings designed to provide the student with all the information needed in the minimum time possible. The use of frequent tables enhances the text and eases the assimilation of information. The material is divided into sections and chapters that provide the student with easily attainable goals for a relatively short period of study.

Pathology Notes is linked to Concise Pathology (Appleton & Lange, 1991) by the same authors. The larger book is designed for use as a textbook during the pathology course in the second year. For those students who have used Concise Pathology as their pathology textbook, this review text will be even easier to assimilate as it represents an outline format of Concise Pathology which presents the facts without the explanations and many of the illustrations.

We believe that this book will provide the most effective mechanism for rapid retrieval of the essential facts needed during preparation for course examinations and for the pathology part of the Board Examination.

—Parakrama Chandrasoma
—Clare R. Taylor
Los Angeles
August 1991

Section I. Effects of Injury on Tissues

Human disease results from the action of various injurious agents on parenchymal cells (Chapter 1) or interstitial connective tissue (Chapter 2), causing biochemical or structural damage.

Cell Degeneration & Necrosis

1

CELLULAR INJURY

LETHAL INJURY

Lethal injuries to the tissues of a living individual cause cell death (**necrosis**). Necrosis is

- Accompanied by biochemical and structural changes.
- Associated with failure of function.
- Irreversible.

NONLETHAL INJURY

Nonlethal injury to a cell may produce cell degeneration, which is

- Manifested as some abnormality of biochemical function, a recognizable structural change, or a combined biochemical and structural abnormality.
- Reversible, but may progress to necrosis if injury persists.

MECHANISMS OF CELLULAR DEGENERATION & NECROSIS

IMPAIRED ENERGY PRODUCTION

Causes
  A. **Hypoglycemia.**
  B. **Hypoxia,** which may result from

- Respiratory obstruction or disease.
- Failure of blood flow, due either to generalized circulatory failure or to local vessel obstruction.
- Anemia, resulting in decreased oxygen carriage by the blood.
- Alteration of hemoglobin (eg, in carbon-monoxide poisoning), making that substance unavailable for oxygen transport.

C. Enzyme inhibition, eg, cyanide, which inhibits cytochrome oxidase.
D. Uncoupling of oxidative phosphorylation, either through chemical reactions or through physical detachment of enzymes from the mitochondrial membrane.

Effects

Generalized failure of energy production first affects brain cells, causing neurologic dysfunction and disturbance of the normal level of consciousness.
  A. Intracellular accumulation of water and electrolytes:

- Accumulation results from dysfunction of the energy-dependent sodium pump in the plasma membrane.
- The earliest microscopic change of water accumulation is **cloudy swelling.**
- **Hydropic change** is a more severe change.
- Changes also occur in the intracellular concentrations of K^+, Ca^{2+}, and Mg^{2+}.

  B. Changes in organelles:

- Swelling of the endoplasmic reticulum interferes with protein synthesis.
- Mitochondrial swelling causes uncoupling of oxidative phosphorylation, which further impairs ATP synthesis.

  C. Switch to anaerobic metabolism, which leads to production of lactic acid and causes a decrease in intracellular pH.

IMPAIRED CELL MEMBRANE FUNCTION

Causes of Plasma Membrane Damage
  A. Free radicals:

- Free radicals are highly unstable particles containing unpaired electrons.
- Their excess energy is released through chemical reactions with adjacent molecules.
- Interaction between oxygen-based free radicals and cell membrane lipids (lipid peroxidation) leads to membrane damage.
- Free radicals are produced in cells exposed to
  - Powerful external energy sources, such as radiation.
  - Chemical poisons, such as carbon tetrachloride.

  B. Activation of the complement system: The final compounds of the activated complement pathway—a complex of C5b, C6, C7, C8, and C9—exert a phospholipaselike effect that can enzymatically damage the plasma membrane.
  C. Lysis by enzymes: Enzymes with lipaselike activity damage cell membranes.

- Pancreatic lipase liberated outside the pancreatic duct in acute pancreatitis causes extensive necrosis.
- Some microorganisms—eg, *Clostridium perfringens,* one of the causes of gas gangrene—produce enzymes that cause extensive necrosis.

Effects of Plasma Membrane Damage
  A. Loss of structural integrity.

B. Loss of function, eg, changes in selective permeability and active transport may result in

- Abnormal entry of water, causing cloudy swelling and hydropic change.
- Electrolyte imbalance in the cell, most commonly increased intracellular sodium and decreased potassium.
- Swelling and disruption of cytoplasmic organelles.

C. Deposition of lipofuscin (brown atrophy): Lipofuscin

- Is a fine, granular, golden-brown pigment composed of phospholipids and proteins.
- Accumulates in the cytoplasm as a result of damage to the membranes of cytoplasmic organelles.
- Is most commonly seen in myocardial cells, liver cells, and neurons.
- Causes no cellular functional abnormalities.
- Is also called "wear and tear" pigment because of its association with aging and chronic diseases.

Note: Accumulation results from a lack of cellular antioxidants that normally prevent lipid peroxidation of organelle membranes.

GENETIC ALTERATION

Causes of DNA Abnormalities
A. Inherited genetic abnormalities.
B. Acquired genetic abnormalities are somatic mutations caused by several agents, including ionizing radiation, viruses, and mutagenic drugs and chemicals.

Effects of DNA Abnormalities
A. Failure of synthesis of structural proteins:

- May cause necrosis due to inhibition of synthesis of vital intracellular structural proteins.
- May cause less severe damage, depending on the severity and type of inhibition of protein synthesis.

B. Failure of mitosis in actively dividing cell lines:

- In the bone marrow, leads to depletion of erythrocytes (anemia) and neutrophils (neutropenia).
- In the intestinal mucosa, causes atrophy of villi.
- In the testis, may result in decreased spermatogenesis, leading to infertility.

C. Failure of growth-regulating proteins may result in cancer (see Chapter 18).
D. Failure of enzyme synthesis:

- Enzyme deficiency in the embryo may result in congenital diseases (inborn errors of metabolism).
- Acquired enzyme defects result in necrosis if a vital biochemical system is affected.
- Enzyme defects involving less vital biochemical reactions result in various sublethal degenerative changes.

METABOLIC DERANGEMENTS

Exogenous Toxic Agents.
Exogenous toxic agents include alcohol, drugs, heavy metals, and infectious agents (see Chapters 8–14).

Endogenous Toxic Substances
Endogenous toxic substances are derived from deranged metabolism
   A. Fatty change (fatty degeneration): Clinically significant fatty degeneration

■ Is the accumulation of triglyceride in the cytoplasm of parenchymal cells due to an acquired defect in the metabolism of triglycerides.
■ Is common in the liver and rare in the kidney and myocardium.

   1. Causes of fatty liver:

■ Increased mobilization of adipose tissue, eg, in starvation and diabetes mellitus.
■ Increased rate of conversion of fatty acids to triglycerides in the liver cell, resulting from overactivity of the involved enzyme systems, eg, alcohol.
■ Decreased rate of oxidation of triglycerides to acetyl-CoA and ketone bodies, eg, in anemia and hypoxia.
■ Deficient synthesis of lipid acceptor proteins, as may occur in protein malnutrition or as a result of exposure to hepatotoxins, eg, carbon tetrachloride and phosphorus.

   2. Types of fatty liver.
      a. Acute fatty liver:

■ Is a rare but serious condition associated with acute liver failure.
■ Occurs in Reye's syndrome, or as a complication of pregnancy, or as a result of tetracycline toxicity.
■ Results in accumulation of *small*, membrane-bound triglyceride droplets in the cytoplasm (microvacuolar fatty change).

      b. Chronic fatty liver:

■ Is much more common than acute fatty liver.
■ Is associated with chronic alcoholism, malnutrition, and several hepatotoxins.
■ Results in accumulation of *large* fat (triglyceride) droplets in the cytoplasm (macrovacuolar fatty change).
■ Is grossly enlarged and yellow, with a greasy appearance when cut.
■ Is rarely associated with clinically detectable liver dysfunction, even when severe.

   3. Fatty change of the myocardium:

■ Triglyceride deposition in myocardial fibers occurs in chronic hypoxic states, notably severe anemia.
■ In chronic fatty change, bands of yellow streaks alternate with red-brown muscle ("thrush breast" or "tiger skin" appearance); this usually causes no clinical symptoms.
■ Acute fatty change occurs in toxic diseases such as diphtheritic myocarditis and Reye's syndrome; the heart is flabby and diffusely yellow; myocardial failure commonly follows.

B. Deposition of iron (hemochromatosis and hemosiderosis):

■ An increase in the total amount of iron in the body is termed **hemochromatosis.** The excess iron accumulates in macrophages and parenchymal cells as ferritin and hemosiderin, and causes parenchymal cell necrosis.

■ Deposition of hemosiderin primarily in tissue macrophages (histiocytes), with or without an increase in total body iron content and without parenchymal cell necrosis, is termed **hemosiderosis.**

1. Localized hemosiderosis (common):

■ Is common and occurs in any tissue that is the site of hemorrhage.

■ Occurs when hemoglobin is broken down and its iron is deposited locally, either in macrophages or in the connective tissue, as hemosiderin.

■ Has no clinical significance; its presence signifies only that hemorrhage has occurred at that site.

2. Generalized hemosiderosis (less common):

■ Occurs with relatively minor iron excess following multiple transfusions, excessive dietary iron, or excess absorption of iron in some hemolytic anemias.

■ Results from hemosiderin deposition in macrophages throughout the body, notably in bone marrow, liver, and spleen.

■ Can be diagnosed in bone marrow and liver biopsies.

■ Has no clinical significance apart from indicating the presence of iron overload to a minor degree.

3. Hemochromatosis (uncommon):

■ Occurs both as an idiopathic (inherited) disease and as a secondary phenomenon following major iron overload.

■ Is distinguished from generalized hemosiderosis by its greater degree of iron overload and the presence of parenchymal-cell damage or necrosis.

■ Acts by accumulation of free ferric iron after intracellular storage mechanisms are exhausted; ferric iron undergoes reduction to produce toxic oxygen-based free radicals.

■ Most severely affects the tissues of the liver, heart, and pancreas.

C. Deposition of copper (Wilson's disease):

■ Copper is a trace mineral that is normally transported in the plasma as ceruloplasmin, and "free" copper.

■ Normally, copper absorption is balanced by excretion, mainly in bile.

■ In Wilson's disease, which is an inherited disorder, excretion of copper into bile is defective and leads to an increase in total body copper.

■ Maximal accumulation of copper occurs in the liver and basal ganglia of the brain (hepatolenticular degeneration).

D. Accumulation of bilirubin: An increase in serum bilirubin is called **jaundice** or **icterus.**
1. Causes of jaundice (See Table 1–1).
a. Hemolytic jaundice:

TABLE 1-1. DIFFERENTIAL FEATURES OF THE DIFFERENT TYPES OF JAUNDICE

	Hemolytic Jaundice	Hepatocellular Jaundice	Obstructive Jaundice
Basic defect	Excessive production of bilirubin	Defective uptake, conjugation or excretion of bilirubin by liver cells	Obstruction of bile ducts
Elevation of serum bilirubin	Mild	Severe	Severe
Type of bilirubin in plasma	Unconjugated	Conjugated and unconjugated	Conjugated
Bile in urine	Absent	Present	Present
Urobilinogen in urine	Increased	Increased	Decreased (absent)
Stercobilin in feces	Increased	Variable	Decreased
Red cell survival	Decreased	Normal	Normal
Liver function tests	Normal	Abnormal	Variable
Bile ducts	May contain pigment stones	Normal	Obstructed, with proximal dilatation

■ Is caused by increased production of bilirubin due to increased erythrocyte breakdown.
■ Is manifested by
  ● Unconjugated bilirubin in serum.
  ● Conjugated bilirubin in bile, with increased incidence of bilirubin gallstones.
  ● Increased fecal stercobilin and urinary urobilinogen levels.
■ Unconjugated bilirubin is not excreted in the urine (**acholuric jaundice**).

  b. Hepatocellular jaundice:

■ Is caused by decreased uptake, conjugation, or excretion of bilirubin by the liver.
■ Is manifested by
  ● Elevated conjugated and unconjugated bilirubin levels in serum.
  ● Excretion of bilirubin in urine (commonly).
  ● Elevated urinary urobilinogen levels (usually), because the liver fails to reexcrete urobilinogen absorbed from the intestine.

  c. Obstructive jaundice:

■ Is caused by decreased excretion of conjugated bilirubin due to biliary tract obstruction, with the result that conjugated bilirubin accumulates proximal to the site of obstruction in the biliary tract and liver (**cholestasis**).

■ Is manifested by
- Elevated conjugated bilirubin in serum.
- Excretion of bilirubin in the urine.
- Decrease in fecal and urinary urobilinogen levels, due to failure of bilirubin to reach the intestine.
- Clay-colored stools (complete biliary obstruction).

2. Effects of deposition of bilirubin.
a. Deposition in connective tissue:

■ Of the skin, scleras, and internal organs, causing yellow-green discoloration.
■ Causes no functional abnormality.

b. Deposition in parenchymal cells:
(1) Kernicterus:

■ Is an uncommon condition in which unconjugated bilirubin is deposited in the basal ganglia (nuclei) of the brain.
■ Occurs only with an increase in unconjugated bilirubin, which is lipid-soluble and can cross the blood-brain barrier.
■ Occurs only in the neonatal period, when the blood-brain barrier is relatively permeable to the entry of bilirubin.
■ Is especially common in premature babies, in whom bilirubin-conjugating enzymes are poorly developed and serum albumin levels low.
■ Is most commonly caused by severe neonatal hemolysis, usually as a result of Rh blood group incompatibility between mother and baby.
■ Is manifested pathologically by intracellular accumulation of bilirubin in brain cells, causing neuronal dysfunction and necrosis, which may cause death in the acute phase.

(2) Liver:

■ Accumulation of bilirubin in liver cells in obstructive jaundice results in cellular swelling.
■ Escape of bilirubin into the liver lobule produces bile "lakes" that may be associated with cell necrosis. Fibrosis ensues that may lead to secondary biliary cirrhosis.

NECROSIS OF CELLS

Morphologic Evidence of Necrosis
A. Early changes:

■ In early necrosis, the cell is morphologically normal.
■ There is a delay of 1–3 hours before changes of necrosis are recognizable on electron microscopy and at least 6–8 hours before changes are apparent on light microscopy.

B. Nuclear changes are the best evidence of cell necrosis:

■ In **pyknosis,** the chromatin of the dead cell clumps into coarse strands, and the nucleus becomes a shrunken, dense, and deeply basophilic mass. In rapidly occurring necrosis, the nucleus undergoes lysis without a pyknotic stage.

- In **karyorrhexis,** the pyknotic nucleus breaks up into numerous small, dense basophilic particles.
- In **karyolysis,** the nucleus undergoes lysis as a result of the action of lysosomal deoxyribonucleases.

C. Cytoplasmic changes:

- About 6 hours after the cell undergoes necrosis, its cytoplasm becomes homogeneous and deeply acidophilic due to denaturation of cytoplasmic proteins and loss of ribosomes.
- When specialized organelles are present in the cell, such as myofibrils in myocardial cells, these are lost early.
- Swelling of mitochondria and disruption of organelle membranes cause cytoplasmic vacuolation.
- Finally, enzymatic digestion of the cell by enzymes released by the cell's own lysosomes causes lysis (**autolysis**).

D. Biochemical changes: The influx of calcium ions into the cell is closely related to irreversible death of the injured cell.

Types of Necrosis
A. Coagulative necrosis:

- The necrotic cell retains its cellular outline, often for several days, appearing as an anucleated mass of coagulated, pink-staining, homogeneous cytoplasm.
- This typically occurs in solid organs, such as the kidney, heart (myocardium), liver, and adrenal gland.

B. Liquefactive necrosis:

- Occurs when lysosomal enzymes released by the necrotic cells cause rapid liquefaction.
- Is typically seen in the brain following ischemia.
- Also occurs during pus formation (**suppurative inflammation**) due to the action of proteolytic enzymes released by neutrophils (**heterolysis**).

C. Fat necrosis:
1. Enzymatic fat necrosis:

- This type characteristically occurs in acute pancreatitis and pancreatic injuries, when pancreatic enzymes are liberated from the ducts into surrounding tissue.
- Lipase acts on the triglycerides in fat cells, breaking these down into glycerol and fatty acids, which complex with plasma calcium ions to form calcium soaps.
- The gross appearance is one of opaque chalky-white plaques and nodules in the peripancreatic adipose tissue.

2. Nonenzymatic fat necrosis:

- This type occurs in the breast, subcutaneous tissue, and abdomen.
- The cause is unknown. Many patients have a history of trauma (**traumatic fat necrosis**) even though trauma is not established as the definitive cause.

D. Caseous and gummatous necrosis: Caseous (cheeselike) and gummatous (gumlike or rubberlike) necrosis occur in infectious granulomas (see Chapter 5).

E. Fibrinoid necrosis:

- Is a type of connective-tissue necrosis seen particularly in autoimmune diseases (eg, rheumatic fever, polyarteritis nodosa, and systemic lupus erythematosus).
- Also occurs in accelerated (malignant) hypertension.
- Especially involves collagen and smooth muscle in the media of blood vessels.
- Is characterized by loss of normal structure and replacement with homogeneous, bright-pink-staining necrotic material that resemble fibrin microscopically.
- Contains varying amounts of immunoglobulins and complement, albumin, breakdown products of collagen, and fibrin.

F. Gangrene: This term denotes a clinical condition in which extensive tissue necrosis is complicated to a variable degree by secondary bacterial infection.

1. Dry gangrene:

- Most commonly occurs in the extremities as a result of ischemic coagulative necrosis of tissues due to arterial obstruction.
- Appears as a black, dry, and shriveled area sharply demarcated from adjacent viable tissue.
- Is associated with secondary bacterial infection, usually insignificant.
- Is treated by surgical removal of dead tissue (debridement).

2. Wet gangrene:

- Results from severe bacterial infection superimposed on necrosis.
- Occurs in the extremities, as well as in internal organs such as the intestine.
- Appears as an area of marked acute inflammation and growth of invading bacteria, causing the necrotic area to become swollen and reddish-black, with extensive liquefaction of dead tissue.
- Is not clearly demarcated from adjacent healthy tissue and is thus difficult to treat surgically.
- Is characterized by bacterial fermentation that produces a typical foul odor.
- Is associated with a high mortality rate.

3. Gas gangrene:

- Is a wound infection caused by *Clostridium perfringens* and other clostridial species.
- Is characterized by extensive necrosis of tissue and production of gas due to fermentation of the bacteria.
- Is manifested by *crepitus*, a crackling sensation on palpation over the site, caused by the presence of gas in the tissues.
- Is associated with a high mortality rate.

Clinical Effects of Necrosis
A. Abnormal function:

- Necrosis of cells leads to functional loss that frequently causes clinical disease.
- The severity of clinical disease depends on the type and extent of tissue destruction in relation to the amount and continued function of surviving tissue.

TABLE 1-2. SERUM ENZYME ELEVATIONS IN CELL NECROSIS

Enzyme	Tissue
Creatine kinase (MB isoenzyme)	Heart
Creatine kinase (BB isoenzyme)	Brain
Creatine kinase (MM isoenzyme)	Skeletal muscle, heart
Lactate dehydrogenase (isoenzyme 1)	Heart, erythrocytes, skeletal muscle
Lactate dehydrogenase (isoenzyme 5)	Liver, skeletal muscle
Aspartate aminotransferase (AST) (glutamic-oxaloacetic transaminase [GOT])	Heart, liver, skeletal muscle
Alanine aminotransferase (ALT) (glutamic-pyruvic transaminase [GPT])	Liver, skeletal muscle
Amylase	Pancreas, salivary gland

■ Abnormal electrical activity originating in areas of cerebral or myocardial necrosis may result in epileptic seizures or cardiac arrhythmias.
■ Failure of peristalsis in an area of intestinal wall necrosis may cause functional intestinal obstruction.
■ Bleeding into necrotic tissue often produces symptoms.

B. Bacterial infection in an area of necrosis or gangrene may disseminate throughout the body via the bloodstream.
C. Release of contents of necrotic cells:

■ Cytoplasmic contents (eg, enzymes) are released into the bloodstream.
■ Elevated enzyme levels often signify cell necrosis. The specificity of the test depends on distribution of the enzyme in various cells of the body (Table 1-2).

D. Systemic effects:

■ Fever due to pyrogens released from necrotic cells.
■ Neutrophil leukocytosis due to acute inflammation.

E. Local effects:

■ Ulceration of epithelial surfaces.
■ Swelling of tissue due to edema.

Abnormalities of Interstitial Tissues

2

MECHANISMS & RESULTS OF INJURY TO THE INTERSTITIUM

Interstitial injury may result from

- Abnormalities in plasma composition.
- Local changes in the tissue (eg, necrosis).

Commonly, abnormalities produce secondary dysfunction of parenchymal cells (eg, as in edema, amyloidosis, electrolyte disorders, etc.).

ACCUMULATION OF EXCESS FLUID (EDEMA)

Edema is the accumulation of excessive amounts of fluid in the interstitium. It

- Is most easily seen in the skin.
- Is evidenced first by pitting of the skin.
- Manifests as visible swelling only when severe.
- Can include accumulation of fluid in body cavities (eg, pleural effusion, pericardial effusion, ascites).
- May be localized (as in inflammation) or generalized (as in sodium and water retention).
- Is called **anasarca** when massive throughout the body.

Note: Distribution of the retained fluid is gravity-dependent.

Localized Edema
A. Inflammatory edema:

- Occurs when acute inflammation causes capillary permeability and increased hydrostatic pressure due to vasodilatation.

Note: Edema is a cardinal sign of acute inflammation (Chapter 3).
B. Allergic Edema:

- Occurs when local release of vasoactive substances (eg, histamine) causes increased capillary permeability and vasodilatation.
- Is common in the skin (wheals, urticaria, "hives").
- Can be (rarely) more widespread (eg, skin, larynx and bronchioles in **angioneurotic edema**).

C. Edema of Venous Obstruction:

- When complete, produces severe edema and hemorrhage.
- When partial, extent of collateral drainage determines degree.

D. Edema of Lymphatic Obstruction:

- Occurs when protein accumulates in the interstitial spaces, leading to increased osmotic pressure.
- Is characterized by pitting in early stages.
- If prolonged, results in fibrosis (non-pitting) and marked epidermal thickening (**elephantiasis**).

Generalized Edema

A. Cardiac Edema: Diminished left ventricular output leads to generalized edema through

- Decreased glomerular filtration pressure.
- Stimulation of the juxtaglomerular apparatus to secrete renin.
- Activation of the angiotensin mechanism.
- Increased aldosterone production by the adrenal (**secondary aldosteronism**).
- Retention of sodium (and water).

Note: In *right* ventricular failure, the central venous pressure is increased, and fluid tends to leak from the systemic circulation (eg, ankle edema). In *left* ventricular failure, the retained water tends to accumulate in the lungs (*see* Pulmonary Edema).

B. Edema of Hypoproteinemia: Generalized edema follows sustained loss of protein with decreases in the plasma osmotic pressure.

- Fluid leaks from systemic capillaries.
- Decrease in plasma volume.
- Vasoconstriction, which leads to hypersecretion of renin and secondary aldosteronism.
- Sodium and water retention by the kidneys.

Note: Causes of hypoproteinemia include

- Insufficient dietary protein (starvation, malnutrition).
- Decreased synthesis of albumin (hepatic disease).
- Increased loss of protein
  - In the urine (nephrotic syndrome).
  - From the intestine (protein-losing enteropathy).

C. Renal Edema:

- Acute glomerulonephritis produces mild edema due to a fall in the glomerular filtration rate.
- Nephrotic syndrome (see Chapter 47) is characterized by massive edema due to hypoproteinemia that follows heavy proteinuria.

Clinical Effects of Edema

In most tissues, edema causes little or no dysfunction. **Edema of the following organs is life-threatening.**

A. Lungs: Pulmonary Edema:

- Is characterized by entry of fluid into the alveoli from the pulmonary capillaries.

■ Manifests when fluid interferes with gas exchange in the lungs.
■ Causes hypoxia and death, if severe.

B. Brain: Cerebral Edema

■ Occurs in many brain disorders (eg, traumatic lesions, infections, neoplasms, and vascular accidents).
■ Causes reversible acute cerebral dysfunction.
■ Is dangerous when associated with increased intracranial pressure that
  ● Produces headache.
  ● Produces edema of the optic disk (papilledema).
  ● May, if severe, force the temporal lobe down into the tentorial opening (tentorial herniation) or the cerebellar tonsil into the foramen magnum (tonsillar herniation).
  ● May cause death due to compression of the cardiorespiratory centers in the brain stem (see Chapter 62).

CHANGES IN BODY TEMPERATURE

■ Changes in body temperature may result from disordered control mechanisms in
  ● Diseases of the brain stem affecting the thermoregulatory center.
  ● Any injury involving necrosis or acute inflammation, due to release of pyrogens such as interleukin-1 and prostaglandins.
  ● Reaction to drugs that affect the thermoregulatory center.
  ● Exposure to extreme environmental conditions.
■ **Fever (hyperthermia)** is an increase in temperature. It results in
  ● Increased metabolic rate, energy and oxygen requirements.
  ● Neuronal dysfunction at temperatures over 42.2 °C (108 °F), which may be followed by delirium, convulsions and death.
■ **Hypothermia** is a decrease in temperature, which has effects opposite to those of fever. Controlled hypothermia is used to reduce the metabolic needs of tissues during prolonged surgery.

ALTERATION IN pH

Maintenance of Normal pH
The pH of the cell is in equilibrium with the pH of the interstitial fluid and plasma. Plasma pH is normally maintained close to 7.4 by

■ Blood buffers, including plasma proteins, hemoglobin, and the bicarbonate-carbonic acid system.
■ Renal control of hydrogen ion excretion.
■ Respiratory control of the amount of CO_2 lost during ventilation.

Causes of Abnormal pH (Table 2–1)
A. Respiratory Disease:

■ The amount of CO_2 lost from the lungs is directly related to total alveolar ventilation.
■ In **respiratory acidosis**
  ● There is decreased alveolar ventilation.
  ● CO_2 is retained.

TABLE 2-1. KEY CHANGES IN SEVERAL ACID-BASE DISORDERS

Acid-Base Disorder	Alveolar Ventilation	Paco2	Serum pH	Serum HCO₃⁻	Urine pH
Respiratory acidosis	Primary decrease	↑	↓	↑	Acid < 6
Respiratory alkalosis	Primary increase	↓	↑	↓	Alkaline > 7
Metabolic acidosis of renal origin	Compensatory increase	↓	↓	↓	Alkaline > 7 (primary)
Metabolic acidosis of nonrenal origin	Compensatory increase	↓	↓	↓	Acid < 6 (compensatory)
Metabolic alkalosis of renal origin	Compensatory decrease	↑	↑	↑	Acid < 6 (primary)
Metabolic alkalosis of nonrenal origin	Compensatory decrease	↑	↑	↑	Alkaline > 7 (compensatory)

- The kidney compensates by excreting acid (hydrogen ion) and retaining bicarbonate.

■ In **respiratory alkalosis**
- There is increased alveolar ventilation.
- CO_2 is lost.
- The kidney compensates by excreting bicarbonate to conserve acid (hydrogen ion).

B. Metabolic Disease:

■ **Metabolic acidosis**
- Results from
  o Failure of the kidney to excrete acid (eg, specific renal tubular defects, renal failure).
  o Loss of alkali due to diarrhea and vomiting.
  o Entry of acid (exogenous or endogenous) into the blood.
- Stimulates the respiratory center.
- Increases ventilation to wash out CO_2 (respiratory compensation).
- Results in acid urine except when acidosis is due to renal disease (then it is alkaline, since the diseased kidney cannot excrete acid).

■ **Metabolic alkalosis**
- Results from
  o Excessive renal excretion of acid.
  o Loss of gastric acid due to vomiting.
  o Ingestion of alkali (antacids).
- Depresses the respiratory center.
- Decreases ventilation, which leads to CO_2 retention.

● Results in alkaline urine, except in patients in whom alkalosis is the result of renal loss of acid.

ELECTROLYTE IMBALANCE

■ **Hypernatremia** (increased plasma sodium)
  ● Occurs with water privation and loss, use of diuretics, steroid excess.
  ● Causes increased extracellular fluid, hypertension.
■ **Hyponatremia** (decreased plasma sodium)
  ● Occurs with water overload, adrenal insufficiency, excess antidiuretic hormone secretion.
  ● Causes hypotension.
■ **Hyperkalemia** (increased plasma potassium)
  ● Occurs in renal failure, adrenal insufficiency, following use of some diuretics, and excess intake of potassium.
  ● Causes high T waves on ECG, cardiac arrhythmias, muscle weakness.
■ **Hypokalemia** (decreased plasma potassium)
  ● Occurs in vomiting, diarrhea, many diuretics, steroid excess.
  ● Causes flat T wave on ECG, cardiac arrhythmias, muscle weakness.
■ **Hypercalcemia** (increased plasma calcium)
  ● Occurs in hyperparathyroidism (including "ectopic" PTH production by tumors), metastatic cancer and myeloma, vitamin D intoxication, sarcoidosis.
  ● Causes cerebral dysfunction, muscle weakness, metastatic calcification, short QT on ECG.
■ **Hypocalcemia** (decreased plasma calcium)
  ● Occurs in hypoparathyroidism, intestinal malabsorption.
  ● Causes tetany, carpopedal spasm, convulsions, long ST on ECG.

DEPOSITION OF CALCIUM (CALCIFICATION)

Metastatic Calcification
Metastatic calcification

■ Is due to an increase in serum calcium or phosphorus levels.
■ Occurs in normal tissues such as arterial walls, kidneys (**nephrocalcinosis**).

Dystrophic Calcification
Dystrophic calcification

■ Is characterized by normal calcium and phosphorus levels.
■ Occurs as a result of local abnormality in tissues, most often in areas of necrosis or degeneration, or tumors.

DEPOSITION OF AMYLOID (Amyloidosis)

■ *Amyloid* denotes a variety of fibrillary proteins deposited in interstitial tissues.
  ● With H&E, it stains homogeneous pink.
  ● With Congo red stain, it appears red (apple-green under polarized light).
  ● On electron microscopy, it appears as nonbranching fibrils 7.5–10 nm wide.

- It has a pleated β-sheet structure.
- Its chemical composition is variable.
- **Amyloid of immunoglobulin origin**
  - Is also called AL amyloid.
  - Is composed of fragments of light chains.
  - Is produced by neoplastic plasma cells (myeloma) and B lymphocytes (B cell lymphomas).
- **Amyloid of other origin**
  - Is composed of fragments of other proteins, including
    - AA amyloid, of serum A protein (a_1-globulin).
    - AE amyloid, of peptide hormone precursors (eg, calcitonin).

Classification

Classification of amyloids is based on protein type and tissue distribution.

A. Systemic Amyloidosis.

1. Primary pattern of distribution:

- Amyloid is found in the heart, gastrointestinal tract, tongue, skin, and nerves.
- The AL type is most common.
- Ninety percent have underlying neoplasm of B lymphocytes (plasma cell myeloma and B cell malignant lymphomas).

2. Secondary pattern of distribution:

- Amyloid is found in the liver, spleen, kidney, adrenals, gastrointestinal tract, and skin.
- The AA type is most common.
- It occurs in chronic inflammatory diseases such as tuberculosis, leprosy, chronic osteomyelitis.

B. Localized Amyloidosis:

- Is characterized by nodular, tumorlike masses.
- Is commonly associated with localized plasma cell neoplasms.

C. Amyloid in Neoplasms:

- Amyloids are found in the stroma of many endocrine neoplasms (eg, medullary carcinoma of the thyroid, pancreatic islet cell neoplasms).
- The amyloid protein is AE (eg, calcitonin).

D. Heredofamilial Amyloidosis:

- This type is rare.
- AF amyloid is deposited in nerves, heart, or kidneys.
- AA amyloid occurs in familial Mediterranean fever.

E. Senile Amyloidosis: Small amounts of AS amyloid are often found in the heart, pancreas, and spleen of the elderly.

Effects of Amyloid Deposition

When amyloid is deposited in basement membranes, especially in small blood vessels, it

- Produces abnormal bleeding.
- Manifests as protein loss from renal glomeruli (a cause of nephrotic syndrome).
- Causes neuropathy.
- Enlarges the tissues (hepatosplenomegaly, cardiomegaly).

ACCUMULATION OF MUCOPOLYSACCHARIDES
Myxoid or **myxomatous degeneration**

- Is an increase in the amount of mucopolysaccharides (glycosaminoglycans) in the interstitium.
- Is common, and usually does not affect function.
- Particularly occurs in
  - Hypothyroidism (myxedema).
  - Joints and tendons, forming a "ganglion."
  - Neoplasms such as neurofibromas.
  - The aorta and cardiac valves in Marfan's syndrome.

INCREASE IN BLOOD & DEPOSITION OF HEMOGLOBIN PIGMENTS

Congestion & Hyperemia
Hyperemia is

- An increase in the amount of blood within dilated vessels.
- Active when acute inflammation occurs.
- Passive following obstruction of venous outflow (also known as congestion).

Hemorrhage
Hemorrhage

- Is the presence of blood in interstitial tissue outside the blood vessels.
- Results in erythrocytes breaking down to release hemoglobin.
- The iron is converted to **hemosiderin,** a brown, granular pigment.
- The porphyrin forms bilirubin, which may be absorbed in the blood or deposited as a golden-yellow, crystalline pigment called **hematoidin.**

Accumulation of Hematin
Hematin

- Is a golden-brown granular pigment derived from hemoglobin.
- Accumulates in reticuloendothelial cells following massive intravascular hemolysis (incompatible blood transfusions and malaria).
- Produces no clinical effects.

Section II. The Host Response to Injury

■ **Phagocytosis** (present in amoebas, hydras, sponges, etc.) involves only simple recognition of damage or of "foreignness."

■ **Acute Inflammation** (present in multicellular animals, worms, mollusks, insects) mobilizes specialized inflammatory cells (phagocytes) to the site of injury, through **chemotaxis** and **microcirculatory changes.**

■ **Immune response** (present in vertebrates) adds specificity, memory, and amplification—functions that are attributable to the presence of lymphocytes.

The sequence of host responses after injury is as follows:

■ The **acute inflammatory response** (Chapter 3) occurs within minutes of injury.

■ The **immune response** (Chapter 4) is triggered at the time of the injury but takes several days to develop.

■ **Chronic inflammation** (Chapter 5) represents a combined inflammatory and immune response against a persistent injury.

■ **Regeneration and repair** (Chapter 6) represent the final steps in the host attempt to restore normal function.

■ **Deficiencies in these responses** are discussed in Chapter 7.

The Acute Inflammatory Response

3

CARDINAL CLINICAL SIGNS
There are five cardinal clinical signs of acute inflammation:

■ **Rubor** (redness).
■ **Calor** (increased heat).
■ **Tumor** (swelling).
■ **Dolor** (pain).
■ **Functio laesa** (loss of function).

MORPHOLOGIC & FUNCTIONAL CHANGES
The two main components of the acute inflammatory response are the microcirculatory response and the cellular response.

Microcirculatory Response
A. Active vasodilatation (hyperemia): Sequential changes include

■ Transient vasoconstriction.

19

TABLE 3–1. DIFFERENCES BETWEEN EXUDATES AND TRANSUDATES

	Ultrafiltrate of Plasma	Transudate	Exudate	Plasma
Vascular permeability	Normal	Normal	Increased	—
Protein content	Trace	0–1.5 g/dL	1.5–6 g/dL[1]	6–7 g/dL[1]
Protein types	Albumin	Albumin	All[2]	All[2]
Fibrin	No	No	Yes	No (fibrinogen)
Specific gravity	1.010	1.010–1.015	1.015–1.027	1.027
Cells	None	None	Inflammatory	Blood

[1]The protein content of an exudate depends on the plasma protein level. In patients with very low plasma protein levels, an exudate may have a lower protein content than 1.5 g/dL.
[2]All = albumin, globulins, complement, immunoglobulins, proteins of the coagulation and fibrinolytic cascades, etc.

■ Dilatation of arterioles, capillaries, and venules.
■ Increased blood flow (**hyperemia**).

B. Increased permeability: Sequential changes manifest in

■ Active contraction of actin filaments in endothelial cells.
■ Separation of intercellular junctions (widening of the pores).
■ Increased amounts of fluid and proteins passing through into the tissues (exudation).
■ Several patterns:
  ● Immediate-transient.
  ● Immediate-sustained (or prolonged).
  ● Delayed-prolonged.

Note: The immediate-transient response is mediated mainly by histamine. Other responses and mediators are less well understood.
C. Exudation of fluid into the interstitial tissue occurs because of

■ Increased capillary permeability.
■ Arteriolar dilatation, which increases the hydrostatic pressure in the microcirculation.

The composition of an exudate

■ Approaches that of plasma (Table 3–1), because the abnormally permeable endothelium permits free passage of plasma proteins.
■ Contains immunoglobulins, complement and fibrinogen (which is rapidly converted to fibrin).

A **transudate,** by contrast,

■ Is formed by passage of fluid across a normally permeable endothelium.

TABLE 3-2. SELECTED CAUSES OF TRANSUDATIVE AND EXUDATIVE PERITONEAL
EFFUSION (ASCITES)

Transudate	Exudate
Cirrhosis of the liver	Bacterial peritonitis
Portal vein obstruction	Tuberculosis peritonitis
Right heart failure	Metastatic neoplasms
Constrictive pericarditis	Mesothelioma (neoplasm of mesothelial cells)
Meigs' syndrome[1]	Connective tissue disease (eg, systemic
Malnutrition (kwashiorkor)	lupus erthyematosus)

[1] Meigs' syndrome is the occurrence of peritoneal and pleural effusion due to transudation of fluid from the surface of an ovarian tumor.

■ Is due to increased hydrostatic pressure or decreased plasma osmotic pressure.
■ Is composed like an ultrafiltrate of plasma.

Note: Distinction of exudate from transudate may be of diagnostic importance (Table 3-2).

D. Changes in blood flow rate: Initial high rate of flow is followed by stagnation as fluid is lost from the vessel by exudation.

E. Changes in lymphatic flow: When lymphatic flow increases,

■ It removes injurious agents and tissue debris.
■ Antigenic agents are passed to the lymph nodes, stimulating a specific immune response.
■ Occasionally virulent agents may spread via the lymphatics, producing **lymphangitis** and **lymphadenitis.**

Cellular Response
A. Types of cells involved:

■ Neutrophils (polymorphonuclear leukocytes) dominate the early phase (first 24 hours).
■ Macrophages, lymphocytes and plasma cells enter the area later (48 hours plus).

B. Margination of neutrophils: Sequentially,

■ The rate of blood flow in dilated vessels decreases.
■ Orderly flow of blood is disturbed.
■ Erythrocytes form aggregates (**rouleaux**).
■ Leukocytes are displaced to the periphery (Fig 3-1).

C. Pavementing of neutrophils describes adherence of marginated neutrophils to the endothelial surface of blood vessels.

D. Emigration of neutrophils occurs, from the blood into the tissues through the widened endothelial pores.

E. Chemotactic factors include complement factor 5a (C5a), and leukotriene B4, which direct the movement of neutrophils along a chemical concentration gradient.

A Normal capillary

B Acute inflammation

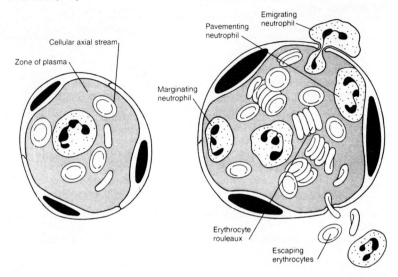

Figure 3–1. Microcirculatory changes in acute inflammation. The capillary in acute inflammation is dilated, has swollen endothelial cells, rouleau formation, and margination and emigration of leukocytes.

F. Movement of other cells:

- Macrophage and lymphocyte emigration is similar to that of neutrophils.
- Chemotactic factors for macrophages are C5a, leukotriene B4, and lymphokines that are liberated by activated lymphocytes.
- **Diapedesis** describes the passage of red cells across the inflamed vessel wall.

G. Phagocytosis involves several steps:
1. Recognition is accomplished

- Directly, or
- After the agent has been coated with immunoglobulin or complement factor 3b (C3b). This is called **opsonization** (Fig 3–2).

Note: Both IgG and C3b are effective **opsonins**. Immune phagocytosis involving opsonins is more efficient.

2. Engulfment:

- A foreign particle engulfed by a cell enters a membrane-bound vacuole called a **phagosome**.
- This fuses with lysosomes to form a **phagolysosome**.
- Lysosomal enzymes, including lactoferrin and lysozyme (muramidase), then degrade the injurious agent.

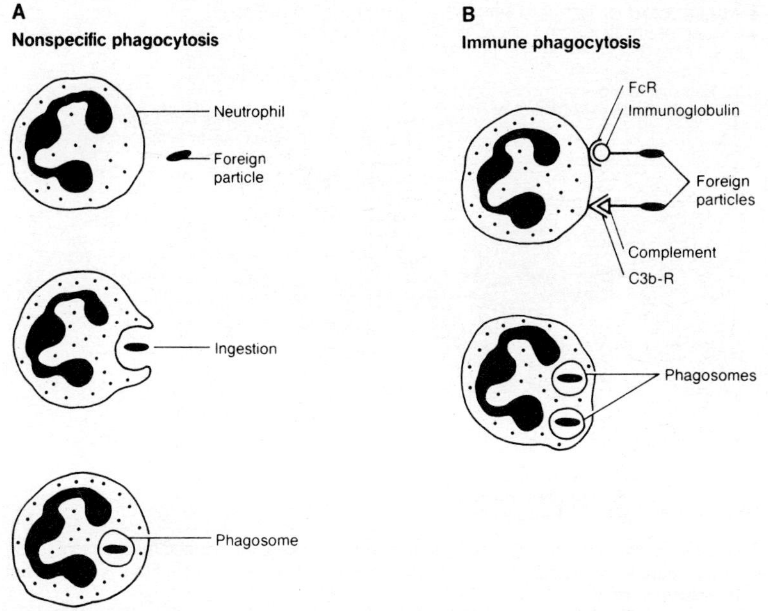

A
Nonspecific phagocytosis

B
Immune phagocytosis

Figure 3–2. Phagocytosis by neutrophil leukocytes. Immune phagocytosis (B) is much more efficient than non-specific phagocytosis (A). The presence on the cell membrane of receptors to the Fc fragment of the immunoglobulin molecule (FcR) and C3b component of the complement (C3b-R) are important in immune phagocytosis. Note that macrophages have similar phagocytic capability.

3. Microbial killing is accomplished through several mechanisms:

- The hydrogen peroxide (H_2O_2)-myeloperoxidase-halide system.
- Hydrogen ions, enzymes, and other bactericidal substances that also exist within lysosomes.
- Macrophage-activating factor, a lymphokine released by sensitized T lymphocytes, assists microbial killing by macrophages.

MEDIATORS OF ACUTE INFLAMMATION

The Triple Response (Fig 3–3)
Described by Sir Thomas Lewis in 1927, a firm stroke of the skin with a blunt instrument evokes

- A "red line" within 1 minute.
- A "red flare."
- A "wheal."

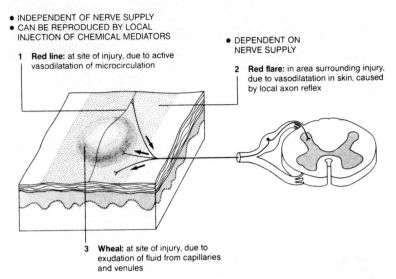

- INDEPENDENT OF NERVE SUPPLY
- CAN BE REPRODUCED BY LOCAL
  INJECTION OF CHEMICAL MEDIATORS

1 **Red line:** at site of injury, due to active
  vasodilatation of microcirculation

- DEPENDENT ON
  NERVE SUPPLY

2 **Red flare:** in area surrounding injury,
  due to vasodilatation in skin, caused
  by local axon reflex

3 **Wheal:** at site of injury, due to
  exudation of fluid from capillaries
  and venules

Figure 3–3. Lewis's triple response. The red line and wheal are caused by chemical mediators: The flare is mediated by a local axon reflex and is the only element that is dependent on the nerve supply.

Removal of the nerve supply to the tissue prevents only the flare, which led Lewis to the conclusion that chemical mediators were involved (Lewis's "H substance," which turned out to be histamine).

Specific Mediators
Many other chemical mediators have been discovered (Table 3–3), but their exact roles are unknown.

A. Vasoactive amines:

- Are histamine and serotonin
- Are released from mast cells and platelets.
- Both cause vasodilatation and increased permeability

B. The kinin system:

- **Bradykinin** is the final product of the kinin system.
- It is formed by the action of **kallikrein.**
- It causes increased vascular permeability and stimulates pain receptors.

C. The coagulation cascade:

- Is activated by injury
- Involves formation of activated factor XII (Hageman factor) and fibrinopeptides, which cause increased vascular permeability and are chemotactic for neutrophils.

TABLE 3–3. MEDIATORS OF ACUTE INFLAMMATION

Mediator	Vasodilation	Increased Permeability		Chemotaxis	Opsonin	Pain
		Immediate	Sustained			
Histamine	+	+++	–	–	–	–
Serotonin (5-HT)	+	+	–	–	–	–
Bradykinin	+	+	–	–	–	+++
Complement 3a	–	+	–	–	–	–
Complement 3b	–	–	–	–	+++	–
Complement 5a	–	++	–	+++	–	–
Prostaglandins	+++	+	+?	+++	–	+
Leukotrienes	–	+++	+?	+++	–	–
Lysosomal pro-teases	–	–	++[1]	–	–	–
Oxygen radicals	–	–	++[1]	–	–	–

[1] Proteases and oxygen-based free radicals derived from neutrophils are believed to mediate a sustained increase in permeability by means of their damage to endothelial cells.

D. The complement system:

- C5a and C3a cause increased vascular permeability by stimulating release of histamine from mast cells.
- C5a is chemotactic for neutrophils and macrophages.
- C3b is an important opsonin.
- C5a activates the lipoxygenase pathway of arachidonic acid metabolism (see following).

E. Arachidonic acid metabolites:

- Phospholipases release arachidonic acid from cell membranes.
- Complex metabolism leads to production of prostaglandins, leukotrienes, and other mediators of inflammation.

F. Neutrophil factors include

- Myeloperoxidase-containing cytoplasmic granules.
- Proteases.
- Acetyl glyceryl ether phosphorylcholine (AGEPC; formerly called **platelet-activating factor**).

G. Inhibitors include

- C1 esterase inhibitor (inhibits the complement cascade).
- α_1-antitrypsin (inhibits proteases).

TABLE 3–4. TYPES OF ACUTE INFLAMMATION

Type	Features	Common Causes
Classic type	Hyperemia: exudation with fibrin and neutrophils; neutrophil leukocytosis in blood.	Bacterial infections; response to cell necrosis of any cause.
Acute inflammation without neutrophils	Paucity of neutrophils in exudate; lymphocytes and plasma cells predominant; neutropenia, lymphocytosis in blood.	Viral and rickettsial infections (immune response contributes).
Allergic acute inflammation	Marked edema and numerous eosinophils: eosinophilia in blood.	Certain hypersensitivity immune reactions (see Chapter 8).
Serous inflammation (inflammation in body cavities)	Marked fluid exudation.	Burns; many bacterial infections.
Catarrhal inflammation (inflammation of mucous membranes)	Marked secretion of mucus.	Infections, eg, common cold (rhinovirus); allergy (eg, hay fever).
Fibrinous inflammation	Excess fibrin formation.	Many virulent bacterial infections.
Necrotizing inflammation, hemorrhagic inflammation	Marked tissue necrosis hemorrhage.	Highly virulent organisms (bacterial, viral, fungal), eg, plague (*Yersinia pestis*), anthrax (*Bacillus anthracis*), herpes simplex encephalitis, mucormycosis.
Membranous (pseudomembranous) inflammation	Necrotizing inflammation involving mucous membranes. The necrotic mucosa and inflammatory exudate form an adherent membrane on the mucosal surface.	Toxigenic bacteria, eg, diphtheria bacillus (*Corynebacterium diphtheriae*) and *Clostridium difficile*.
Suppurative (purulent) inflammation	Exaggerated neutrophil response and liquefactive necrosis of parenchymal cells; pus formation. Marked neutrophil leukocytosis in blood.	Pyogenic bacteria, eg, staphylococci, streptococci, gramnegative bacilli, anaerobes.

SYSTEMIC CLINICAL SIGNS
Systemic clinical signs include

- **Fever** due to pyrogens and prostaglandins.
- **Changes in the peripheral white blood cell count:**
  - **Neutrophil leukocytosis** with "shift to the left"—less mature forms with fewer nuclear lobes (band forms)—and **toxic granulation.**

Note: Viral infections tend to produce neutropenia and lymphocytosis.

- Changes in Plasma Protein Levels
  - So called acute-phase reactants increase, including C-reactive protein, α_1-antitrypsin, fibrinogen, haptoglobin, and ceruloplasmin. This leads to an **increased erythrocyte sedimentation rate.**

TYPES OF ACUTE INFLAMMATION
The various types of acute inflammation are summarized in Table 3-4.

COURSE OF ACUTE INFLAMMATION
The course of acute inflammation is as follows:

- **Resolution:** In uncomplicated acute inflammation the tissue returns to normal (Chapter 6).
- **Repair** occurs after more severe damage; it involves regeneration, fibrosis, and scar formation (Chapter 6).
- Virulent bacterial infections may go on to liquefactive necrosis (**suppurative inflammation, pus formation, abscess**).
- An **immune response** (Chapter 4) develops, and may lead to
  - **Chronic inflammation** if the injury persists (Chapter 5).

The Immune Response 4

There are two main types of immune response:

- **Cell-mediated immunity**
  - Is a function of T lymphocytes.
  - Leads to the production of effector (killer or cytotoxic) T cells, and lymphokines that mediate cell interactions.
  - Is modulated by two subtypes of T cells:
    - ○ Helper T cells enhance it.
    - ○ Suppressor T cells have the opposite effect.
- **Humoral immunity**
  - Is a function of B cells.
  - Leads to the production of plasma cells that secrete immunoglobulins (antibodies).

CHARACTERISTICS OF THE IMMUNE RESPONSE
The immune response is characterized by:

- **Specificity** (reactivity restricted to the inducing agent, or **antigen**).
- **Amplification** (an enhanced response on repeated exposure to the same antigen).
- **Memory** (the ability to mount an enhanced response against the same antigen on subsequent exposure).

Tolerance to Self Antigens
The concepts of self and nonself (foreignness) are central to immunologic reactivity:

- **Tolerance** is specific nonresponsiveness to self antigens.
- There are two proposed mechanisms:
  - Deletion in embryo of those clones of lymphocytes capable of recognizing self antigens.
  - Production of specific suppressor cells (lymphocytes) that inhibit an immune response to self antigens.

Specificity
The specificity of the immune response is dependent on the ability of the immune system to produce an almost unlimited number of antibodies and T lymphocytes.

- An antigen evokes a response from a specific B or T lymphocyte that is preprogrammed to react against it (ie, the lymphocyte bears receptors with appropriate specificity for the antigen).
- The antigen receptor is immunoglobulin on B cells and an immunoglobulinlike molecule on T cells.
- A **B cell** stimulated by antigen multiplies to produce a clone of **plasma cells** that produce antibody.
- A T cell stimulated by antigen multiplies to produce a clone of specific cytotoxic T cells.

■ The net effect is usually protective (**immunity**).
■ Occasionally adverse reactions develop (**hypersensitivity**) (Chapter 8).

ANTIGENS

Antigens are molecules that evoke an immune response when introduced into a host that recognizes them as nonself. They are large "rigid" molecules (proteins or polysaccharides) with MW greater than 5000. Smaller molecules that may be antigenic are called **haptens:**

■ These include lipids, carbohydrates, oligopeptides, nucleic acids, and drugs.
■ They are not large enough in themselves to act as antigens.
■ They may, however, bind specifically with an antibody.
■ They may be antigenic when combined with larger-molecular-weight "carriers."

Antigenic Determinant (Epitope)

The **epitope** is that part of the antigen or hapten that reacts with the immune system. It is composed of only a few (4–8) amino acids or sugar residues. A single antigenic molecule may bear several different epitopes.

Types of Antigens
A. Extrinsic Antigens:

■ Are introduced into the body from outside.
■ Include microorganisms, foreign cells, and particles.
■ Are ingested, inhaled, or injected into the body.

B. Intrinsic Antigens are derived from molecules in the body altered by

■ Addition of hapten.
■ Partial denaturation of native molecules.
■ Transformation in the development of cancer cells.

C. Sequestered Antigens:

■ Are anatomically hidden from the immune system beginning in early embryonic life (eg, lens protein and spermatozoa).
■ Consequently, they do not develop tolerance.
■ Their release into the circulation in later life may result in an immune response (autoimmunity).

Recognition of Antigens

An optimal immune response to most antigens occurs only after interaction of the antigen with macrophages, T lymphocytes, and B lymphocytes.

■ Macrophages acting in this role are termed antigen-processing cells.
■ Dendritic reticulum cells in lymphoid follicles (Fig 4–1) process antigens for B cells
■ Interdigitating reticulum cells in the paracortical zone of lymph nodes process antigen for T cells.
■ "Processing" involves internalization of antigen by the macrophage, and re-expression on the cell surface in conjunction with MHC (major histocompatibility complex) molecules.

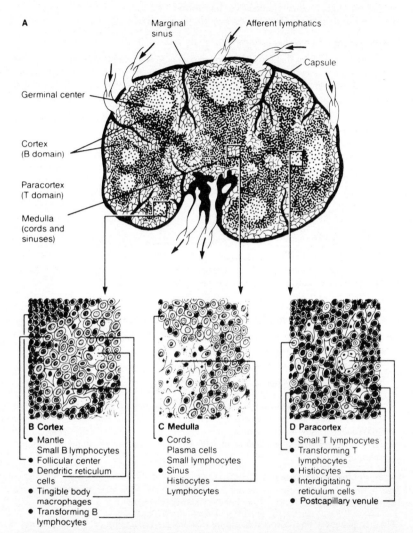

A

Marginal sinus

Afferent lymphatics

Capsule

Germinal center

Cortex (B domain)

Paracortex (T domain)

Medulla (cords and sinuses)

B Cortex
- Mantle
  Small B lymphocytes
- Follicular center
- Dendritic reticulum cells
- Tingible body macrophages
- Transforming B lymphocytes

C Medulla
- Cords
  Plasma cells
  Small lymphocytes
- Sinus
  Histiocytes
  Lymphocytes

D Paracortex
- Small T lymphocytes
- Transforming T lymphocytes
- Histiocytes
- Interdigitating reticulum cells
- Postcapillary venule

Figure 4–1. Diagram of lymph node showing an outer cortex containing follicles or germinal centers (B cell zone), a subjacent paracortex (T cell zone), and central medullary sinuses and cords. Antigen processing for B cells occurs in the follicles (by dendritic reticulum cell, and for T cells in the paracortex (by interdigitating reticulum cells). Macrophages are concentrated in the sinuses.

■ Antigen receptors on T cells recognize the combination of antigen-MHC molecules on the macrophage, leading to T cell activation.
  ● Helper T cells recognize antigen in association with MHC class II molecules.
  ● Suppressor T cells recognize MHC class I molecules.
■ For most antigens (T cell-dependent) the response involves macrophages, B cells and T cells.
■ Some multivalent antigens (T cell-independent) may activate B cells directly.

CELLULAR BASIS OF THE IMMUNE RESPONSE

LYMPHOID TISSUE

Central Lymphoid Tissue
Central lymphoid tissue is composed of the thymus and bone marrow, and is the site in which primitive lymphoid cells of the fetus are developed and primed. **Priming** refers to the early period of lymphocyte development when diversity occurs and tolerance develops (Fig 4–2).

Peripheral Lymphoid Tissue
Peripheral lymphoid tissue is composed of lymph nodes (Fig 4–1), spleen, Waldeyer's ring (the tonsils), and gut-associated lymphoid tissue. It is the site wherein reside the mature lymphocytes that respond to antigenic stimuli. Lymphocytes continuously recirculate through the lymphoid tissues via the peripheral blood and lymphatics.

LYMPHOCYTES
Lymphocytes are derived from **lymphoid stem cells** in the fetal bone marrow, and are classified on the basis of their site of development in the fetus (Fig 4–2):

■ **T (thymus-dependent) lymphocytes** develop in the thymus.
■ **B lymphocytes** develop in the bursa of Fabricius in birds (hence B cells). The functional bursal equivalent in humans is the fetal liver or bone marrow.
■ All resting lymphocyte subpopulations resemble one another morphologically and can be distinguished only by immunologic methods (Table 4–1).

T Lymphocytes (T Cells)
A. Distribution of T cells in the body:

■ T cells develop in the fetal thymus.
■ After maturation, they are distributed to the T cell domains of the peripheral lymphoid tissue, including
  ● The **paracortex of the lymph nodes,** between the lymphoid follicles (Fig 4–1); 70% of lymphocytes in lymph nodes are T lymphocytes.)
  ● The periarterial lymphoid sheath in the **splenic white pulp** (40% of splenic lymphocytes are T cells.)
  ● The peripheral blood (80–90% of peripheral blood lymphocytes are T cells).

  B. T cell transformation follows stimulation (activation) either by a specific antigen or by nonspecific agents such as mitogens, eg, phytohemagglutinin (PHA, a plant extract).

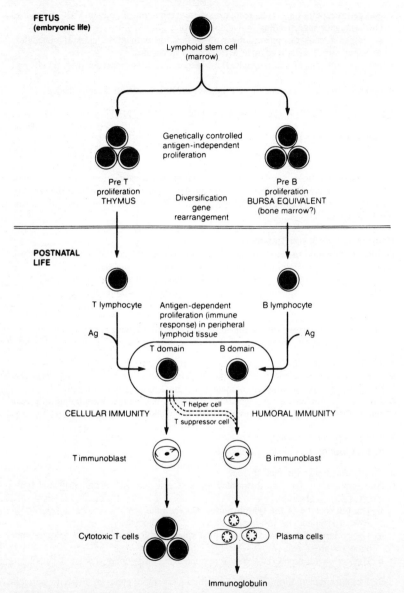

Figure 4–2. Lymphocyte development into B cells and T cells, plus diversification of receptor specificity, occurs in the embryo. In postnatal life, individual lymphocytes are driven to proliferate by antigen (transformation), with the net result of "humoral immunity" (B cells) and "cellular immunity" (T cells).

TABLE 4–1. SELECTED MONOCLONA ANTIBODIES EMPLOYED FOR LEUKOCYTE IDENTIFICATION AND THEIR CORRESPONDING CD ANTIGENS[1]

CD Antigen	Corresponding Monoclonal Antibodies	Principal Leukocytes Expressing the Antigen
CD1	OKT6, Leu6	Thymocytes
CD2	OKT11	T cells and NK cells (E rosette receptor)
CD3	OKT3, Leu4	Mature T cells (Pan-T)
CD4	OKT4, Leu3	"Helper-inducer" T cells
CD5	OKT1, Leu1[2]	T cells (Pan-T)[2]
CD8	OKT8, Leu2	"Suppressor-cytotoxic" T cells
CD9	Ba-2	Subset of B cells
CD10	CALLA	Cells of common acute lymphoblastic leukemia
CD11	OKM1, Mo-1	Monocytes, granulocytes, NK cells (C3b receptor)
CD15	Leu M1	Monocytes, granulocytes
CD20	B1	Most B cells
CD24	BA-1	Early B cells
CD45	CLA	Most leukocytes (common leukocyte antigen)
CD57	NK-1, Leu7	Natural killer cells
CD71	OKT9	Monocytes, early lymphocytes (transferrin receptor)
CD75	LN-1	B cells in follicular center phase
None assigned	PC-1	Plasma cells

[1]The CD (cluster differentiation) terminology for leukocyte antigens has been recommended by the World Health Organization following a series of international workshops.
[2]Note that as new data become available, it is apparent that expression of many of these antigens is not wholly restricted to a single cell lineage, eg, the Pan-T cell antibodies OKT1 and Leu1 (CD5) also react with a subset of normal B cells and with B cell lymphocytic leukemia.

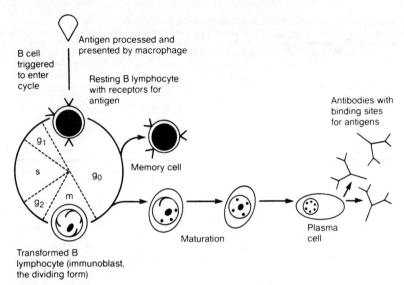

Figure 4–3. B cell transformation, showing binding of antigen with receptor, leading to proliferation of the B cell and eventual production of antibody-producing plasma cells. Note that T cells undergo a similar process, leading to production of effector T cells.

- T lymphocytes transform into large, actively dividing cells known as **transformed T lymphocytes** or **immunoblasts** (see Fig 4–3).
- These divide to produce effector T cells.
- Effector T lymphocytes morphologically resemble resting small lymphocytes and are often termed **sensitized, cytotoxic,** or **killer** T cells.

Note: This process of T cell transformation constitutes the **amplification phase** of the immune response (Fig 4–4), during which the few T cells bearing receptors that recognize the particular antigen form a clone of numerous **effector T cells** reactive against the same antigen.

   C. Functions of effector T cells: Effector T cells play important roles in three functions of the immune system.

     1. Cell-mediated immunity

      a. Cytotoxicity occurs in immunologic response to antigens on the surface of neoplastic cells, transplanted tissues, and virus-infected cells. Cytotoxic T cells apparently cause lysis by producing holes in the surface membranes of antigen-positive cells.

      b. Production of lymphokines that regulate the functions of macrophages and other lymphocytes (Table 4–2).

     2. Regulation of B lymphocyte activity:

- **Helper T cells** (CD4 antigen-positive) assist in activation and transformation of B lymphocytes and in immunoglobulin production.

TABLE 4–2. LYMPHOKINES (CYTOKINES)[1]

Lymphokine	Action	Source
MIF (migration inhibitory factor)	Inhibits random macrophage migration.	T cells
MAF (macrophage-activating factor)	Enhances lytic action of macrophages.	T cells
γ-Interferon	Enhances lytic action of macrophages.	T cells
Fibroblast-activating factor	Induces proliferation of fibroblasts.	T cells
B cell growth factor (BCGF)	Stimulates B cell proliferation.	T cells
B cell differentiation factor (BCDF)	Induces differentiation of B cell progeny to plasma cells.	T cells
Interleukin-2 (T cell growth factor)	Stimulates T cell proliferation.	T cells
Interleukin-3 (similar to colony-stimulating factor)	Supports monocyte proliferation.	T cells
Interleukin-1 (endogenous pyrogen)	Promotes immunoglobulin production by B cells and differentiation of T cells; may enhance NK activity plus other cell types affected.	Macrophages[2]
β-Interferon	May inhibit growth of several cell types, including tumor cells.	Macrophages
Angiogenesis factor	Stimulates new capillary formation.	Macrophages

[1]Strictly speaking, only factors released by T lymphocytes can be called lymphokines; however, the term is sometimes used loosely to include the products of macrophages. "Cytokines" is a more general term denoting hormonelike mediators secreted during immune and inflammatory reactions.
[2]Macrophages = monocytes in blood; histiocytes in tissue.

- **Suppressor T cells** (CD8 antigen-positive) inhibit B cell activation and regulate immunoglobulin synthesis.
- The normal ratio of helper T lymphocytes to suppressor T lymphocytes (CD4:CD8 ratio) in peripheral blood is 0.9–2.7.
- This ratio may be greatly decreased in certain diseases, including immunodeficiency states and AIDS.

    3. Delayed hypersensitivity: See Chapter 8.
    D. Identification of T cell subpopulations:

- T and B lymphocytes and their subsets cannot be distinguished morphologically.
- They are usually identified by cell-surface antigens that act as immunologic markers.
- These antigens are detected by specific monoclonal antibodies (Table 4–1), using

either immunofluorescence or immunoperoxidase methods on tissue sections, or flow cytometry.
■ Genetic techniques detecting rearrangement of T cell receptor genes are also useful in recognizing T cells.
■ Other markers such as the E rosette test are obsolete.

B. Lymphocytes
A. Distribution of B cells in the body:

■ B cells develop in the functional equivalent of the avian bursa of Fabricius (fetal liver or marrow in mammals). (See Fig 4–2).
■ After maturation, B cells are distributed to the B cell domains of the peripheral lymphoid tissue, including
  ● The primary and reactive (secondary or germinal) follicles or centers of lymph nodes (Fig 4–1; 30% of lymphocytes in the lymph nodes are B cells).
  ● The reactive centers in the malpighian bodies of the splenic white pulp (40% of splenic lymphocytes are B cells).
  ● The recirculating pool of lymphocytes between peripheral blood and the lymphatics (10–20% of peripheral blood lymphocytes are B cells).

  B. B cell transformation follows stimulation by either a specific antigen or a non-specific mitogen such as pokeweed mitogen.

■ B lymphocytes are transformed into large actively dividing **transformed B lymphocytes** or **B immunoblasts** (Fig 4–3).
■ These divide to produce plasma cells (which are the effector B cells).
■ The plasma cells secrete a specific antibody (immunoglobulin).
■ This is known as **humoral immunity.**

C. Identification of B cells:

■ Plasma cells have a distinctive morphologic appearance, with abundant basophilic cytoplasm and an eccentrically placed nucleus, with chromatin distributed in coarse clumps at its periphery ("cartwheel" or "clockface" pattern).
■ Plasma cells can be shown to contain large amounts of cytoplasmic immunoglobulin, using immunofluorescence or immunoperoxidase methods.
■ Other B lymphocytes must be identified by
  ● The presence of surface immunoglobulin.
  ● Membrane markers detected using monoclonal antibodies (Table 4–1).
  ● Genetic techniques for rearrangement of the immunoglobulin genes.

Null Cells (NK Cells & K Cells)
Null Cells are a heterogeneous group of lymphocytes defined by a lack of the usual markers (hence nonmarking or "null" cells). Null cells account for 5–10% of peripheral blood lymphocytes. They include various cell types:

■ Cells early in the T or B cell differentiation pathways prior to expression of many surface markers.

- **Natural killer (NK) cells,** which are cytotoxic and can lyse some foreign cells even if the organism has never been exposed to the inciting antigen. NK cells are identifiable by monoclonal antibodies anti-NK-1 and Leu-7 (CD57).
- **K cells,** which are cytotoxic with the aid of an antibody (antibody-dependent cell-mediated cytotoxicity [ADCC]).

MACROPHAGES (Monocytes of Blood; Histiocytes of Tissues)

Distribution in the Body
Macrophages are derived from monocyte precursors in bone marrow. They are found in all tissues of the body as tissue histiocytes, including

- Lymph node sinuses (Fig 4–1).
- The sinusoids in the red pulp of the spleen.
- The liver (Kupffer cells).
- The lung (alveolar macrophages).
- Brain tissue as microglial cells.
- Peripheral blood and bone marrow, where they appear as monocytes and their precursors.
- Possibly **dendritic reticulum cells** in the lymph node follicles and **interdigitating reticulum cells** in the paracortical zone, because they handle antigen for B and T lymphocytes.

Note: In the past the term *reticuloendothelial system* was used to encompass all of these cell types.

Identification of Macrophages
Macrophages may be identified by

- Histochemical staining for several enzymes (eg, nonspecific esterase).
- Immunohistochemical methods staining for other cell products (eg, muramidase or lysozyme).
- Monoclonal antibodies (Leu M1 [CD15], OKM1, Mo-1 [CD11]; see Table 4–1).

Functions of Macrophages
A. Phagocytosis.
1. Nonimmune phagocytosis:

- Macrophages phagocytose foreign particulate matter in the absence of an immune response.
- Microbial phagocytosis and killing are greatly facilitated when immunity is present (see Fig 3–2).

2. Immune phagocytosis:

- Macrophages have surface receptors for C3b and the Fc fragment of immunoglobulins (Ig).
- Particles coated with Ig or C3b (opsonins) are more easily phagocytosed.

B. Processing of antigens: (See T and B cells.)
C. Interaction with lymphokines:

■ Macrophages interact with lymphokines produced by T lymphocytes (macrophage-activating factor, macrophage inhibitory factor, gamma-interferon). (See Table 4–2).
■ Formation of granulomas is a typical result of such interaction.
■ Macrophages also produce lymphokinelike factors, including interleukin-1, beta-interferon, and T and B cell growth-promoting factors (Table 4–2).
■ The interactions of lymphocytes and macrophages in the tissues are manifested morphologically as chronic inflammation (see Chapter 5).

IMMUNOGLOBULINS (Antibodies)

Synthesis of Immunoglobulins
Immunoglobulins are synthesized by plasma cells that differentiate from B lymphocytes (B immunoblasts):

■ All immunoglobulin molecules synthesized by a single plasma cell are identical.
■ All plasma cells derived through transformation and proliferation of a single B lymphocyte precursor are identical; ie, they constitute a clone (Fig 4–4).
■ Immunoglobulin molecules synthesized by members of different clones of plasma cells have different specificities (react with different antigens).
■ These differences in specificity are due to changes in the amino acid sequences in the so-called V (variable) region of the immunoglobulin molecule (Fig 4–5).

Structure of Immunoglobulins (Fig 4–5)
The basic immunoglobulin molecule is composed of two heavy (H) chains and two light (L) chains connected by disulfide bonds.

■ **Light chains** consist of either two κ chains or two λ chains.
■ **Heavy chains** fall into five classes (IgA, IgG, IgM, IgD, IgE). Several subclasses also exist.
■ Antibodies produced against human Ig chains in animals may be used to recognize and distinguish the different light and heavy chains in humans (**isotypes**).
■ Each chain has a constant and a variable part:
  ● The **constant part** remains relatively constant in amino acid sequence.
  ● The **variable part** is characterized by widely divergent amino acid sequences.
  ● The antigen-combining (binding) sites are formed by the paired variable regions of the L and H chains.
■ Each IgG molecule consists of two paired chains that form two binding sites (Fig 4–5).
■ Specificity is determined by the sequence of amino acids in the hypervariable regions of the L–H chain pairs.
■ These hypervariable regions may also serve as antigens (**idiotypes**) if injected into other animals under suitable conditions.
■ The anti-idiotype antibody produced against the hypervariable region combines only with immunoglobulin molecules having that exact specificity (hypervariable region).
■ Other immunoglobulin classes show the same basic structure—except that IgM is a pentamer and IgA commonly exists as a dimer.

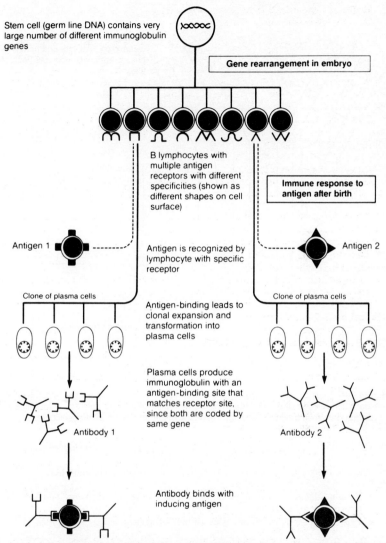

Stem cell (germ line DNA) contains very large number of different immunoglobulin genes

Gene rearrangement in embryo

B lymphocytes with multiple antigen receptors with different specificities (shown as different shapes on cell surface)

Immune response to antigen after birth

Antigen 1

Antigen is recognized by lymphocyte with specific receptor

Antigen 2

Clone of plasma cells

Antigen-binding leads to clonal expansion and transformation into plasma cells

Clone of plasma cells

Plasma cells produce immunoglobulin with an antigen-binding site that matches receptor site, since both are coded by same gene

Antibody 1

Antibody 2

Antibody binds with inducing antigen

Figure 4–4. Diagram of the B cell response, showing selection by antigen of B cells (two different B cells) with the appropriate "receptor fit." The transformation process (not shown) leads to production of plasma cells (two different clones shown) that produce antibody that also "fits" the antigen (ie, is specific to it). Note that the huge range of B cells, each bearing a different receptor (diversification), is generated early in embryonic development by the gene-"shuffling" mechanism. T cells undergo a similar process, producing multiple effector T cells.

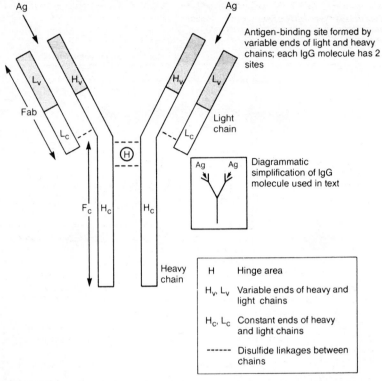

Figure 4–5. Diagram of an immunoglobulin molecule (IgG). The two antigen-binding sites are each composed of the V (variable) regions of a light-heavy chain pair. The differences in V regions determined by the "shuffled" genes account for the different specificities.

- The **constant region** has receptors for **complement** and is the **Fc fragment** that binds with those cells having Fc receptors (macrophages, NK cells etc.).
- Inherited antigenic differences between heavy chains constitute **allotypes.**
- Ig molecules may be cleaved by
  - **Papain digestion,** which produces 2 Fab (antibody) fragments and one Fc (crystallizable) fragment.
  - **Pepsin digestion,** which produces a F(ab)$'_2$ fragment and an Fc fragment.

Regulation of Antibody Production

Antibody production is initiated by activation of responsive B cells by antigen. Serum levels peak in 1 or 2 weeks and then begin to decline.

- **Helper T cells** (CD4-positive) augment antibody production due, at least in part, to release of lymphokines such as BCGF and BCDF (Table 4–2; B cell growth and differentiation factors, respectively).

■ **Suppressor T cells** (CD8-positive) have the opposite effect, serving to down-regulate the immune response.

Note: The **anti-idiotype network theory** proposes that the production of a particular specific antibody inevitably is followed by production of second (anti-idiotype) antibody that competes for the B cell antigen receptor, thereby down-regulating production of that specific antibody.

ANTIGEN RECOGNITION & GENERATION OF ANTIGENRECEPTOR DIVERSITY

Lymphocytes express receptors for antigen on their surfaces (Fig 4–4). Numerous receptors, with differing specificities, exist. Each individual lymphocyte expresses receptors for only a single antigen. Therefore, numerous (about 10^6–10^9) different lymphocytes exist, each expressing a single type of receptor.

■ **The antigen receptor of B lymphocytes is immunoglobulin.**
■ A gene-shuffling mechanism (see following) produces the many different surface immunoglobulin molecules that serve as antigen receptors on B cells.
■ In simplistic terms (see also Fig 4–4):
  ● The antigen selects lymphocytes that express receptors (ie, surface immunoglobulin of B cells) with reciprocal fit.
  ● This interaction induces the B cell to divide and transform.
  ● Subsequently it produces a clone of plasma cells that secrete antibody molecules essentially the same as those expressed on the surface of the initial antigen-recognizing lymphocyte.
■ **T cell receptor consists of a pair of polypeptide chains:**
  ● Including an alpha and a beta chain, each having a variable and constant region, thereby showing close resemblance to the B cell receptor (surface immunoglobulin).
  ● Thus it is regarded as a member of the "immunoglobulin super family," and shows a similar degree of diversity.
  ● Diversity of the T cell receptor is generated early in embryonic life by a gene-shuffling mechanism very similar to that occurring in B cells.
■ In simplistic terms:
  ● Antigen selects T cells bearing receptors with the appropriate specificity.
  ● This induces proliferation of a specific set of T cells.
  ● The net result is the generation of numerous effector T cells of identical specificity.
■ Antigen recognition by T cells is complex:
  ● For helper T cells, MHC class II molecules participate.
  ● For suppressor and cytotoxic T cells, MHC class I molecules participate.
  ● T cells bearing a receptor composed of gamma and delta chains have also been described.

Generation of Diversity: Gene-"Shuffling" Mechanisms

The diversity of antigen receptors on B and T cells is generated at the DNA level during differentiation of lymphoid precursors in embryonic life.

■ The genes involved are situated on
  ● Chromosome 2 (κ chain).
  ● Chromosome 22 (λ chain).

- Chromosome 8 (heavy chains).
- Chromosome 14 (α chain of T cell receptor).
- Chromosome 7 (β chain of T cell receptor).
- The heavy chain "multigene" contains
  - 200 different V (variable) gene segments each coding for a variable region of an immunoglobulin heavy chain.
  - Multiple D (diversity), J (joining), and C (constant region) segments.
- A splicing deletion mechanism brings together different combinations, thereby producing different functional genes and different antibodies.
- Light chains are similarly constituted except that they lack D segments.
- The alpha and beta chain (T receptor) genes also are similar.

ANTIGEN-ANTIBODY INTERACTIONS
Antibodies react with antigens with differing effects:

- **Precipitation** with small sized antigens.
- **Agglutination** with cellular antigens.
- **Neutralization** of certain toxins.
- **Opsonization** with certain particulate and cellular antigens, facilitating phagocytosis.
- **Activation of complement,** which occurs when certain IgG or IgM antibodies react with antigen.

COMPLEMENT

Activation of Complement
Complement is a system of plasma proteins (C1–C9) that exist in serum in an inactive form: activation leads to cell membrane lysis. Activation may occur in one of two ways.
   A. Classic pathway is initiated by the interaction of IgM or IgG with an antigen.

- C3 convertase is formed by activation of C1,4,2.
- Proceeds in cascade fashion (Fig 4–6).
- Its overall sequence is 1, **4**, 2, 3, 5, 6, 7, 8, 9).

   B. Alternate pathway (**properdin pathway**) differs from the classic pathway only in its mechanism of activation. The alternate pathway

- Does not require antigen-antibody interaction or the early (C1, C4, C2) complement factors.
- Cascade is initiated by aggregated IgG complexes, complex carbohydrates, and bacterial endotoxins.
- Forms C3 convertase by the interaction of properdin (a serum globulin), two other serum factors (B and D), and magnesium ions (Fig 4–6).

Effects of Complement Activation
Complement activation is associated with an acute inflammatory response characterized by vasodilation, increased vascular permeability, and fluid exudation mediated by C3a and C5a.

- Both C3a and C5a are strongly chemotactic for neutrophils (anaphylatoxic effect).
- C3b acts as an opsonin enhancing phagocytosis.
- **Membrane lysis** is the key immunologic effect.

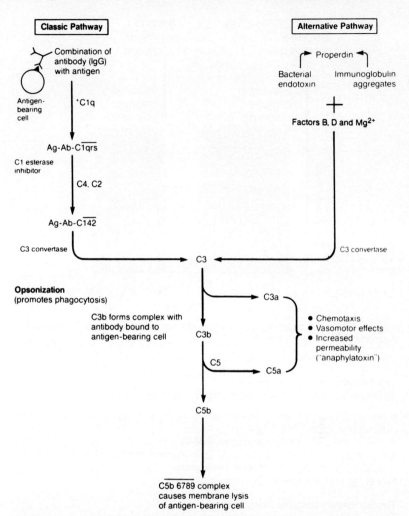

Figure 4–6. Activation of complement. The activated complement factors remain attached to the antigen-antibody complex on the surface of the antigen-bearing cell. Soluble complement fragments such as C3a and C5a are split off and pass into the surrounding interstitial tissue.

TYPES OF IMMUNE RESPONSE

Two types of immune response can be recognized, based on whether the immune system has been previously exposed to the antigen or not.

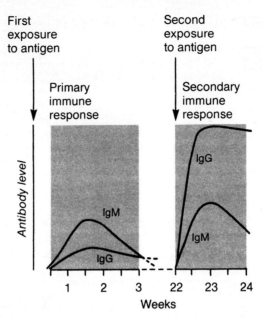

Figure 4–7. Primary and secondary immune responses, showing the rates of rise and fall of specific AgG and IgM antibodies.

The Primary Immune Response

The Primary immune response follows the first exposure to a particular antigen.

- Several days elapse before enough immunoglobulin is produced to be detected as an increase in serum levels (Fig 4–7).
- IgM is produced first; IgG production follows.
- The change from IgM to IgG or other Igs is a normal event in B cell activation and involves "switching" of the heavy chain genes.
- Ig levels peak and then decline over several days.

The Secondary Immune Response

The secondary immune response follows repeat exposure to an antigen.

- Production of a detectable increase in serum Ig occurs much more rapidly (2–3 days).
- IgG is the principal immunoglobulin secreted.
- Peak levels are higher and the decline occurs much more slowly (months).
- **Immunologic memory** is the ability to mount a specific secondary response:
  - It should be distinguished from a nonspecific increase in Ig levels (**anamnestic response**) that probably represents incidental stimulation of several B cells by lymphokines generated during the specific response.

CLINICAL USES OF THE IMMUNE RESPONSE

Serologic Diagnosis of Infection

After the first week of a primary response to an infectious agent, IgM becomes detectable in serum. **Caution:** Negative results of serologic tests do not rule out the possibility of early disease (ie, the first week).

- Since IgM typifies the primary response, increased specific IgM indicates active or recent disease.
- Levels increase rapidly but decline swiftly during convalescence.
- Rising levels of specific IgM or IgG on paired serum samples drawn several days apart are diagnostic of active infection (increase greater than fourfold).
- In contrast to IgM, IgG levels remain high for long periods, and elevated specific IgG levels signify only past infection, not necessarily recent.

Immunization

Passive immunization is the administration of antibody to an individual to protect against infection.

- The antibody may consist of
  - Pooled human serum (hepatitis A, rubella).
  - Serum from an animal specifically immunized against an antigen (tetanus toxin).
- Protection is short lived.
- A newborn baby has natural passive immunity due to the transplacental transfer of maternal antibodies that lasts about 6 months.

Active immunization is the administration of antigens of the infectious agent, often repeatedly, to produce a powerful immune response.

- Protection is long lived.
- Childhood vaccines use this principle.

Note: The term *vaccination* is derived from Edward Jenner's use of cowpox vaccinia virus to prevent smallpox in 1796.

Chronic Inflammation

5

Chronic inflammation is the sum of the responses mounted by the tissues against a persistent injurious agent: bacterial, viral, chemical, immunologic, etc. The tissues involved show evidence of several overlapping pathologic processes:

- Immune response, both cell-mediated and humoral, is characterized by the presence of lymphocytes, plasma cells, and macrophages.
- **Phagocytosis** is mediated by macrophages that have been activated by T cell lymphokines.
- **Repair** is characterized by new blood vessel formation, fibroblastic proliferation, and collagen deposition (fibrosis).

Chronic inflammation

- May follow an acute inflammatory response that fails to vanquish the agent, or may occur without a clinically apparent acute phase.
- Is distinguished from acute inflammation by the absence of cardinal signs such as redness, swelling, pain, and increased temperature.
- Is associated with agents that cause insidious but progressive (and often extensive) **tissue necrosis** accompanied by ongoing **repair by fibrosis.**

CHRONIC INFLAMMATION IN RESPONSE TO ANTIGENIC INJURIOUS AGENTS

Mechanisms
Chronic inflammation usually occurs in response to an injurious agent that is antigenic (eg, a microorganism), although some antigens may also be released from damaged tissues.

- Persistence of the antigen leads to accumulation of activated T lymphocytes, plasma cells, and macrophages at the site of injury.
- Because these cells are the prominent cell types in chronic inflammation, they are also called **chronic inflammatory cells.**
- Although triggered at the time of injury, the immune response takes several days to develop; chronic inflammatory cells thus take several days to appear.

Morphologic Types
Differentiation of the various types of chronic inflammation is based on the nature of the inciting agent and the subsequent immune response against it.
   A. Granulomatous chronic inflammation.
   1. Characteristic features:

- **Epithelioid cell granulomas,** which are composed of activated macrophages having abundant pale, foamy cytoplasm. They are called *epithelioid* cells because of a superficial resemblance to epithelial cells (Fig 5–1).

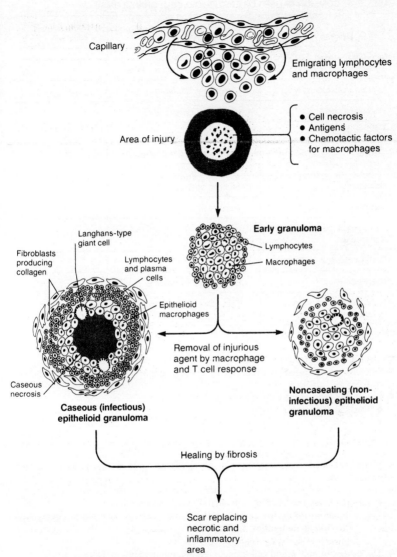

Figure 5–1. Phases in formation of epithelioid granulomas during chronic inflammation. Caseous necrosis occurs especially in those cases in which an infectious agent is responsible for the injury (eg, tuberculosis).

TABLE 5–1. COMMON CAUSES OF EPITHELIOID CELL GRANULOMAS

Disease	Antigen	Caseous Necrosis
Infectious diseases Tuberculosis	*Mycobacterium tuberculosis*	+ +
Leprosy (tuberculoid type)	*Mycobacterium leprae*	–
Histoplasmosis	*Histoplasma capsulatum*	+ +
Coccidioidomycosis	*Coccidiodies immitis*	+ +
Q fever	*Coxiella burnetti* (rickettsial organism)	–
Brucellosis	*Brucella* species	–
Syphilis	*Treponema pallidum*	+ +[1]
Noninfectious diseases Sarcoidosis	Unknown	–
Crohn's disease	Unknown	–
Berylliosis	Beryllium (? + protein)	–
Foreign body (eg, in intravenous drug abuse)	Talc, fibers (? + protein)	–

[1] Termed *gummatous necrosis* in syphilis.

- Macrophage aggregation, induced by lymphokines produced by activated T cells.
- Granulomas are usually surrounded by lymphocytes, plasma cells, fibroblasts, and collagen.
- **Langhans-type giant cells** may be present. They are
  - Derived from macrophages.
  - Characterized by 10–50 nuclei around the periphery of the cell.

2. **Causes:** Epithelioid granulomas form when

- Macrophages have successfully phagocytosed the injurious agent but it survives inside them.
  - An active T lymphocyte-mediated cellular immune response occurs.
  - Lymphokines produced by activated T lymphocytes include
    - **Migration-inhibiting factor (MIF),** which causes macrophage aggregation.
    - **Macrophage-activating factor (MAF),** which increases the ability of macrophages to destroy phagocytosed particles.
- The causes of epithelioid cell granulomas are summarized in Table 5–1.

3. **Changes in affected tissues:**

- Individual granulomas expand and fuse to form large masses.

■ In infectious granulomas, central **caseous** (cheesy) **necrosis** is a common feature (Fig 5–1).

■ A similar form of necrosis called **gummatous** (rubbery or gumlike) **necrosis** occurs in syphilis.

■ Both result from a T lymphocyte-mediated hypersensitivity reaction (type IV hypersensitivity). (See Chapter 8.)

B. Nongranulomatous chronic inflammation.
   1. Characteristic features:

■ Sensitized lymphocytes (specifically activated by antigen), plasma cells, and macrophages accumulate in the injured area.

■ These are scattered diffusely, and do not form focal granulomas.

■ Necrosis and fibrosis are common.

   2. Causes and changes in affected tissues: Simple nongranulomatous chronic inflammation may follow several types of immune processes.
   a. Chronic viral infections, eg, chronic viral hepatitis.
   b. Chronic autoimmune diseases, eg, atrophic gastritis, Hashimoto's thyroiditis.
   c. Chronic chemical intoxications, eg, alcoholic hepatitis.
   d. Chronic nonviral infections, eg, lepromatous leprosy where the T cell response is poor. When the T cell response is vigorous, granulomas form (tuberculoid leprosy).
   e. Chronic metazoan infections: Mast cells and eosinophils are additional features of chronic inflammation caused by metazoan parasites.

CHRONIC INFLAMMATION IN RESPONSE TO NONANTIGENIC INJURIOUS AGENTS

Foreign body granulomas form in response to large nonantigenic particles, such as sutures, talc particles, and inert fibers. **Foreign body giant cells** are often present, and are characterized by numerous nuclei dispersed throughout the cell rather than around the periphery (as in Langhans-type giant cells). Foreign material is usually identifiable in granuloma, particularly if viewed under polarized light.

FUNCTION & RESULT OF CHRONIC INFLAMMATION

Chronic inflammation serves to contain and, over a long time, remove an injurious agent that is not otherwise easily eradicated. Several mechanisms play a part:

■ Direct killing by activated lymphocytes.

■ Interaction with antibodies produced by plasma cells.

■ Activation of macrophages by lymphokines.

■ **Tissue necrosis** is often a feature; and if extensive may be associated with serious clinical illness.

■ **Associated fibrosis** is the major repair mechanism, but if extensive the scarring may itself contribute to the disease (eg, constrictive pericarditis).

■ When healing occurs, an acellular fibrous scar marks the site of injury.

MIXED ACUTE & CHRONIC INFLAMMATION

Acute and chronic inflammation represent different types of host response to injury; their features may overlap:

- **Chronic suppurative inflammation** often becomes walled off by chronic inflammation and fibrosis when large amounts of pus are present in the area (eg, chronic abscess, chronic suppurative osteomyelitis, and pyelonephritis).
- **Recurrent acute inflammation** may occur if there is a predisposing cause (eg, in the gallbladder when there are gallstones, or in a scarred heart valve).
- The term **subacute inflammation** is often used to denote this pattern.

Healing & Repair   6

RESOLUTION
Resolution is the ideal outcome of healing. It occurs when the tissue is, in effect, restored to its preinjury state. Fibrinous inflammatory exudate and debris are removed via the lymphatics, or by neutrophils and macrophages. Because there is little or no cell necrosis, regeneration is not necessary, and there is no scar formation.

REGENERATION
When cell loss is extensive, regeneration can still restore injured tissue to normal. The extent to which this occurs depends on

- The regenerative capacity of involved cells (ie, their ability to divide).
- The number of surviving viable cells.
- The presence of surviving connective tissue to provide a framework for restoration.

Before regeneration can occur, the necrotic cells must be removed by the inflammatory response. The cells of the body can be divided into three groups on the basis of their regenerative capacity (Table 6–1).

Labile Cells (Intermitotic Cells)
A. Characteristics:

- Labile cells normally divide actively throughout life to replace cells that are continually being lost from the body.
- Mature differentiated cells in these tissues cannot divide; their numbers are maintained by division of their parent labile (stem) cells.

B. Healing in tissues with labile cells:

- Following injury, surviving labile cells proliferate rapidly to replace cells lost by necrosis:
  - For example, loss of endometrium during menstruation is followed by complete regeneration within days.
  - Hemolysis is followed by rapid replacement from erythroid precursors in bone marrow.

Note: Regeneration can only occur if sufficient labile stem cells survive the injury; eg, regeneration does not occur after heavy radiation to the marrow, which destroys stem cells (aplastic anemia).

Stable Cells (Reversibly Postmitotic Cells)
A. Characteristics: Stable cells typically have a long life span and a low rate of division, but retain the capacity to enter the mitotic cell cycle after injury (Fig 6–1). Cells in this category include

- The parenchymal cells of most solid glandular organs (liver, pancreas).
- The mesenchymal cells (fibroblasts, endothelial cells).

TABLE 6–1. CLASSIFICATION OF CELLS ON THE BASIS OF THEIR REGENERATIVE CAPACITY

Cell Types	Mitotic Capacity	Examples

Labile (intermitotic)	Short G_0 phase; almost always in mitotic cell cycle	Hematopoietic stem cells
		Basal cells
		  Epidermis
		  Genitourinary tract
		Crypt cells of gut mucosa
		Hair follicle cells
		Seminiferous germ cells
		Epithelium of ducts

Stable (reversibly postmitotic)	Long G_0 phase; can divide actively when stimulated	Parenchymal cells
		  Liver
		  Kidney (renal tubules)
		  Lung (alveoli)
		  Pancreas
		  Breast
		  Endocrine glands
		Mesenchymal cells
		  Osteoblast
		  Chondrocyte
		  Fibroblast
		  Endothelial cell
		  Adipocyte

Permanent (irreversibly postmiotic)	None (cannot divide)	Neurons in central nervous system Ganglion cells in peripheral nervous system Cardiac muscle cells[1] Skeletal muscle cells[1]

[1]Cardiac and skeletal muscle cells demonstrate limited mitotic capability in experimental settings. In humans, they are functionally permanent cells.

B. Healing in tissues with stable cells:

■ Enough viable cells must remain to provide a source of parenchymal cells for regeneration.
■ There must be an intact connective tissue framework. This is exemplified in the kidney:
  ● Selective necrosis of renal tubular cells (acute renal tubular necrosis) with sparing of the renal tubular framework is rapidly followed by regeneration from the surviving tubular epithelial cells.
  ● But when necrosis of both the parenchyma and the connective tissue framework occurs (renal infarct), no regeneration is possible and healing occurs by scar formation.

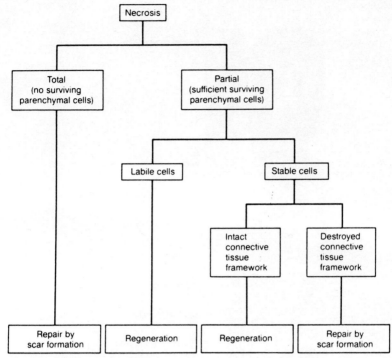

Figure 6-1. Factors influencing regeneration and repair by scar formation after injury to tissues containing labile and stable cells. Note that permanent cells have no capability of regeneration and always heal by scar formation.

Permanent Cells (Irreversibly Postmitotic Cells)

A. Characteristics: Permanent cells have no capacity for mitotic division in postnatal life.

B. Healing in tissues with permanent cells: Injury to permanent cells is always followed by **scar formation.** No regeneration is possible.

REPAIR BY SCAR FORMATION

A **scar** is a mass of collagen that is the end result of repair by **organization and fibrosis.** It occurs when

■ Resolution fails to happen in an acute inflammatory process.
■ There is ongoing tissue necrosis in chronic inflammation.
■ Parenchymal cell necrosis cannot be repaired by regeneration.

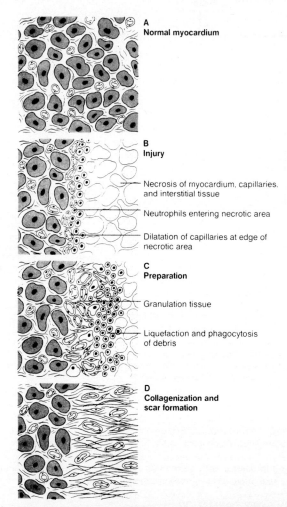

A
Normal myocardium

B
Injury

Necrosis of myocardium, capillaries, and interstitial tissue

Neutrophils entering necrotic area

Dilatation of capillaries at edge of necrotic area

C
Preparation

Granulation tissue

Liquefaction and phagocytosis of debris

D
Collagenization and scar formation

Figure 6–2. Repair of a myocardial infarct by scar formation. A normal myocardium is shown in **A.** The infarct evokes an acute inflammatory response and is invaded from the periphery by neutrophils (**B**), which liquefy the necrotic tissue. This is followed by entry of macrophages and granulation tissue (**C**), which removes the necrotic debris and leads to replacement of the necrotic zone by scar (**D**).

The **process of repair** by scar formation can be divided into several overlapping phases (Fig 6–2):

■ **Preparation** includes removal of the inflammatory exudate and debris, as in resolution or regeneration.

■ **Granulation tissue**
  ● Grows into the injured area from healthy surrounding tissues as necrotic debris is being removed.
  ● Consists of newly formed capillaries, proliferating fibroblasts, and residual inflammatory cells.
  ● Process is controlled by a variety of growth-factors, including lymphokines, platelet-derived growth factor, and macrophage-derived growth factor.
  ● On gross examination, is soft, fleshy, and deep red because of the numerous capillaries.
  ● Eventually replaces all of the injured area, in a process termed **organization.**
■ Accompanied by **production of fibronectin,** a glycoprotein
  ● Apparently plays a key role in the formation of granulation tissue.
  ● Is derived from plasma, and also is synthesized by fibroblasts and endothelial cells.
  ● Is chemotactic for fibroblasts and promotes organization.
■ **Collagenization**
  ● Synthesized by fibroblasts in the form of a precursor, tropocollagen (procollagen).
  ● Tropocollagen (MW 285,000) is composed of three separate alpha polypeptide chains wrapped together to form a tight triple helix.
  ● After secretion these molecules polymerise, overlapping one another by about ¼ of their length to produce the characteristic 67-nm-periodicity–transverse striations seen in collagen fibrils under the electron microscope.
  ● Under the light microscope, collagen stains pink with hematoxylin and eosin (H&E) stain, and green or blue with special trichrome stains.
  ● The terms **fibrous tissue** and **scar tissue** are synonymous with collagen.
  ● Synthesis of tropocollagen by fibroblasts requires ascorbic acid (vitamin C); major deficiency of vitamin C (scurvy) leads to defective collagen formation.
  ● There are at least five types of collagen (types I–V), based on the minor variations in the structure of their polypeptide chains.
■ **Maturation** occurs as the young, pink scar, consisting of granulation tissue and collagen, becomes less cellular and less vascular, and turns white in color.
■ **Contraction** and **Strengthening** constitute the final phase of repair.
  ● Contraction decreases the size of the scar. It is due in the early stages to active contraction of actomyosin filaments in fibroblasts (myofibroblasts). Later contraction is a property of the collagen molecule itself.
  ● Strengthening is due to formation of increasing amounts of collagen and changes in the type of collagen.

HEALING OF SKIN WOUNDS
Understanding the mechanisms involved in the healing of skin wounds provides insight into healing in general.

Types of Skin Injury

Skin injuries are classified on the basis of severity and the nature of the involvement.

A. Abrasion ("scrape") is defined as removal of the superficial part of the epidermis only.

■ Regeneration occurs from labile cells that survive in the underlying basal germinative layer.
■ There is no scarring.

B. Incision ("cut") and laceration ("tear"):

■ Both epidermis and dermis are disrupted but with minimal loss of germinative cells.
■ If the defect is small, and there is no infection and no foreign material, healing is rapid (healing by first intention; see following).

C. Wounds with epidermal defects:

■ More severe injuries (eg, crush injuries, extensive lacerations, burns) cause loss of large areas of the complete epidermis, including the basal germinative cells, plus variable necrosis of underlying dermis.
■ In such cases, a phase of inflammation precedes the repair process (healing by second intention; see following).

Healing Processes

A. Healing by first intention (primary union).
    1. Process of primary union:

■ Clean wounds, in which the edges of the wound are in close apposition, heal by first intention (Fig 6–3).
■ The small defect fills with clotted blood, which forms a scab and seals the wound.
■ The epidermis regenerates from basal cells at the edges of the wound.
■ In the subjacent dermis, the wound fills with clotted blood and heals by scar formation.

    2. The scar: The young scar that becomes visible when the scab separates from the skin is initially pink, but soon becomes white and progressively smaller.
    3. Tensile strength:

■ Is poor in the first week; a surgical incision is artificially held together by sutures, clips, or tape for this period (longer would be better, but risk of wound infection increases).
■ Increases to about 30–50% of normal skin by 4 weeks and to 80% after several months.

    B. Healing by second intention (secondary union): Wounds that fail to heal by first intention heal by second intention (secondary union). See Fig 6–4.
    1. Reasons for failure of primary union:

■ Physical inability to achieve apposition of wound margins.
■ The presence of foreign material or necrotic tissue.

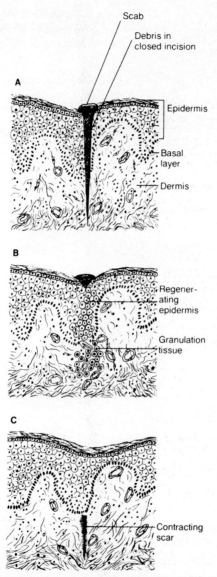

A:
Scab

Debris in closed incision

Epidermis

Basal layer

Dermis

B:
Regenerating epidermis

Granulation tissue

C:
Contracting scar

Figure 6–3. Healing of a surgical incision by first intention. **A:** Debris in the narrow gap between apposed skin edges is removed by neutrophils and macrophages. **B:** The epidermis regenerates rapidly, and granulation tissue in the dermal gap becomes collagenized to form a thin dermal scar (**C**).

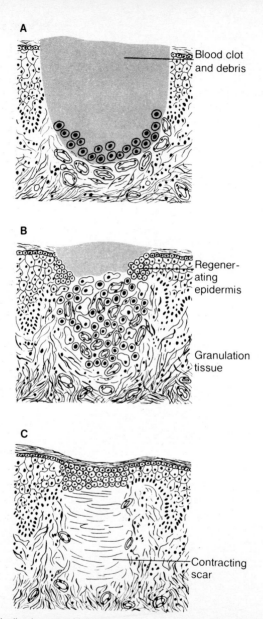

Figure 6–4. Healing by second intention of a large would with extensive necrosis. **A:** The large area of tissue necrosis evokes acute inflammation with entry of neutrophils from the periphery. Slow liquefaction of debris and ingrowth of granulation tissue from the base (**B**) leads to scar formation (**C**). The epidermis regenerates slowly from the edges.

■ Infection, suppuration.
■ Large epidermal defects

2. Process of secondary union is essentially the same as that of healing by first intention, but take much longer because of more extensive damage (Fig 6–4).

■ Surgical debridement (removal of necrotic tissues) and skin transplantation may help speed the process in severe cases.
■ Skin appendages such as hair follicles and glands are regenerated if enough residual labile cells remain.

C. Causes of defective wound healing: The presence of any of these factors may greatly increase the risk of surgery.
   1. Failure of collagen synthesis, which may result from vitamin C, protein, or zinc deficiency.

■ **Ehlers-Danlos syndrome** is a group of rare inherited diseases with defects in the tropocollagen synthetic pathway.
   ● Abnormalities include impaired wound healing, easy bruisability, and fragile skin.
   ● One interesting effect is hyperextensibility of joints due to laxity of collagen in joint capsules.

2. Excessive collagen production results in formation of abnormal nodular masses (keloids) at the sites of skin injury. This is more common in blacks, with familial tendency.
   3. Local factors.
      a. Foreign or necrotic tissue or blood, if present in the wound.
      b. Infection with persisting inflammation and (commonly) abscess formation.
      c. Abnormal blood supply: Ischemia due to arterial disease and impaired venous drainage both hinder wound healing.
      d. Decreased viability of cells following irradiation or administration of chemotherapy.
   4. Diabetes mellitus, possibly due in part to poor blood supply.
   5. Excessive levels of adrenal corticosteroids, whether due to administration of exogenous corticosteroids or to endogenous adrenal hyperactivity (Cushing's syndrome).

Deficiencies of the Host Response   **7**

The nonspecific inflammatory response and the immune response act synergistically. Deficits in either may result in increased susceptibility to attack by microorganisms, including organisms of low virulence that do not cause disease in a normal host (**opportunistic infections**).

DEFICIENCIES OF THE INFLAMMATORY RESPONSE

DEFICIENCY OF THE VASCULAR RESPONSE
Deficiencies of the vascular response include **diabetes mellitus,** which is characterized by thickening of the basement membrane of small vessels that increases susceptibility to infection. With **vascular disease (ischemia),** arterial narrowing is a factor, especially in the elderly.

ABNORMAL NEUTROPHIL FUNCTION
Quantitative disorders of neutrophil function include neutropenia (decreased numbers of neutrophils), which is associated with a defective cellular response in acute inflammation. Neutropenia

- Is critical when the peripheral-blood neutrophil count is less than $100/\mu L$.
- Is most commonly caused by cytotoxic drugs and radiation therapy (Chapter 26).

Qualitative Disorders of neutrophil motility include:

- **Lazy leukocyte syndrome,** in which neutrophil emigration is abnormal.
- **Chédiak-Higashi syndrome,** in which defective degranulation of neutrophils is associated with the presence of cytoplasmic inclusions (enlarged lysosomes).
- Extrinsic inhibitors of leukocyte motility, which occur with rheumatoid arthritis and related disorders.
- Complement deficiency.

Disorders of phagocytosis include

- Deficiency of opsonins (eg, hypogammaglobulinemia, and complement factor 3 (C3) deficiency).
- Chédiak-Higashi syndrome.
- Use of antimalarial drugs and corticosteroids.

Disorders of Microbial Killing
   A. **Chronic granulomatous disease of childhood** is an X-linked recessive disorder (ie, it affects males). It is characterized by

- Decreased ability of neutrophils to produce hydrogen peroxide.

■ Recurrent infections of skin, lungs, bone, and lymph nodes.
■ Particular susceptibility to diseases caused by staphylococci and *Serratia* that produce catalase.
■ Diagnosis through
  ● Nitroblue tetrazolium dye test.
  ● Decreased bacterial killing curves.
  ● Histologic examination of involved tissue, which shows granuloma formation.

B. Myeloperoxidase deficiency is a rare cause of failure of neutrophil function.

C. Granulocytic leukemia: Neutrophils, monocytes, or both are increased in number in granulocytic leukemias (Chapter 26), but they usually function abnormally.

DEFICIENCIES OF THE IMMUNE RESPONSE

CONGENITAL (PRIMARY)
All types of congenital immunodeficiency are rare.

Severe Combined Immunodeficiency (SCID)
SCID is one of the most severe forms of congenital immunodeficiency. It is characterized by a defect of lymphoid stem cells (① in Fig 7–1) that leads to **failure of development of both T and B lymphocytes:**

■ The thymus fails to descend normally.
■ Lymphoid tissues are almost devoid of lymphocytes.
■ Immunoglobulins are absent in serum (Table 7–1).
■ Viral, fungal, bacterial, or protozoal infections occur.
■ Most patients have the autosomal recessive form (Swiss-type); a few have the X-linked recessive form.
■ The enzyme **adenosine deaminase** is commonly lacking, thereby inhibiting cell division.
■ Treatment is bone marrow transplantation.
■ Severe infections occur early in life, with death usual in the first year.

Thymic Hypoplasia (DiGeorge Syndrome)
In thymic hypoplasia, congenital failure of development of the thymus (② in Fig 7–1) results in lack of T lymphocytes in the blood and T cell areas of lymph nodes and spleen. Patients show signs of

■ Deficient cell-mediated immunity.
■ Viral, mycobacterial, and fungal infections in infancy.
■ B lymphocyte development near normal.
■ Serum immunoglobulin levels near normal.

Thymic hypoplasia is part of a more severe abnormality of development of the third and fourth pharyngeal pouches. Parathyroid glands may be absent, leading to hypocalcemia and early death.

T Lymphopenia (Nezelof's Syndrome)
T lymphopenia, or Nezelof's syndrome is thought to result from abnormalities of T cell maturation in the thymus.

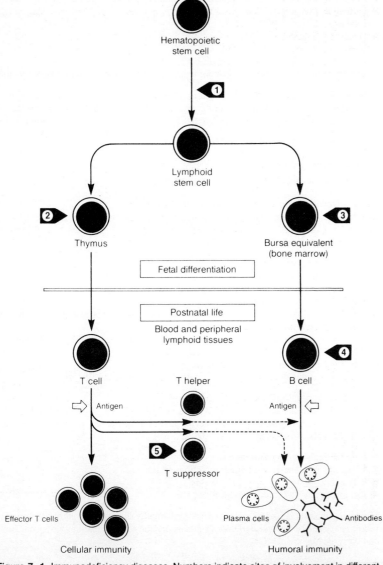

Figure 7–1. Immunodeficiency diseases. Numbers indicate sites of involvement in different disorders and correspond to discussion in text.

TABLE 7–1. IMMUNODEFICIENCY DISEASES

	Peripheral Blood Lymphocytes	Peripheral Blood T Cells	Peripheral Blood B Cells	Tissue Lymphoid Cells	Serum Immunoglobulin	Other Features
Severe combined immunodeficiency	↓	↓	↓	Absent	↓	Lack of adenosine deaminase in 50% of patients with autosomal recessive form of disease.
Thymic aplasia (DiGeorge syndrome)	↓	↓	N¹	T cells depleted in thymus-dependent areas of lymph nodes and spleen	N	Abnormal development of pharyngeal pouches; parathyroids absent.
T lymphopenia (Nezelof's syndrome)	↓	↓	N	N	N/↓	Heterogenous group; immunoglobulins may also be decreased.
Bruton's congenital agammaglobulinemia	N	N	↓	Absence of follicles and plasma cells in lymph nodes	↓	Neutropenia.

(continued)

TABLE 7-1. (Continued)

	Peripheral Blood Lymphocytes	Peripheral Blood T Cells	Peripheral Blood B Cells	Tissue Lymphoid Cells	Serum Immunoglobulin	Other Features
Variable immunodeficiency	N	N	N/↓	Decrease in plasma cells	↓	Associated autoimmune disease; occasionally, lymphadenopathy with follicular hyperplasia.
Selective IgA deficiency	N	N	N	N	↓ IgA only	Common (1 :1000 general population).
Wiskott-Aldrich syndrome	N/↓	N/↓	N	N	↓ (Especially helper IgM)	Involuted thymus, thrombocytopenia, eczema.
Ataxia-telangiectasia	↓	N/↓	N	Variable	↓ (Especially IgA)	Embryonic-type thymus; lymphomas common.
HIV infection (AIDS)	N/↓	↓ (Especially helper T cells)	N	Abnormal follicular hyperplasia or lymphocyte depletion	N	Decreased helper:suppressor T cell ratio; Kaposi's sarcoma; β cell lymphomas.
Epitheloid thymoma (Good's syndrome)	↓	↓	N	Decreased or absent plasma cells	N/↓	Decreased eosinophil count; red cell aplasia.

¹N = normal.

Bruton's Congenital Agammaglobulinemia

Bruton's agammaglobulinemia is an X-linked recessive seen mostly in male infants. It is characterized by

- Failure of development of B lymphocytes (③ in Fig 7–1).
- Absence of B lymphocytes in the peripheral blood and in the B cell domains of lymph nodes and spleen.
- Absence of reactive follicles and plasma cells in lymph nodes.
- Marked decrease or absence of serum immunoglobulins, but the thymus and T lymphocytes develop normally.
- Infections in the infant after passively transferred maternal antibody levels decrease (age 6 months or so).
- Recurrent infections of the lungs, meninges, middle ear, and sinuses caused by *Streptococcus pneumoniae* and *Haemophilus influenzae* are characteristic.

Common Variable Immunodeficiency

Common variable immunodeficiency is characterized by decreased levels of some or all of the immunoglobulin classes.

- Peripheral blood lymphocytes, including B cells, are usually normal.
- In some cases, an excess of suppressor T cells has been described (⑤ in Fig 7–1), particularly in an acquired form of the disease that develops in adult life.
- Inheritance patterns are variable.
- Bacterial infections and giardiasis recur.

Isolated IgA Deficiency

Selective deficiency of IgA is the most common immunodeficiency, occurring in about 1 in 1000 individuals. It

- Is due to a defect in the terminal differentiation of IgA-secreting plasma cells (④ in Fig 7–1).
- May be associated with abnormal suppressor T lymphocytes (⑤ in Fig 7–1).
- Is often asymptomatic in patients, or they may demonstrate increased incidence of pulmonary and gastrointestinal infections (since they lack mucosal IgA).

Note: They may develop anti-IgA antibodies that react with IgA in transfused blood (type I hypersensitivity; Chapter 8).

Immunodeficiency Associated With Inherited Diseases
A. Wiskott-Aldrich syndrome:

- Is X-linked recessive.
- Is characterized by eczema, thrombocytopenia, and immunodeficiency.
- Exhibits low T cells and serum IgM levels.
- Patients develop recurrent viral, fungal, and bacterial infections.

B. Ataxia-telangiectasia:

- Is autosomal recessive.
- Is characterized by cerebellar ataxia, skin telangiectasia, and deficiencies of T lymphocytes, IgA, and IgE.

Complement Deficiency

Deficiencies of various complement factors has been described; all are rare. C2 and C3 deficiencies are the most common.

SECONDARY & ACQUIRED IMMUNODEFICIENCY

Secondary immunodeficiency occurs as a common consequence of certain conditions, including

- Malignancy: Hodgkin's disease, lymphoma, advanced cancer.
- Iron or protein calorie deficiency.
- Chronic diseases: diabetes mellitus, renal failure.
- Use of cytotoxic drugs, steroids, radiotherapy.
- Aging.

Acquired Immune Deficiency Syndrome (AIDS)
A. Incidence:

- It is increasingly common.
- By 1988, there were about 60,000 cases in the USA.
- 2 million individuals are estimated to be infected with HIV (human immunodeficiency virus).

B. Definition:
AIDS is defined by criteria set forth by the US Centers for Disease Control (CDC). Simplified, the criteria for diagnosis include a combination of tests for serum HIV antibody status and the presence of indicator diseases. To be diagnosed as having AIDS, the patient

- **Must be HIV-positive.**
- **Must exhibit the presence of indicator diseases** such as
  - Recurrent opportunistic infections (including pneumocystis, mycobacterial species, and candida).
  - High-grade lymphomas, especially of brain.
  - Kaposi's sarcoma.
- **In an HIV results-equivocal or status-unknown patient,** AIDS is diagnosed by **both**
- The presence of any of the above "indicators."
- The absence of any other cause of immunodeficiency, such as cytotoxic therapy, preexisting lymphoma, or congenital immunodeficiency.
- **In an HIV test negative patient,** AIDS is excluded **unless** indicator diseases persist and the CD4 (helper T cell) count falls to less than 400/μL.

Note: Patients may take variable (unknown) time to convert to HIV positivity following initial infection.
C. Etiology and pathogenesis:

- Etiologic agent is an RNA retrovirus called **human immunodeficiency virus (HIV)**—previously called human T cell lymphotropic virus type III (HTLV III) and lymphadenopathy-associated virus (LAV).
- Virus attacks helper (CD4/OKT4-positive) T lymphocytes.

■ Other cells that share common epitopes with CD4 cells—such as macrophages and cells in the central nervous system—are also susceptible.

■ Entry of HIV into T lymphocytes results in

● Cell death.

● Latent infection.

● Appearance of anti-HIV antibodies in the serum. Antibodies are not protective, and HIV viremia persists.

■ **Diagnostic tests** include:

● The ELISA test, which detects anti-HIV antibody, but gives a small number of false-positive and false-negative results.

  ○ All positive ELISA tests must therefore be followed by a highly specific confirmatory test—Immunoblot (Western blot)—to detect HIV protein.

● HIV culture tests (growing the virus), P24 antigen assays (detecting viral antigens), and HIV PCR tests (detecting HIV nucleic acid by the polymerase chain reaction), are available in some specialized centers.

D. Transmission:

■ Sexual contact.

■ Direct injection into the blood (transfusion or IV drug abuse).

■ Risk of transmission by other body fluids such as saliva and tears is very low.

■ Rare cases have been reported after accidental blood spills and needle sticks.

■ The risk of infection by casual contact with an infected person is almost nil.

■ Testing for HIV antibody in blood donors has greatly reduced the risk of HIV transmission by transfusion of blood and blood products (eg, factor VIII concentrate that is used to treat hemophilia).

E. Individuals at high risk for HIV infection:

■ Male homosexuals and bisexuals, who account for over 70% of cases of AIDS in the USA.

■ Intravenous drug abusers, who account for about 15% of cases.

■ Heterosexual female contacts of male bisexuals and IV drug abusers.

■ Patients transfused with blood products—especially hemophiliacs and infants.

■ Central Africans (common among heterosexuals, plus vertical transmission from mother to fetus).

F. Manifestations and stages of HIV infection: See Table 7–2.
1. Incubation period:

■ Post transfusion appears to be a median of about 8 years in adults (2 years in infants) to overt AIDS.

■ Following infection, the percentage of asymptomatic HIV-positive individuals who go on to develop AIDS is still unknown.

2. Changes in the immune system:

■ Decrease in the number of helper/inducer (CD4/OKT4-positive) T cells in the blood.

■ Decreased helper T cell:suppressor T cell ratio in the blood.

TABLE 7–2. CLASSIFICATION OF STAGES OF HIV INFECTION:
CDC (CENTERS FOR DISEASE CONTROL) STAGING

CDC I	Asymptomatic infection (may be brief flulike illness).
CDC II	Conversion to HIV-positive serology (ELISA test).
CDC III	Onset of immunologic defects, generalized lymphadenopathy (also known as ARC [AIDS-related complex]).
CDC IV	Overt AIDS with opportunistic infections and neoplasms.

Mean incubation period (time from infection to overt AIDS):
  Children < age 5 years: 2 years
  Adults (and older children): 8 years

Adverse prognostic indications include constitutional symptoms (fever, weight loss, diarrhea), low CD4 lymphocytes, low anti-P24 antibody, circulating P24 antigen, persisting viremia.

- These changes lead to functional immunodeficiency.
- The decreased helper:suppressor T cell ratio is not diagnostic of HIV infection and may occur in several other immunodeficiency states.

3. AIDS-related complex (ARC):

- ARC patients are HIV-positive.
- They are symptomatic, but have none of the indicator diseases that are used to define AIDS.
- Symptoms include fatigue, weight loss, night sweats, and diarrhea.
- Biopsied lymph nodes show marked reactive follicular hyperplasia with characteristic histologic features (Chapter 28)—a condition called **persistent generalized lymphadenopathy (PGL).**
- The percentage of patients with ARC who go on to develop AIDS is not known for certain.

4. AIDS is the final phase of HIV infection.

- The HIV-positive patient develops one of many opportunistic infections or neoplasms that define the disease (see preceding).
- Once present, AIDS relentlessly and invariably progresses to death.
- Drugs such as azidothymidine (AZT) and ribavirin have been shown to prolong life to a degree, but do not appear curative.

EFFECTS OF IMMUNE DEFICIENCY

Infections
T cell deficiency predisposes to infections with viruses, mycobacteria, fungi, and protozoa such as *Pneumocystis carinii* and *Toxoplasma gondii*. B cell deficiency predisposes to pyogenic bacterial infections.

Malignant Neoplasms
Kaposi's sarcoma and B cell lymphomas are the most common neoplasms in immunodeficient individuals. They occur in HIV infection, Wiskott-Aldrich syndrome, and ataxia-telangiectasia, and after long-term immunosuppressive therapy (eg, in renal transplantation).

Autoimmune Diseases
Autoimmune diseases tend to develop in patients with congenital immunodeficiency (Bruton's agammaglobulinemia, common variable immunodeficiency, selective IgA deficiency, and complement factor deficiency). They include rheumatoid arthritis, systemic lupus erythematosus, autoimmune hemolytic anemia, and thrombocytopenia.

Graft vs. Host Disease
Graft vs. host disease occurs in severely T cell-deficient patients who receive viable "foreign" immunocompetent cells (eg, in blood transfusions and bone marrow transplants). Foreign lymphocytes proliferate and react against the host. It is usually fatal.

DIAGNOSIS OF IMMUNE DEFICIENCY
In diagnosing immune deficiency, useful studies include

- Determination of serum immunoglobulin and complement levels.
- Blood lymphocyte count, T and B cell number.
- Helper/suppressor ratio.
- Special tests, such as viral culture and serologic studies (in HIV infection) and enzyme determinations (in severe combined immunodeficiency disease). See Table 7–1.

Section III. Agents Causing Tissue Injury

Immunologic Injury   8

IMMUNOLOGIC HYPERSENSITIVITY

Immunologic hypersensitivity is defined as an abnormal exaggerated immune reaction to a foreign agent, with resulting injury to host tissues. An initial exposure to antigen (sensitization) is followed by hypersensitivity on subsequent exposure (challenge dose).

Type I (Immediate) Hypersensitivity (Atopy; Anaphylaxis)
A. Mechanism (Table 8–1):

- Initial exposure to the antigen (allergen) causes production of **IgE antibodies** (reagins).
- IgE attaches to the surface membrane of mast cells and basophils.
- Subsequent exposure to the same antigen causes degranulation of mast cells and release of vasoactive substances (histamine, serotonin, leukotrienes).
- Chemotactic factors cause accumulation of neutrophils and eosinophils.

B. Disorders resulting from type I hypersensitivity.
1. Localized type I hypersensitivity:

- Is also termed atopy.
- Is associated with an inherited predisposition.
- May involve different tissues.

a. Skin:

- Contact with allergen causes immediate reddening, swelling, itching, etc.
- Reactions include acute dermatitis, eczema, urticaria, hives.
- The antigen may come in contact with skin **directly,** by injection, or through insect bites or stings.
- Or, it may be **ingested** (eg, food or drug allergies that produce cutaneous reactions).

b. Nose:

- Allergen may be inhaled (most commonly, pollens).
- May manifest as allergic rhinitis or hay fever.

c. Lung:

- Allergens may be inhaled (pollen, dust).
- May manifest as bronchospasm or allergic asthma.

TABLE 8–1. HYPERSENSITIVITY MECHANISMS

Type	Antibody	Mechanism	Effect	Examples of Diseases
Type I (immediate, anaphylactic)	IgE		Edema, bronchospasm	Local (eczema, hay fever, asthma)
			Anaphylaxis	Systemic
Type II (cytotoxic)	IgG or IgM		Lysis, phagocytosis	Transfusion and drug reactions
			Stimulation	Thyrotoxicosis
			Inhibition	Myasthenia gravis

Type III (immune complex)	IgG or IgM		Arthus-type reaction	Local reactions (hypersensitivity pneumonitis)
			Serum sickness-type reaction	Systemic serum sickness (Table 8–4)
Type IV (delayed, cell-mediated)	No antibody		Delayed-type hypersensitivity	Contact dermatitis

d. Intestine:

■ Allergen may be ingested (eg, nuts, seafood).
■ May manifest as abdominal cramps and diarrhea (allergic gastroenteritis).

2. Systemic type I hypersensitivity reaction (Anaphylaxis):

■ This is rare—but immediately life-threatening.
■ Release of vasoactive amines into the circulation leads to circulatory failure (**anaphylactic shock**). Death may occur in minutes.
  ● **Angioneurotic edema** is a less severe form that may produce fatal edema of the larynx.
■ Anaphylaxis
  ● Typically results from injected allergens (eg, penicillin, foreign serum, local anesthetics, radiographic contrast dyes).
  ● Rarely, may follow ingested allergens (seafood, egg, berries) or cutaneous allergens (bee and wasp stings).
  ● May require only a small amount of allergen in sensitized individuals.

Type II Hypersensitivity
A. Mechanism (Table 8–1):

■ Initial exposure produces IgG or IgM antibodies.
■ These react with antigen on the surface of cells.
■ The antigen involved may be
  ● Intrinsic, as is some autoimmune diseases.
  ● Extrinsic and attached to the cell surface (eg, a drug bound to the cell and acting as a hapten).
  ● This interaction causes cell damage in several ways.

  1. Lysis is by activation of complement.
  2. Phagocytosis by macrophages, which recognize the antigen-antibody complex on the cell.
  3. Antibody-dependent cell-mediated cytotoxicity (ADCC) by natural killer (NK) cells. This is sometimes classified separately as type VI hypersensitivity.
  4. Change in cellular function: Binding of antibody causes increase or inhibition of cell function (see Stimulation and Inhibition in Hypersensitivity, following). Some authorities classify this separately as type V hypersensitivity.
B. Disorders resulting from type II hypersensitivity.
  1. Antigens on erythrocytes.
  a. Blood transfusion reactions (see Chapter 25).
  b. Hemolytic disease of the newborn: Maternal antibodies destroy fetal erythrocytes. This is more common in Rh incompatibility (usually IgG antibodies that cross the placenta); and rarer in ABO incompatibility, since the antibodies are IgM and do not cross the placenta.
  c. Other hemolytic reactions occur due to drugs acting as haptens on red cells, or infections associated with the development of antierythrocyte antibodies (eg, infectious mononucleosis, mycoplasmal pneumonia).

2. Antigens on neutrophils:

■ Neonatal leukopenia results from passage of maternal antibodies across the placenta.
■ Posttransfusion reactions may result from activity of host serum against donor leukocyte HLA system.

3. Antigens on platelets:

■ Are associated with neonatal thrombocytopenia.
■ Result in posttransfusion febrile reactions through mechanisms similar to those described for leukocytes.
■ Idiopathic thrombocytopenic purpura is an autoimmune disease with antiplatelet antibodies.

4. Antigens on basement membrane are associated with Goodpasture's syndrome (Chapter 48), which results from antibodies against renal and pulmonary basement membranes.

5. Stimulation and inhibition in hypersensitivity: Some authors classify inhibition or stimulation of cells by antibody as type V hypersensitivity.

a. Stimulation (Graves disease; primary hyperthyroidism):

■ Stimulatory IgG antibodies bind to surface antigens on thyroid follicular cells.
■ This leads to secretion of increased amounts of thyroid hormone (Chapter 58).

b. Inhibition:

■ **Myasthenia gravis,** wherein an IgG antibody is directed against acetylcholine receptors at the motor-end plate, blocking neurotransmission.
■ **Pernicious anemia,** wherein antibodies may bind to intrinsic factor and inhibit absorption of vitamin B_{12}.

Type III Hypersensitivity (Immune Complex Injury)

A. Mechanism (Table 8–1): Interaction of antigen and antibody results in the formation of immune complexes, either locally or systemically. Two types of immune complex injury are recognized.

1. Arthus-type reaction:

■ This is a local reaction with necrosis at the entry site of the antigen.
■ It is uncommon.
■ It can be seen in the skin after repeated injection of antigen (eg, in rabies vaccination, which involves multiple doses of vaccine).
■ Type III hypersensitivity is also believed to be responsible for **hypersensitivity pneumonitis** (Table 8–2).

2. Serum sickness-type reaction is more common. Sequentially,

■ Injection of large doses of antigen, such as foreign serum proteins, leads to formation of circulating immune complexes.
■ These activate complement and produce necrotizing vasculitis, which
   ● May be generalized (eg, in serum sickness; or in systemic lupus erythematosus).
   ● May affect a single organ (eg, in poststreptococcal glomerulonephritis).

TABLE 8-2. DIFFERENT ANTIGENS CAUSING HYPERSENSITIVITY PNEUMONITIS

Disease	Exposure	Antigen Source
Farmer's lung	Moldy hay	Micropolyspora faeni
Bagassosis	Moldy sugar cane	Thermophilic actinomycetes
Air conditioner pneumonitis	Humidifiers, air conditioners	Thermophilic actinomycetes
Redwood, maple, red cedar pneumonitis	Moldy bark, moldy sawdust	Thermophilic actinomycetes, Cryptostroma corticale, sawdust
Mushroom worker's lung	Mushrooms, compost	Thermophilic actinomycetes
Cheese worker's lung	Moldy cheese	Penicillium casei
Malt worker's lung	Malt dust	Aspergillus clavatus
Bird fancier's lung	Bird excreta and serum	Avian serum proteins
Enzyme lung	Enzyme detergents	Alcalase derived from Bacillus subtilis
Drug-induced hypersensitivity pneumonitis	Drugs, industrial materials	Nitrofurantoin, cromolyn, hydrochlorothiazide, toluene diisocyanate
"Sauna" lung	Contaminated steam in saunas	Aspergillus pullulans

Note: Serum sickness-type immune complex injury may occur in a large number of diseases (Table 8-3), as the major pathogenic mechanisms or as a minor complication.

B. Diagnosis of immune complex disease: Diagnosis may be accomplished by

- Visualization of the immune complexes in tissues by electron microscopy.
- Use of immunofluorescence or immunoperoxidase techniques for detection of tissue-bound immune complexes or complement, eg, the granular (lumpy) deposits in glomerulonephritis.
- Tests for circulating immune complexes.

Type IV (Delayed) Hypersensitivity
A. Mechanism (Table 8-1):

- It is mediated by cells, not antibody.
- Sensitized T lymphocytes are directly cytotoxic or secrete lymphokines that activate macrophages, etc. (Chapter 4).
- Reaction is "delayed" 24-72 hours after exposure of a sensitized individual to the offending antigenin—contrast to type I hypersensitivity, which develops within minutes.

TABLE 8–3. DISEASES IN WHICH IMMUNE COMPLEX FORMATION HAS BEEN SHOWN TO PLAY A ROLE

Infections
  Poststreptococcal glomerulonephritis[1]
  Subacute infective endocarditis
  Mycoplasma pneumonia
  Syphilis
  Viral hepatitis (acute and chronic)
  Guillain-Barré syndrome
  Malaria
  Leishmaniasis

Malignant diseases
  Lymphocytic leukemias (acute and chronic)
  Hodgkin's disease
  Various cancers (especially of lung or breast; melanoma)

Autoimmune diseases
  Systemic lupus erythematosus[1]
  Rheumatoid arthritis
  Polyarteritis nodosa[1]
  Hashimoto's disease (thyroiditis)
  Celiac disease
  Henoch-Schönlen purpura
  Rheumatic fever

Drug reactions
  Serum sickness[1]
  Penicillamine toxicity[1]

[1]The main clinical manifestations of these diseases are the result of immune complex deposition in tissues. In the other diseases in this list, immune complexes have been demonstrated but their deposition usually plays a secondary and less important role.

- T cell-mediated cytotoxicity is involved in
  - Contact dermatitis.
  - The responses against cancer cells, virus-infected cells, and transplanted cells bearing foreign antigens.
  - Autoimmune diseases.
- Histologically, involved tissue shows
  - Necrosis of affected cells.
  - Lymphocytic infiltration.
  - Granulomatous inflammation (see Chapter 5).
  - Occasionally, caseous necrosis, especially when hypersensitivity develops to certain infectious agents, such as fungi and mycobacteria.

Note: T cell–mediated hypersensitivity is the basis for skin tests used in the diagnosis of infection by mycobacteria (**tuberculin** and **lepromin** tests) and fungi (**histoplasmin** and **coccidioidin** tests).

B. Disorders resulting from type IV hypersensitivity.

1. Infections:

■ Particularly those caused by facultative intracellular organisms, eg, mycobacteria and fungi.

■ Epithelioid cell granulomas, often with caseous necrosis.

2. Autoimmune diseases:

■ Hashimoto's thyroiditis.

■ Autoimmune gastritis associated with pernicious anemia.

3. Contact dermatitis:

■ Type IV hypersensitivity response is limited precisely to the area of contact of antigen with skin (eg, back of a watch, buckle of a suspender, bracelet).

■ Common antigens are nickel, dichromate compounds (in leather), drugs, dyes in clothing, and plants (including poison ivy and poison oak).

■ Sensitization is detected by patch tests.

4. Graft rejection: See following.

TRANSPLANT REJECTION

The only absolute limitations upon tissue transplantation are the immunologic reactions against the transplanted cells and the availability of appropriate donor organs.

■ **Autografts (autologous)**—transplantation of the host's own tissues from one part of the body to another (eg, skin, bone, venous grafts)—do not cause immunologic rejection reactions.

■ **Isografts**—exchange of tissue between genetically identical (monozygotic) twins—likewise do not evoke an immune response.

■ **Allografts**—transplants between genetically dissimilar members of the same species. Normally the grafted tissue is rejected.

■ **Xenografts (heterologous grafts)**—transplants obtained from a species different from the recipient. Such grafts evoke a severe immunologic reaction.

Note: Allografts or xenografts of avascular tissues (cornea, heart valves) may be successful.

Transplantation (Histocompatibility) Antigens
A. Antigens on erythrocytes:

■ Antigens of the ABO, Rh, MNS, and other blood-group systems are not histocompatible antigens per se.

■ Compatibility between donor erythrocytes and recipient serum is essential both in blood transfusions and in tissue transplantation.

■ Erythrocyte antigen compatibility is determined by typing and cross-matching of erythrocytes.

B. Antigens on the surface of nucleated cells.
HLA (human leukocyte antigen) complex:

■ Includes the histocompatibility antigens.

- In humans, the corresponding genes form the major histocompatibility complex (MHC) on the short arm of chromosome 6.
- Four major loci (HLA-A, HLA-B, HLA-C, and HLA-D) are recognized.
- A fifth, closely related to the HLA-D locus and called HLA-DR, has also been proposed.
- Each locus contains two alleles (alternative forms of a gene) that code for two HLA antigens.
- The five loci are so close together that they are generally inherited as a unit of five (**haplotype**); ie, five maternal and five paternal.
- There are a large number of possible alleles for each locus, each coding for a different antigen.
- The huge number of possible HLA antigen combinations makes it unlikely that any two unrelated individuals will share the identical HLA type.
- Since the five HLA loci are usually inherited as a haplotype, there is an approximately 1:4 chance of a complete (2-haplotype) HLA match among siblings.
- In **HLA typing**, peripheral-blood lymphocytes are typed using panels of antisera with antibodies of known HLA specificity. HLA-D that cannot be determined serologically is typed by the mixed-lymphocyte culture technique.
- The survival of renal allograft is highest when donor and recipient are closely matched for HLA-D and HLA-DR.

Mechanisms of Transplant Rejection (Table 8–4)
Both humoral and cell-mediated mechanisms play a role in transplant rejection.
A. Humoral Mechanisms:

- Antibodies against transplanted antigens may be present in the recipient's serum before transplantation, or may develop subsequently.
- Humoral rejection is equivalent to types II and III hypersensitivity reactions.
- Antibody-antigen interactions on the surface of transplanted cells result in cell necrosis (type II).
- Immune complex deposition in blood vessels activates complement and causes acute necrotizing vasculitis or chronic intimal fibrosis with narrowing of the vessels (type III).

B. Cell-mediated mechanisms:

- T lymphocytes become sensitized to transplanted antigens.
- Injury results from direct cytotoxicity and secretion of lymphokines.
- Acute and chronic necrosis of parenchymal cells is accompanied by lymphocytic infiltration and fibrosis.
- Cellular mechanisms are more important than humoral mechanisms in the rejection process.

Clinical Types of Transplant Rejection
A. Hyperacute rejection:

- Occurs within minutes after transplantation.
- Is characterized by severe necrotizing vasculitis with diffuse ischemic damage to the transplanted organ.

TABLE 8–4. IMMUNOLOGIC MECHANISMS INVOLVED IN TRANSPLANT REJECTION

Active Immunologic Factor in Recipient	Type of Hypersensitivity	Target Sites in Transplant	Pathologic Effect	Type of Clinical Rejection
Preformed antibody against donor transplantation antigens	Type II cytotoxic Type III immune complex formation (local, Arthus-type)	Small blood vessels in donor tissue	Fibrinoid necrosis and thrombosis of small vessels; ischemic necrosis of parenchymal cells.	Hyperacute rejection
Circulating antibody formed due to humoral immune response against donor transplantation antigens	Type II cytotoxic	Parenchymal cells	Acute necrosis of parenchymal cells.	Acute rejection
	Type III immune complex formation (local, Arthus-type)	Small blood vessels	Fibrinoid necrosis and thrombosis in acute phase; intimal fibrosis and narrowing in chronic phase.	Acute rejection, chronic rejection
Activated T cells elicited by cellular immune response against donor transplantation antigens	Type IV	Parenchymal cells	Progressive, slow loss of parenchymal cells.	Chronic rejection

- Is due to the presence in the recipient's serum of high levels of preformed antibodies against the graft.
- Mechanism is an **Arthus-type immune complex injury.**
- Has become rare since development of direct tissue cross-matching.

B. Acute Rejection:

- Is common.
- Occurs within days to months after transplantation.
- Is "acute" because, even though it may take some time to appear, it progresses rapidly once it has begun.
- Is characterized by acute cellular destruction.

■ Mechanism involves both humoral and cell-mediated mechanisms.
■ In **immune complexes,** cause acute vasculitis, leading to ischemia.
■ **Cell-mediated T cell cytotoxicity** leads to parenchymal-cell necrosis and lympho-cytic infiltration (eg, in renal grafts, acute tubular necrosis with lymphocytes).
■ Treatment is by immunosuppressive drugs such as corticosteroids (eg, prednisone) and cyclosporine, or with antilymphocyte serum to ablate the patient's T cells.

C. Chronic rejection:

■ Is present to some degree in most transplanted tissues.
■ Causes slowly progressive cell loss and fibrosis with deterioration of function over a period of years.
■ Mechanism is principally cell-mediated type IV, sometimes with the addition of immune complex deposition (type III).

AUTOIMMUNE DISEASE

Immunologic Tolerance to Self Antigens

The immune system recognizes the body's own antigens as self antigens (natural toler-ance). See Chapter 4. Autoimmune diseases occur when a breakdown of this natural tolerance leads to an immune response against a self antigen. Two theories have been proposed to explain the mechanism of natural tolerance.

A. Clonal deletion theory:

■ Postulates that lymphocyte clones that have receptors for antigens encountered in fetal life (self antigens) are deleted.
■ Adults therefore lack self-reactive clones.
■ Autoimmunity is then explained by the emergence of forbidden clones of lympho-cytes that are reacting to self antigens. These are presumably the result of a new B or T cell gene rearrangement (shuffling) at the stem cell level.

B. Specific cell suppression theory:

■ Postulates that tolerance is due to active suppression of self-reactive cells.
■ Mechanism is not clear, but possibilities include
   ● Action of T suppressor cells.
   ● The presence of suppressor factors in blood.

Breakdown of Natural Tolerance (Autoimmunity)

Injury in autoimmune diseases is caused by both humoral and cell-mediated hypersen-sitivity (types II, III, and IV). Several different mechanisms have been proposed for the breakdown of tolerance (see Table 8–5).

Types of autoimmune disease (Table 8–6)

There are two major types, according to whether the antigens involved are

■ On a specific cell type (**organ-specific** autoimmune disease).
■ Universal cellular components such as nucleic acids and nucleoproteins (**systemic,** autoimmune disease).
   ● The presence of the various antibodies may be of diagnostic value (Table 8–6).

TABLE 8–5. PROPOSED MECHANISMS OF AUTOIMMUNE DISEASES

Proposed Mechanism	Antigens Involved in Pathogenesis	Reason for or Cause of Mechanism	Resulting Autoimmune Disease
1. Emergence of sequestered antigen	Thyroglobulin (?)	Antigen sequestered in thyroid follicle	Hashimoto's thyroiditis
	Lens protein	Antigen sequestered from bloodstream	Sympathetic ophthalmitis
	Spermatozoal antigens	Antigen developed in adult life	Infertility (male)
2. Alteration of self antigens	Drugs, viruses, other infections	Attachment of hapten, partial degradation	Hemolytic anemias, ?systemic lupus erythematosus, ?rheumatic fever
3. Loss of serum suppressor antibodies	Many types	B cell deficiency; congenital Bruton's agammaglobulinemia	Many types
4. Loss of suppressor T cells	Many types	T cell deficiency; postviral infection	Rare
5. Activation of suppressed lymphocyte clones	Epstein-Barr virus; ?other viruses	B cell stimulation	?Rheumatoid arthritis
6. Emergence of "forbidden" clones	Many types	Neoplastic transformation of lymphocytes; malignant lymphoma and lymphocytic leukemias	Hemolytic anemia, thrombocytopenia
7. Cross-reactivity between self and foreign antigens	Antistreptococcal antibody and myocardial antigens	Antibody against foreign antigen reacts against self antigen	Rheumatic fever
8. Abnormal immune response genes (Ir genes)	Many types	Loss of control of the immune response due to lack of Ir genes.	Many types[1]

[1]Immune response (Ir) genes are closely linked to HLA antigens. Those autoimmune diseases in which Ir gene abnormalities play a part are associated with an increased incidence of certain HLA types.

TABLE 8–6. AUTOIMMUNE DISEASES

Diseases	Autoantibodies[1]
Systemic multiorgan diseases Systemic lupus erythematosus	Antinuclear Anti-DNA (double-stranded) Anti-DNA (single-stranded) Anti-Sm Antiribonucleoprotein Others
Mixed connective tissue disease (MCTD)	Antinuclear Antiribonucleoprotein
Progressive systemic sclerosis	Antinuclear Anticentromere
Dermatomyositis	Antinuclear Antimyoglobin
Rheumatoid arthritis (and Sjögren's syndrome)	Anti-immunoglobulin (rheumatoid factor)
Restricted organ-specific diseases Myasthenia gravis	Antiacetylcholine receptor
Hashimoto's thyroiditis	Antithyroglobulin
Graves' disease (toxic goiter)	Thyroid-stimulating immunoglobulin
Insulin-resistant diabetes	Anti-insulin receptor
Juvenile insulin-dependent diabetes	Anti-insulin Anti-islet cell
Goodpasture's syndrome	Antilung basement membrane Antiglomerular basement membrane
Pernicious anemia	Antiparietal cell Anti-intrinsic factor
Addison's disease	Antiadrenal cell
Bullous pemphigoid	Anti-skin basement membrane
Pemphigus vulgaris	Anti-skin intercellular matrix
Hypoparathyroidism	Antiparathyroid cell
Primary biliary cirrhosis	Antimitochondrial
Chronic active hepatitis	Antinuclear Antihepatocyte Anti-smooth muscle

(continued)

TABLE 8–6. (*Continued*)

Diseases	Autoantibodies[1]
Vitiligo	Antimelanocyte
Infertility (male)	Antispermatozoal
Infertility (female)	Antiovarian (corpus luteum)
Hemolytic anemia	Antierythrocyte
Neutropenia	Antileukocyte
Thrombocytopenia	Antiplatelet

[1]The antibodies named are those typical of each disease state, and not all patients with the disease will demonstrate them. In addition, the presence of these various antibodies is not necessarily limited to a particular disease state (eg, antithyroglobulin antibody is present in Hashimoto's disease [90%], myxedema [70%], Graves' disease [40%], nontoxic goiter and thyroid cancer [30%], pernicious anemia [25%], and normal controls [5–10%].

- Many autoimmune diseases are familial (eg, systemic lupus erythematosus, Hashimoto's thyroiditis, pernicious anemia).
- Others are associated with specific HLA antigens (eg, HLA-D3 with systemic lupus erythematosus; HLA B27 with ankylosing spondylitis.

Mechanisms of Cell Injury in Autoimmune Diseases

Mechanisms of cell injury in autoimmune diseases include types II, III, and IV hypersensitivity.

- Many organ-specific diseases are the result of type II and/or type IV mechanisms:
  - Stimulatory type II antibodies are important in Graves' disease.
  - Inhibitory type II antibodies are important in myasthenia gravis.
- Many of the multi-organ autoimmune diseases result from type III mechanisms.

Abnormalities of Blood Supply   9

Local failure of blood supply to a tissue leads to **infarction** (ischemic necrosis). Generalized failure of blood supply leads to a systemic decrease in perfusion and **shock.**

CAUSES OF TISSUE ISCHEMIA

ARTERIAL OBSTRUCTION

Atherosclerosis—plus thrombosis (Chapter 20)—is the commonest cause of arterial obstruction in developed countries today. Four million Americans have clinical atherosclerosis. A million and a quarter have heart attacks each year. Five hundred thousand have strokes.

Factors Influencing the Effect of Arterial Obstruction

A. Availability of collateral circulation: In tissues having no collateral arterial supply, obstruction of the end artery supplying the tissue leads to complete cessation of blood flow and infarction.

B. Integrity of collateral arteries: Narrowing of arteries decreases the effectiveness of any available collateral circulation. This is more of a problem in the elderly because of generalized atherosclerosis.

C. Rate of development of obstruction: Sudden obstruction produces more severe ischemic changes because there is less time for enlargement of potential collateral vessels.

D. Tissue susceptibility to ischemia: Brain and heart are highly susceptible; infarction occurs within minutes. Skeletal muscle, bone, and cartilage are more resistant.

E. Tissue metabolic rate: Cooling reduces metabolic requirements and delays the onset of ischemic damage.

VENOUS OBSTRUCTION

Venous obstruction is common, but symptoms are usually minimal because of good collateral drainage.

Effect of Venous Obstruction

When collateral drainage is inadequate, obstruction leads to severe venous congestion, capillary rupture, and hemorrhage. In extreme cases, venous infarction may result.

Venous Congestion in Heart Failure

A. Pulmonary venous congestion:

- Left heart failure causes congestion of the pulmonary circulation.
- If severe and acute, pulmonary edema results.
- If chronic, pulmonary fibrosis follows, with hemosiderin-laden macrophages ("heart failure cells") in the alveoli.

B. Hepatic venous congestion:

- Right heart failure causes congestion of the systemic circulation.
- This is first manifested in the liver (acute hepatic congestion, or nutmeg liver).
- In longstanding cases, hypoxia leads to focal necrosis and fibrosis (cardiac cirrhosis).

Venous Infarction

Venous infarction occurs with total occlusion of all venous drainage (eg, superior sagittal sinus thrombosis, renal vein thrombosis, superior mesenteric vein thrombosis).

- Venous infarcts are always hemorrhagic.
- Special types of venous infarcts include
  - **Strangulation**—constriction of the neck of a hernial sac.
  - **Torsion**—twisting of the pedicle of an organ (eg, the testis).

EFFECTS OF TISSUE ISCHEMIA

INFARCTION

Infarction is the development of an area of localized necrosis that results from sudden reduction of its blood supply. Infarction is due to

- Arterial obstruction by thrombosis or embolism.
- More rarely, venous obstruction.

Classification of Infarcts
A. Pale versus red:

- Pale (white, anemic) infarcts occur as a result of arterial obstruction in organs such as the heart, kidney, and brain that lack significant collateral circulation.
- Red (or hemorrhagic) infarcts occur when there is a dual blood supply—eg, lung and liver—or when collaterals permit some ongoing, but inadequate, blood flow.
- Venous infarcts are always red, due to congestion.

B. Solid versus liquefied:

- Infarcts are solid in all tissues except the brain, due to coagulative necrosis.
- Liquefactive necrosis occurs in brain, often producing a cystic cavity.

C. Sterile versus septic:

- Most infarcts are sterile.
- Septic infarcts occur when
  - The occluding embolus is infected (eg, in bacterial endocarditis).
  - Infarction occurs in a tissue (eg, intestine) that normally contains bacteria.
  - Bacteria arrive in the bloodstream (unusual, since blood is normally sterile).

Morphology of Infarcts

Infarcts in kidney, spleen, and lung are **wedge-shaped,** with the occluded artery being situated near the apex. Cerebral and myocardial infarcts are **irregular,** their shape determined by the distribution of the occluded artery and the collateral supply.

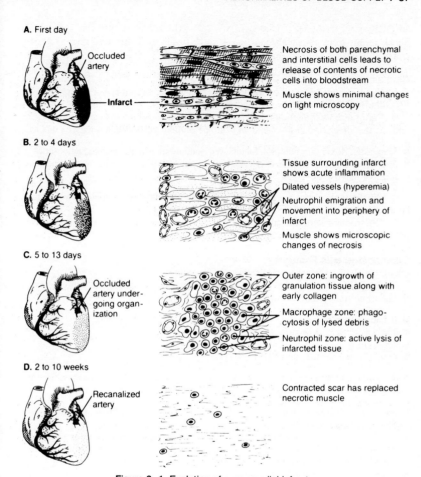

A. First day

Occluded artery

Infarct

Necrosis of both parenchymal and interstitial cells leads to release of contents of necrotic cells into bloodstream

Muscle shows minimal changes on light microscopy

B. 2 to 4 days

Tissue surrounding infarct shows acute inflammation

Dilated vessels (hyperemia)

Neutrophil emigration and movement into periphery of infarct

Muscle shows microscopic changes of necrosis

C. 5 to 13 days

Occluded artery undergoing organization

Outer zone: ingrowth of granulation tissue along with early collagen

Macrophage zone: phagocytosis of lysed debris

Neutrophil zone: active lysis of infarcted tissue

D. 2 to 10 weeks

Recanalized artery

Contracted scar has replaced necrotic muscle

Figure 9–1. Evolution of a myocardial infarct.

Evolution of Infarcts

Necrosis is followed by heterolysis of dead cells, phagocytosis of debris, ingrowth of granulation tissue, and fibrosis (scarring). (See Fig 9–1).

- In the brain, liquefied cells are phagocytosed by special macrophages (microglia), and the cystic cavity becomes walled off by astrocytes (a process termed *gliosis,* the cerebral analogue of fibrosis).
- The time required for healing varies with size:
  - Small infarcts heal in 1–2 weeks.
  - Large ones heal in 1–2 months.

SHOCK

Shock results from a generalized decrease in perfusion of tissues associated with decrease in effective cardiac output.

Causes

A. Hypovolemia (decreased blood volume) is due to hemorrhage or excessive fluid loss (diarrhea, vomiting, burns, dehydration, heat stroke).

B. Peripheral Vasodilatation, when excessive pooling of blood in peripheral vessels reduces the effective blood volume and cardiac output. Vasodilatation may be due to

- Metabolic, toxic, or humoral factors (eg, endotoxic shock, anaphylactic shock).
- Rarely, neurogenic stimuli in anesthesia or spinal-cord injury. Simple fainting is a form of neurogenic shock.

C. Cardiogenic shock results from severe reduction in cardiac output due to primary cardiac disease (eg, acute myocardial infarction, arrhythmias).

D. Obstructive shock results from major obstruction to blood flow, as in massive pulmonary embolism, left atrial thrombus, or cardiac tamponade.

Clinicopathologic Features

Shock develops in stages as outlined in the following.

A. Stage of compensation: Initial decrease in cardiac output triggers reflex increase in heart rate (tachycardia) and peripheral vasoconstriction

- It maintains blood pressure in vital organs (brain and myocardium).
- There is a rapid, low-volume (thready) pulse.
- The skin is cold and clammy.
- Oliguria is due to reduced GFR.

B. Stage of impaired tissue perfusion: Prolonged compensatory vasoconstriction and sludging of red cells impairs tissue perfusion, with several adverse effects:

- Anaerobic glycolysis, leading to production of lactic acid and **lactic acidosis** in the blood.
- Cell necrosis, especially in the kidney, followed by **acute renal tubular necrosis.**
- **Shock lung** (adult respiratory distress syndrome, or ARDS), with edema, hemorrhage, and formation of hyaline membranes).
- Anoxic necrosis of the liver.
- Ischemic necrosis in the intestines.

C. Stage of decompensation: Eventually reflex peripheral vasoconstriction fails, leading to

- Progressive hypotension.
- Myocardial hypoxia, cerebral hypoxia, loss of consciousness, and death.

Prognosis

Death occurs if the underlying cause cannot be treated (eg, massive myocardial infarct) or extensive tissue damage occurs prior to instituting treatment (so-called irreversible shock).

CAUSES OF VASCULAR OCCLUSION

The causes of vascular occlusion include

- **Extramural compression** by fibrosis or a neoplasm.
- **Diseases of the vessel wall,** including atherosclerosis and vasculitis.
- **Arterial spasm** (rare).
- **Thrombosis and embolism**—the most common causes of vessel obstruction.

THROMBOSIS

Normal Hemostasis

Normally there is a balance between thrombus formation and dissolution (**fibrinolysis**). Following injury, there is simultaneous activation of both the coagulation and fibrinolytic systems.

A. Formation of hemostatic platelet plug:

- Injury to endothelium exposes collagen, which results in the **adherence of platelets,** forming a hemostatic plug.
- **Platelet aggregation** in turn releases granules containing serotonin, ADP, ATP, and thromboplastic substances from platelets.
- Layers of platelets alternating with fibrin in a thrombus appear on microscopic examination as pale lines (lines of Zahn).

B. Coagulation of blood: Activation of Hageman factor (factor XII) initiates the intrinsic coagulation pathway (Fig 9–2; see also Chapter 27).

Abnormal Hemostasis

Abnormal hemostasis results from a disturbance of the normal balance that exists between thrombus formation and fibrinolysis.

- A shift towards thrombus formation leads to thrombosis and vascular occlusion.
- A shift towards fibrinolysis, or deficiency of coagulation factors, leads to hemorrhagic disorders (Chapter 27).

Factors in Thrombus Formation

Factors in thrombus formation include

- **Endothelial damage,** which stimulates platelet adhesion and coagulation.
- **Changes in blood flow,** turbulence.
- **Changes in the blood** (eg, increased fibrinogen or platelets).
- Entry of thromboplastic substances into the blood (eg, snake venoms, amniotic fluid, neutrophil granules, and mucin from cancer cells).

Types of Thrombi

Two types of thrombi are

- Pale thrombi, composed of fibrin and platelets, with few entrapped erythrocytes. Usually they occur in arteries.
- Red thrombi, which contain large numbers of erythrocytes trapped in the fibrin mesh. Usually they occur in veins.

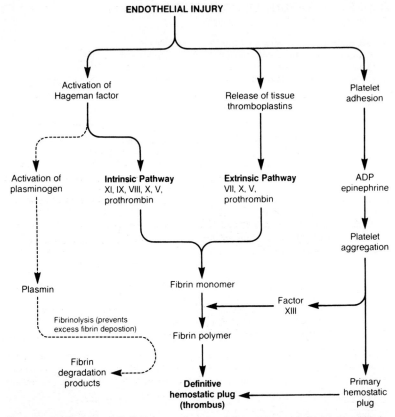

Figure 9–2. Effect of endothelial injury on the coagulation system and platelets, resulting in formation of the definitive hemostatic plug or thrombus. Note that simultaneous activation of the opposing fibrinolytic system provides a degree of control over the extent of thrombus formation.

Sites of Thrombosis
A. Arterial thrombosis (Fig 9–3):

- Is common.
- It typically occurs after endothelial damage and local turbulence caused by atherosclerosis (Chapter 20).
- Large- and medium-sized arteries such as the aorta, carotid arteries, circle of Willis, coronary arteries are mainly affected.
- Less commonly, it follows polyarteritis nodosa, giant-cell arteritis, or thromboangiitis obliterans (Chapter 20).

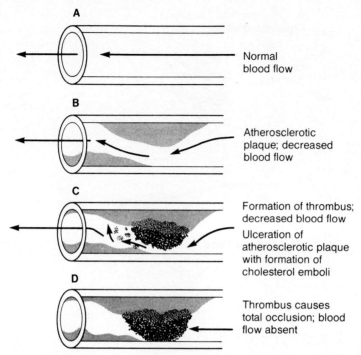

Normal
blood flow

Atherosclerotic
plaque; decreased
blood flow

Formation of thrombus;
decreased blood flow

Ulceration of
atherosclerotic plaque
with formation of
cholesterol emboli

Thrombus causes
total occlusion; blood
flow absent

Figure 9–3. Thrombosis is an atherosclerotic artery. A: Normal artery, showing typical laminar blood flow. B: Atherosclerotic artery, showing atherosclerotic plaques. The endothelium is intact, but the vessel lumen is narrowed. Decreased blood flow and increased turbulence are present. C: Ulcerated atherosclerotic plaque from which fragments of the plaque have become detached and passed distally as cholesterol emboli. Blood flow is further decreased and turbulence increased. Thrombosis has occurred over the ulcerated area. D: Extension of thrombosis has caused total occlusion of the artery, and there is no blood flow in the vessel.

B. Cardiac thrombosis: Thrombi form within the chambers of the heart in the following circumstances.

1. Inflammation of cardiac valves: Endocarditis and valvulitis lead to local turbulence and deposition of platelet/fibrin thrombi (**vegetations**) on the valves.

2. Damage to mural endocardium: Endocardial thrombi form following infarction of the subjacent myocardium.

3. Turbulence and stasis in atrial chambers: Large ball thrombi may form in atrial fibrillation.

Note: In all of the above, fragments of thrombus may detach to form emboli (see following).

A
Thrombophlebitis

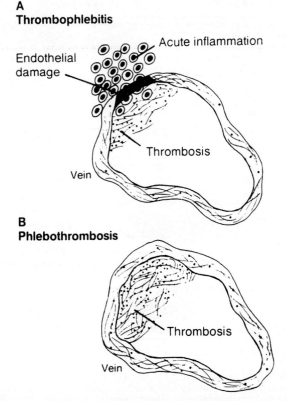

B
Phlebothrombosis

Figure 9–4. Venous thrombosis. A: In thrombophlebitis, acute inflammation of the venous wall leads to endothelial damage and thrombosis. The thrombus is adherent to the vein wall, and embolism is rare. B: In phlebothrombosis, inflammation and venous endothelial damage are typically minimal. Sluggish blood flow and altered blood coagulability play an important role in thrombus formation. The thrombus is loosely attached to the vein wall and commonly becomes detached to cause embolism.

C. Venous thrombosis (Fig 9–4).
1. Thrombophlebitis:

- Denotes venous thrombosis occurring secondary to acute inflammation.
- Involves the superficial veins of the extremities.
- Is characterized by the thrombus being firmly attached to the vessel wall, and rarely forming emboli.

Note: Thrombophlebitis migrans is the occurrence of multiple thrombi in patients with visceral cancers, most commonly pancreatic or gastric (Trousseau's sign).

2. Phlebothrombosis:

- Denotes venous thrombosis occurring in the absence of obvious inflammation.
- Occurs mostly in the deep veins of the leg (deep-vein thrombosis).

Note: The large thrombi are only loosely attached and often form emboli (eg, pulmonary embolism).

a. Causes:

- In phlebothrombosis, endothelial injury is usually minimal.
- Sluggish blood flow is an important causative factor.
  - In the venous plexus of the calf muscles, blood flow is normally maintained by calf muscle contraction (the muscle pump).
  - Thus, immobilization in bed favors thrombosis.
- Changes in the composition of blood in postoperative or postpartum patients favor thrombosis because of the increased levels of some coagulation factors (fibrinogen and factors VII and VIII).
- Oral contraceptives may have similar effects.

Evolution of Thrombi
A. Fibrinolysis:

- Lysis of the thrombus (fibrinolysis) accompanied by reestablishment of the lumen is the ideal end result.
- The fibrinolytic system is activated at the same time as the clotting sequence (Fig 9–2).
- Drugs such as streptokinase and tissue plasminogen activator (TPA) may be effective when used immediately after thrombosis.

B. Organization and recanalization:

- Occur in large thrombi.
- Phagocytosis of the thrombus is followed by ingrowth of granulation tissue and fibrosis (organization). The vessels in the granulation tissue may establish new channels across the thrombus (recanalization).

C. Thromboembolism: A fragment of thrombus may become detached and carried in the circulation to lodge at a distant site (see following).

DISSEMINATED INTRAVASCULAR COAGULATION (DIC)
The widespread development of small thrombi in the microcirculation throughout the body is serious and often fatal.

Causes
In many cases, the cause of disseminated intravascular coagulation is unknown. It occurs as a complication of many diseases (Table 9–1).

Effects
A. Decreased tissue perfusion: Due to multiple occlusions of small vessels, disseminated intravascular coagulation may lead to microinfarction and shock.

TABLE 9-1. DISORDERS ASSOCIATED WITH DISSEMINATED INTRAVASCULAR
COAGULATION

Infectious diseases
  Gram-negative bacteremia
  Meningococcal sepsis
  Gram-positive bacteremia
  Disseminated fungal infections
  Rickettsial infections
  Severe viremias (eg, hemorrhagic fevers)
  Plasmodium falciparum malaria
  Neonatal and intrauterine infections
Obstetric disorders
  Amniotic fluid embolism
  Retained dead fetus
  Abruptio placentae
Liver diseases
  Massive liver cell necrosis
  Cirrhosis of the liver
Malignant diseases
  Acute promyelocytic leukemia
  Metastatic carcinoma, mainly adenocarcinoma
Miscellaneous disorders
  Small vessel vasculitides
  Massive trauma
  Burns
  Heat stroke
  Surgery with extracorporeal circulation
  Snakebite (Russell's viper)
  Severe shock
  Intravascular hemolysis

B. Bleeding is due to exhaustion of clotting factors (consumption coagulopathy), excess fibrinolysis, and release of fibrin degradation products, which have anticoagulant properties. Often the main clinical effect is hemorrhage.

Treatment
Heparin is administered to inhibit the formation of thrombi. Infusion of platelets and plasma can restore the depleted coagulation factors.

EMBOLISM
Embolism is the occlusion or obstruction of a vessel by an abnormal mass (solid, liquid, or gaseous) transported from a different site by the circulation.

- Most emboli are detached fragments of thrombi (**thromboembolism**).
- Other types include fat, amniotic fluid, bone marrow, tumor cells, parasites, debris from atheromatous plaques, and foreign particulate matter.

Origin of Emboli
A. Origin in systemic veins:

- Emboli that originate in systemic veins and the right side of the heart lodge in the pulmonary arterial system unless

- They are so small (eg, fat globules) that they can pass through the pulmonary capillaries.
- There is a patent foramen in the heart allowing the emboli to lodge in a systemic artery (**paradoxic embolism**).
- Emboli that originate in the portal vein lodge in the liver.

B. Origin in heart and systemic arteries: Emboli originating in the left side of the heart and systemic arteries lodge in a distal systemic artery in brain, heart, kidney, extremity, intestine, etc.

Types & Sites of Embolism
A. Thromboembolism: Detached fragments of thrombi are the commonest form of embolus.
    1. Pulmonary embolism.
        a. Causes and incidence:

- Pulmonary emboli are the most serious form of thromboembolism.
- They affect about 600,000 patients per year in the USA; about 100,000 die.
- *Over 90% of pulmonary emboli originate in the deep veins of the leg (phlebothrombosis).*
- They are more common with certain states that predispose to phlebothrombosis:
  - Postoperative and postpartum periods.
  - Cardiac failure.
  - Oral contraceptives.

        b. Clinical effects: Size is the factor most influencing the clinical effects of pulmonary embolism.
            (1) Massive emboli may lodge in the main pulmonary artery, where they cause circulatory obstruction and **sudden death.**
            (2) Medium-sized emboli:

- In otherwise healthy lung, medium-sized emboli cause local gas exchange deficits but not infarction, because lung has a second blood supply from the bronchial arteries.
- In patients with chronic left heart failure or pulmonary vascular disease, local infarcts may occur.

            (3) Small emboli have little effect unless numerous or sustained, when **pulmonary hypertension** may result.
    2. Systemic arterial embolism.
        a. Causes, origins of emboli:

- Infective endocarditis—emboli arise from vegetations on the mitral and aortic valves.
- Mural endocardial thrombi in patients who have suffered myocardial infarction.
- Atrial thrombi in patients with atrial fibrillation.
- Mural thrombi in patients with aortic and ventricular aneurysms.

Note: Thromboemboli from any of these locations pass distally to lodge in some smaller artery.
        b. Clinical effects depend on the size, the site, and the collateral supply. **Infarction** is

■ Common in brain, heart, kidney, and spleen.
■ Less common in intestine and limbs, unless collaterals are compromised.

  B. Air embolism is rare. About 150 mL of air causes death.
  1. Causes.
    a. Surgery of or trauma to internal jugular vein: The negative pressure in the thorax tends to suck air into the jugular vein.
    b. Childbirth or abortion via the ruptured placental venous sinuses.
    c. Blood transfusions are a risk if positive pressure is used to transfuse the blood.
    d. Therapeutic pneumothorax, a procedure formerly used to treat pulmonary tuberculosis.
    e. Uterotubal insufflation, an obsolete procedure once used to investigate infertility.
  C. Nitrogen gas embolism (decompression sickness is also called "**the bends**" or **caisson disease.**
  1. Cause:

■ Air breathed at high underwater pressure equilibrates with the tissues (nitrogen is selectively soluble in adipose tissue).
■ If decomposition is too rapid, nitrogen comes out of solution and forms bubbles in the tissues and bloodstream.
■ The bubbles act as emboli.
■ Scuba divers who ascend rapidly from depths as shallow as 10 m are at risk.

  2. Clinical effects:

■ Platelets adhere to nitrogen bubbles, leading to disseminated intravascular coagulation.
■ Impaction of gas bubbles in capillaries adds to the ischemia.
■ Involvement of the brain in severe cases may cause death.
■ Nerve and muscle involvement causes pain ("the bends").
■ Lung emboli cause difficulty in breathing ("the chokes").

  D. Fat embolism.
  1. Cause: Typically follows fractures of large bones (eg, femur) that expose the fatty bone marrow.
  2. Clinical effects:

■ Large fat globules (>20 μm) are arrested in the lung and cause respiratory distress.
■ Smaller fat globules pass into the systemic circulation, and may produce a hemorrhagic skin rash or acute diffuse neurologic dysfunction.
■ About 10% of patients with clinical fat embolism die. Fat can be demonstrated in vessels at autopsy.

  E. Bone marrow embolism: Fragments of bone marrow may also form emboli after trauma, but produce little clinical effect.
  F. Atheromatous (cholesterol) embolism:

■ Ulcerated plaques often release atheromatous material into the circulation.

- Such emboli lodge in small systemic arteries.
- In the brain they produce **transient ischemic attacks.**

G. Amniotic fluid embolism:

- This is rare, but with a mortality rate of about 80%.
- Thromboplastic substances in amniotic fluid induce disseminated intravascular coagulation.
- Emboli composed of fetal hair or squamous cells may be found in the lungs at autopsy.

H. Tumor embolism:

- These are usually too small to constitute significant emboli.
- Renal carcinoma has a propensity to grow into the inferior vena cava, and may form larger emboli.

Nutritional Disease

NUTRITIONAL DEFICIENCY

Nutritional deficiency may be broad based (eg, protein calorie deficiency), or may be restricted to deficiency of one specific factor (eg, B_{12} deficiency).

Primary Malnutrition

Primary malnutrition is due to inadequate food intake.

Secondary Malnutrition

Secondary malnutrition is due to

- Failure of intestinal absorption.
- Increased metabolic demand.
- Antagonists (eg, folic-acid antagonists such as methotrexate, which is used in cancer chemotherapy.

NUTRITIONAL EXCESS

Excessive intake of food results in obesity. More rarely, clinical disease occurs with excessive intake of specific food substances (eg, vitamins A and D and iron).

PROTEINS & CALORIES

PROTEIN-CALORIE MALNUTRITION (Marasmus; Kwashiorkor)

Causes

Protein-calorie malnutrition is usually associated with general malnutrition arising out of economic factors.

- Children tend to be most affected.
- Marasmus and kwashiorkor are now thought to be part of a spectrum of protein-calorie malnutrition, kwashiorkor being the more severe.

Clinical Features

    A. **Developmental Effects.**

        1. **Growth retardation.**

        2. **Intellectual impairment,** if severe during the first 2 years of life.

        3. **Immunologic deficiency:** Defects in both humoral and cellular immunity result in a high incidence of infections.

    B. **Marasmus:**

- Represents the compensated phase of protein-calorie malnutrition, in which the dietary deficiencies are compensated for by catabolism of the body's "expendable" tissues—adipose tissue and skeletal muscle.

- Leads to extreme wasting.
- Marasmic children are alert and will eat and absorb food normally.

C. Kwashiorkor:

- Represents the decompensated phase of protein-calorie malnutrition.
- As compensatory mechanisms fail, the metabolism slows, and decreased synthesis of enzymes and proteins occurs.
- Results include lethargy and somnolence, malabsorption (deficient digestive enzyme production), edema and ascites (decreased serum albumin), hepatomegaly (fatty liver and cirrhosis due to abnormal lipid metabolism), and loss of pigmentation of skin and hair.
- Anemia develops as a result of deficiencies of iron and folic acid and decreased erythropoietin production.

EATING DISORDERS
Eating disorders arise from psychiatric disorders.

Anorexia Nervosa
Anorexia nervosa occurs chiefly in teenage girls:

- Severe self-restriction of food intake leads to protein-calorie malnutrition, similar in many ways to marasmus.
- Patients show abnormal hypothalamic-pituitary function, failure of ovulation and amenorrhea.

Bulimia
Bulimia occurs chiefly in young women:

- It is characterized by episodes of overeating (binges) followed by induced vomiting, laxative abuse, fasting, etc. (binge-purge cycles).
- Induced vomiting may produce esophageal tears (Mallory-Weiss syndrome).

OBESITY
While definitions vary, obesity is usually defined as **body weight 20% greater than ideal weight** for the population as a whole.

Cause

- Obesity is caused by long-term caloric intake in excess of requirements.
- Excess calories are converted into stored adipose tissue.
- In the USA, obesity affects 20% of middle-aged men and 40% of middle-aged women.

Clinical Features
A. **Hypoventilation syndrome** is due to increased fat in the chest wall (pickwickian syndrome).
B. **Diseases associated with obesity:** The increased mortality rate associated with

TABLE 10–1. DISEASES ASSOCIATED WITH OBESITY

Disease	Mechanism	Clinical Effects
Adult-onset diabetes mellitus	Obesity leads to increased resistance to insulin action, which leads to glucose intolerance. Diabetes mellitus occurs in genetically susceptible individuals.	B cell (pancreatic islet) hyperplasia followed by atrophy. Complications of diabetes mellitus (eg, retinopathy, neuropathy). Risk factor for atherosclerosis.
Hypertension	Statistical association with obesity but no clear mechanism elucidated. Increased secretion of adrenal glucocorticosteroids is a minor factor.	Risk factor for atherosclerosis. Cerebral hemorrhage (stroke).
Hyperlipidemia	Increased fat mobilization from adipose stores results in increased lipoprotein synthesis in liver.	Risk factor for atherosclerosis. Hypertriglyceridemia, hypercholesterolemia, increased very low density lipoprotein (VLDL).
Atherosclerotic arterial disease	Statistical association with obesity along with other risk factors (diabetes, hypertension, hyperlipidemia).	Myocardial infarction (ischemic heart disease) (heart attack); cerebral thrombosis and infarction (stroke).
Cholelithiasis (gallstones)	Increased cholesterol excretion in bile.	Acute and chronic and cholecystitis.
Osteoarthrosis	Increased body weight causes cartilage degeneration in weight-bearing joints.	Lumbar spine, hips, and knees most commonly affected.

obesity is mainly due to a dramatic increase in the incidence of certain diseases (Table 10–1).

VITAMINS

Vitamins are complex organic substances required as coenzymes for many metabolic processes. They are classified as

- Fat-soluble (A, D, E, and K).
- Water-soluble (B vitamins and vitamin C). The B group includes thiamine, riboflavin, nicotinamide, pyridoxine, folic acid, and cyanocobalamin.

VITAMIN A

Vitamin A is a group of compounds that includes vitamin A alcohol (retinol) and the provitamin A carotenes. Vitamin A occurs in liver and dairy products; as carotene in leafy green and yellow vegetables.

Vitamin A Deficiency (Hypovitaminosis A)

A. Causes: Deficiency may be dietary (malnutrition) or due to malabsorption states.

B. Clinical features.

1. Visual impairment: Failure of night vision (**nyctalopia**) is due to decreased production of rhodopsin.

2. Abnormal maturation of squamous epithelium:

■ Hyperplasia and excessive keratinization of squamous epithelia involves
  - The conjunctiva (xerophthalmia and Bitot's spots).
  - The cornea; opacities and erosions (keratomalacia). Vitamin A deficiency is one of the commonest causes of blindness in Asia.
  - The skin (follicular hyperkeratosis).
  - Glandular epithelium; such as the bronchial mucosa, which undergoes squamous metaplasia. Increased susceptibility to respiratory tract and enteric infections may be attributable to epithelial changes.

Vitamin A Toxicity (Hypervitaminosis A)

Vitamin A toxicity produces cerebral dysfunction, raised intracranial pressure, liver enlargement, and bone changes.

VITAMIN D

Vitamin D (cholecalciferol) is the active form of 1,25 dihydrocholecalciferol (Fig 10–1). It is derived in two ways:

■ From the diet.
■ From the skin by the action of sunlight.

Vitamin D Deficiency

A. Causes:

■ Primary dietary deficiency occurs when malnutrition coexists with minimal exposure to sunlight.
  - Vitamin D fortification of milk has made deficiency uncommon in developed countries.
  - Deficiency still occurs in strict vegetarians who eat no dairy products.
■ Secondary deficiency may occur in intestinal malabsorption, chronic renal disease (failure of α-hydroxylation of 25-cholecalciferol at the 1 position), or in liver failure (failure of α-hydroxylation at the 25 position).

B. Clinical features.

1. Pathophysiology:

■ Deficiency results in reduced intestinal absorption of calcium.
■ This leads to a negative calcium balance with failure of calcification of osteoid in bone (**rickets** or **osteomalacia**).

2. Rickets:

■ A disease of children characterized by failure of mineralization of osteoid in bone, with abnormalities of bone growth.

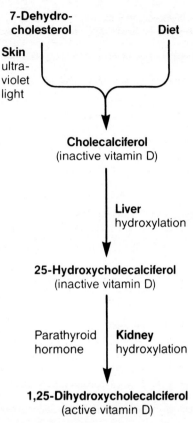

Figure 10–1. Metabolism of vitamin D.

■ Failure of mineralization occurs when the plasma level of either **calcium or phosphate** is decreased over a prolonged period.

   a. Causes and principal clinical types
      (1) Nutritional deficiency occurs through a dietary deficiency of vitamin D or, less often, calcium, or through fat malabsorption.
      (2) Vitamin D-resistant rickets:

■ Is refractory to treatment with vitamin D.
■ Is an X-linked dominant trait.
■ Is characterized by increased phosphate loss from the renal tubules (hypophosphatemic rickets).

(3) End-organ insensitivity to vitamin D: Target cell receptors are insensitive to the action of 1,25-dihydrocholecalciferol. This is very rare, inherited, and resistant to treatment with vitamin D.

(4) Vitamin D-sensitive rickets:

■ Includes various conditions with failure of conversion of precursors to active 1,25-dihydrocholecalciferol.
■ Responds to treatment with vitamin D.

b. Clinical features:

■ Rickets occurs in children.
■ Failure of mineralization results in
  ● Inadequate new bone formation at the epiphyses.
  ● Growth retardation.
  ● Widening of the epiphyses of bones of the wrists and knees.
  ● Osteoid growths at the costochondral junctions ("rachitic rosary").
  ● Various deformities, such as bowing of the tibias and abnormal curvatures in vertebrae and the pelvis.
■ Microscopic changes at the epiphysis include masses of disorganized cartilage, uncalcified osteoid, and abnormal calcification of trabeculae.

3. Osteomalacia is the adult analogue of rickets. Since bone growth is complete, growth retardation does not occur, but remodeling is abnormal and excess osteoid is formed.

Vitamin D Toxicity (Hypervitaminosis D)

Vitamin D toxicity occurs only with extreme overdose. Increased calcium absorption and bone resorption cause hypercalcemia, which leads to metastatic calcification, nephrocalcinosis, and chronic renal failure.

VITAMIN K

Vitamin K is a cofactor in the synthesis of blood coagulation factors II (prothrombin), VII, IX, and X in the liver. The main source of vitamin K in humans is the intestinal bacterial flora.

Vitamin K Deficiency
A. Causes:

■ Intestinal malabsorption of fat.
■ Lack of intestinal bacterial flora—in newborns, or after prolonged broad-spectrum antibiotic therapy.
■ Vitamin K antagonists, eg, coumarin anticoagulants. Many rat poisons are also vitamin K antagonists.

Note: Dietary deficiency is rare because the vitamin occurs in many foods.
B. Clinical features:

■ Decreased plasma levels of coagulation factors II (hypoprothrombinemia), VII, IX, and X.

- Bleeding tendency manifested as bruises, gastrointestinal tract hemorrhage (usually melena), and hematuria.
- Increased prothrombin time.

Vitamin K Toxicity
Vitamin K toxicity is rare; it results in hemolytic anemia.

VITAMIN E
Vitamin E (tocopherol) acts as an antioxidant. It is fat soluble, and present in many foods. No specific deficiency disease has been identified in humans.

VITAMIN C
Vitamin C (ascorbic acid) is a water-soluble vitamin present in fresh fruit and leafy vegetables. It is required for the synthesis of collagen,and osteoid.

Vitamin C Deficiency
A. Causes:

- Dietary deficiency causes scurvy.
- Seen in infants on certain powdered milks, in elderly people whose diets lack fresh fruit or vegetables, and in malnutrition. It was formerly seen in long-distance sailors.

B. Clinical features:

- Collagen types with the highest hydroxyproline content (eg, those in blood vessels) are most severely affected.
- One of the early clinical features is bleeding and bruising.
- Wound healing is also abnormal.
- The gums become swollen and bleed easily.
- Bone growth at the epiphysis is impaired, leading to growth retardation.
- Microscopically, in contrast to rickets, scurvy is associated with deficient osteoid and much calcified cartilage.

Vitamin C Toxicity
Megadoses of Vitamin C increase the incidence of urinary calculi.

THIAMINE (Vitamin B₁)
Thiamine is a coenzyme in the decarboxylation of pyruvate and α-ketoglutarate, which produces acetyl-CoA. **Thiamine excess is not toxic.**

Thiamine Deficiency
A. Causes: Dietary deficiency generally uncommon, except where polished rice is the staple food, and in chronic alcoholics.
B. Clinical features.
1. Wet beriberi: Cardiac failure produces massive peripheral edema, from which the term *wet* is derived.
2. Dry beriberi:

- Dry beriberi is characterized by changes in the nervous system:
  - **Peripheral neuropathy,** due to segmental demyelination.

- **Korsakoff's syndrome** (loss of memory and confabulation), due to neuronal loss.
- **Wernicke's encephalopathy** (abnormalities in fine motor activity), due to hemorrhages in the mamillary bodies, the periventricular region of the brain stem, and the occulomotor nuclei.

RIBOFLAVIN (Vitamin B_2)

Riboflavin is one of the flavoproteins, which participate in electron transfer in the respiratory chain.

- It is widely distributed in both animal and plant foods; deficiency occurs only with significant malnutrition.
- Excessive intake causes no ill effects.
- Clinical manifestations of deficiency include:
  - **Cheilosis** (inflammation of the lips).
  - **Angular stomatitis** (fissures at the corners of the mouth).
  - Atrophy of mucous membranes, especially the tongue.
  - Corneal opacities, ulceration, and blindness.

NICOTINIC ACID (NIACIN) & NICOTINAMIDE (NIACINAMIDE)

Niacin is an integral part of nicotinamide adenine dinucleotide (NAD) and NAD phosphate (NADP).

Niacin Deficiency

A. Causes: Niacin is present in many foods, and deficiency occurs only with significant malnutrition.

B. Deficiency causes pellagra, characterized by dermatitis, diarrhea, and dementia ("the 3 D's").

    1. Dermatitis involves mainly sun-exposed skin, which is reddened, pigmented, and excessively keratinized.

    2. Diarrhea is due to mucosal atrophy, affecting mouth, tongue, and gastrointestinal tract.

    3. Dementia is due to progressive degeneration of neurons in the cerebral cortex.

Niacin Toxicity

Very large doses of niacin produce vasodilation and a burning sensation, especially of the head and neck.

PYRIDOXINE (Vitamin B_6)

Pyridoxine forms the coenzyme pyridoxal 5-phosphate. It is found in virtually all foods, and pure dietary deficiency is rare.

Pyridoxine Deficiency

A. Causes:

- The commonest cause of clinical pyridoxine deficiency is the ingestion of drugs that are pyridoxine antagonists; these include isoniazid (INH), oral contraceptives, methyldopa, and levodopa.
- Infants who are fed processed-milk preparations deficient in pyridoxine develop convulsions.

B. Clinical features:

- Seborrheic dermatitis.
- Blepharitis.
- Cheilosis, glossitis, and angular stomatitis.
- Convulsions in infants and peripheral neuropathy in adults.
- Hypochromic and sideroblastic anemia, due to abnormal hemoglobin synthesis.

FOLIC ACID & VITAMIN B₁₂

Folic acid and vitamin B_{12} (cyanocobalamin) deficiencies are among the commonest vitamin deficiencies in industrialized societies.

- Folate and B_{12} are coenzymes in synthesis of nucleic acids.
- Deficiency of one or both produces **megaloblastic anemia** (for discussion, see Chapter 24).

MINERALS

The body requires many trace minerals in addition to iron, calcium, magnesium, and phosphate. These include zinc, copper, selenium, iodine, fluoride, manganese, cobalt, molybdenum, vanadium, chromium, and nickel.

IRON

Iron has several functions, and deficiency is common:

- It is due to inadequate intake, impaired absorption, or blood loss.
- Its result is failure of hemoglobin synthesis, leading to **hypochromic anemia** (Chapter 24).
- Iron excess may lead to **hemochromatosis** (Chapters 1 and 43).

TRACE ELEMENTS

Iodine

A deficiency of iodine causes a decrease in thyroid hormone output and leads to thyroid hyperplasia (goiter). See Chapter 58.

Fluoride

Deficiency of fluoride is associated with development of dental caries. Excess fluoride intake causes mottling of tooth enamel.

Calcium & Phosphate

Calcium and phosphate levels in blood and their absorption from the intestine are regulated by parathyroid hormone and vitamin D (Chapter 59).

- Most abnormalities of calcium and phosphate metabolism result from parathyroid disease or vitamin D-related disease (eg, rickets, osteomalacia).
- Excessive intake of calcium occurs in **Milk alkali syndrome,** due to chronic ingestion of milk and antacids.
- **Malabsorption syndrome** may lead to hypocalcemia (decreased absorption of vitamin D and calcium).

Magnesium
Deficiency of magnesium results in tetany similar to that seen with hypocalcemia. Causes include malabsorption, malnutrition, and diuretics.

Zinc
Manifestations of zinc deficiency include anemia, growth retardation and gonadal atrophy, diarrhea and skin rashes.

Copper
Deficiency of copper may lead to anemia and neutropenia, decreased bone production (resulting in osteoporosis), and neurologic abnormalities. For abnormal storage of copper see Wilson's disease (hepatolenticular degeneration).

Selenium
Deficiency of selenium has been implicated as a cause of congestive cardiomyopathy.

Disorders Due to Physical Agents

11

MECHANICAL TRAUMA

Abrasion (Scrape)
Abrasions are minor injuries, with loss of superficial layers of the epidermis. Regeneration is complete; there is no scarring.

Contusion (Bruise)
Contusions are characterized by extravasation of blood into the tissue.

- Breakdown products of hemoglobin are responsible for the change in color from red through purple, black, green, and brown.
- Hemosiderin-laden macrophages provide microscopic evidence of injury.
- Major bleeding may produce a distinct lump (hematoma).
- In patients with bleeding disorders, minor injury may lead to massive bleeding and hematoma.

Laceration & Incision (Tearing & Cutting)
With lacerations or incisions, bleeding due to disruption of blood vessels may be severe.

- Cutting of a vital tissue may produce critical deficits (eg, spinal cord transection causes complete motor and sensory failure below the level of injury).
- Avulsion refers to complete severance of a tissue from the body.

Fracture
The word *fracture* denotes a break or rupture of bone.

PRESSURE INJURIES

Increase in Atmospheric Pressure
A. Blast injuries act on the body in one of two ways:

- Pressure waves may enter the body through any orifice (eg, mouth or anus) to damage lungs or intestine.
- Pressure waves acting on the surface of the body may rupture the diaphragm or liver.

B. Undersea diving: Undersea divers are subject to decompression sickness (bends) due to the formation of nitrogen bubbles in the blood when they surface too quickly (Chapter 9).

Decrease in Atmospheric Pressure

A. Hypoxia can occur due to sudden decompression of an aircraft cabin at high altitudes.

B. Middle ear pressure changes are caused by failure of equilibration with atmospheric pressure through the auditory (eustachian) tubes.

■ Respiratory infection or allergic rhinitis exacerbates the problem.

■ Chronic inflammation (barotitis) may follow recurrent changes (eg, with airline personnel).

INJURIES DUE TO HEAT & COLD

Localized Cold Injury

Two distinct conditions are recognized as deriving from localized cold injury.

A. Immersion foot (trench foot) is so called because it was a complication of trench warfare during World War I.

■ It is the result of long exposure to mud or water at cold but nonfreezing temperatures.

■ Subsequent vasoconstriction and thrombosis lead to ischemia and gangrene.

B. Frostbite is the result of exposure to freezing temperatures. Ischemic necrosis may occur within a few hours.

Generalized Cold Injury (Hypothermia)

In hypothermia, the entire body is exposed to low temperatures.

■ Reflex vasoconstriction conserves body heat for a while, but eventually core temperature falls.

■ Cellular metabolism is reduced, blood pools in the periphery, and circulatory failure results.

■ It is more common in elderly individuals.

Localized Heat Injury (Burns)

Burns are a major cause of death in the USA. Their severity is determined by several factors (Table 11-1).

A. Evaluation of burns.

   1. Depth:

■ **First-degree burn** is minor, affecting only superficial epidermis.

  ● It shows erythema and edema.

■ **Second-degree burn** affects the full thickness of the epidermis and part of the dermis, but spares the adnexa of the skin (hair follicles, etc.).

  ● It shows vesiculation (blister formation) in addition to erythema and edema.

Note: First- and second-degree burns are also called **partial-thickness burns.**

■ **Third-degree (full thickness) burns** involve the entire epidermis and dermis, including adnexal structures.

  ● Third-degree burns heal very slowly by regeneration of epithelium from the edges. Scarring is usually severe.

TABLE 11–1. CLASSIFICATION OF BURNS ACCORDING TO SEVERITY[1]

Major burns
 Second-degree, > 25% body surface area in adults
 Second-degree, > 20% body surface area in children
 Third-degree, > 10% body surface area
 Burns involving hands, face, eyes, ears, feet, perineum[2]
 Burns associated with smoke inhalation, electrical injury, and other major trauma
 Burns in patients at poor risk (elderly, very young children)
Moderate burns
 Second-degree, 15–25% body surface area in adults
 Second-degree, 10–20% body surface area in children
 Third-degree, 2–10% body surface area
Minor burns
 First-degree, burn of any surface area
 Second-degree, < 15% body surface area in adults
 Second-degree, < 10% body surface area in children
 Third-degree, < 2% body surface area

[1]Modified and reproduced, with permission, from Mills J et al (editors): *Current Emergency Diagnosis & Treatment,* 2nd ed. Lange, 1985.
[2]This category does not by itself threaten life, but it threatens vital structures and therefore requires special management.

2. Surface area: When more than 10% of body surface area is covered with full-thickness burns, the loss of protein-rich fluid from the surface of the burn may be so great that hypoproteinemia and hypovolemia occur.

3. Site: Burns in contaminated areas (eg, perineum) are prone to infection.

4. Smoke inhalation: Most deaths in fires result from smoke inhalation and hypoxia. Toxic fumes from burning plastics are especially dangerous.

B. Complications.

1. Hypovolemia results from fluid exudation on the surface of the burn. If severe, it leads to shock and acute renal failure.

2. Necrosis of erythrocytes: Release of hemoglobin and red-cell stroma into the plasma may cause acute renal failure.

3. Necrosis of epidermis and dermis: If extensive, scab formation (eschar) may lead to contraction and ischemia of underlying tissues.

4. Infection:

■ Burned skin no longer serves as a barrier to infection.

■ Organisms commonly involved include staphylococci and *Pseudomonas* species, and fungi such as *Candida albicans* and *Aspergillus.*

5. Peptic ulcers: acute ulcers of the stomach and duodenum (Curling's ulcer) may occur following major burns; the cause is unknown.

6. Scarring may be extensive with third degree burns.

Generalized Heat Injury

Generalized heat injury results from exposure to a hot environment. Sweating usually prevents increase in body core temperature.

A. Heat cramps are due to loss of water and salt in sweat.

B. Heat exhaustion:

■ Is characterized by weakness, headache, nausea, and vertigo, followed by collapse, which is usually brief.

■ Is due to hemoconcentration resulting from water and electrolyte loss in sweat, and to peripheral vasodilatation, which occurs as a compensatory mechanism.
  ● The skin is gray and wet.
  ● The blood pressure may be low.

■ Is not dangerous, and most patients recover when removed to a cool area.

C. Heat pyrexia (heat stroke):

■ Is a severe, life-threatening condition.

■ Represents failure of heat regulation, preceded by cessation of sweating.

■ Is accompanied by confusion, delirium, loss of consciousness, peripheral circulatory failure, and shock.

■ Treatment is to cool patient rapidly.

D. Malignant hyperthermia:

■ This is an inherited disease of skeletal muscle.

■ Hyperpyrexia occurs upon administration of certain drugs used in anesthesiology, eg, halothane and muscle relaxants.

Note: Malignant hyperthermia is not caused by exposure to a hot external environment.

ELECTRICAL INJURIES

The severity of electrical injuries is related to the amount of current that flows through the body, which in turn is related directly to the voltage difference and inversely to the resistance.

■ Severe injuries are more common in countries that use a 220- to 240-volt domestic supply than in those that use a 110-volt supply.

■ Wet skin, which has a much lower resistance than dry skin, predisposes to more severe electrical injury.

■ Severity of damage in a particular tissue is dependent on the following factors:
  ● The electrical resistance of the tissue.
  ● The exact path taken by the current through the body. For example, cardiac arrhythmias may develop if the current passes across the heart.
  ● The duration. Alternating current (AC) is more dangerous than direct current (DC) because it causes tetanic contraction of muscles that may prevent the victim from letting go of the contact source.

■ The passage of electricity through the body has two main effects:
  ● Interference with the generation of electrical action potentials, causing cardiorespiratory arrest, cardiac arrhythmias, and heart block.
  ● Generation of heat (electrical burns).

IONIZING RADIATION INJURY

Exposure of Humans to Ionizing Radiation

Ionizing radiation includes electromagnetic waves (x-rays and gamma rays) and certain types of particulate radiation (Table 11–2).

TABLE 11–2. IONIZING RADIATION

Type of Radiation	Description	Features
Particulate radiation Alpha particle	Nature: helium nucleus Charge: +2 Mass number: 4	Shallow penetration in tissue; causes dense ionization and damage. Causes little harm externally but dangerous if used internally as an alpha particle-emitting isotope.
Beta particle	Nature: electron Charge: −1 Mass number: negligible mass	Penetrates up to 1 cm of soft tissue. Dense ionization. Used to treat skin cancer; dangerous if used internally.
Neutron	Nature: neutron Charge: no charge Mass number: 1	Exists in low- and high-energy forms; the latter penetrates tissues and causes dense ionization.
Proton	Nature: proton Charge: +1 Mass number: 1	Not used routinely in medicine.
Deuteron	Nature: deuterium (heavy hydrogen) nucleus Charge: +1 Mass number: 2	Can be used for radiolabeling of compounds.
Waveform radiation X-rays Gamma rays	Waves of varying lengths. Behave as photons (discrete units of radiant energy) in tissue. No mass or charge.	Deep penetration of tissues; low density of ionization, so tissue damage is minimal compared with alpha and beta particles.

- **Natural radiation** is derived from radioactive elements in the environment and cosmic rays.
- Manmade radiation comes from isotopes used in nuclear medicine, nuclear power plants, nuclear weapons, etc.
- Diagnostic tests use very small doses of radiation that are generally not harmful.
- Higher doses are used in the treatment of cancer (**radiotherapy**).
- The unit of measure for radiation absorbed by tissues is the **gray (Gy)**—formerly it was the rad. **1 Gy = 100 cGy = 100 rads.**

Mechanism of Radiation Injury
The two principal mechanisms of radiation injury are shown in Fig 11–1.

Effects of Radiation Injury
In radiation injury, DNA represents the main target:

- High doses of radiation produce extensive DNA injury and cellular necrosis.
- Smaller doses cause functional abnormalities of DNA and interfere with mitosis.
- These DNA changes are permanent and may be associated with the later development of cancer.
- The severity of tissue damage depends on several factors.

    A. Dose.
    B. Penetration:

- Alpha particles have a limited ability to penetrate.
- Smaller beta particles (electrons) penetrate more deeply.
- X-rays and gamma rays also penetrate deeply, often passing through the body with little dissipation of energy, and therefore little damage.

    C. Sensitivity of tissues: This varies with different tissues (Table 11–3).
    D. Duration of exposure.

Total Body Irradiation
    A. Causes: It is generally the result of nuclear fallout.
    B. Effects:

- Are dose-dependent (Table 11–4).
- If long-term, as seen in survivors of Hiroshima and Nagasaki, there is an increased incidence of cancer (particularly leukemia), cataracts, infertility, and bone-marrow aplasia. Even the offspring appear to be at increased risk.

Localized Irradiation

- Localized irradiation is used in the treatment of cancer, based on the rationale that cancer cells (which are rapidly proliferating) are more sensitive to radiation than are the normal (nonproliferating or slowly proliferating) cells.

    A. Sensitivity of tissues.
        1. Cancer cells (malignant neoplasms) may be classified as radiosensitive or radioresistant (Table 11–3).
        2. Normal tissues also vary in sensitivity (Table 11–3).

Radiation source

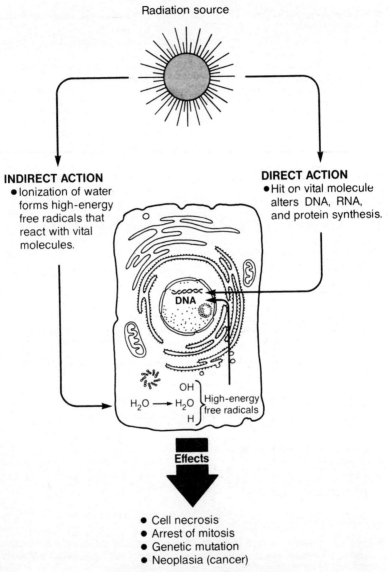

INDIRECT ACTION
- Ionization of water forms high-energy free radicals that react with vital molecules.

DIRECT ACTION
- Hit on vital molecule alters DNA, RNA, and protein synthesis.

DNA

$H_2O \longrightarrow H_2O$ OH H } High-energy free radicals

Effects

- Cell necrosis
- Arrest of mitosis
- Genetic mutation
- Neoplasia (cancer)

Figure 11–1. Effects of radiation on cells.

TABLE 11–3. RADIOSENSITIVITY OF CELLS[1]

	Permanent Cells (No or Very Low Mitotic Activity)	Stable Cells (Little Mitotic Activity)	Labile Cells (Rapidly Proliferating Tissues)
	Radioresistant	Intermediate radiosensitivity	Radiosensitive
Normal cells and tissues	Adult neurons	Muscle Connective tissue Liver Endocrine organs Glial cells	Bone marrow Intestinal epithelium Hair follicles Gonads Skin
Tumors	Ganglioneuroma (tumor of neurons) Benign neoplasms of connective tissue	Sarcoma (cancer of connective tissue cells) Glioma (tumor of glial cells) Liver cell cancer	Leukemia and lymphoma (of marrow and lymphocytes) Germinoma (neoplasm of gonads)

[1] Radiosensitivity correlates with the degree of mitotic activity of the tissue or tumor. Radioresistant and radiosensitive are relative terms, since all tissues are radiosensitive if the dose is high enough. Sensitivity also varies in different species: cockroaches can survive doses of several thousand rads; bacteria, doses of 10,000 rads or more.

TABLE 11–4. EFFECT OF TOTAL BODY IRRADIATION

Dose (Gy)	Syndrome	Latent Period	Clinical Features	Mortality Rate
0–0.5 Gy (0–50 rads)	None[1]	—	—	—
0.5–2 Gy (50–200 rads)	Acute radiation syndrome	Weeks–months	Fatigue, nausea, vomiting	0%
2–6 Gy (200–600 rads)	Hematopoietic syndrome	1–2 weeks	Leukopenia, thrombocytopenia	20–50%
3–10 Gy (300–1000 rads)	Gastrointestinal syndrome	1 day–2 weeks	Mucosal necrosis, diarrhea, fluid and electrolyte loss	50–100%[2]
10+ Gy (1000+ rads)	Cerebral syndrome	Hours–2 days	Ataxia, convulsions, delirium, coma	100%

[1] Though there are no immediate effects, low-level exposure of an individual to radiation is associated with an increased long-term incidence of cancer and low-level exposure of a population produces an increased mutation rate, with the possibility of birth defects.
[2] The mortality rate associated with gastrointestinal syndrome is almost 100% at doses over 6 Gy (600 rads). With exposure to lower doses (between 3 and 6 Gy [300–600 rads]), patients have features of both the gastrointestinal and hematopoietic syndromes and the mortality rate is lower.

B. Radiation damage of normal tissues:

- Tissues exposed to radiation demonstrate various abnormalities.
- In all tissues there is disruption of collagen, hyalinization of blood vessels and atypia of cells and nuclei.
- In addition, specific changes occur in various organs.

1. Skin:

- Early changes include erythema, swelling, and desquamation (acute radiodermatitis).
- Later, chronic radiodermatitis occurs, with epidermal atrophy, atypical cytologic features, fibrosis, telangiectasias, and loss of hair.
- Cancer may occur years later.

2. Bone marrow:

- Marked hypoplasia may occur within hours.
- Granulocytopenia may occur at about the end of the first week.
- Anemia may develop after 2–3 weeks.
- Regeneration is rapid if stem cells survive.

3. Lymphoid tissues are extremely radiosensitive, leading to lymphopenia.

4. Lungs are quite radio-resistant, but high doses cause radiation pneumonitis, with pulmonary edema and formation of hyaline membranes. Chronic changes include interstitial fibrosis.

5. Intestines: The mucosa of the intestine is radiosensitive. Radiation colitis causes diarrhea with blood and mucus.

6. Long-term effects are difficult to predict.

a. Carcinogenic effect: There may be development of radiation-induced neoplasms in patients who have been successfully treated for cancer.

b. Genetic effect: Genetic abnormalities (mutations) may be passed to subsequent generations.

C. Methods to minimize injury of normal tissues.

1. Shielding: Lead shields permit radiation to enter the body only through predetermined ports, or windows.

2. Radioisotope implants deliver the dose locally to the tumor.

3. Selective uptake is exemplified by the administration of radioactive iodine in the treatment of well-differentiated thyroid carcinoma.

4. Monoclonal antibodies targeted at tumor-associated antigens, carry small amounts of radioactive isotopes to the tumor site.

5. Fractionated doses: Multiple graded doses administered over time permit normal cells to recover in the interval between doses.

Ultraviolet Radiation

Ultraviolet radiation is present in sunlight. It has very low penetrating capability. Light-skinned individuals exposed to excessive sunlight are at risk for:

- Erythema and severe pain (sunburn).
- Various types of cancer of the skin, particularly basal-cell carcinoma, squamous carcinoma, and malignant melanoma.

Disorders Due to Chemical Agents

CLASSIFICATION OF CHEMICALS CAUSING INJURY

Chemicals of Abuse
Common drugs of abuse include ethyl alcohol, tobacco, and psychotropic drugs such as narcotics, cocaine, amphetamines, sedatives, and marihuana.

Therapeutic Drugs
Prescribed drugs may also cause injury through side effects, drug interactions, overdosage, or improper use.

Industrial & Agricultural Chemicals
Metals, insecticides, herbicides, industrial chemicals, toxic waste constitute a major public health hazard.

MECHANISMS OF HUMAN EXPOSURE

Voluntary Abuse
Addicts voluntarily use habituating substances because of physiologic or psychologic dependence.

Suicide or Homicide
Drugs may be taken or surreptitiously administered with suicidal or homicidal intent.

Accidental Ingestion
Toxic chemicals, particularly household products, may be accidentally ingested; young children are especially at risk.

Occupational Exposure
Exposure to toxic chemicals is common in agricultural and industrial workers.

Incidental Unrecognized Inadvertent Exposure
Exposure to trace levels of toxic chemicals in food, water and air (pollutants, passive smoking) is a major potential cause of disease.

ETHYL ALCOHOL ABUSE (Alcoholism)

Incidence
Abuse of alcohol is a major worldwide health problem, estimated to affect about 10% of the US population.

Clinical Syndromes
A. Acute alcoholic intoxication.
1. Blood alcohol concentration:

■ Acute intoxication correlates with the blood alcohol concentration (BAC).
■ Clinical evidence of intoxication appears at a BAC of about 100 mg/dL, although in some legal jurisdictions the presumption is 80 or even 50 mg/dL.
   ● Coma occurs when the BAC reaches 300–500 mg/dL.
   ● Chronic alcoholics develop tolerance.
■ Correlation of intake with blood levels is only approximate (Fig 12–1).
■ The following factors influence BAC:

a. The type of alcoholic beverage: Alcohol content varies from one beverage to another (Fig 12–1).
b. The rate of ingestion.
c. The rate of absorption:

■ Is greatest when the stomach is empty.
■ Decreases with the presence of fat in the stomach.

d. The rate of tissue distribution is related to body weight; obese persons have lower blood levels.
e. The rate of metabolism may vary considerably. Alcohol is metabolized in the liver by alcohol dehydrogenase.
f. The rate of excretion: Excretion of alcohol in urine and exhaled air is usually a small but constant amount that correlates with BAC; thus urine and breath testing correlates with blood testing.
2. Clinical features:

■ Ethyl alcohol (ethanol) is a central nervous system depressant.
■ The highest cortical brain centers are affected first; inhibitions are relaxed.
■ At relatively low blood levels (about 50 mg/dL), alcohol impairs fine judgment, fine motor skills, and reaction time.
■ Alcohol has been implicated as a contributing cause in about 50% of fatal traffic accidents.
■ Acute alcohol ingestion may also be associated with focal liver-cell necrosis (Chapter 43), accompanied by fever, jaundice, and painful enlargement of the liver.

B. Chronic alcoholic intoxication.
1. Chronic alcoholic liver disease: Chronic liver disease (cirrhosis) is a common cause of death in alcoholics (see Chapter 43).
2. Chronic pancreatitis: (See Chapter 45.)
3. Alcoholic cardiomyopathy is uncommon, but may lead to cardiac failure.
4. Nervous system abnormalities: Peripheral neuropathy is a prominent manifestation associated with alcohol.
5. Associated malnutrition:

■ Alcoholics tend to forego food in favor of drink.
■ Vitamin deficiency is common; this includes deficiencies of
   ● Thiamine (**Wernicke's encephalopathy, Korsakoff's psychosis**).

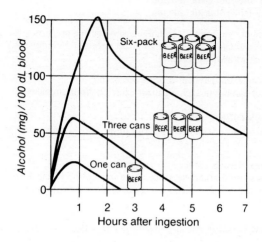

Equivalents	Alcohol content
Can of beer 360 mL	3–8%
Measure of spirits 35 mL	40–60%
Glass of wine 120 mL	8–15%
Glass of sherry or port 80 mL	15–23%

Figure 12–1. Approximation of blood alcohol concentrations following alcohol ingestion for a 70-kg individual.

- Folic acid (**megaloblastic anemia**).
- Pyridoxine (**sideroblastic anemia**).

C. Fetal alcohol syndrome: Alcohol ingestion during pregnancy causes dose-related fetal growth retardation and increased infant perinatal mortality rates.

D. Alcohol withdrawal syndrome:

- Both psychologic and physical dependence occur.
- Withdrawal of alcohol in such a patient causes delirium tremens.

CIGARETTE SMOKING

Cigarette smoking increases the overall risk of death by as much as 70% compared to nonsmokers.

- Smokers die 5–8 years earlier than nonsmokers.
- Many diseases occur at increased incidence in smokers (Table 12–1).
- Smoking low-tar and low-nicotine cigarettes decreases this risk by only a small amount.
- Use of snuff and chewing tobacco increases the risk of oral cancer.
- Although lung cancer (especially squamous and small-cell) is most often associated

TABLE 12–1. PHARMACOLOGY AND PATHOLOGY OF CIGARETTE SMOKING[1]

Pharmacology	
Active ingredient:	Nicotine ($C_{10}H_{14}N_2$)
Addictive agent:	Nicotine
Dose per inhalation:	50–150 μg
Dose per cigarette:	1–2 mg
Lethal dose:	50 mg
Absorption:	From lungs (instantaneous); more slowly from buccal mucosa
Half-life:	Levels fall rapidly, requiring new dose every 30–40 minutes in addicts
Other toxic substances:	Numerous carcinogens

Diseases of increased incidence and severity in smokers[2]
Cancer of the lung (X 10)
Chronic obstructive pulmonary disease (X 10)
  (chronic bronchitis and emphysema)
Atherosclerotic arterial disease (X 2)
  Ischemic heart disease (angina and infarction)
  Cerebral thrombosis and infarction
Thromboangiitis obliterans (Buerger's disease) (X 100)
Chronic peptic ulcer (X 2–3)
Cancer of the oral cavity and tongue (X 5)
Cancer of the urinary bladder (X 5)
Cancer of the larynx and pharynx (X 5)
Cancer of the esophagus (X 5)

[1]Modified from Christen AG, Cooper KH: Strategic withdrawal from cigarette smoking. *CA* 1979; **29**:96.
[2]Figures in parentheses = increased risk compared to the nonsmoking population.

with smoking, smokers are at increased risk for other cancers as well: bladder, oral cavity, larynx, esophagus.

■ Obstructive airways disease and atherosclerosis also occur at increased frequency in smokers.

PSYCHOTROPIC DRUG ABUSE

Types of Drugs Abused

Abuse of drugs is a worldwide problem. Drugs may be ingested, smoked, sniffed, injected into the skin (popping), or injected intravenously (mainlining). Types of drugs include

■ Stimulants such as cocaine and amphetamines.
■ Depressants such as heroin, barbiturates, and benzodiazepines (eg, diazepam).
■ Hallucinogens such as marihuana, lysergic acid diethylamide (LSD), and phencyclidine (PCP).

Effects
A. Direct effects:

■ All of the psychotropic drugs affect the nervous system.
■ Drugs available on the street contain unknown and variable concentrations of active drug and contaminants.
■ Alteration in mental function increases the risk of traffic accidents, criminal behavior, and acts of violence, including suicide.
■ Withdrawal symptoms may be severe.

B. Indirect effects:

■ Street drugs are often "cut" (diluted) with contaminants such as cotton fibers, talc, sugars, etc.
■ Infection may be transmitted by nonsterile needles shared by IV drug abusers. These include
  ● Staphylococcal abscesses and endocarditis.
  ● Hepatitis B virus.
  ● Human immunodeficiency virus (HIV, the cause of AIDS).

C. Long-term effects:

■ From **marihuana,** chronic bronchitis.
■ From **cocaine** sniffing, perforation of the nasal septum.
■ From **heroin,** focal glomerulonephritis.

METALS

Lead Poisoning

A. Causes: Lead is used in the manufacture of batteries and paints, and as a gasoline additive. It is a pervasive environmental pollutant.

■ When ingested or inhaled, lead is deposited in tissues such as bone and kidney.

■ At particular risk are industrial workers and children in older homes with leaded paintwork.

B. **Effects** are usually due to chronic accumulation.
   1. **Erythrocytes:** Lead inhibits several enzymes in the hemoglobin synthetic pathway.

■ Serum free erythrocyte protoporphyrin, urinary coproporphyrin III, and δ-aminolevulinic acid levels are increased, serving as tests for lead poisoning.
■ Impairment of hemoglobin synthesis leads to **anemia,** with hypochromia and basophilic stippling.

   2. **Nervous system:**

■ **Lead encephalopathy** is characterized by necrosis of neurons, demyelination, and astrocytosis.
■ In very young children, mental development is impaired.
■ In adults, demyelination produces a motor neuropathy characterized by footdrop and wristdrop.

   3. **Kidney:**

■ Damage to the proximal renal tubular cells causes aminoaciduria and glycosuria.
■ On histologic examination, tubular epithelial cells contain pink intranuclear inclusions.

   4. **Gastrointestinal tract:** The patient experiences colicky pain due to muscle spasm (**lead colic, "painter's cramps"**).
   5. **Other affected areas:**

■ A blue line appears along the margins of the gums.
■ Deposition in epiphyses in children produces diagnostic dense lines on X-ray.

Mercury Poisoning

Ingestion of small amounts of mercury is not as dangerous as exposure to lead, because mercury is more easily excreted. Mercury combines with sulfhydryl groups of enzymes and interferes with ATP production.

A. **Acute mercury poisoning:**

■ Usually seen in suicide attempts, inhalation of mercury vapors on the job, or use of insecticides.
■ Major toxicity manifests as acute renal tubular necrosis.
■ Ulcerations of the mouth, stomach, and colon also occur.

B. **Chronic mercury poisoning:**

■ Is due to industrial pollution or eating fish from polluted coastal waters.
■ Predominant clinical effects are
   ● Cerebral and cerebellar atrophy (neuronal loss) with dementia, emotional instability, and visual and auditory disturbances.
   ● Nephrotic syndrome.

Aluminum Poisoning
Aluminum toxicity causes osteomalacia by blocking normal calcification.

Arsenic Poisoning

- Arsenic is a constituent of many agricultural pesticides.
- It binds to sulfhydryl groups, blocking many enzymes.
- Acute poisoning is rare and almost always with suicidal intent.
- Death may be rapid, with circulatory collapse, renal necrosis and severe abdominal pain.
- Chronic poisoning leads to accumulation in hair, skin, and nails; examination of hair and nail samples for arsenic content is a sensitive diagnostic technique.
- Clinically there are changes in many tissues:
  - The skin shows increased pigmentation and thickening (arsenical keratosis).
  - Dysplasia predispose to the development of skin cancer (squamous carcinoma).
  - Nails show abnormal transverse ridges (Mees' lines).
  - Peripheral nerves demonstrate demyelinating neuropathy.
  - There is increased incidence of hepatic angiosarcoma.

INSECTICIDES & HERBICIDES
Insecticides are widely available for agricultural and home use. They are thus often used in suicide attempts and may also contaminate the environment and food sources.

- Insecticides may be absorbed from the skin (direct contact), lungs (inhalation), or intestine (ingestion).
- Farm workers are at high risk.
- Accidental ingestion by children is common.

Chlorinated Hydrocarbons
Chlorinated hydrocarbons such as DDT and dieldrin are widely used.

- They cause mostly neurologic effects—delirium and convulsions followed by coma and death.
- Chronic exposure leads to fatty liver.

Organophosphates
These compounds were initially developed as nerve gases.

- Malathion is an acetylcholinesterase inhibitor.
- Large doses are rapidly fatal, due to inhibition of neuromuscular impulses, with resulting paralysis.
- Pupillary constriction, blurring of vision, abdominal cramps, diarrhea, salivation, sweating, and bronchoconstriction are early signs of toxicity.

Paraquat
Paraquat is a herbicide that is extremely dangerous if ingested.

- It produces ulceration of the oral mucosa, and necrosis of the liver, renal tubular cells, and lung (hyaline membrane formation, pulmonary hemorrhage, and edema).
- Survivors develop progressive pulmonary fibrosis.

INDUSTRIAL CHEMICALS

Methyl Alcohol (Methanol)
Methyl alcohol is a highly toxic solvent. It is often added to laboratory-grade ethyl alcohol to make it undrinkable.

- It produces a profound metabolic acidosis.
- It also causes irreversible degeneration of the retina and optic nerve.

Ethylene Glycol
Ethyline glycol is a common ingredient in antifreeze.

- Ingestion causes severe metabolic acidosis.
- It is metabolized to calcium oxalate, which is deposited as crystals, causing acute renal failure.

Carbon Tetrachloride
Carbon tetrachloride is a solvent used in dry cleaning. Inhalation or ingestion leads to convulsions or coma, hepatic necrosis (centrilobular), and renal tubular necrosis.

Carbon Monoxide
Carbon monoxide is found in automobile exhausts, natural gas, and with improper combustion in household gas and paraffin heaters.

- Carbon monoxide combines with hemoglobin to form carboxyhemoglobin, which cannot carry oxygen.
- Poisoning produces hypoxia involving the brain (eg, headache, confusion, visual disturbances, dizziness, convulsions, and coma).
- Poisoning can be recognized clinically by the cherry-red color of the blood, skin, and lips.
- Diagnosis is confirmed by finding of carboxyhemoglobin in the blood.

Cyanide
One of the most powerful poisons known, the lethal dose of cyanide is around 0.1 mg.

- It is used for electroplating and metal cleaning and in the manufacture of batteries.
- An industrial accident in India in 1984 released fumes of a cyanide compound that caused over 2000 deaths.
- Cyanide inactivates cytochrome oxidase.
- Acute poisoning causes rapid death.

THERAPEUTIC AGENTS (Drugs)

Prescription Drugs
No drug is free from adverse effects.

    A. Dose-related toxic effects: The therapeutic dose must be titrated against any toxic effect; eg, cytotoxic drugs are predictably toxic to cancer cells, but also kill normal bone marrow.

    B. Idiosyncratic side effects: This type of toxicity is not predictable. It is dangerous, since it occurs unexpectedly. Examples include:

- Massive liver-cell necrosis with use of halothane or isoniazid.
- Acute interstitial renal disease and renal failure with use of methicillin, sulfonamides, and other drugs.
- Bone-marrow suppression with use of chloramphenicol, phenylbutazone, and gold salts.
  - Note that chloramphenicol also produces a less severe dose-related form of bone marrow suppression.
- Lung fibrosis with bleomycin, methotrexate, and nitrofurantoin.
- Acute cardiac dysfunction with local anesthetics such as procaine.

C. Allergic or hypersensitivity reactions: Allergic reactions are also unpredictable, though a history of sensitization may sometimes be elicited.

- Mechanisms of sensitization are described in Chapter 8.
- Clinical manifestations include **anaphylaxis, rashes, hemolytic anemia, thrombocytopenia, glomerulonephritis,** and various autoimmune diseases.

Commonly Used Drugs

Nonprescription (over-the-counter) drugs also may produce adverse reactions.
  A. Aspirin:

- Aspirin (and other salicylates) can be fatal in large doses (fatal dose for an adult is 15 g).
- Children are much more susceptible than adults.
- Aspirin stimulates respiration and produces an initial **respiratory alkalosis.**
- As aspirin accumulates, it produces a severe **metabolic acidosis.**
- Other effects include
  - Bleeding tendency (altered platelet function).
  - Erosive acute gastritis (may cause gastric bleeding).
  - **Reye's syndrome** in children, characterized by acute fatty liver and encephalopathy, and a high mortality rate.

B. Abuse of phenacetin-containing analgesics: Chronic abuse of phenacetin analgesics produces renal papillary necrosis.
  C. Acetaminophen (paracetamol): Overdosage causes massive dose-related hepatic necrosis that is often fatal.
  D. Oral contraceptives:

- These are prescription drugs, but freely available.
- Early preparations contained high levels of estrogen; adverse effects included
  - Thrombosis, pulmonary embolism.
  - Liver lesions: focal nodular hyperplasia, liver cell adenoma.
  - Gallstones.
- Today's oral contraceptives have low levels of estrogen, which may result in lowered risk.

Infectious Diseases: I. Mechanisms of Tissue Changes in Infection

13

The outcome of infection is determined by opposing groups of factors. On one hand are the ability of the agent to overcome host defenses, the site of infection, the dose of organisms, and their pathogenicity. On the other are the ability of the host to resist infection, the host's natural defenses, and the host's immune response.

CLASSIFICATION OF INFECTIOUS AGENTS

Classification According to Structure

For purposes of study, infectious agents are arranged in order of increasing structural complexity, beginning with viruses and proceeding through rickettsiae, chlamydiae, mycoplasmas, bacteria, fungi, algae, and protozoa to metazoa (Table 13–1).

Classification According to Pathogenicity

The ability to cause disease is called **pathogenicity.**

- Agents can be subdivided into nonpathogens, low-grade pathogens and high-grade pathogens (the latter are said to be **virulent**).
- Virulent organisms readily cause disease.
- Low-grade pathogens cause disease only in immunocompromised hosts (**opportunistic infections**).

Classification According to Site of Multiplication

The site of multiplication of the agent largely determines the types of inflammatory and immune response.

A. Obligate intracellular organisms:

- Grow and multiply only in living host cells.
- Require living cell systems for successful culture.
- Include viruses, rickettsiae, chlamydiae.

B. Facultative intracellular organisms:

- Are capable of both extracellular and intracellular growth (often in macrophages).
- Include mycobacterial species, actinomyces and some fungi.

C. Extracellular organisms:

- Include most bacteria, and some fungi.
- Generally can be cultured on artificial media.

TABLE 13–1. INFECTIOUS AGENTS OF HUMANS, CLASSIFIED ACCORDING TO STRUCTURE

Group	Cellular Complexity	Additional Classification Criteria	Major Pathogenic Types	Culture Requirements
Viruses[1]	Virion	DNA or RNA Size Morphology Immunologic	Adenovirus, herpesvirus, poxvirus, papovavirus, arbovirus, myxovirus, retrovirus, picornavirus, etc	Grow only in tissue culture.
Rickettsiae	Simple cells (prokaryotes)	Immunologic	*Rickettsia prowazekii, Rickettsia tsutsugamushi, Rickettsia rickettsii, Coxiella burnetii*	Grow only in tissue culture.
Chlamydiae	Simple cells (prokaryotes)	Immunologic	*Chlamydia psittaci, Chlamydia trachomatis*	Grow only in tissue culture.
Bacteria (including mycoplasmas, spirochetes, vibrios)	Simple cells (prokaryotes)	Morphology (cocci, bacilli, spirochetes, etc) Gram stain Oxygen requirement Biochemical reactions Immunologic	*Staphylococcus, Streptococcus, Neisseria, Clostridium, Corynebacterium,* enterobacteria, *Brucella, Haemophilus, Yersinia, Salmonella, Mycobacterium, Bacteroides, Vibrio, Mycoplasma,* etc	Most grow on artificial media.

(continued)

TABLE 13-1. (Continued)

Group	Cellular Complexity	Additional Classification Criteria	Major Pathogenic Types	Culture Requirements
Fungi	Complex cells (eukaryotes)	Morphology Type of spores	Dermatophytes, Aspergillus, Mucor, Candida, Coccidioides, Histoplasma, Cryptococcus, Blastomyces	Most grow on artificial media.
Algae	Complex cells (eukaryotes)		Rarely infect humans	Not routinely cultured; many cannot be cultured.
Protozoa	Complex cells (eukaryotes)	Morphology Sexual cycle	Amebas, Giardia, Trichomonas, Trypanosoma, Leishmania, Toxoplasma, Plasmodium, Pneumocystis, Cryptosporidium, Isospora	Not routinely cultured; a few cannot be cultured.
Metazoa Helminths and flukes	Multicellular parasites	Morphology (flat and round worms)	Taenia, Ascaris, Enterobius, Trichuris, Necator, Strongyloides, Echinococcus, Trichinella, Clonorchis, Schistosoma, Wuchereria, Brugia	Cannot be cultured.
Insecta, Arachnida	Multicellular parasites	Morphology	Sarcoptes scabiei, fleas, and ticks	Cannot be cultured.

[1]Viruses contain either DNA or RNA: All other organisms contain both DNA and RNA.

TISSUE CHANGES IN INFECTION
Infection may be

- Latent (ie, no overt disease).
- Followed by pathologic changes (disease), due to the direct effects of the organism or due to the effects of the inflammatory and immune responses.

Tissue Damage Caused by Infectious Agents
The extent of direct tissue damage is a function of virulence (high pathogenicity).
A. Obligate intracellular organisms: Viruses, rickettsiae and chlamydiae may produce a variety of changes in infected cells.
    1. Cell necrosis:

- Different viruses have affinity for different parenchymal cells (ie, they are organotropic). For example, they may be
  - **Neurotropic,** such as poliovirus, or arborviruses (cause encephalitis).
  - **Dermatotropic,** such as pox viruses or papilloma virus.
  - **Hepatic and enterotropic,** as in rotavirus or hepatitis viruses.
- Acute extensive necrosis may cause death (eg, due to encephalitis, myocarditis, or massive liver necrosis).
- Slow cell necrosis over a long period constitutes **persistent viral infection.** This can occur
  - In the liver (chronic persistent and chronic active viral hepatitis).
  - In the brain (**slow viral infections** include subacute sclerosing panencephalitis—caused by measles virus, kuru, and Creutzfeldt-Jakob disease).

    2. Cell swelling is the result of sublethal injury, and may affect many cell types.
    3. Inclusion body formation: Inclusion bodies are composed either of assembled viral particles or of remnants of viral nucleic acid synthesis. They occur in the nucleus or the cytoplasm, are visible microscopically, and may aid diagnosis (Table 13–2).
    4. Giant cell formation: Multinucleated giant cells occur in some viral infections, including measles (Warthin-Finkeldey giant cells), herpes simplex, and varicella-zoster.
    5. Latent viral infection: Viruses can remain latent in the infected cell for life.
      a. Reactivation:

- Herpes simplex and varicella-zoster viruses may remain latent in sensory ganglia.
- Upon reactivation (due to stress, coexistent disease), the virus then migrates via the nerves to the skin or mucosa, where cell necrosis occurs.
- Herpes simplex type-1 infection causes cold sores.
- Varicella-zoster virus causes chickenpox in childhood, but may reactivate many years later as shingles.

      b. Oncogenesis (production of neoplasms): Certain viruses appear to be oncogenic in animals and in man. (See Chapter 19.)
B. Facultative intracellular organisms: Damage attributed to the inflammatory (granuloma formation) and immune (delayed hypersensitivity) responses.
C. Extracellular organisms can cause cell injury in one of several ways.
    1. Release of locally acting enzymes, including

- *Staphylococcus aureus,* which produces:
  - Coagulase, which converts fibrinogen to fibrin—

TABLE 13-2. CHARACTERISTIC HISTOLOGIC CHANGES PRODUCED IN CELLS
INFECTED BY OBLIGATE INTRACELLULAR AGENTS

Infectious Agents	Histologic Features
Cytomegalovirus	Enlargement of cell (cytomegaly). Eosinophilic, large intranuclear inclusion surrounded by a halo.[1] Small, multiple, granular, basophilic cytoplasmic inclusions.
Herpes simplex virus and varicella-zoster virus	Large, eosinophilic intranuclear inclusion surrounded by a halo.[1] Nuclei with ground-glass appearance. Multinucleated (3-8 nuclei) giant cells.
Variola (smallpox) virus	Multiple, granular, round, eosinophilic cytoplasmic inclusions (Guarnieri bodies).
Rabies virus	Round, 2-10 μm, eosinophilic cytoplasmic inclusions (Negri bodies).
Hepatitis B virus	Cytoplasm with ground-glass appearance.
Measles virus	Multinucleated (10-50 nuclei) Warthin-Finkeldey giant cells. Small eosinophilic intranuclear inclusions.
Molluscum contagiosum virus	Homogeneous eosinophilic cytoplasmic inclusion that fills the cell, pushing the nucleus aside.
Chlamydia	Small, multiple, eosinophilic cytoplasmic inclusions.

[1]Also called Cowdry A inclusions. Though most commonly seen in herpesvirus infections, Cowdry A inclusions are not pathognomonic for herpesviruses; they may occasionally be produced by other viruses.

- An effect which is closely linked to virulence.
■ Streptococcus pyogenes, which produces:
  - Hyaluronidase and streptokinase, which facilitate the spread of infection.
  - Several hemolysins.
■ *Clostridium perfringens* produces lecithinase, hyaluronidase, collagenase, and hemolysins. The result is gas gangrene.

    2. Production of local vasculitis: Highly virulent organisms—eg, (*Bacillus anthracis*), *Aspergillus,* and *Mucor*—cause thrombosis and ischemia.
    3. Production of remotely acting toxins.
        a. Endotoxins:

■ Are lipopolysaccharide components of the cell walls of gram-negative bacteria.
■ Are released into the bloodstream after the death and lysis of bacteria.
■ Activate coagulation and complement systems.
■ Cause generalized peripheral vasodilatation, disseminated intravascular coagulation, and fever (endotoxic or gram-negative shock).

        b. Exotoxins:

■ Are substances (often proteins) actively secreted by living bacteria.

TABLE 13–3. DISEASES CAUSED BY BACTERIAL TOXINS

Bacterium	Disease	Toxin	Mechanism of Disease
Staphylococcus aureus	Staphylococcal gastroenteritis	Enterotoxin	Toxin preformed in food outside body; probably acts on neural receptors in intestine to stimulate vomiting. Self-limited illness; low mortality rate.
	Toxic shock syndrome	Hemolysin (exotoxin [TSST-1])	Toxin produced in tampons, infected wounds; causes diffuse erythematous skin rash. Serious disease with high mortality rate.
	Neonatal bullous impetigo	Exfoliatin (epidermolysin)	Toxin causes epidermal necrosis ("scalded skin syndrome"). Serious disease with high mortality rate.
Streptococcus pyogenes	Scarlet fever	Erythrogenic toxin	Toxin causes erythemic diffuse skin rash; associated with streptococcal pharyngitis; low mortality rate.
Corynebacterium diphtheriae	Diphtheria	Diphtheria toxin	Exotoxin absorbed into blood from site of bacterial multiplication in upper respiratory tract. Inhibits polypeptide synthesis in cells; causes myocarditis and peripheral neuritis; high mortality rate.
Clostridium tetani	Tetanus	Tetanus toxin	Exotoxin produced in wound is absorbed into blood stream and nerves; blocks release of an inhibitory mediator in spinal neurons and thereby leads to muscle spasm and seizures; binds to gangliosides in the central nervous system; high mortality rate.

(continued)

TABLE 13–3. (Continued)

Bacterium	Disease	Toxin	Mechanism of Disease
Clostridium botulinum	Botulism	Botulinus toxin	Toxin preformed in food; interferes with acetylcholine release at neuromuscular end plate to produce muscle paralysis. High mortality rate.
Vibrio cholerae	Cholera	Enterotoxin	Enterotoxin produced by multiplying vibrios in intestinal lumen attaches to mucosal cell receptors, causing activation of adenyl cyclase, increased cyclic AMP production, and secretion of electrolytes and water by the cell. Severe secretory diarrhea. High mortality rate.
Clostridium difficile	Pseudomembranous enterocolitis	C difficile toxin	Broad-spectrum antibiotics (especially clindamycin) favor overgrowth of C difficile in gut lumen. Toxin produced causes necrosis of epithelial cells. High mortality rate; good response to vancomycin.
Clostridium perfringens	Gastroenteritis	Enterotoxin	Toxin has unknown mechanism; causes secretory diarrhea; self-limited disease with low mortality rate.
Toxigenic Escherichia coli	Traveler's diarrhea	Enterotoxins	Several toxins described; one has action similar to that of V cholerae. Self-limited mild disease with low mortality rate.
Shigella dysenteriae type I	Dysentery	Exotoxin	Affects central nervous system, leading to coma. May affect endothelial cells and cause disseminated intravascular coagulation. These changes compli-

(continued)

TABLE 13–3. (*Continued*)

Bacterium	Disease	Toxin	Mechanism of Disease
			cate acute colitis caused by direct infection.
Neisseria menigitidis Gram-negative bacilli	Meningococcemia Gram-negative bacteremia	Endotoxin	Endotoxins are cell wall constituents of gram-negative bacteria. In the blood they cause fever; activate complement; activate factor XII (Hageman factor), leading to disseminated intravascular coagulation; and have vasoactive effects leading to shock.

- Actions cause specific effects (Table 13–3).
- Are highly antigenic, inducing the formation of antitoxins.
- Are heat-labile, destroyed by cooking or heating to above 60°C. (By contrast, endotoxins are relatively heat-stable.)

    c. Enterotoxins are special exotoxins that act on intestinal mucosal cells (Table 13–3).

Tissue Changes Caused by Host Response to Infection
The host response frequently causes many of the clinical signs and symptoms associated with the infection and may sometimes cause tissue damage and even death.
    A. Acute inflammation:

- With many infections, acute inflammation results in **pain, redness, warmth,** and **swelling.**
- **Fever** is mediated by exogenous pyrogens (factors released by the organisms) or endogenous pyrogens, including interleukin-1.
- **Extracellular organisms** (most bacteria) typically induce acute inflammation with large numbers of neutrophils.
- **Facultative intracellular organisms** typically induce a response with numerous macrophages.
- **Obligate intracellular organisms** (mainly viruses and rickettsiae) induce an acute cellular response with lymphocytes, plasma cells, and macrophages but few neutrophils.

    B. Suppurative inflammation:

- Suppuration (pus formation) is characterized by liquefactive necrosis; an **abscess** is a walled-off area of suppuration.
- It is likely to develop when anatomic abnormalities or foreign materials interfere with resolution of acute inflammation.

1. Acute suppuration is due to certain kinds of bacteria that are relatively resistant to phagocytosis, eg, *S. aureus, Klebsiella, Pseudomonas, Escherichia* species, and type-3 pneumococci.

2. Chronic suppuration:

■ May follow persistent acute suppurative inflammation (eg, chronic osteomyelitis)
■ May occur as a primary phenomenon due to infection with *Actinomyces* or *Nocardia* species) or certain mycelial fungi. Small yellow colonies of organisms (sulfur granules) may be visible in the pus.

C. Chronic inflammation:

■ Is best regarded as evidence of an immune response occurring in infected tissue.
■ Antigen may be released by damaged host tissues, although the inciting antigens are mostly derived from the infectious agent.
■ May follow an unresolved acute response.
■ May occur de novo if the initial phase of infection fails to excite an acute inflammatory response (as with many viruses and intracellular bacteria).

1. Chronic granulomatous inflammation: (See Chapter 5.)

■ Epithelioid-cell granulomas represent T cell–mediated immunity and associated type IV hypersensitivity.
■ They may be associated with extensive necrosis and fibrosis.
■ Responsible agents include:
 ● Mycobacteria (*Mycobacterium tuberculosis, M. leprae,* atypical mycobacteria).
 ● Fungi that grow as nonmycelial forms in tissues (*Coccidioides immitis, Histoplasma capsulatum, Cryptococcus neoformans, Blastomyces dermatitidis.*
 ● *Brucella* species.
 ● *T. pallidum.* (Note that this is the only one of these organisms that grows extracellularly).
■ Identification of the causative agent is by culture, or with special stains for mycobacteria (acid-fast stain) or fungi (methenamine silver stain).

2. Chronic inflammation with diffuse proliferation of macrophages is characterized by a deficient cell-mediated immune response.

■ Lymphokines are absent, macrophages do not aggregate to form granulomas, and delayed hypersensitivity is absent.
■ Responsible organisms include:
 ● Mycobacteria (*M. leprae, M. tuberculosis*) and atypical mycobacteria, especially when in immunodeficient (including elderly) patients.
 ● *Klebsiella rhinoscleromatis.*
 ● *Leishmania* species.
■ A common feature is the presence of numerous organisms in the macrophages, which phagocytose but show limited ability to kill the organisms.

3. Chronic inflammation with lymphocytes and plasma cells:

■ Typically occurs in response to persistent infection caused by intracellular organisms (eg, viruses).

■ Represents a combined humoral and cell-mediated immune response.
■ Is associated with cell necrosis that is followed by fibrosis.

D. Combined suppurative and granulomatous inflammation:

■ Is commonly seen in deep fungal infections (eg, histoplasmosis) and as **stellate granulomas** (star-shaped granulomas with central acute necrosis) in certain other rare conditions, including
  ● Lymphogranuloma venereum (LGV), caused by *Chlamydia trachomatis*.
  ● Cat scratch disease, caused by a small gram-negative bacterium (not yet characterized).
  ● Tularemia (caused by *Francisella tularensis*).
  ● glanders (caused by *Pseudomonas mallei*), and
  ● Melioidosis (caused by *Pseudomonas pseudomallei*).
■ The specific diagnosis of these infectious diseases depends on culture or immunologic tests.

Infectious Diseases: II. Mechanisms of Infection

14

INCIDENCE OF INFECTIOUS DISEASES

Incidence varies throughout the world, reflecting differences in geographic and socioeconomic conditions, public health measures and medical care. Effective public-health measures include immunization, health education, sanitation, and vector control (mosquitoes etc.).

Infectious Disease in the USA

A. In hospital practice: About 40% of infections in hospitals are acquired in the hospital itself (**nosocomial infections**) (Table 14–1).

- They are mostly bacterial, and especially involve the lungs or the genitourinary tract.
- **Hospital-acquired pneumonia** is the most serious such infection, with a mortality rate of 20%.

　　1. Increased susceptibility occurs with concurrent illness and use of immunosuppressive drugs.

　　2. Use of invasive procedures: Surgery, catheterization, phlebotomy etc., provide possible routes and vehicles for entry of microorganisms.

　　3. Numerous sources of infection: Hospitals harbor sources of infection—mainly other patients, but also dust containing organisms and spores.

　　4. Use of antibiotics: The widespread use of antibiotics promotes overgrowth of antibiotic-resistant strains, including *Escherichia coli, Pseudomonas aeruginosa, Proteus* species, *Klebsiella* species, *Serratia* species and *Staphylococcus aureus*.

B. In community practice:

- Viral infections are common, especially those involving the upper respiratory tract (eg, coryza, influenza) and the gastrointestinal tract (eg, viral gastroenteritis).
- The most common bacterial infections are sexually transmitted diseases (eg, gonorrhea, syphilis), and respiratory infections (eg, streptococcal pharyngitis, sinusitis, otitis, pneumonia).

Infectious Disease in Developing Countries

Infectious disease is the major health care problem in developing countries. The total number of cases dwarfs the number from developed countries (billions of cases per year, as compared with millions). See Table 14–2.

- Protozoal and helminthic infections are very common; minor bacterial diseases are vastly underreported.

TABLE 14-1. COMMON INFECTIONS SEEN IN HOSPITALS IN THE USA[1]

Infection	Community-Acquired	Hospital-Acquired
Number of Cases/Year	*3 Million*	*2 Million*
Breakdown according to type of infectious agent (%) Bacteria	93	90
Viruses	6	Rare
Fungi	<1	10
Parasites (ie, protozoa, metazoa)	<1	Rare
Breakdown according to site (%) Genitourinary tract[2]	38	41
Lung	20	12
Upper respiratory tract	8	<1
Gastrointestinal tract	3	<1
Central nervous system	<1	<1
Disseminated infection[3]	<1	9
Others	29[4]	37[5]

[1]Note that this table represents only those infections serious enough to warrant hospitalization. The pattern of infectious diseases encountered in general medical practice outside hospitals differs greatly, with mild viral infections of the upper respiratory and gastrointestinal tracts accounting for a great number and percentage of cases.
[2]Common genitourinary tract infections in the community include sexually transmitted infections such as gonorrhea.
[3]Disseminated infections, commonly caused by bacteria and fungi, occur in immunocompromised patients, usually those being treated for cancer.
[4]Includes a wide variety of other sites.
[5]Includes infections of surgical wounds which are responsible for a majority of this group of hospital-acquired infections.

■ Associated problems include:
  ● Lack of means or facilities for treatment, so that relatively minor infections such as viral gastroenteritis produce significant mortality.
  ● Lack of childhood immunization.
  ● Lack of public health programs such as health education, vector control, and sanitation.
  ● Malnutrition.
■ Note that success can be achieved; public health immunization has eradicated smallpox.

TABLE 14–2. ANNUAL INCIDENCE OF MAJOR INFECTIONS IN ASIA, AFRICA, AND LATIN AMERICA[1]

Disease	Number of Cases per Year	Number of Deaths per Year
Diarrhea	5 billion	5–10 million[2]
Malaria	150 million[3]	1–2 million
Measles	80 million	900,000
Schistosomiasis	20 million[3]	750,000
Tuberculosis	7 million	400,000
Whooping cough	20 million	250,000
Amebiasis	1.5 million	30,000
Typhoid	500,000	25,000
Hookworm	1.5 million[3]	50,000
Ascariasis	1 million[3]	20,000
Filariasis	3 million[3]	. . .

[1]These are estimates based on available statistics, which are inexact.
[2]Most deaths from diarrhea occur in young children, in whom fluid and electrolyte loss has serious effects. The cause of diarrhea is frequently a self-limiting rotavirus infection.
[3]The prevalence of these infections is much higher: 1 billion people are believed to harbor *Ascaris* without symptoms; 900 million have hookworm, 800 million have malaria, 250 million have filariasis, and 200 million have schistosomiasis.

METHODS & PATHWAYS OF INFECTION

■ Humans encounter many microorganisms every day, but few enter the tissues, and most that do are destroyed by defense mechanisms. Organisms of low pathogenicity colonize the skin, upper respiratory tract, genitourinary tract, and gastrointestinal tract (resident, commensal) and may exclude more virulent forms by competition.

Portals of Entry of Infectious Agents
The various routes of entry of organisms into the body are all protected to a degree by defense mechanisms that are breached in some way when infection occurs. Once within the body, spread may occur directly or via blood or lymphatics.
   A. Skin:

■ The keratinized epithelium forms an effective physical barrier to infection.
■ Sweat and sebum provide additional chemical barriers.
■ Macerated, burned, or ischemic skin is not effective as a barrier and may be associated with an increased incidence of infection.

1. Direct contact: A few skin infections are acquired by direct physical contact, eg, herpes simplex, dermatophyte fungi (tinea or ringworm), and impetigo caused by *Staphylococcus aureus* or *Streptococcus pyogenes.*

2. Wound infections: Once the integrity of the skin is disrupted, infection is common through many organisms, including *Clostridium perfringens* (gas gangrene) and *Clostridium tetani* (tetanus).

3. Injection by vectors: Skin is penetrated by an arthropod vector carrying an infectious agent.

■ Examples include leishmaniasis, trypanosomiasis (sleeping sickness), and typhus.

■ The vector may act as a simple carrier or may be an integral part of the life cycle of the agent (Table 14–3).

■ Viruses transmitted by arthropod vectors are called **arboviruses** (arthropod-borne viruses).

4. Injection by humans:

■ Includes transfusion of infected blood and blood products, though screening of donors, blood, and blood products decreases the risk.

■ Contaminated needles used by drug abusers provide another method of infection.

■ Organisms include human immunodeficiency virus (HIV), hepatitis B virus, hepatitis non-A non-B virus, and *Treponema pallidum.*

5. Active larval penetration includes hookworm larvae, cercariae of *Schistosoma* species, larvae of *Strongyloides stercoralis.*

B. Respiratory tract:

■ Mucus moved upward by the beating action of the ciliary epithelium provides some protection.

■ Lysozyme (in nasal passages, derived from tears), and IgA (in the respiratory passages) provide additional defense.

■ Oropharyngeal lymphoid tissue (tonsils, Waldeyer's ring) provides a local immunologic barrier.

■ Inhalation of droplets carrying infectious agents is the usual mechanism of transmission:

  ● Viruses are common (influenza, measles, rubella, varicella-zoster, mumps).

  ● Bacteria are less so (streptococci, *Haemophilus influenzae,* diphtheria, mycobacteria).

■ Entry of organisms into the bronchi and lungs is facilitated by defective local defense mechanisms:

  ● Depression of the cough reflex by narcotic drugs, general anesthesia, coma, or alcohol intoxication.

  ● Interference with ciliary transport, as with alcoholism or cold.

  ● Loss of ciliated cells, as occurs in squamous metaplasia due to smoking.

  ● Bronchial obstruction.

C. The gastrointestinal tract:

■ Entry is often through infected food and drink; this would include fecal contamination (the fecal-oral route).

TABLE 14-3. ARTHROPOD VECTORS OF HUMAN INFECTIONS

Disease	Infectious Agent	Vector
Simple transmission by vector		
Plague	*Yersinia pestis*	Fleas (rarely ticks, lice)
Relapsing fever	*Borrelia recurrentis*	Lice, ticks
Lyme disease	*Borrelia burgdorferi*	Ixodid ticks
Typhus, spotted fever	*Rickettsia* species	Fleas, ticks, mites, lice
Epidemic encephalitides	Togaviruses, bunyaviruses	Mosquitoes, ticks
Yellow fever	Togavirus group B	Mosquitoes
Dengue fever	Togavirus group B	Mosquitoes
Hemorrhagic fevers	Bunyaviruses	Mosquitoes, ticks
Colorado tick fever	Reovirus (genus *Orbivirus*)	Ticks
Vector is intrinsic part of parasite life cycle		
Malaria	*Plasmodium* species	*Anopheles* mosquitoes
Leishmaniasis	*Leishmania* species	Sandflies (*Phlebotomus* in Old World; *Lutzomyia* and *Psychodopygus* in New World)
Sleeping sickness	*Trypanosoma* species	Tsetse flies (*Glossina*)
Chagas' disease	*Trypanosoma cruzi*	Reduviid bugs
Babesiosis	*Babesia microti*	Ticks
Filariasis	*Wuchereia, Brugia* species	Mosquitoes
Onchocerciasis	*Onchocerca volvulus*	*Simulium* flies
Loiasis	*Loa loa*	*Chrysops* flies

- It includes rotavirus gastroenteritis, amebiasis, giardiasis, salmonellosis (food poisoning, as well as typhoid), shigellosis, hepatitis A virus and poliovirus.
- Important defense mechanisms are:
  - The mucosal lining.
  - The acidity of the stomach.

- The continuous flow of the contents of the intestinal lumen. (Stagnation, as in diverticula and intestinal obstruction, leads to bacterial overgrowth.)
- The mucus, which contains IgA.
- The submucosal lymphoid tissue.
- Commensal intestinal flora (particularly in the colon). Broad-spectrum antibiotics that destroy the commensal flora may lead to infection of the gut by pathogens (eg, *Clostridium difficile* enterocolitis).

D. Genitourinary tract is normally sterile. Risk of infection is increased by

- Obstruction of urinary flow.
- Alteration in the normal vaginal flora following administration of broad-spectrum antibiotics.
- Instrumentation, or catheterization.
- Sexual activity. Note that ascending infection from the perineum is more common in the female, probably due to the shorter urethra.

Infection of the Bloodstream
The presence of microorganisms in the blood (bacteremia, viremia, parasitemia, fungemia) is always abnormal. Diagnosis is established by blood cultures, or blood smears for some parasites (eg, malaria).

A. Transient bacteremia:

- Is relatively common, found in persons with infected teeth and gums, etc.
- Is rapidly removed by defenses.
- Rarely produces disease, except:
  - In immunocompromised hosts.
  - In patients with chronic cardiac valve disease or cardiac prostheses (organisms are able to grow in damaged or prosthetic valves), in whom infective endocarditis may develop.

B. Severe bacteremia (septicemia):

- Denotes serious infection with large numbers of microorganisms actively multiplying in the bloodstream.
- Is associated with toxemia, high fever, chills, tachycardia, and hypotension (shock). Death may result.

TRANSMISSION OF INFECTION
Successful parasitism requires not only the abilities to infect and multiply in a host, but also transmission from one host to another.

- Prevention of transmission is a mechanism for disease control (eg, eradication of the mosquito vector for malaria).
- In some instances, transmission involves complex life cycles.

Transmission of Agents with Simple Life Cycles (Fig 14–1)
Transmission of most microorganisms (viruses, chlamydiae, rickettsiae, mycoplasmas, and bacteria) is either

- Direct—eg, by physical contact, inhalation, injection, or ingestion (Fig 14–1).

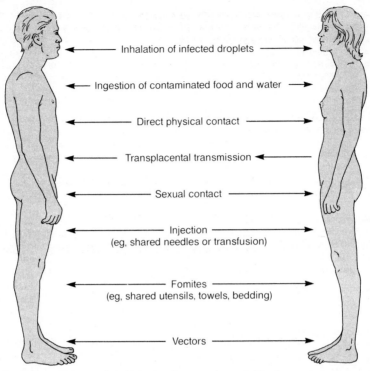

Figure 14–1. Simple cycles of infection (human to human). Simple organisms that require no developmental stage during transmission (eg, viruses, bacteria) are transmitted in this manner.

- Or, by simple passage in vectors (Table 14–3).
- **Spores, cysts** and **ova** are resistant to adverse conditions and thus facilitate transmission of certain organisms, including
  - Some bacteria (C tetani, B anthracis).
  - Many fungi.
  - Some protozoa (E histolytica, G lamblia).
  - Some metazoa (intestinal helminths, schistosomes).

- These structures may lie dormant in soil or water and become reactivated under favorable conditions.
- For viruses, transmission may be
  - **Horizontal,** denoting transmission from one host to another—directly or by vectors.
  - **Vertical,** in which viral nucleic acid is transmitted in genetic material from parent to offspring.

Transmission of Agents with Complex Life Cycles

Complex life cycles, frequently with a sexual as well as a nonsexual (or vegetative) cycle of multiplication, are found in

- Some protozoa.
- All metazoa (worms, etc.).

When the life cycle of an organism includes more than one host species:

- The **definitive host** is the one in which the sexual cycle takes place.
- The **intermediate host** contains the vegetative part of the cycle (eg, for schistosomiasis, man is the definitive host, a snail, the intermediate host).
- Humans may be infected with parasites whose natural (usual) host is an animal. For example:
  - Hydatid cyst (larval form of dog tapeworm, *Echinococcus granulosus*).
  - Cysticercosis (larval form of pork tapeworm, (*Taenia solium*) (Table 14–4).

Note: Individual life cycles are described in the Organ Systems section.

Reservoirs of Infection

Most human infectious diseases are caused by agents that selectively parasitize humans.

- Such infections must be acquired from a human source—either an infected individual or an asymptomatic carrier.
- A few diseases are acquired from animal reservoirs (Table 14–4).
- A history of exposure to the animal reservoir is helpful in diagnosis, eg,
  - Ingestion of infected meat (clonorchiasis, trichinosis).
  - Contact with infected carcass (anthrax).
  - Ingestion of animal urine or feces (leptospirosis, brucellosis).
  - Animal bite or scratch (cat-scratch disease, rabies).
  - Bite of arthropod vector that has bitten an infected animal (eg, plague, arbovirus encephalitis).

DIAGNOSIS OF INFECTIOUS DISEASE

The aim of diagnosis in infectious diseases is to recognize that a sick patient is ill with an infectious disease and to identify the specific agent responsible.

Clinical Examination

A few infectious agents produce highly characteristic clinical illnesses, eg, herpes zoster, malaria. In most infectious diseases, one of several agents may be responsible.

Microbiologic Examination

Demonstration of the agent through microscopic examination or culture of tissues and fluids is the most common means of arriving at an etiologic diagnosis of infectious disease.

- Most organisms can be identified by suitable culture:
  - Exceptions include *T. pallidum, Mycobacterium leprae*, most protozoa, and metazoa.
- Culture also permits assessment of sensitivity to drugs where appropriate.

TABLE 14–4. INFECTIONS HAVING ANIMAL RESERVOIRS

Disease	Infectious Agent	Animal Reservoir
Plague	*Yersinia pestis*	Wild rats, ground squirrels, chipmunks
Tularemia	*Francisella tularensis*	Rabbits, ground squirrels
Anthrax	*Bacillus anthracis*	Cattle, sheep
Glanders	*Pseudomonas mallei*	Horses, mules, donkeys
Leptospirosis	*Leptospira* species	Rats, dogs, pigs, cattle
Brucellosis	*Brucella* species	Cattle, goats, pigs
Cat-scratch disease	*Unknown bacteria*	Cats
Psittacosis	*Chlamydia psittaci*	Birds
Encephalitis	*Arboviruses*	Horses, wild primates
Rabies	*Rabies virus*	Dogs, cats, bats, foxes, skunks, raccoons
Cryptococcosis	*Cryptococcus neoformans*	Birds
Toxoplasmosis	*Toxoplasma gondii*	Cats
Larva migrans (visceral and cutaneous)	Animal helminths	Cats, dogs
Hydatid cyst (echino-coccosis)	*Echinococcus granulosus*	Cattle, sheep
Trichinosis	*Trichinella spiralis*	Carnivores (pigs, bears)
Beef or pork tapeworms	*Taenia* species	Pigs, cattle
Fish tapeworm	*Diphyllobothrium latum*	Fish
Schistosomiasis	*Schistosoma* species	Snails (particular species)
Clonorchiasis	*Clonorchis sinensis*	Fish

Immunologic Techniques

A fourfold increase in antibody titers is diagnostic in most instances. (This compares an early serum sample with a later one.) IgM rises first (in days) and falls first; IgG rises later, but remains elevated for years.

Histologic Examination

Certain fungi, protozoa, and metazoal parasites may be identified by the presence of ova, cysts, yeast, spherules, hyphae, and so forth. Some viruses produce characteristic inclusions (eg, cytomegalovirus, herpes simplex virus, and measles virus). See Chapter 13.

Section IV. Disorders of Development & Growth

Disorders of Development

15

ABNORMAL FETAL DEVELOPMENT

Definitions

- **Agenesis:** Complete absence of the organ due to failure of formation of primitive precursor cell mass (the *anlage*).
- **Dysgenesis:** Abnormal differentiation leads to a structurally abnormal organ (eg, in renal dysgenesis, epithelium-lined cysts and cartilage are found instead of a normal kidney).
- **Hypoplasia:** Structurally normal, but small, organ.
- **Aplasia:** Organ is completely absent; differs from agenesis in that the primitive anlage is formed, but fails to develop further.
- **Congenital:** Disorder present at birth, regardless of cause.
- **Mutation:** Denotes any stable heritable genetic change, whether or not associated with detectable structural abnormalities of the chromosomes.

Causes of Fetal Abnormalities

The known causes of fetal abnormalities fall into two major groups:

- Those affecting the genome (genetic).
- Those affecting the proliferating cells of the embryo or fetus.

Most causes of injury to a child or adult may also act on the fetus (Table 15–1).

- The most severe abnormality of embryo or fetus is death.
  - This is termed *abortion* in the first 14 weeks.
  - It is called *intrauterine death* thereafter.

FETAL ABNORMALITIES CAUSED BY GENETIC DISORDER

Chromosomal Aberrations
A. Normal chromosomal complement:

- The normal human cell has 46 chromosomes: 22 pairs of **autosomes** and 2 **sex chromosomes.**

TABLE 15–1. FACTORS CAUSING FETAL (CONGENITAL) ABNORMALITIES OR INJURY

Genetic disorders
  Chromosomal aberrations[1]
  Single gene abnormalities
  Polygenic abnormalities
External agents (teratogens)
  Ionizing radiation
  Infection (eg, rubella, cytomegalovirus, toxoplasmosis, syphilis)[1]
  Drugs and poisons
  Alcohol and smoking
  Mechanical trauma
Abnormalities of placentation (Chapter 55)
  Vascular insufficiency[1]
  Placental separation[1]
Maternal-fetal transfer of IgG antibodies
  Hemolytic disease of the newborn (Chapter 25)[1]
  Neonatal myasthenia gravis (Chapter 66)
  Neonatal thyrotoxicosis (Chapter 58)
Other associated factors
  Nutritional deficiency
  Diabetes mellitus[1]
  Socioeconomic status
  Maternal and paternal age
  Premature delivery[1]

---

[1]Common causes of fetal death. Spontaneous abortion occurs in 20–25% of all conceptions; lethal congenital abnormalities occur in 1–2% of all births; and nonlethal abnormalities (which may become manifest in later life) occur in 2% of all live births.

- One of each pair of chromosomes is derived from each parent.
- The **karyotype** describes the chromosomes of an individual.
  - A normal male is 46, XY.
  - A normal female, 46, XX.
- When two X chromosomes are present in a cell, as in a normal female, one of them becomes inactivated and condensed on the nuclear membrane (Barr body).
- Absence of Barr bodies indicates that the cell has only one X chromosome (normal male, XY; Turner's syndrome, XO).

B. Mechanisms of chromosomal aberrations.
1. Nondisjunction in meiosis:

- Leads to the production of gametes (ova and spermatozoa) that contain both (gamete has 24 chromosomes) or neither (gamete has 22 chromosomes) member of the chromosome pair.
- Union of such a gamete with a normal gamete leads to a zygote that has either three of the involved chromosomes (**trisomy**) or only one (**monosomy**).
  - Trisomy and monosomy involving the sex chromosomes are generally compatible with life.
  - Autosomal trisomy and monosomy are usually incompatible with life, or produce severe abnormalities.

2. Nondisjunction in mitosis:

■ Nondisjunction in the early zygote produces **mosaicism,** the presence in an individual of two or more genetically different cell populations.
  ● This most often affects sex chromosomes.
  ● Mosaic individuals manifest phenotypic abnormalities that are less severe than when every cell is affected.

3. Deletion is loss of part of a chromosome due to breakage. It is usually lethal in the embryo.

4. Translocation is the transfer of broken segments between chromosomes.

■ In **balanced translocations,** all genetic material is present and functional, and the individual may be phenotypically normal, although gametes and offspring may be abnormal (as in one form of Down's syndrome—see following).

5. Other chromosomal rearrangements: Inversion and ring chromosome formation may occur after breakage or abnormal division, producing various effects.

C. Causes of chromosomal aberrations: Most occur at random without known cause. Contributing factors include the following.

1. Increasing maternal age: For example, in **trisomy 21** (Down's syndrome), the risk is 1:2000 live births in women under 30 years, and 1:50 for women over 45 years.

2. Ionizing radiation: Since there is no "safe" low dose, diagnostic abdominal X-rays should be avoided if possible in pregnant women.

3. Drugs: Especially when used in early pregnancy; chromosomal abnormalities can result from use of anticancer agents, thalidomide, and other drugs.

D. Common Autosomal Abnormalities.

1. Down's syndrome (trisomy 21): This is the most common autosomal disorder.

■ The affected infant has upward-slanting eyes, and prominent epicanthal folds (a purported resemblance to Asian facial features, hence the older term *mongolism*).
■ Mental retardation is a constant feature.
■ Congenital heart anomalies are present in 30%; ventricular septal defect is most common.
■ There is an increased susceptibility to acute leukemia.
■ Three types of Down's syndrome are recognized.

a. Nondisjunction Down's syndrome:

■ Most cases (95%) are due to this mechanism.
■ It is associated with increasing maternal age.
■ The child has an extra 21 chromosome (47,XX,+21 or 47,XY,+21).
■ The parents have normal karyotypes.

b. Translocation Down's syndrome:

■ In 5% of cases it is due to inheritance of a balanced translocation from one of the parents—commonly a 14, 21 and more rarely a 21, 22 translocation.
■ One parent carries the abnormal chromosome.
■ The affected infant has 46 chromosomes, one of which has the extra 21 linked to it.
■ This is not associated with increased maternal age.
■ The carrier parent is at risk of producing further affected offspring.

c. Mosaic Down's syndrome is very rare.
2. Edwards' syndrome (trisomy 18) is rare.

- It is usually lethal before 1 year of age.
- It entails severe mental retardation, and is characterized by "rocker bottom" feet, overlapping fingers, etc.

3. Patau's syndrome (trisomy 13) is rare.

- Most affected infants die soon after birth.
- Abnormal development of the forebrain and facial structures, with single central eye (cyclops).

4. Cri du chat (cat cry) syndrome:

- Occurs through deletion of the short arm of chromosome 5.
- Is characterized by a mewing, catlike cry; entails severe mental retardation.

5. Acquired chromosomal abnormalities after birth manifest as somatic mutations in children and adults and are associated with a variety of neoplasms (Chapter 18). The germ cells are usually not involved, and these anomalies are therefore not heritable.

E. Common sex chromosomal abnormalities.

1. Klinefelter's syndrome (testicular dysgenesis):

- Is common, occurring at a rate of 1:600 live male births.
- Is usually caused by nondisjunction of the X chromosome in the mother, resulting in an extra X chromosome (47, XXY).
- The phenotype is male, but at puberty the testes remain small and secondary sex characteristics fail to develop.
- Patient may be tall, due to delayed closure of epiphyses.
- Seminiferous tubules contain mainly Sertoli cells and undergo progressive atrophy.
- Patients are usually infertile.
- The diagnosis may be made by finding Barr bodies in a buccal scraping or by performing karyotypic analysis.

2. Turner's syndrome (ovarian dysgenesis):

- This occurs at a rate of 1:2500 live female births.
- It is caused by either
  - Nondisjunction of the X chromosome in one parent, leading to absence of one X chromosome in all cells of the affected individual (45, XO).
  - Or, mosaicism (some cells 45, XO; others 46, XX) due to nondisjunction in a postzygotic mitotic division.
- Patients show webbing of the neck, congenital cardiac anomalies (most commonly coarctation of the aorta), short stature, obesity, and skeletal abnormalities.
- Phenotypically they are female, but ovaries are rudimentary ("streak ovaries"), and there is amenorrhea, with poor development of female secondary sex characteristics.
- The diagnosis may be made by the absence of Barr bodies in the buccal smear and karyotypic analysis.

3. XXX syndrome ("superfemale"): Most such patients appear normal; some show mental retardation, some have menstrual problems.

4. XYY syndrome:

- Most patients appear as normal males.
- Reports of antisocial behavior in this patient group await confirmation.

Single-Gene (Mendelian) Disorders

A. Dominant and recessive genes: Single-gene disorders are inherited in a manner predicted by mendelian laws, depending on whether

- The abnormal gene is on a sex chromosome or an autosome.
- It is dominant or recessive.
- The gene has two alleles (alternative forms of the gene) **A and a.** Three genotypes (AA, Aa, and aa) are possible.

Note that

- In **homozygous** genotypes (AA and aa) the two alleles are identical.
- In **heterozygous** genotypes (Aa), the alleles are different.
- Inheritance is **dominant** if only one abnormal allele is required for phenotypic expression of the disease (genotypes **Aa, AA**): ie, if the allele **A** is abnormal, both **AA and Aa** individuals show the disease, and **aa** is normal.
- A **recessive** trait, on the other hand, requires the presence of *two* abnormal alleles for expression of disease (genotype **aa**): ie, if the allele **a** is abnormal only **aa** individuals show the disease; **Aa** individuals are heterozygous carriers of the trait (they do not express the disease); and **AA** is normal.

B. Autosomal dominant diseases: (Table 15–2.)

- There is characteristically a family history (Table 15–3).
- Transmission of the abnormal gene to the next generation only occurs following reproduction by affected individuals.
- Variation occurs in
  - The frequency with which the abnormal gene produces disease (penetrance).
  - The degree of abnormality seen in different individuals (expressivity).

TABLE 15–2. COMMON AUTOSOMAL DISORDERS[1]

Autosomal Dominant	Autosomal Recessive
Achondroplasia (dwarfism)	Cystic fibrosis (mucoviscidosis)
Marfan's syndrome	Alpha$_1$-antitrypsin deficiency
Neurofibromatosis	Phenylketonuria
Von Willebrand's disease	Wilson's disease
Hereditary hemorrhagic telangiectasia	Tay-Sachs disease
Osteogenesis imperfecta	Sickle cell anemia
Acute intermittent porphyria	Glycogen storage diseases
Huntington's chorea	Galactosemia
Hereditary spherocytosis	
Adult renal polycystic disease	
Hereditary angioedema	
Familial hypercholesterolemia	

[1] Approximately 750 autosomal dominant disorders have been described.

TABLE 15–3. FEATURES OF AUTOSOMAL DOMINANT AND RECESSIVE INHERITED DISEASES

Autosomal Dominant	Autosomal Recessive
1. A = abnormal dominant gene.	1. a = Abnormal recessive gene.
2. Patient with disease is Aa heterozygote; AA homozygote is usually not compatible with life.	2. Patient with disease is aa homozygote. AA is normal; Aa is symptomless carrier.
3. Males and females are equally affected.	3. Males and females are equally affected.
4. At least one parent (Aa) shows overt disease.	4. Both parents are symptomless carriers (Aa); neither parent shows overt disease.
5. Overt disease is present in every generation.	5. Disease skips generations.
6. Higher incidence of overt disease among siblings; 50% chance of disease in children when one parent is affected.	6. Lower incidence of overt disease among siblings; 25% chance of disease in children of 2 symptomless carriers.
7. Cannot be transmitted by an individual without disease.	7. Can be transmitted by an individual without disease (carrier); offspring of a parent with overt disease (aa) and of a normal individual will all be carriers.
8. No association with consanguineous marriages.	8. Associated with consanguineous marriages.

C. **Autosomal recessive diseases: (Table 15–2.)**

■ Family history is characteristic (Table 15–3).
■ In many instances the result is deficiency of a single enzyme, ie, **inborn errors of metabolism** (see following).
■ Overall, autosomal recessive traits are rare, except in societies that discourage mating outside the group (eg, Tay-Sachs disease is virtually restricted to Ashkenazic Jews).

D. **Sex chromosome–linked Diseases (Table 15–4)** are characterized by an unequal incidence of the disease in males and females.

■ **X-linked recessive diseases:**
  ● Are common.
  ● Are expressed in the male (only one X chromosome).
  ● Are transmitted by asymptomatic female heterozygous carriers.
  ● Half of the male offspring of a mating between a carrier female and a normal male will manifest the disease.
  ● If an affected male mates with a normal female, all of the daughters will be carriers and the sons will be unaffected.
■ **X-linked dominant diseases:**
  ● Are uncommon.
  ● Are more common in females (two X chromosomes).

TABLE 15–4. COMMON SEX-LINKED DISORDERS

X-linked recessive
Hemophilia A
Christmas disease (hemophilia B)
Bruton's agammaglobulinemia
G6PD deficiency
Testicular feminization
Duchenne muscular dystrophy
Chronic granulomatous disease
Red-green color blindness[1]
X-linked dominant
Hypophosphatemic (vitamin D-resistant) rickets
Y-linked
None known

---

[1] Total color blindness is autosomal recessive and very rare.

E. Inborn errors of metabolism:

■ Inherited single-gene abnormalities:
  ● Cause failure of synthesis of an enzyme.
  ● Cause a subsequent block in a metabolic pathway.
  ● May involve amino acid, lipid, carbohydrate, or mucopolysaccharide metabolism.
■ These diseases are all rare.
  ● Most are autosomal-recessive.
  ● A few occur as X-linked recessive.

　　1. Abnormal amino-acid metabolism (Table 15–5) is characterised by accumulation of abnormal amounts of an amino acid, the detection of which is of diagnostic value (eg, phenylketonuria—excess phenylalanine in serum and urine).
　　2. Abnormal lipid metabolism (lipid storage diseases) (Table 15–6):

■ Is characterised by accumulation of abnormal amounts of complex lipids in cells, especially in lysosomes, hence the term **lysosomal storage diseases.**
■ Are all autosomal-recessive, excepting Fabry's disease.
■ Storage of lipid occurs in different cells in the various diseases, accounting for the differing signs and symptoms.
■ Is **diagnosed** by
  ● Clinical features:
    ○ Tay-Sachs disease—cherry red macula.
    ○ Gaucher's disease—hepatosplenomegaly.
  ● Light microscopic examination:
    ○ Distribution of abnormal, lipid-distended cells.
    ○ Foamy cytoplasm in Tay-Sachs and Niemann-Pick disease.
    ○ Fibrillary or crinkled cytoplasm in Gaucher's cells.
  ● Electron microscopic inclusions:
    ○ Whorled distended lysosomes in Tay-Sachs disease.
    ○ Parallel lamellas (zebra bodies) in Niemann-Pick disease.
    ○ Linear stacks in Gaucher's disease.
  ● Demonstration of the enzyme deficiency in cultured skin fibroblasts.

TABLE 15-5. EXAMPLES OF INHERITED ENZYME DEFICIENCY CAUSING ABNORMAL AMINO ACID METABOLISM

Disease	Amino Acids Affected	Enzyme Deficiency	Inheritance Pattern	Clinical Features
Phenylketonuria	Phenylalanine	Phenylalanine hydroxylase	AR[1]	Mental retardation; musty or mousy odor; eczema; increased plasma phenylalanine levels.
Hereditary tyrosinemia	Tyrosine	Hydroxyphenylpyruvic acid oxidase	AR	Hepatic cirrhosis, renal tubular dysfunction; elevated plasma tyrosine levels.
Histidinemia	Histidine	Histidase	AR	Mental retardation; speech defect.
Maple syrup urine disease (branched-chain ketoaciduria; ketoaminoacidemia)	Leucine, valine, isoleucine	Branched-chain ketoacid oxidase	AR	Postnatal collapse; mental retardation; characteristic "maple syrup" odor in urine.
Homocystinuria	Methionine, homocystine	Cystathionine synthase	AR	Mental retardation; thromboembolic phenomena; ectopia lentis.

[1] AR = autosomal recessive.

TABLE 15–6. INBORN ERRORS OF LIPID METABOLISM: LYSOSOMAL (OR LIPID) STORAGE DISEASES

Disease	Enzyme Defect	Accumulated Lipid	Tissues Involved
Tay-Sachs disease	Hexosaminidase A	G_{M2} ganglioside	Brain, retina
Gaucher's disease	β-Glucosidase (glucocerebrosidase)	Glucocerebroside	Liver, spleen, bone marrow, brain
Neimann-Pick disease	Sphingomyelinase	Sphingomyelin	Brain, liver, spleen
Metachromatic leukodystrophy	Arylsulfatase A	Sulfatide	Brain, kidney, liver, peripheral nerves
Fabry's disease	α-Galactosidase	Ceramide trihexoside	Skin, kidney
Krabbe's disease	Galactosylceramidase	Galactocerebroside	Brain

3. Abnormal glycogen metabolism (glycogen storage disease) (Table 15–7):

- Is caused by deficiency of an enzyme involved in the metabolism of glycogen.
- In most cases is autosomal-recessive, with onset in infancy.

a. Accumulation of glycogen occurs when glycogen accumulates as granules in the cytoplasm; cells appear pale and distended.

b. Dysfunction of involved cells:

- Hepatic involvement causes hepatomegaly and liver failure.
- Myocardial involvement causes heart failure.

TABLE 15–7. GLYCOGEN STORAGE DISEASES

Type	Enzyme Defect	Severity of Disease	Involved Tissues
I (von Gierke's disease)	Glucose-6-phosphatase	Severe	Liver, kidney, gut
II (Pompe's disease)	α-1,4 Glucosidase	Lethal	Systemic distribution but heart most affected
III (Cori's disease)	Amylo-1,6 Glucosidase (debranching enzyme)	Mild	Systemic distribution; liver commonly affected
IV (Andersen's disease)	Amylo-1,4–1,6-transglucosidase (branching enzyme)	Lethal	Systemic distribution but liver most affected
V (McArdle's disease)	Muscle phosphorylase	Mild	Skeletal muscle
VI (Hers' disease)	Liver phosphorylase	Mild	Liver
VII–XII	Extremely rare diseases	Variable	Variable

TABLE 15-8. MUCOPOLYSACCHARIDOSES (MPS SYNDROMES)

Type	Enzyme Defect	Accumulated Mucopolysaccharide	Tissues Involved	Mode of Inheritance[1]	Severity
I (Hurler's syndrome)	α-L-Iduronidase	Heparan sulfate, dermatan sulfate	Skin, cornea, bone, heart, brain, liver, spleen	AR	Severe
II (Hunter's syndrome)	L-Iduronosulfate sulfatase	Heparan sulfate, dermatan sulfate	Skin, bone, heart, ear, retina	XR	Moderate
III (Sanfilippo's syndrome)	Many types	Heparan sulfate	Brain, skin	AR	Moderate
IV (Morquio's syndrome)	N-Acetylgalactosamine 6-sulfatase	Keratan sulfate, chondroitin sulfate	Skin, bone, heart, eye	AR	Mild
V–VII	Rare diseases characterized by many types of enzyme defects	Variable	Variable	AR	Mild

[1]AR = autosomal recessive; XR = X-linked recessive.

c. Abnormal glucose delivery: With severe liver involvement (eg, type I), **hypoglycemia** occurs.

4. Abnormal mucopolysaccharide metabolism (mucopolysaccharidoses) (Table 15–8):

- Occurs in rare inherited lysosomal storage diseases.
- Mucopolysaccharides (glycosaminoglycans) accumulate in a variety of cells.
- This leads to hepatosplenomegaly and deformities in skin and bones (*gargoylism* is the outmoded name for Hurler's syndrome).
- Affected cells are distended (balloon cells).
- Peripheral blood cells may contain large purple cytoplasmic granules (Alder-Reilly bodies).
- Dysfunction of affected parenchymal cells causes mental retardation, heart failure, etc.

F. Detection of heterozygous carrier state in recessive traits:

- Heterozygous carriers of a recessive trait do not show overt disease, but may display biochemical changes that provide a means of detecting the carrier state:
- For example, in **hemophilia A,** female carriers do not bleed abnormally, but do show some reduction in levels of factor VIII (see Chapter 27).

Polygenic (Multifactorial) Inheritance
Multifactorial inheritance is believed important in diseases such as high blood pressure and diabetes mellitus, but it is not predictable on the basis of genetic laws.

FETAL ABNORMALITIES CAUSED BY EXTERNAL AGENTS (TERATOGENS)
Congenital anomalies affect about 2% of newborns. Some are due to genetic disorders (see preceding). Some are due to teratogenic (defect-causing) agents (see following). The cause of most is unknown.

Ionizing Radiation
Ionizing radiation effects DNA and the genetic apparatus of the cell. It is also directly cytotoxic to the developing embryo. There is no "safe" low dose, therefore it should be avoided during pregnancy if possible.

Teratogenic Viral Infections
Teratogenic viral infections include **rubella** in the first trimester of pregnancy, which produces congenital heart disease, deafness, and cataracts. Influenza, mumps, and varicella have also been implicated, but the evidence is not conclusive.

Drugs
A. Thalidomide causes a distinctive fetal anomaly—phocomelia, or malformed limbs—when used in pregnancy.

B. Diethylstilbestrol (DES) was used in the past to treat threatened abortion, but is now known to be followed by a high incidence of clear-cell adenocarcinoma of the vagina in female offspring, often at an early age.

Alcohol (Fetal Alcohol Syndrome)
The severity of fetal alcohol syndrome correlates with the amount of alcohol consumed by the mother.

- The syndrome occurs in 1:1000 live births in the USA and in 30–50% of infants born to women who consume over 125 g of alcohol (about 450 mL of whisky) per day.
- It is characterized by growth retardation, abnormal facies, cardiac defects, vertebral anomalies (including spina bifida), and metal retardation.

Cigarette Smoking
Cigarette smoking has been demonstrated to lead to fetal growth retardation.

POSTNATAL DEVELOPMENT

NORMAL POSTNATAL DEVELOPMENT
Most tissues are fully developed and functional at birth.

- Liver and kidney are less well-developed and many newborn infants develop transient jaundice due to immaturity of liver enzyme systems.
- The lungs mature late in fetal life and are immature in premature infants.
  - Lung maturity may be assessed by estimating the lecithin, sphingomyelin, and phosphatidylglycerol levels in amniotic fluid.
- The brain undergoes considerable development after delivery, including extensive myelination in the central nervous system.
- Lymphoid tissues show maximum growth during childhood, after which involution occurs.
- Genital tissues show final development at puberty.

DISEASES OF INFANCY & CHILDHOOD
The risk of death is greatest during the neonatal period, with a mortality rate of 6.4:1000 live births in the United States.

- Most neonatal deaths result from complications of pregnancy and labor (Table 15–9).
- The infant mortality rate is regarded as a sensitive indicator of the quality of health care, and is much higher in developing countries.
- The risk of death falls dramatically after the first year of life. From 1 to 4 years it is about 0.6:1000 population, and from 5 to 14 years it is about 0.3:1000 (US figures).

Disorders Associated with Low Birth Weight
Normal infants at term weigh 2700–3900 g. A premature infant is defined as one with a birth weight of less than 2500 g, regardless of gestational age.

- Birth weights low for gestational age may result from congenital anomalies, fetal infections, placental insufficiency, maternal hypertension, or heavy substance abuse.
- The mortality rate for infants under 1000 g is 90%.
- The survival rate improves rapidly when infants achieve a weight of 1500 g.

A. Respiratory distress syndrome (RDS):

- Causes 7000 infant deaths a year in the USA.
- Affects infants under 34 weeks of gestational age.
- Results when type II pneumocytes in immature lungs fail to secrete adequate surfactant. This manifests in alveolar collapse in the first hour after delivery.

TABLE 15–9. LEADING CAUSES OF DEATH DURING CHILDHOOD; USA, 1980

Neonatal period; 6.4 deaths per 1000 live births.
  Complications of prematurity
    Respiratory distress syndrome
    Intracranial hemorrhage
    Necrotizing enterocolitis
  Birth trauma
  Birth asphyxia
  Neonatal infections
  Hemolytic disease of the newborn
  Congenital anomalies
First year
  Congenital anomalies
  Sudden infant death syndrome
  Infectious diseases
  Accidents
  Neurologic diseases
  Malignant neoplasms
Age 1–4 years
  Accidents
  Congenital anomalies
  Malignant neoplasms (including leukemia)
  Infectious diseases
Age 5–14 years
  Accidents
  Malignant neoplasms (including leukemia)

- Is associated with progressive respiratory distress, hypoxemia, and cyanosis.
- Microscopically, lungs show loss of alveolar epithelium and exudation of protein-rich fluid into alveoli (so-called hyaline membrane disease—see Chapter 34).
- Mortality rate remains around 30%.

B. Intraventricular hemorrhage:

- Occurs in preterm infants.
- Begins in the periventricular region of the cerebral hemispheres and extends into the ventricles.
- The cause is unknown.
- Mortality rate is about 75%.

C. Necrotizing enterocolitis:

- This is a dangerous condition seen in neonatal intensive care units.
- Hypoxia and bacterial infection—notably *Escherichia coli*—probably contribute to the cause.

D. Perinatal Infections:

- Are caused by
  - Transplacental infection in late pregnancy.
  - Infection of the fetus by contagion during delivery.

- Are called *TORCHS*, an acronym for *t*oxoplasmosis, *o*ther (viruses), *r*ubella, *c*ytomegalovirus, *h*erpes simplex, and *s*yphilis.

A. Toxoplasma gondii and cytomegalovirus infections:

- These are third-trimester fetal infections.
- They involve chiefly the brain and eyes.
- Survivors may show dystrophic calcification, microcephaly, mental retardation, and chorioretinitis.

B. Treponema pallidum infection (congenital syphilis):

- Due to transplacental infection of the fetus born to a mother with early active syphilis.
- When infection is severe, intrauterine death occurs.
- Congenital syphilis is a less severe form; it may manifest as fever, skin rashes, mucosal lesions, osteochondritis, lymph-node enlargement, abnormally formed teeth (Hutchinson's teeth, Moon's teeth), bone defects, nerve deafness, or blindness due to interstitial keratitis.

C. Rubella virus infection:

- Infection in the first trimester produces growth abnormalities as described earlier.
- Infection in late pregnancy may lead to fever, petechial skin rash, and liver enlargement.

D. Infections acquired in the birth canal:

- Herpes simplex is the most important.
- The infected newborn infant may develop viremia or encephalitis.
- Mortality is high; survivors may show neurologic deficits.
- Active genital herpes infection of the mother is an absolute indication for cesarean section.
- Other infections acquired during passage through an infected birth canal include gonorrhea and lymphogranuloma venereum, both of which cause conjunctivitis.

Sudden Infant Death Syndrome (SIDS; "Crib Death")

- This is common; there are about 10,000 deaths a year in the USA.
- It occurs predominantly during sleep in the age group from 2 to 4 months.
- There are many theories, but the cause is unknown.

Congenital Anomalies, Inborn Errors of Metabolism, & Hemolytic Disease of the Newborn
Congenital anomalies and inborn errors of metabolism have been considered earlier in this chapter. For hemolytic disease of the newborn, see Chapter 25.

Malignant Neoplasms
Malignant neoplasms are less common overall in children than in adults, but account for over 10% of deaths in the age group from 5 to 14 years. The major types are: acute lymphoblastic leukemia, lymphomas, neuroblastoma, nephroblastoma, retinoblastoma and central nervous system tumors (Chapter 17).

SEXUAL DEVELOPMENT

ABNORMAL SEXUAL DEVELOPMENT
Abnormal sexual development leads to:

- Ambiguous genitalia ("intersex") in infants.
- Abnormalities of secondary sex characteristics.
- Infertility (Table 15–10).

True Hermaphroditism
True hermaphroditism is a condition in which both testicular and ovarian tissue develop in the same individual (Table 15–10). It is rare.

Pseudohermaphroditism
Pseudohermaphroditism is relatively common.

- The gonads correspond to the genetic sex, but the external genitalia differ to varying degrees.
- Classification as a male or female is based on genetic sex (Table 15–10).
- Ambiguous genitalia also occur in females with adrenogenital syndromes (see Chapter 60).

Testicular Feminization Syndrome
This syndrome manifests as a genetic male (46, XY) but phenotypic female.

- It is inherited (X-linked recessive).
- The absence of receptors for androgens (end-organ insensitivity) results in female form.
- Patients appear to be normal young females, but have primary amenorrhea.
- Testes are present, but undescended, and should be removed because of increased incidence of testicular neoplasms.

AGING

THEORIES OF AGING

Programmed Aging Theory
Programmed aging theory postulates that the genome of every cell is programmed at conception to cease mitotic division after a certain time.

- Errors in transcription of nucleic acids lead to cell death.
- Some rare diseases, such as **progeria,** seems to support the theory of programmed aging.:
  - Progeria appears to accelerate the aging process.
  - In infantile progeria, a young child resembles a wizened old person, with loss of hair, fusion of epiphyses, atherosclerosis, and arterial calcification.

DNA Damage Theory
DNA damage theory postulates that aging is the result of DNA damage, due either to somatic mutations or to failure of DNA repair mechanisms in aging cells.

TABLE 15–10. ABNORMALITIES OF SEXUAL DEVELOPMENT

Syndrome	Karyotype	Barr Bodies	Gonads	External Genitalia
True hermaphroditism	Variable; 46XX, 46XY, mosaicism	+ or −	Both ovarian and testicular tissue are present.	Variable; male or female or both.
Sex chromosome defects Klinefelter's syndrome	47, XXY	+	Dysgenetic testes	Male (eunuchoid; poorly developed secondary sex characteristics; infertile).
Turner's syndrome	45, XO	−	Dysgenetic (streak) ovaries	Female (poorly developed secondary sex characteristics; infertile; amenorrhea).
Male pseudohermaphroditism Testicular feminization	46, XY	−	Testes (immature)	Female; end-organ failure to androgen action; no uterus (infertile, amenorrhea); secondary sex characteristics well developed and female because of presence of adrenal estrogens.
Failure of development of external genitalia	46, XY	−	Testes	Male; ambiguity caused by undescended testes, bifid scrotum, hypospadias poor penile development.
Bilateral cryptorchidism	46, XY	−	Testes	Failure of testicular development; infertility.

(*continued*)

TABLE 15–10. (*Continued*)

Syndrome	Karyotype	Barr Bodies	Gonads	External Genitalia
Female pseudo-hermaphroditism Primary (idiopathic)	46, XX	+	Ovaries	Male (unknown cause).
Androgens in utero	46, XX	+	Ovaries	Female; variable masculinization at birth.
Adrenogenital syndromes	46, XX	+	Ovaries	Female: masculinization at birth due to excess adrenal androgenic hormones.

Neuroendocrine Theory
Neuroendocrine theory postulates that the aging process is programmed into brain cells (eg, the hypothalamus), much as puberty and menopause are "programmed."

Immune Theory
Immune theory postulates that a decline in immunologic reactivity predisposes the individual to development of infections, autoimmune diseases, and neoplasia. This does not explain other features of aging.

Free Radical Theory
Free radical theory postulates that oxygen-based free radicals produce increasing injury with age; lipofuscin is one visible manifestation of such damage.

Cumulative Injury Theory
Cumulative injury theory postulates that aging merely represents the aggregate effect of pathologic insults sustained over the years.

CHANGES ASSOCIATED WITH AGING
A. Cellular changes
1. Cell loss:

- With age there is atrophy of organs, most evident in the brain and heart, in which replacement of lost cells does not occur.
- Cell loss in the brain is selective, with the greatest loss occurring in the basal ganglia, substantia nigra, and hippocampus.

2. Organelle changes:

- There is disorganization of endoplasmic reticulum, ribosomes mitochondria.

■ **Lipofuscin** (Chapter 1)—a brown pigment believed to be derived from degraded organelle membranes—accumulates in heart, brain, and liver.

    3. **DNA abnormalities** are more common in aged cells as a result of a progressive failure of DNA repair mechanisms.

    B. Connective tissue changes include:

■ Deposition of calcium and amyloid.
■ Fragmentation of elastic fibers, accelerated by sunlight.
■ Changes in the ground substance.
■ Erosion and fibrillary breakdown of cartilage and bone (osteoarthrosis) (Chapter 68).
■ Diffuse loss of bone (osteoporosis).

    C. Hair changes: Hair becomes thin and sparse and loses its pigment.
    D. Reproductive system changes such as menopause.

Changes in Host Defense Mechanisms

The thymus begins to atrophy even in childhood. Immunodeficiency and autoimmune connective tissue diseases increase in the elderly.

DISEASES ASSOCIATED WITH AGING

Older individuals are susceptible to many diseases, particularly atherosclerosis and its complications (Chapter 20), cancer (Chapters 17, 18 and 19), and degenerative diseases of the central nervous system and connective tissue (Chapters 64 and 68).

Disorders of Cellular Growth, Differentiation, & Maturation

16

ABNORMAL GROWTH: ATROPHY, HYPERTROPHY, & HYPERPLASIA

Definitions

- **Atrophy** is a decrease in the size of a tissue or organ, resulting from a decrease in the
  - Size of individual cells.
  - Number of cells composing the tissue.
- **Hypertrophy** is an increase in the size of a tissue due to increased size of individual cells, eg, increased thickness of the left ventricle resulting from increased size of the constituent myocardial fibers in patients with high blood pressure.
- **Hyperplasia** is an increase in the size of a tissue due to increased numbers of component cells, eg, increased breast size during pregnancy resulting from increase in the total number of epithelial cells and lobules.

Causes of Atrophy

A. Atrophy of disuse occurs, for example, in immobilized skeletal muscle and bone when a fractured limb is put in a cast.

- Initially there is a rapid decrease in cell size (reversible) but, if disuse is prolonged, muscle fibers also decrease in number (nonreversible).
- Immobilized bone shows decrease in size of the trabeculae, leading to osteoporosis.

B. Denervation atrophy: Damage to the lower motor neuron leads to rapid atrophy of muscle fibers supplied by that nerve.

C. Atrophy due to loss of trophic hormones:

- Endometrium, breast, and many endocrine glands are dependent on trophic hormones.
- Withdrawal of these hormones leads to atrophy of the target cells; eg, atrophy of ovaries at the menopause.

D. Atrophy due to lack of nutrients:

- Malnutrition (marasmus) results in generalized atrophy of body tissues such as skeletal muscle.
- Ischemia produces atrophy of the affected tissue due to progressive cell loss.

TABLE 16–1. HYPERTROPHY AND HYPERPLASIA OF ORGANS

Tissue	Cause of Increased Demand
Skeletal muscle hypertrophy	Physical activity, weight lifting
Cardiac muscle hypertrophy	Increased pressure load (high blood pressure, valve stenosis) or increased volume load (valve incompetence causing regurgitation of blood)
Smooth muscle (wall of intestine, urinary bladder) hypertrophy	Obstructive lesions
Bone marrow hyperplasia Erythroid hyperplasia	Increased destruction of erythrocytes (hemolytic process); prolonged hypoxia (living at high altitudes).
Megakaryocytic hyperplasia	Increased destruction of platelets in the periphery
Myeloid hyperplasia	Increased demand for neutrophils (as in inflammation)
Lymph node hyperplasia	Antigenic stimulation (proliferative immune response)
Uterine myometrial hypertrophy	Pregnancy (hormone-induced)
Breast hyperplasia	Pregnancy and lactation (hormone-induced)
Renal hypertrophy	Unilateral disease of one kidney; removal of one kidney

E. Senile atrophy is most apparent in tissues populated by permanent cells, eg, the brain and heart; is frequently compounded by ischemia.

F. Pressure atrophy is caused by prolonged compression of tissue, probably due to ischemia.

Causes of Hypertrophy & Hyperplasia

A. Physiologic hypertrophy and hyperplasia are adaptations to increased demand (Table 16–1). If the demand is removed, the tissues revert toward normal.

B. Pathologic hypertrophy and hyperplasia occur in the absence of an appropriate stimulus of increased functional demand. Examples include:

- **Myocardial hypertrophy,** which is without recognizable cause (eg, in the absence of hypertension or valvular or congenital heart disease). (See Cardiomyopathy, Chapter 23.)
- **Endometrial hyperplasia,** particularly when estrogens are not opposed by progesterone secretion, as at menopause (see Chapter 53).
- **Bilateral adrenal hyperplasia,** following excessive production of ACTH (see Chapter 60).
- **Thyroid hyperplasia (goiter),** which results from increased TSH stimulation of the thyroid.
- **Hyperplasia of the prostate,** believed to be due to hormonal imbalances in elderly males (see Chapter 51).

ABNORMAL GROWTH PRINCIPALLY INVOLVING DIFFERENTIATION: METAPLASIA

Metaplasia is an abnormality of cellular differentiation in which one type of mature cell is replaced by a different type of adult cell.

- The "new" metaplastic tissue appears structurally normal.
- The process is reversible.
- Metaplasia most commonly involves epithelium.
- **Squamous metaplasia** is the most common type, especially affecting endocervix and bronchial mucosa, as a result of chronic irritation.
- **Glandular metaplasia** occurs in the esophagus, usually as a result of acid reflux (Chapter 37), and in stomach and intestine.
- Metaplasia rarely occurs in mesenchymal tissue.
- Most metaplasia is of little clinical significance, although loss of cilia and of mucus production in the bronchi may predispose to infection.
- Metaplasia of itself carries no increased risk of cancer; however, dysplasia is often present concurrently, and it does (see following).

ABNORMAL GROWTH INVOLVING BOTH DIFFERENTIATION & MATURATION: DYSPLASIA

Characteristics of Dysplasia

Dysplasia is an abnormality of both differentiation and maturation. The term *dysplasia* is often used loosely but, strictly interpreted, dysplasia shows the following characteristics.

A. Nuclear abnormalities:

- Increased size of nucleus, both absolute and relative (increased nuclear:cytoplasmic ratio).
- Increased chromatin content (hyperchromatism).
- Abnormal chromatin distribution (coarse clumping).
- Nuclear membrane irregularities such as thickening and wrinkling.

B. Cytoplasmic abnormalities result from failure of normal differentiation, eg,

- Lack of keratinization in squamous cells.
- Lack of mucin in glandular epithelium.

C. Increased rate of cell multiplication:

- Is manifested by increased mitotic rate, with mitotic figures occurring away from the normal stem cell zone (eg, above the germinal layer in squamous epithelium).
- Individual mitoses are morphologically normal in dysplasia.

D. Disordered maturation:

- Dysplastic epithelial cells retain a resemblance to basal stem cells as they move upward in the epithelium; ie, normal differentiation (keratin production) fails to occur.
- Dysplasia is usually graded as mild, moderate, or severe.

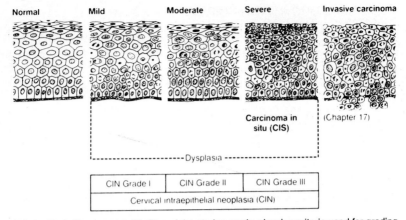

Figure 16–1. Squamous epithelium of the uterine cervix, showing criteria used for grading dysplasia (cervical intraepithelial neoplasia). The maturation defect, the nuclear:cytoplasmic ratio, and the nuclear chromatin abnormalities progressively increase as the grade of dysplasia increases. Note that infiltration of the neoplastic cells through the basement membrane distinguishes invasive carcinoma from dysplasia and carcinoma in situ.

Significance of Dysplasia

When it is defined in this manner, epithelial dysplasia is a **premalignant lesion.**

- In simple terms, dysplasia is a step short of cancer (Chapter 17).
- In the uterine cervix, the relationship of dysplasia to cervical cancer is so intimate that the term *cervical intraepithelial neoplasia* (CIN) is used synonymously with the term *dysplasia* (Fig 16–1).
- Severe dysplasia of the cervix and carcinoma in situ (ie true cancer in all respects except for lack of invasion) have the same clinical significance and are treated similarly.
- The risk of developing invasive cancer varies with
  - The grade of dysplasia—the more severe, the greater the risk.
  - The duration of dysplasia—the longer the duration, the greater the risk.
  - The site. Dysplasia in the urinary bladder is associated with a more imminent risk of cancer than is cervical dysplasia, in which several years may elapse before invasive carcinoma develops.

Differences Between Dysplasia & Cancer
A. Lack of invasiveness:

- The abnormal cellular proliferation in dysplasia (and carcinoma in situ) does not invade the basement membrane.
- Complete removal of the dysplastic area is therefore curative.
- Cancer, in contrast, invades the basement membrane and spreads from the local (primary) site via lymphatics and blood vessels, so that excision of the primary site may not be curative.

B. Reversibility:

■ Dysplastic tissue, particularly that affected by the milder grades of dysplasia, may sometimes spontaneously return to normal.
■ Cancer is an irreversible process.

Diagnosis of Dysplasia
A. Gross examination:

■ Patient is usually asymptomatic.
■ In many cases gross examination shows no abnormality.
■ The **Schiller test** for cervical dysplasia exploits the lack of cellular differentiation of the dysplastic epithelium; when the cervix is painted with iodine solution, normal squamous epithelium turns brown, owing to its glycogen content; dysplastic epithelium remains unstained.

B. Microscopic examination:

■ Smears made from material scraped from the suspect epithelium may be used for cytologic diagnosis.
■ Tissue obtained by biopsy is used for histologic diagnosis, which generally is more reliable.
■ Microscopic examination of the nuclear and cytoplasmic features provides evidence for both diagnosis and grading of dysplasia.
■ Dysplasia must be distinguished from other epithelial changes associated with inflammation and regeneration (which may show some cellular disorganization, or so-called atypia, that is not premalignant).
■ Routine cytologic screening of Papanicolaou (Pap) cervical smears has permitted early detection and treatment of cervical dysplasia, and resulted in a decreased incidence of invasive cancer of the cervix some 20 years later.

Neoplasia: I. Classification, Nomenclature, & Epidemiology of Neoplasms

Neoplasia ("new growth") is an abnormality of

- Cellular differentiation.
- Maturation.
- Control of growth.

Neoplasms

- Commonly form masses of abnormal tissue (tumors).
  - Note that not all tumors are neoplasms.
- Are **benign** or **malignant** depending on several features, chiefly the ability of malignant neoplasms to spread or metastasize.
- When malignant are called **cancers.**
- Are defined (as proposed in the early 1950s by Rupert Willis):
  - "A neoplasm is an abnormal mass of tissue, the growth of which exceeds and is uncoordinated with that of the surrounding normal tissues and persists in the same excessive manner after cessation of the stimuli that evoked the change" (see Chapter 18).

CLASSIFICATION OF NEOPLASMS

Classification of neoplasms has major implications for prognosis and therapy.

- Two major approaches are employed:
  - Biologic behavior—benign versus malignant.
  - Cell or tissue of origin (histogenesis).
- Other features such as site, embryologic derivation, or gross features are employed in some instances.

BIOLOGIC BEHAVIOR OF NEOPLASMS

Types of Biologic Behavior

The biologic behavior of neoplasms constitutes a spectrum with two extremes.

A. Benign: At one extreme, a benign neoplasm grows slowly, is encapsulated, and does not spread to distant sites (ie, no metastasis). (See Table 17–1.)

B. Malignant: At the other extreme, malignant neoplasms grow rapidly, infiltrate surrounding tissues, metastasize, and are often lethal (Table 17–1).

C. Intermediate: Between these two extremes is a smaller third group of neoplasms that are locally invasive but rarely metastasize.

TABLE 17–1. SUMMARY OF FEATURES DIFFERENTIATING BENIGN AND MALIGNANT NEOPLASMS[1]

Benign	Malignant
Gross features	
Smooth surface with a fibrotic capsule; compressed surrounding tissues.	Irregular surface without encapsulation; destruction of surrounding tissues.
Small to large, sometimes very large.	Small to large.
Slow rate of growth.	Rapid rate of growth.
Rarely fatal (except in central nervous system) even if untreated.	Usually fatal if untreated.
Microscopic features	
Growth by compression of surrounding tissue.	Growth by invasion of surrounding tissue.
Highly differentiated, resembling normal tissue of origin microscopically.	Well or poorly differentiated. Most malignant neoplasms do not resemble the normal tissue of origin (anaplasia).
Cells similar to normal and resembling one another, presenting a uniform appearance.	Cytologic abnormalities,[2] including enlarged, hyperchromatic, irregular nuclei with large nucleoli; marked variation in size and shape of cells (pleomorphism).
Few mitoses;[3] those present are normal.	Increased mitotic activity; abnormal, bizarre mitotic figures often present.
Well-formed blood vessels.	Blood vessels numerous and poorly formed; some lack endothelial lining.
Necrosis unusual; other degenerative changes may be present.	Necrosis and hemorrhage common.
Distant spread (metastasis) does not occur.	Metastasis to distant sites.
Investigative techniques	
DNA content usually normal.	DNA content of cells increased, additional chromosomes commonly present.
Karyotype usually normal.	Karyotypic abnormalities, including aneuploidy and polyploidy, are common.[4]

[1]None of these features are absolute; metastasis, invasion, and anaplasia are the most helpful.
[2]Note that the cytologic abnormalities of malignant neoplasms resemble those of dysplasia but are more extreme.
[3]Note that some nonneoplastic states have numerous mitotic figures (eg, normal bone marrow, lymph nodes undergoing an immune response).
[4]Subtle gene deletions or translocations are being recognized with increased frequency.

Identification of Biologic Behavior by Pathologic Examination

The pathologist classifies a neoplasm as benign or malignant on the basis of histologic and cytologic features. The characteristics listed in Table 17–1 serve only as general guidelines.

A. Rate of growth:

- Malignant neoplasms generally grow more rapidly than benign ones.
- Assessment of the growth rate is based upon
  - Clinical observation.
  - Microscopic examination—the number of mitotic figures and primitive appearance of nuclei (enlarged, dispersed chromatin, large nucleoli).

B. Size: The size of a neoplasm generally has no bearing on its biologic behavior.

C. Degree of differentiation:

- The term *differentiation,* applied to neoplasms, denotes the degree to which the neoplasm resembles the normal adult cells of the tissue in question.
  - Benign neoplasms are usually fully differentiated.
  - Malignant neoplasms usually are not.
  - **Anaplasia** describes the state where there is no morphologic resemblance whatsoever to normal tissue (ie, it is very poorly differentiated).
- Malignant neoplasms are usually more cellular, have a higher mitotic rate, and display the cytologic features of malignancy (Table 17–1).

D. Changes in DNA:

- Abnormalities in DNA content increase with the degree of malignancy.
- Malignant cells are **hyperchromatic,** showing more dense staining of the nucleus, reflective of the increased content of DNA.
- Cytogenetic studies demonstrate **aneuploidy** and **polyploidy** in malignant tumors.

E. Infiltration and invasion:

- Benign neoplasms are surrounded by a capsule of compressed and fibrotic normal tissue.
- Malignant neoplasms, on the other hand, have infiltrating margins, and show invasion.
- There are several exceptions to this rule.

F. Metastasis: The occurrence of metastasis (noncontiguous or distant growth of tumor; Chapter 18) is absolute evidence of malignancy.

CELL OR TISSUE OF ORIGIN (Histogenesis)

Neoplasms are classified and named chiefly on the basis of their presumed cell of origin.

- A first order of classification is based upon differing potentials for further development—totipotent, pluripotent, and differentiated or unipotent.
- A second-order division is based upon cell type (Table 17–2).

Neoplasms of Totipotent Cells

In postnatal life the only totipotent cells—ie, cells that are capable of differentiating (maturing) into any cell type—are the **germ cells.**

TABLE 17-2. CLASSIFICATION OF COMMON NEOPLASMS

Differentiation Potential and Cell Type	Cell or Site	Benign Neoplasm	Malignant Neoplasm
Totipotent cells	Germ cell	Teratoma (mature)	Teratoma (immature), seminoma (dysgerminoma), embryonal carcinoma, yolk sac carcinoma, choriocarcinoma
Pluripotent cells (embryonic blast cells of organ anlage)	Retinal anlage Renal anlage Primitive (peripheral) nerve cells Primitive neuroectodermal cells		Retinoblastoma Nephroblastoma (Wilms's tumor) Neuroblastoma Medulloblastoma
Differentiated cells Epithelial cells Squamous	Skin, esophagus, vagina, mouth, metaplastic epithelium	Squamous papilloma	Squamous carcinoma Basal cell carcinoma
Glandular	Gut, respiratory tract, secretory glands, bile ducts, ovary, endometrium of uterus	Adenoma Cystadenoma	Adenocarcinoma Cystadenocarcinoma
Transitional	Urothelium	Papilloma	Transitional cell carcinoma
Hepatic	Liver cell	Adenoma	Hepatocellular carcinoma (hepatoma)
Renal	Tubular epithelial cell	Adenoma	Adenocarcinoma
Endocrine	Thyroid, parathyroid, pancreatic islets	Adenoma	Adenocarcinoma
Mesothelium	Mesothelial cells	Benign mesothelioma	Malignant mesothelioma

(continued)

TABLE 17-2. (Continued)

Differentiation Potential and Cell Type	Cell or Site	Benign Neoplasm	Malignant Neoplasm
Placenta	Trophoblast cells	Hydatidiform mole	Choriocarcinoma
Mesenchymal cells Fibrous tissue	Fibroblast	Fibroma	Fibrosarcoma
Cartilage	Chondrocyte	Chondroma	Chondrosarcoma
Nerve	Schwann cell	Schwannoma	Malignant peripheral nerve sheath tumor
	Neural fibroblast	Neurofibroma	Malignant peripheral nerve sheath tumor
Bone	Osteoblast	Osteoma	Osteosarcoma
Fat	Lipocyte	Lipoma	Liposarcoma
Notochord	Primitive mesenchyme		Chordoma
Vessels	Endothelial cells	Hemangioma Lymphangioma	Hemangiosarcoma, Kaposi's sarcoma Lymphangiosarcoma

	Meningeal cells	Meningioma	Malignant meningioma
Pia and arachnoid	Meningeal cells	Meningioma	Malignant meningioma
Muscle	Smooth muscle cells Striated muscle cells	Leiomyoma Rhabdomyoma	Leiomyosarcoma Rhabdomyosarcoma
Melanocytes	Melanocytes[1]	Nevi (various types)	Melanoma (malignant)
Glial cells	Astrocytes		Astrocytomas Glioblastoma multiforme
	Ependymal cells Oligodendroglial cells		Ependymoma Oligodendroglioma
Hematopoietic tissue (marrow)	Erythroblasts[2] Myeloblasts[2] Monoblasts[2]		Erythroblastic leukemia[2] (Di Guglielmo) Myeloid leukemia[2] Monocytic leukemias[2]
Lymphoid tissue	Lymphoblasts Lymphocytes[2]		Malignant lymphomas, lympho-cytic leukemias, myeloma
	Histiocytes[2]		Malignant histiocytosis

[1] The origin of melanocytes is still controversial; we have placed them with mesenchymal tissues on the basis of their content of vimentin intermediate filaments (like other mesenchymal cells) as opposed to keratin (as in epithelial cells).

[2] The cells of origin, nomenclature, and relationships of these neoplasms are complex and are discussed fully in Chapters 26 and 29.

- Germ-cell neoplasms may
  - Show minimal differentiation (seminoma and embryonal carcinoma).
  - Develop into a variety of tissues, including trophoblast (choriocarcinoma), yolk sac (yolk sac carcinoma), somatic structures (teratoma).
  - **Teratomas**
    - ○ Show somatic differentiation and contain elements of all three germ layers: entoderm, ectoderm, and mesoderm.
    - ○ Are further classified as mature (well-differentiated, usually benign) or immature (made up of fetal-type tissues, malignant).
- See also chapters 51 (Testis) and 52 (Ovary).

Neoplasms of Embryonic Pluripotent Cells

Pluripotent cells can mature into a limited number of different cells types.

- The corresponding neoplasms have the potential for formation of diverse structural elements; eg, nephroblastoma commonly contains structures resembling renal tubules, plus muscle, cartilage, and bone.
  - These neoplasms are generally called **embryomas** or **blastomas.**
  - They usually occur in early childhood and include nephroblastoma, neuroblastoma, retinoblastoma, medulloblastoma, and embryonal rhabdomyosarcoma.

Neoplasms of Differentiated (Unipotent) Cells

Differentiated, adult-type cells make up most of the cells in the body during postnatal life. Most neoplasms of adults are derived from differentiated cells.

- Classification is based upon a combination of several criteria (Table 17–2):
  - Epithelial versus mesenchymal.
  - Benign versus malignant.
  - Tissue of origin.

A. Nomenclature of neoplasms of differentiated cells (Fig 17–1).
1. Epithelial neoplasms: Benign epithelial neoplasms are called

- **Adenomas**—arising from epithelium within a gland.
- **Papillomas**—arising from the surface of squamous, glandular, or transitional epithelium, and growing upward in a papillary structure.
- Malignant epithelial neoplasms are called **carcinomas,** which include
  - Adenocarcinomas—from glandular epithelia.
  - Squamous carcinomas—from squamous epithelia.
  - Transitional cell carcinomas—from transitional epithelia.

2. Mesenchymal neoplasms:

- Benign mesenchymal neoplasms are named after the cell of origin followed by the suffix *-oma* (Table 17–2; eg, fibroma).
- Malignant mesenchymal neoplasms are named after the cell of origin followed by the suffix *-sarcoma* (eg, fibrosarcoma).

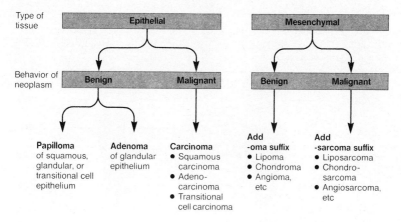

Figure 17–1. Nomenclature of neoplasms arising from differentiated (adult-type) cells.

B. Exceptions to these rules: Several neoplasms do not conform to this system.

1. Neoplasms that "sound benign" but are really malignant: Lymphoma, plasmacytoma, melanoma, glioma, and astrocytoma are all malignant, yet have the suffix *-oma.*

2. Neoplasms that "sound malignant" but are really benign: Two rare bone neoplasms, osteoblastoma and chondroblastoma, may sound malignant because of the suffix *-blastoma,* but are benign.

3. Leukemias: Leukemias are classified on the basis of their clinical course (acute or chronic) and cell of origin (lymphocytic, granulocytic, etc.; Chapter 26). They rarely produce localized tumors.

4. Mixed tumors are neoplasms composed of more than one neoplastic cell type.

5. Neoplasms whose cell of origin is unknown: Such neoplasms often are named after the person who first described them (eg, Hodgkin's disease, Kaposi's sarcoma, Ewing's sarcoma.)

Hamartomas & Choristomas

■ These tumorlike growths are thought to be the result of developmental anomalies.
■ They are not true neoplasms (ie, they do not show continuous excessive growth).
  ● A **hamartoma** is composed of tissues that are normally present in the organ in which the tumor arises; eg, a hamartoma of the lung consists of a disorganized mass of bronchial epithelium and cartilage.
  ● A **choristoma** contains tissues that are not normally present in its site of origin; eg, a disorderly mass of smooth muscle and pancreatic acini in the wall of the stomach.

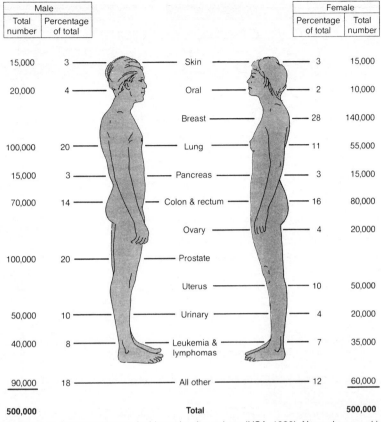

Male				Female	
Total number	Percentage of total			Percentage of total	Total number
15,000	3	Skin		3	15,000
20,000	4	Oral		2	10,000
		Breast		28	140,000
100,000	20	Lung		11	55,000
15,000	3	Pancreas		3	15,000
70,000	14	Colon & rectum		16	80,000
		Ovary		4	20,000
100,000	20	Prostate			
		Uterus		10	50,000
50,000	10	Urinary		4	20,000
40,000	8	Leukemia & lymphomas		7	35,000
90,000	18	All other		12	60,000
500,000		**Total**			**500,000**

Figure 17–2. Estimated cancer incidence by site and sex (USA, 1989). Nonmelanoma skin cancer and carcinoma in situ have been excluded. There are approximately 500,000 cases of nonmelanoma skin cancer per year in the USA. (Modified and reproduced, with permission, from CA 1988;38:5.)

INCIDENCE & DISTRIBUTION OF CANCER IN HUMANS

Incidence & Mortality Rates

- Cancer is the second overall leading cause of death (after ischemic heart disease) in the USA.
- It caused 460,000 deaths (accounting for 22% of all deaths) in 1985.
- Its incidence is rising.

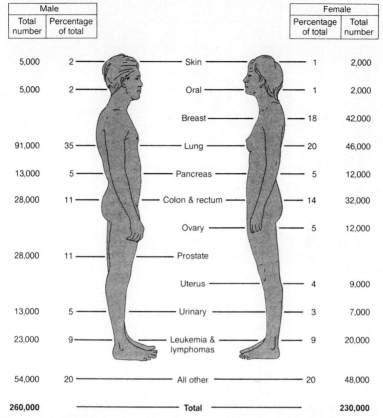

Male				Female	
Total number	Percentage of total			Percentage of total	Total number
5,000	2	Skin		1	2,000
5,000	2	Oral		1	2,000
		Breast		18	42,000
91,000	35	Lung		20	46,000
13,000	5	Pancreas		5	12,000
28,000	11	Colon & rectum		14	32,000
		Ovary		5	12,000
28,000	11	Prostate			
		Uterus		4	9,000
13,000	5	Urinary		3	7,000
23,000	9	Leukemia & lymphomas		9	20,000
54,000	20	All other		20	48,000
260,000		**Total**			**230,000**

Figure 17–3. Estimated cancer deaths by site and sex (USA, 1989). Nonmelanoma skin cancer has been excluded. The incidence of lung cancer in women is increasing rapidly; in 1986, lung cancer replaced breast cancer as the leading cause of cancer deaths in women.

- Both the incidence (Fig 17–2) and the death rate (Fig 17–3) of cancer must be considered. Note that the latter reflects the success of therapy.
- For example, skin cancer (not included in Figures 17–2 and 17–3) has the highest incidence, more than 500,000 cases per year, but a very low death rate, due to early diagnosis and effective treatment.

Major Factors Affecting Incidence

A. Sex: Prostate cancer in men and uterine cancer and breast cancer in women are obviously sex-specific. For other cancers, differences may reflect greater occupational

TABLE 17-3. THE GEOGRAPHY OF CANCER

Incidence per 100,000 Males per Site[1]

	Total	Nasopharynx	Tongue	Esophagus	Stomach	Colon	Liver	Lung	Prostate	Leukemia
Africa (Natal)	200	0	2	[40][2]	12	2	[28]	[40]	25	4
South America (Colombia)	200	0	3	5	[60]	4	4	20	25	5
Singapore (Chinese)	[250]	[20]	2	[20]	[45]	10	[32]	[54]	4	4
India and Sri Lanka	130	1	[14]	13	10	4	1	13	7	3
USA	[260]	1	3	6	15	[27]	4	[44]	23	10
UK	[240]	1	1	3	25	15	1	[73]	18	10
Japan	190	1	3	5	[60]	15	2	[36]	5	5

[1]These statistics are the 1979 figures for men. In women, the mortality rate from breast cancer varies between high rates of 33.8 : 100,000 in the United Kingdom and 27.1 in the USA to low rates of 6.0 in Japan, 2.7 in Hong Kong, and 1.2 in Thailand.
[2]Particularly high incidence figures are bracketed [ ].

TABLE 17–4. DISEASES ASSOCIATED WITH INCREASED RISK OF NEOPLASIA

Nonneoplastic or Preneoplastic Condition	Neoplasm
Mongolism (trisomy 21)	Acute myeloid leukemia
Xeroderma pigmentosum (plus sun exposure)	Squamous carcinoma of skin
Gastric atrophy (pernicious anemia)	Gastric carcinoma
Tuberous sclerosis	Cerebral gliomas
Café au lait skin patches	Neurofibromatosis (dominant inheritance); acoustic neuroma, pheochromocytoma
Actinic dermatitis	Squamous carcinoma of skin; malignant melanoma
Glandular metaplasia of esophagus (Barrett's esophagus)	Adenocarcinoma of esophagus
Dysphagia plus anemia (Plummer-Vinson syndrome)	Esophageal carcinoma
Cirrhosis (alcoholic, hepatitis B)	Hepatocellular carcinoma
Ulcerative colitis	Colon carcinoma
Paget's disease of bone	Osteosarcoma
Immunodeficiency states	Lymphomas
AIDS	Lymphoma, Kaposi's sarcoma
Autoimmune diseases (eg, Hashimoto's thyroiditis)	Lymphoma (eg, thyroid lymphoma)
Dysplasias (eg, cervical dysplasia)	Cancer (see Chapter 16)

exposure (dye and rubber industries for bladder cancer; mining and asbestos for lung cancer) and smoking habits.

B. Age: Most neoplasms have a predilection for particular age groups.

- In children
  - Carcinoma is rare.
  - Leukemias, malignant lymphomas, and various "blastomas" (eg, neuroblastoma, retinoblastoma) are relatively common.
- In adults, carcinomas make up by far the largest group of malignant tumors.

C. Occupational, social, and geographic factors: Because the risk is so high in certain industries, an occupational history is an essential part of a full medical examination (see Chapter 18).

- The social habit of cigarette smoking—and to a lesser extent pipe and cigar smoking, snuff taking, and tobacco chewing—represent risk factors for development of several types of cancer.
- Sexual and childbearing histories are important:
  - Women who have breastfed have a lower incidence of breast cancer.
  - Women who began sexual activity early and had multiple partners are at greater risk for cervical cancer.
  - Circumcised men have a lower incidence of carcinoma of the penis than their uncircumcised counterparts.
- Herpesvirus and papovavirus infections (Chapter 53) have been implicated as factors.
- Geographic variations also occur from one country to another (Table 17–3), and from urban to rural areas.
- In some cases, variations are due to differences in occupations (eg, shipyard workers, asbestosis, and mesothelioma), diet (eg, moldy food, aflatoxin, and liver cancer), or endemic viruses (eg, Epstein-Barr virus and Burkitt's lymphoma).

D. Family history:

- A few cancers have a simple pattern of genetic inheritance (Chapter 18; eg, retinoblastoma, polyposis coli and carcinoma of the colon, medullary carcinoma of the thyroid).
- For other cancers, the genetic link is not as strong (eg, breast cancer) or is almost nonexistent (eg, lung cancer).

E. History of associated diseases:

- A history of previous cancer greatly increases the chances that the current illness represents either a metastasis (which may be delayed many years) or a second primary tumor.
- In addition, certain nonneoplastic diseases carry an associated higher risk of development of cancer (Table 17–4).

Neoplasia: II. Mechanisms & Causes of Neoplasia

18

Neoplasia is an abnormality of cell growth and multiplication characterized by

- Excessive cellular proliferation that usually produces an abnormal mass, or tumor.
- Uncoordinated growth.
- Persistence of this excessive cell proliferation—ie, neoplasia is an irreversible process.

THEORIES OF ORIGIN OF NEOPLASIA

- The viral theory of neoplasia coincided with the demonstration that certain animal neoplasms are transmitted by ultrafiltrable agents (Rous sarcoma, 1908; Shope papilloma, 1933; Bittner milk factor, 1935).
- Immunologic theories came to the fore after experiments involving tumor transplantation in animals (Ehrlich, 1908; immune surveillance, Burnet, 1950s).
- DNA mutations as a cause of neoplasia were proposed after the discovery of DNA structure and function (Watson and Crick, 1950s).

Multifactorial Origin of Neoplasia

An **initiator** produces the first in a series of changes leading to neoplasia (initiation). This is followed by prolonged action of one or more **promoters** that eventually lead to neoplasia.

- The requirement of successive insults (multiple hit theory) accounts for the long latent period between the action of a cancer-causing agent and the appearance of a cancer.
- This concept of multiple hits combines several of the theories listed in the following material, and is illustrated by the role of Epstein-Barr virus and subsequent chronic immune stimulation in the induction of African Burkitt's lymphoma in humans (Fig 18–1).

Genetic Mutation Theory

Neoplasia may follow changes in growth-regulating genes due to spontaneous mutation or the action of external mutagens.

- Abnormal production of regulatory proteins alters the pattern of cell growth or differentiation.
- Many different oncogenic agents, including chemical carcinogens and viruses, may exert their effects through this mechanism.

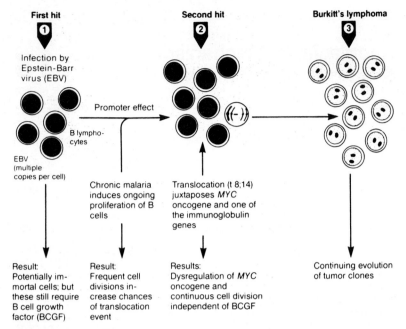

Figure 18–1. Oncogenesis in Burkitt's lymphoma. The first "hit" is infection of B lymphocytes with Epstein-Barr virus. Chronic malaria induces proliferation of B lymphocytes, increasing the likelihood of the second event, which is a chromosomal translocation that activates a cellular oncogene and leads to malignant lymphoma.

A. Neoplasia associated with constant genetic abnormalities:

■ Retinoblastoma:
- Families with a high incidence show partial deletion of the long arm of chromosome 13.
- It is postulated that the missing genetic material (the Rb gene) controls the growth of retinal cells.
- Retinoblastoma develops when the second Rb gene is also lost due to mutation or abnormal mitosis of the residual normal chromosome 13.
- The Rb gene is thus a recessive tumor suppressor gene.

■ Chronic granulocytic leukemia:
- In over 90% of patients, there is a reciprocal translocation between chromosome 22 and chromosome 9 (the resulting small 22 is known as the Philadelphia chromosome, Ph[1]. See Chapter 19).
- Translocation of the *C-ABL* oncogene from chromosome 9 to 22 leads to production of a novel growth-regulating protein (a tyrosine protein kinase), which is believed to cause neoplastic proliferation of granulocytes.

■ As techniques become more refined, genetic abnormalities are being identified in many tumors.

B. Neoplasia associated with chromosomal instability:

■ Certain rare syndromes associated with chromosomal instability and abnormal DNA repair mechanisms have a high risk of cancer.
■ These conditions include Bloom's syndrome, Fanconi's syndrome, ataxia telangiectasia, and xeroderma pigmentosum.
■ In **xeroderma pigmentosum** the action of ultraviolet light (the promoter) produces multiple skin cancers, due to inherited failure of DNA repair mechanisms (the initiator).

C. Neoplasia associated with aging: The increased incidence of cancer in the aged may be due to faulty DNA repair.

Virogene Oncogene Theory

■ Specific DNA sequences (**cellular oncogenes** [*C-ONC*]) are present in normal cells and produce growth factors that regulate normal growth.
■ These oncogenes may be abnormally activated (or de-repressed) by various carcinogens, including viruses, radiation, and chemicals, producing cancer.
■ Certain RNA oncogenic viruses contain **viral oncogenes** (*V-ONC*) that are essentially identical to cellular oncogenes. They are found in certain experimental animal neoplasms (Table 18–1), and in humans (see Table 18–2).
■ Cellular oncogenes are inherited as part of the cell genome.

TABLE 18–1. REPRESENTATIVE ONCOGENES

Viral Oncogene	Species Origin	Tumor Type	Virally Determined DNA in Host Cell	Tyrosine Phosphorylase Product
V-*src*	Chicken	Sarcoma	Yes	Yes
V-*yes*	Chicken	Sarcoma	Yes	Yes
V-*myc*	Chicken	Carcinoma, sarcoma, leukemia	Yes	?
V-*myb*	Chicken	Leukemia	Yes	?
V-*abl*	Mouse	Leukemia	Yes	Yes
V-*mos*	Mouse	Sarcoma	Yes	?
V-*ras*	Rat	Sarcoma, leukemia	Yes	?
V-*fes*	Cat	Sarcoma	Yes	Yes
V-*sis*	Monkey	Sarcoma	Yes	?

TABLE 18–2. ONCOGENIC VIRUSES

Group	Virus	Host	Tumor
RNA viruses (retroviruses) Type C	Avian leukemia-sarcoma complex	Chicken	Leukosis, Rous sarcoma
	Murine leukemia-sarcoma complex	Mouse, rat, hamster	Leukemia, sarcoma (lymphoma)
	Feline leukemia-sarcoma complex	Cat/dog	Leukemia, sarcoma
Type B	Murine mammary tumor virus (Bittner milk factor)	Mouse	Breast cancer
Type C-like	HTLV-I	Human	T cell leukemia
	Human immunodeficiency virus (AIDS virus)	Human	AIDS-related lymphomas
DNA viruses Papovavirus	Papilloma virus	Human, rabbit, cow, dog	Papilloma (laryngeal), condylomata acuminata, verruca vulgaris, ?carcinoma of cervix
	Polyoma virus	Mouse	Many tumors in newborn hamsters
	SV-40	Monkey	Tumors in hamsters only
Herpesvirus	Herpes simplex type 2	Human	?Carcinoma of cervix
	Epstein-Barr virus	Human	Carcinoma of nasopharynx, Burkitt's lymphoma
	Avian	Chicken	Marek's disease
	Rabbit	Rabbit	Lymphoma
Poxvirus	Fibroma-myxoma	Rabbit	Fibromyxoma
	Molluscum contagiosum	Human	Molluscum contagiosum[1]
Parapoxvirus	Hepatitis B	Human, rodent, duck	Hepatocellular carcinoma

[1]A self-limited proliferative disease of the epidermis: not a true neoplasm.

- Many oncogenes tested to date code for either
  - A protein kinase (tyrosine phosphorylase) with growth-regulating properties, or
  - A cell surface receptor for known growth factors (eg, erb B and epidermal growth factor.)
- DNA oncogenic viruses also appear to contain oncogene segments.

Theory of Failure of Immune Surveillance
Immune surveillance encompasses several concepts:

- Neoplastic changes frequently occur in the body.
- Neoplastic cells produce new molecules (neoantigens, tumor-associated antigens).
- The immune system reacts against these new antigens.
- Clinically detectable neoplasms appear only if they escape recognition and destruction by the immune system.
- Failure of immune surveillance has been invoked to explain the higher incidence of neoplasia in immunodeficiency states, in transplant recipients, and in the elderly.

AGENTS CAUSING NEOPLASMS (Oncogenic Agents; Carcinogens)

- Carcinogens are substances that are known to cause cancer—or at least produce an increased incidence of cancer—in an animal or human population.
- Except for cigarette smoking, the agents discussed in the following have been implicated in only a small percentage of cases.
- The marked geographic variation in the incidence of different cancers (Chapter 17) is thought to result more from the action of different carcinogens than from variations in genetic makeup.

Chemical Oncogenesis
One of the major problems associated with the identification of chemical carcinogens is the long lag phase, sometimes 20 years or more between exposure and the development of cancer (Chapter 19).

- Data from in vitro assays (such as the Ames test) or animal studies provide current guidelines, but are difficult to extrapolate to humans.
- Most chemical carcinogens act by producing changes in DNA.
  - A small number act by epigenetic mechanisms, ie, they cause changes in growth-regulating proteins without producing changes in DNA.
  - Others may serve as promoters for viruses or other carcinogens.

   A. Polycyclic hydrocarbons: The first recognized carcinogen in humans was soot, which caused scrotal cancer in chimney sweeps (Sir Percivall Pott, 1775). Later it was shown that the active carcinogens in soot were polycyclic hydrocarbons—benzo(α)pyrene and dibenzanthracene.
   B. Cigarette smoking:

- Cigarette smoking—and to a lesser extent, cigar and pipe smoking—is associated with an increased risk of cancer of the lung, bladder, oropharynx, and esophagus.
- Smoking accounts for more cancer deaths than all other known carcinogens combined.

- Cigarette smoke contains numerous carcinogens, the most important of which are polycyclic hydrocarbons (tars).
- The risk of developing cancer is about 10 times higher in someone who smokes a pack of cigarettes a day for 10 years (10 "pack years") than in a nonsmoker.
- If a smoker stops smoking, the risk drops almost to that of a nonsmoker after 10 years.

C. Aromatic amines:

- Exposure to benzidene and naphthylamine is associated with bladder cancer (first recognized in workers in the leather and dye industries).
- Aromatic amines are procarcinogens that enter the body through the skin, lungs, or intestine and are converted to carcinogenic metabolites that are excreted in the urine.

D. Cyclamates and saccharin: These artificial sweeteners cause bladder cancer in experimental animals. No carcinogenic effect has been demonstrated in humans.

E. Azo dyes: These dyes were used as food coloring agents ("scarlet red" and "butter yellow"); they cause liver tumors in rats, and have been withdrawn from commercial use.

F. Aflatoxin: Aflatoxin is produced by the fungus *Aspergillus flavus*, which grows on improperly stored food, particularly grain, groundnuts, and peanuts, and causes liver necrosis and, in the long-term, liver cancer.

G. Nitrosamines:

- Small amounts of these compounds are carcinogenic in animals.
- Nitrosamines are produced in the stomach from nitrites, which are commonly used as food preservatives.
- The high incidence of gastric cancer in Japan is thought to be related more to high intake of smoked fish (containing polycyclic hydrocarbons) than to high nitrosamine levels.

H. Betel leaf: The chewing of betel leaf in Sri Lanka and parts of India is responsible for an extremely high incidence of cancers of the oral cavity.

I. Anticancer drugs: Alkylating agents interfere with nucleic-acid synthesis and may cause oncogenic mutations (leukemia is a common complication of cancer chemotherapy).

J. Asbestos:

- Has been widely used as an insulating material and fire retardant.
- Is inhaled into the lung, where it produces chronic pulmonary fibrosis and fibrous proliferation of the pleura.
- It also is associated with two types of cancer.

1. Malignant mesothelioma: Nearly all patients who develop malignant mesothelioma give a history of asbestos exposure.

2. Bronchogenic carcinoma:

- Patients with asbestos exposure also have a risk of lung cancer about twice that of the general population.
- This risk is greatly magnified by smoking.
- Family members of shipyard workers also are at risk.

K. Other industrial carcinogens include heavy metals such as nickel, chromium, and cadmium (lung cancer), arsenic (skin cancer), and vinyl chloride (angiosarcoma of the liver).

Radiation Oncogenesis
A. Ultraviolet radiation:

- Sunlight is associated with various kinds of skin cancer, including squamous carcinoma, basal-cell carcinoma, and malignant melanoma.
- Skin cancer is the most common type of cancer in the USA; it is seen more often in the elderly.
- UV radiation is especially a problem for fair-skinned individuals in sunny climates who are continually exposed to the sun.

B. X-ray radiation:

- Early radiologists developed radiation dermatitis, with a high incidence of skin cancer.
- With the use of penetrating X-rays, radiologists suffered an increased incidence of leukemia.
- Today the risk is minimized by effective protective measures against X-rays: diagnostic X-rays deliver very small doses.
- Radiation-induced malignant neoplasms, commonly sarcomas, occur 10–30 years after radiation therapy.

C. Radioisotopes:

- Osteosarcoma once occurred among factory workers who used radium-containing paints to produce luminous watch faces; trace amounts of radium were ingested and deposited in bone.
- Exposure of miners to radioactive minerals is associated with an increased incidence of lung cancer.
- Thorotrast, a dye formerly used in diagnostic radiology, is deposited in the liver, leading to an increased risk of angiosarcoma, liver-cell carcinoma, and cholangiocarcinoma.
- Radioactive iodine is associated with an increased risk of thyroid cancer developing 15–25 years later.

D. Nuclear fallout:

- The Japanese of Hiroshima and Nagasaki who survived the atomic bomb have shown an increased incidence of leukemia and carcinoma of the breast, lung, and thyroid.
- Inhabitants of the Marshall Islands, who were accidentally exposed to fallout following atomic testing, showed a high incidence of thyroid neoplasms.

Viral Oncogenesis (Table 18–2)

- Both DNA viruses and RNA viruses can cause neoplasia.
- DNA viruses insert their nucleic acid directly into the genome of the host cell.
- RNA viruses utilize a RNA-directed DNA polymerase (reverse transcriptase) to produce a DNA copy of the RNA viral genome (provirus), which is inserted into the host genome.

■ Some RNA viruses contain a "built-in" oncogene that directly activates the cell; others insert adjacent to an endogenous cellular oncogene, which is thereby activated.

■ The presence of a viral genome in a cell can be demonstrated in various ways:
● Reciprocal hybridization studies using DNA probes.
● Recognition of virus-specific antigens on infected cells.
● Detection of virus-specific mRNA.

A. Oncogenic RNA viruses: These retroviruses (formerly called *oncornaviruses*) cause many neoplasms in experimental animals (Tables 18–1 and 18–2). They have been implicated in only a few human neoplasms.

1. Japanese T cell leukemia: First described in Japan, a retrovirus (human T lymphocyte virus type I [HTLV-I]) has been cultured from tumor cells.

2. Infection with HIV: Human immunodeficiency virus (HIV) is a retrovirus that causes acquired immune deficiency syndrome (AIDS), and possibly also B cell lymphomas.

3. Breast carcinoma: In mice, breast carcinoma is caused by the mouse mammary tumor virus (MMTV), an RNA virus transmitted in breast milk. A similar virus may play a role in human breast cancer.

B. Oncogenic DNA viruses (Table 18–2).

1. Papilloma viruses:

■ Cause benign papillomas in skin and mucous membranes, including
● The common wart (verruca vulgaris).
● The venereal wart (condyloma acuminatum).
● Recurrent laryngeal papillomas in children.

■ Types 16, 18, 31, and 32 have been implicated in invasive carcinoma of the cervix.
■ Types 6 and 11, by contrast, are found in benign venereal warts.

2. Molluscum contagiosum causes self-limited wartlike squamous tumors in the skin—probably not true neoplasms.

3. Epstein-Barr virus (EBV) causes infectious mononucleosis, and plays a role in the development of two separate neoplasms:

■ Burkitt's lymphoma in Africa (Fig 18–1).
■ Nasopharyngeal carcinoma in the Far East.

4. Herpes simplex virus (HSV) type 2: Found in association with cancer of the uterine cervix, it may have an etiologic role, or may simply be an opportunistic pathogen.

5. Cytomegalovirus (CMV): Found in Kaposi's sarcoma (AIDS), it may have an etiologic role in causing the sarcoma, or may be an opportunist.

6. Hepatitis B virus is common in Africa and the Far East, where it induces sustained liver-cell proliferation (regeneration) leading to a high incidence of hepatocellular carcinoma.

7. Adenoviruses cause cancer in animals, but have not been shown to be carcinogenic in humans.

Nutritional Oncogenesis
Except for the presence of known carcinogens (described in the preceding), there is little hard evidence linking cancer to diet. It has been suggested that a high fiber diet (as in

native Africans) promotes rapid passage of food through the intestines, and minimises the risk of colon cancer.

Hormonal Oncogenesis
A. Induction of neoplasms by hormones.
1. Estrogens: Sustained high levels of estrogen cause endometrial hyperplasia, followed by dysplasia and carcinoma of the endometrium.

2. Hormones and breast cancer: Oral contraceptives (the high-estrogen variety) carry a slightly increased risk of breast cancer. The low-estrogen varieties do not.

3. Diethylstilbestrol (DES) leads to a high incidence of adenocarcinoma of the vagina in girls exposed to the drug as fetuses, when the mother was given the drug to prevent a miscarriage.

4. Steroid hormones: Oral contraceptives and anabolic steroids are, rarely, associated with development of benign **liver cell adenomas.**

B. Hormonal dependence of neoplasms: The cells of some neoplasms have receptors for hormones on their cell membranes, and depend on the presence of the hormone for optimal growth.
1. Prostatic cancer is almost always dependent on androgens. Removal of both testes, or administration of estrogens, slows growth (temporarily).

2. Breast cancer:

- Frequently is dependent on estrogens and/or progesterone.
- Oophorectomy or treatment with the estrogen-blocking drug tamoxifen causes regression (temporary) in such cases.
- Testing breast cancer for receptor status is part of the diagnostic process.

3. Thyroid cancer:

- Well-differentiated thyroid cancers are dependent on TSH.
- Administration of thyroid hormone suppresses TSH secretion and may slow tumor growth.

Genetic Oncogenesis (The Role of Inheritance in Oncogenesis)
Many animals show a genetic susceptibility for development of neoplasms. In humans the situation is complex.

A. Neoplasms with Mendelian (single-gene) inheritance:

- Cancer-causing genes may act in a dominant or recessive manner.
- If dominant, they may produce a molecule that directly causes neoplasia.
- If recessive, lack of both normal genes may lead to failure to produce a factor necessary for control of normal growth.

1. Retinoblastoma:

- Forty percent of cases are inherited.
- The morphologic appearance of familial and sporadic forms is identical. However, the familial form displays other distinguishing features:
  - It is commonly bilateral.
  - It shows inherited deletion of the Rb gene on the long arm of chromosome 13 (the other 13 is normal at birth—heterozygous);

- Spontaneous regression is common, allowing some carriers of the gene to survive to reproductive age.
- Actual oncogenesis requires a second event, namely, deletion of the corresponding part of the long arm of the remaining chromosome 13, producing a homozygous state and development of retinoblastoma.
- In sporadic cases, two mutational deletions, involving both chromosomes 13, must occur.
- The result is an apparent dominant pattern of inheritance due to the high rate of conversion of the heterozygous state (lacks one Rb gene) to the homozygote (lacks both Rb genes), in which the recessive change is expressed.
- A similar abnormality of chromosome 13 occurs in small-cell undifferentiated carcinoma of the lung (Chapter 36).

2. Wilms's tumor (nephroblastoma):

- Many cases are associated with deletion of part of chromosome 11.
- Both sporadic and familial cases occur, by mechanisms thought to resemble those described for retinoblastoma.

3. Other inherited neoplasms with an apparent autosomal dominant inheritance pattern include:

- Neurofibromatosis (von Recklinghausen's disease).
- Multiple endocrine adenomatosis, manifested by benign neoplasms in the thyroid, parathyroid, pituitary, and adrenal medulla.
- Familial polyposis coli, characterized by innumerable adenomatous polyps in the colon; cancer eventually develops in all patients unless they undergo colectomy.
  - Gardner's syndrome is a variant, associated with benign neoplasms in bone, soft tissue, and skin.
- Nevoid basal-cell carcinoma syndrome is characterized by dysplastic melanocytic nevi and basal cell carcinomas in the skin.

B. Neoplasms with polygenic inheritance: Many common human neoplasms are familial, without a clear pattern of inheritance.

1. Breast cancer: First-degree female relatives of a premenopausal woman with breast cancer have a fivefold risk of developing breast cancer.

2. Colon cancer:

- Cancer of the colon occurs both as a complication of inherited familial polyposis coli and independently.
- Some "cancer families" exist, with abnormally high incidences of multiple cancers, including colon, endometrium and breast.
- This the result of inheritance of multiple genes, some of which may be oncogenes.

C. Neoplasms occurring more frequently in inherited diseases:

- Inherited diseases with a high risk of neoplasia include
  - Syndromes characterized by increased chromosomal fragility (eg, xeroderma pigmentosum, Bloom's syndrome, Fanconi's syndrome, and ataxia telangiectasia).
- Syndromes of immunodeficiency (Chapter 7).

Biologic & Clinical Effects of Neoplasms

19

ORIGINS OF NEOPLASIA
Two types of origins have been proposed for neoplasms.

Monoclonal Origin
The monoclonal origin theory proposes that the neoplastic change occurs in single cell, which then multiplies and gives rise to a clone (the neoplasm).

- A monoclonal origin has been clearly shown in neoplasms of B lymphocytes (lymphomas and plasma cell myelomas) that produce immunoglobulin.

Field Origin
The field origin theory proposes that the action of a carcinogen produces a field of potentially neoplastic cells, several of which progress to overt neoplasia.

- Multifocal (field) neoplasms occur in skin, urothelium, liver, breast, and colon.
- These theories are not mutually exclusive.

CHARACTERISTICS OF NEOPLASIA

The Lag Period
The lag period is the interval between exposure (to the carcinogen) and development of the neoplasm.

- For atomic fallout (Hiroshima and Nagasaki) the lag period ranges from 10 to 20 years; following asbestos exposure it may be as long as 40 years.
- The lag period probably represents the sum of
  - The time from **initiation** through the period of action of one or more **promoters** to the first neoplastic cell.
  - The time it then takes for the neoplasm to become clinically evident.

Precancerous (Premalignant) Changes (Table 19–1)
In most instances, no abnormality is apparent during the lag period. However, in some instances overt neoplasia is preceded by an intermediate abnormal, nonneoplastic growth pattern—a precancerous lesion. It is important to recognize precancerous lesions, because surgical excision is curative.

Occult Cancer
Occult cancers are so named because they remain undiscovered during life (eg, up to 80% of males dying of other causes at age 80 show occult carcinoma of the prostate).

TABLE 19–1. PRECANCEROUS (PREMALIGNANT) LESIONS

Precancerous Lesion	Cancer
Hyperplasia	
Endometrial hyperplasia	Endometrial carcinoma
Breast—lobular and ductal hyperplasia	Breast carcinoma
Liver—cirrhosis of the liver	Hepatocellular carcinoma
Dysplasia[1]	
Cervix	Squamous carcinoma of cervix
Skin	Squamous carcinoma
Bladder	Transitional cell carcinoma
Bronchial epithelium	Lung carcinoma
Metaplasia[2]	
Glandular metaplasia of esophagus	Adenocarcinoma of esophagus
Inflammatory lesions	
Ulcerative colitis	Carcinoma of colon
Atrophic gastritis	Carcinoma of stomach
Autoimmune (Hashimoto's) thyroiditis	Malignant lymphoma, thyroid carcinoma
Benign neoplasms	
Colonic adenoma	Carcinoma of colon
Neurofibroma	Malignant peripheral nerve sheath tumor (malignant schwannoma)

[1] These are de novo dysplasias; dysplasia also usually precedes malignancy in the other conditions listed.
[2] Note that metaplasia of itself is usually not preneoplastic—in the lung, squamous cell metaplasia is followed by dysplasia and then neoplasia.

Changes in Structure & Function of Neoplastic Cells (Fig 19–1)

A. Surface membrane alterations: Changes include alterations in the activity level of membrane enzymes, and loss of **contact inhibition,** wherein cancer cells in culture grow over the top of one another (normal cells do not).

B. Immunologic Alterations.

1. Appearance of tumor-associated antigens: Most neoplastic cells express new antigens (neoantigens, tumor-associated antigens).

a. Common viral antigens: In viral-induced neoplasms, new antigens are frequently coded by the virus. All neoplasms caused by a particular virus will show the same new antigen.

b. Unique antigens: Neoplasms induced by chemicals or radiation manifest new antigens that are distinctive for each different neoplasm induced.

c. Oncofetal antigens are expressed both in cancer (onco) and fetal tissues; they include **carcinoembryonic antigen (CEA)** and **α-fetoprotein (AFP).**

■ Most tumor-associated antigens are only weakly immunogenic but may evoke humoral and cellular immune responses, including a lymphocytic infiltrate surrounding the neoplastic cells.

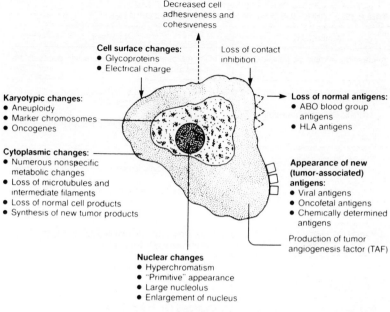

Figure 19–1. Changes in neoplastic cells.

2. Loss of antigens normally present: Neoplastic cells also frequently lack antigens that are present in normal cells (eg, loss of blood-group antigens in invasive bladder cancer).

C. Karyotypic abnormalities: Many malignant cells show major chromosomal abnormalities such as aneuploidy and polyploidy. In addition, some neoplasms show distinctive changes of diagnostic value (Table 19–2):

■ The first to be identified was the **Philadelphia chromosome** (Ph¹), an abnormally small chromosome 22 resulting from reciprocal translocation of genetic material between chromosome 22 and chromosome 9.

■ Ninety percent of patients with chronic granulocytic leukemia have Ph¹; the 10% who do not have a worse prognosis.

D. Tumor cell products:

■ The secretion of various tumor cell products is important for two reasons:
  ● They act as tumor markers.
  ● They may produce clinical effects (paraneoplastic syndromes) unrelated to direct involvement of tissue by the tumor.

1. Oncofetal antigens:

■ **Carcinoembryonic antigen** is found in most malignant neoplasms arising from tissues that develop from the embryonic entoderm (eg, colon and pancreatic cancer and some cases of gastric and lung cancer).

TABLE 19–2. CHROMOSOMAL ABNORMALITIES IN NEOPLASMS

Abnormality	Neoplasm
Aneuploidy, tetraploidy, polyploidy	Many malignant neoplasms, especially poorly differentiated and anaplastic types
Translocation[1] 9 ⇌ 22 t(9;22) (Philadelphia chromosome)	Chronic myeloid leukemia (90%) Acute myeloid leukemia Acute lymphocytic leukemia (FAB types L_1 and L_2 [Chapter 26])
8 ⇌ 14 t(8;14)	Burkitt's lymphoma[3] Acute lymphocytic leukemia (FAB type L_3 [Chapter 26])[3] Immunoblastic B cell lymphoma
15 ⇆ 17 t(15;17)	Promyelocytic leukemia (Chapter 26)
4 ⇌ 11 t(4;11)	Acute lymphocytic leukemia (FAB type L_2)[3] Immunoblastic B cell lymphoma
11 ⇆ 14 t(11;14)	Chronic lymphocytic leukemia
14 ⇌ 18 t(14;18)	Some B cell lymphomas
6 ⇌ 14 t(6;14)	Cystadenocarcinoma of ovary
3 ⇌ 8 t(3;8)	Renal adenocarcinoma Mixed parotid tumor (benign)
Deletions[1,2] Deletion of 8 and 17	Blast crisis of chronic myeloid leukemia
5q− and 7q−	Acute myeloid leukemia Acute monocytic leukemia
3p−	Small cell carcinoma of lung
1p−	Neuroblastoma[3]
13q−	Retinoblastoma[3]
11p−	Nephroblastoma[3]
−22	Meningioma
Trisomy Trisomy 12	Chronic lymphocytic leukemia

[1]Many of these translocations and deletions occur at the point of insertion of an oncogene.
[2]Note p = short arm and q = long arm of designated chromosome.
[3]Mainly tumors of childhood.

- It is not specific for cancer, since slight increases in serum levels also occur in several nonneoplastic diseases (eg, ulcerative colitis and cirrhosis of the liver).
- **α-fetoprotein** is synthesized by primitive gonadal germ-cell neoplasms (embryonal or yolk sac carcinomas) and liver cell carcinoma.
- Mildly elevated levels may be seen in cirrhosis.

2. Enzymes: Elevated serum levels of **prostate-specific acid phosphatase** occur in invasive prostate cancer.

3. Immunoglobulins:

- Neoplasms of B lymphocytes (some B cell lymphomas, myeloma) frequently synthesize immunoglobulins that may be detected as a monoclonal band on serum protein electrophoresis (see Chapter 30).

4. Excessive hormone secretion:

- Well-differentiated neoplasms of endocrine cells may produce excess hormones. For example:
  - Parathyroid tumors—parathormone.
  - Medullary carcinoma of the thyroid—calcitonin.
  - Pituitry adenoma—prolactin, growth hormone, etc.
  - Pheochromocytoma—catecholamines.
  - Islet cell adenomas—insulin, glucagon, gastrin.

5. Ectopic hormone production:

- Malignant neoplasms derived from cells that normally do not secrete hormones may sometimes do so (ectopic hormone production), eg,
  - Small cell carcinoma of the lung—ACTH, antidiuretic hormone.
  - Squamous carcinoma of the lung—parathormone.
  - Renal cell carcinoma—erythropoietin.

Changes in Growth Pattern of Neoplastic Cells

A. Excessive cell proliferation: Neoplastic cells usually multiply more rapidly than their normal counterparts. They usually accumulate to form a tumor. (Except for leukemias, which are spread throughout the bone marrow and blood).

1. Rate of growth and malignancy: As a general rule, the degree of malignancy of a neoplasm correlates with its rate of growth: the more rapid, the more malignant.

2. Assessment of growth rate:

- Clinically, the **doubling time** is a crude measure: For Burkitt's lymphoma, it is a few days; for some slow-growing cancers, a few years.
- The **mitotic count** provides a rough histologic assessment of aggressiveness.

B. Abnormal differentiation and anaplasia:

- Benign and slow-growing malignant neoplastic cells tend to differentiate normally and resemble their normal counterparts (ie, they are **well-differentiated**).
- As the degree of malignancy increases, the degree of differentiation decreases, and they show less resemblance to normal cells (**poorly differentiated**).
- When the differentiation is so slight that there is no resemblance to normal, a neoplasm is said to be **undifferentiated** or **anaplastic**.

- Cytologic abnormalities that increase in degree in proportion to malignancy include
  - Pleomorphism (in appearance of cells).
  - Increased nuclear size.
  - Increased nuclear:cytoplasmic ratio.
  - Hyperchromatism.
  - Prominent large nucleoli.
  - Abnormal chromatin distribution.
  - Nuclear membrane abnormalities.
  - Failure of cytoplasmic differentiation.

C. Invasion (infiltration):

- Benign neoplasms do not invade—they compress the surrounding normal tissue forming a fibrous capsule.
- Malignant neoplasms invade or infiltrate normal tissues.
- Invasion of the basement membrane distinguishes invasive cancer from intraepithelial (or in situ) cancer.
  - Having penetrated the basement membrane, malignant cells gain access to the lymphatics and blood vessels.
  - This leads to distant **metastasis** (secondary growths).
- Microscopic examination during surgery of rapidly frozen tissue sections is helpful in determining the extent of spread and the margins of excision.

D. Metastasis: Secondary neoplasms (metastases) arising by dissemination of malignant cells from the primary tumor to distant sites occurs only in malignant neoplasms.

1. Lymphatogenous metastasis:

- Metastasis via the lymphatics occurs early in carcinomas and melanomas.
- Sarcomas tend to spread mainly via the bloodstream.
- Lymphatic spread is first to the regional nodes, which thus present an important site for clinical or surgical examination.

2. Hematogenous metastasis:

- Entry of cancerous cells into the bloodstream is a common event with many malignant neoplasms.
- Most of these malignant cells do not survive to grow into metastases.
- The most common site of metastasis is the first capillary bed encountered by blood draining from the primary site, eg,
  - Liver, for intestinal cancers draining via the portal vein.
  - Lung, for cancers draining into systemic veins.
- Skeletal metastases are common in cancer of the prostate, thyroid, lung, breast, and kidney.

3. Metastasis in body cavities (seeding): Less often, malignant cells may spread via the body cavities (eg, pleura, peritoneum, or pericardium) or the subarachnoid space.

4. Dormancy of metastases:

- Cancerous cells that spread to distant sites may remain dormant there (or at least undetected) for many years.
- This makes it difficult to pronounce a patient cured even after many years.

TABLE 19-3. LOCAL EFFECTS OF TUMOR

Local Effect	Cause/Result
Mass	Presentation as tissue lump or tumor
Ulcer (nonhealing)	Destruction of epithelial surfaces (eg, stomach, colon, mouth, bronchus)
Hemorrhage	From ulcerated area or eroded vessel
Pain	Any site with sensory nerve endings; tumors in brain and many viscera are initially painless
Seizures	Tumor mass in brain; seizure pattern often localizes the tumor
Cerebral dysfunction	Wide variety of deficits depending on site of tumor
Obstruction	Of hollow viscera by tumor in the wall; bronchial obstruction leads to pneumonia; obstruction of bile ducts causes jaundice
Perforation	Of ulcer in viscera; in bowel may produce peritonitis
Bone destruction	Pathologic fracture, collapse of bone
Inflammation	Of serosal surface, pleural effusion, pericardial effusion, ascites
Space-occupying lesion	Raised intracranial pressure in brain neoplasms; anemia due to displacement of hematopoietic cells by metastases to the bone marrow
Localized loss of sensory or motor function	Compression or destruction of nerve or nerve trunk; classic example is involvement of recurrent laryngeal nerve by lung or thyroid cancer, with resulting hoarseness
Edema	Due to venous or lymphatic obstruction

EFFECTS OF NEOPLASIA ON THE HOST

Neoplasia may be the underlying cause of almost any sign or symptom anywhere in the body.

Direct Effects of Local Growth of Primary Tumors

The signs and symptoms arising from local growth of a benign neoplasm or a primary malignant neoplasm vary with the site of the lesion. The growing tumor may compress or destroy adjacent structures, and cause inflammation, pain, vascular changes, and varying degrees of functional deficits (Table 19–3).

Direct Effects of Growth of Metastases

Metastases may compress and destroy adjacent tissues in the same way that a primary lesion does, but effects may become manifest at multiple sites.

TABLE 19–4. DISTANT EFFECTS OF TUMORS AND PARANEOPLASTIC SYNDROMES

Clinical Effect	Causative Factors
Various hormonal effects, eg, hypoglycemia, Cushing's syndrome, gynecomastia, hypertension	Hormone produced by endocrine tumors; so-called "ectopic" hormones produced by nonendocrine neoplasms.
Anemia	Chronic blood loss or unknown toxic effects cause iron deficiency type. Replacement of marrow by tumor causes leukoerythroblastic type (see Chapter 24). Thymoma may be associated with spontaneous aplastic (hypoplastic) type; such anemia may also be iatrogenic. Autoantibodies (especially from lymphoma) cause hemolytic type. Fragmentation of erythrocytes in abnormal vessels of neoplasms.
Immunodeficiency	Lymphoma especially.
Hyperviscosity syndrome, Waldenström's macroglobulinemia, Raynaud's phenomenon	Monoclonal immunoglobulin (usually IgM) from lymphoma or myeloma (see Chapter 30).
Purpura	Various causes, usually decreased platelets due to marrow involvement or effects of therapy; decreased levels of coagulation factors, especially if liver is extensively involved.
Acanthosis nigricans	Thirty percent of cases are associated with visceral carcinoma (especially of the stomach); cause is unknown.
Dermatomyositis	In adults, 50% of cases are associated with underlying cancer; mechanism is unknown.
Pruritus	Hodgkin's disease (mechanism unknown); any tumor with obstructive jaundice.
Disseminated intravascular coagulation	Widespread cancer (probably due to release of thromboplastic substances by dying tumor cells; see Chapter 27).
Polycythemia	Renal cancer, hepatoma, uterine myoma, and cerebellar hemangioblastoma; in some instances due to erythropoietinlike substance produced by tumor.
Gout	Hyperuricemia due to excess nucleic acid turnover; may be precipitated by cytotoxic therapy.
Myasthenia gravis, myasthenic (Eaton-Lambert) syndrome	Thymoma especially; autoantibodies (see Chapter 66); other tumors; mechanism unknown.

(continued)

TABLE 19–4. (Continued)

Clinical Effect	Causative Factors
Clubbing of fingers and hypertrophic pulmonary osteoarthropathy	Lung cancer and other intrathoracic neoplasms especially; mechanism unknown.
Peripheral neuropathy (sensory and motor)	Various cancers.
Myopathy (especially of proximal muscles)	Mechanism unknown.
Cerebral and cerebellar degeneration	Lung and breast cancer; mechanism unknown.
Migratory thrombophlebitis (especially in leg veins)	Carcinoma of stomach, pancreas, lung, and other organs; release of thromboplastins by necrotic tumor.
"Marantic" (nonbacterial thrombotic) endocarditis	Various cancers (see Chapter 22); mechanism unknown.
Hypercalcemia	Parathyroid hormone (including ectopic production), release of calcium from lysed bone (metastases), or lytic factors (as in myeloma).
Cachexia, hypoalbuminemia, fever	Advanced cancer; possible autoimmune, toxic, and nutritional mechanisms.

Paraneoplastic (Nonmetastatic) Syndromes

Cancer may also cause various signs and symptoms, distant from the primary lesion, that are unassociated with metastases.

- These effects are termed *paraneoplastic* (or nonmetastatic) syndromes (Table 19–4). The mechanisms are largely unknown.

APPROACH TO CANCER DIAGNOSIS

Clinical Suspicion

The diagnosis of cancer is particularly difficult because of its protean manifestations. A thorough clinical history is essential. This includes

- Family history (for genetic predisposition or disorders associated with a high cancer rate).
- Social history (eg, smoking).
- Occupational history (eg, shipyard worker, miner).
- Diet and geographic origin (eg, smoked fish, aflatoxin, high incidence of hepatitis B).
- Sexual and childbearing history, eg,
  - Nuns have a high rate of breast cancer, in contrast to women who have borne and breast-fed several children.
  - Carcinoma of the cervix is more common in women who begin sexual activity at an early age and have many different partners.

■ Physical examination is directed toward discovery of a lesion that may be sampled by biopsy or aspiration for a histologic diagnosis.

Early Diagnosis
When symptoms and signs associated with cancer first appear, the disease is usually already advanced.

■ Screening examinations attempt to uncover presymptomatic disease.
■ Routine cytologic screening in the form of annual cervical smears (Papanicolaou smears) in all women age 35 and over constitutes the best example of this approach.

Cytologic Diagnosis
Samples for cytologic examination—exfoliated cells in sputum, urine, cerebrospinal fluid, and body fluids; bone marrow aspirates—may be obtained by a variety of techniques, including

■ Brushing or scraping of epithelium, or of a lesion that has been visualized by endoscopy (bronchoscopy, gastroscopy, coloscopy). Papanicoulaou smears of the cervix are included in this group.
■ Fine-needle aspiration of material directly from a mass.
■ In most instances, cytologic diagnosis is confirmed by biopsy and histologic examination before radical treatment is undertaken.

Histologic Diagnosis
Histologic diagnosis is considered the definitive method of establishing the diagnosis of a neoplasm.

■ When the histologic features alone do not permit conclusive diagnosis, ancillary techniques such as immunohistology, special stains, and electron microscopy are necessary (Table 19–5).
■ Diagnosis may be based on examination of the entire neoplasm removed at surgery (excisional biopsy) or examination of a sample of the neoplasm obtained either by incisional biopsy or with a large-bore cutting needle.
  A. Techniques.
    1. Frozen section method:

■ Frozen sections are prepared and examined within minutes of surgery.
■ This provides information while the patient is still on the operating table.
■ The disadvantage of this method is that the cytologic details are poor, and the diagnosis is less sure.

    2. Paraffin section method:

■ Small blocks of formalin-fixed tissue are embedded in paraffin to provide a rigid matrix for cutting sections.
■ This process takes about 24 hours, but provides good material for microscopic diagnosis.
■ Hematoxylin and eosin (H&E) stain is the standard stain for these sections; the hematoxylin stains the nuclei blue, and the eosin stains cytoplasm and extracellular material pink.
■ Special stains may be needed (Table 19–5).

TABLE 19–5. COMMON SPECIAL STAINS

Stain	Clinical Usefulness
Histochemical	
Reticulin stain	Pattern in carcinoma differs from that of lymphoma or sarcoma.
Fontana stain	Most melanomas are positive.
Trichrome, phosphotungstic acid-hematoxylin (PTAH)	Tumors of muscle origin, glial neoplasms.
Periodic acid-Schiff (PAS) after diastase digestion; mucicarmine	Adenocarcinomas are positive.
Grimelius' silver stain	Carcinoid tumors are positive.
Immunoperoxidase	
Antibodies to keratins	Present in epithelial cells only, including carcinomas.
Antibody to vimentin	Present in mesenchymal cells, including sarcomas.
Antibody to carcinoembryonic antigen	Present in many carcinomas, especially of colon and gastrointestinal tract.
Antibody to α-fetoprotein	Most hepatomas and some germ cell tumors are positive.
Antibody to prostatic acid phosphatase	Stains only prostatic epithelium, including metastatic prostatic cancer.
Antibodies to immunoglobulins	Stains certain B cell lymphomas and multiple myeloma; monoclonal pattern identifies neoplastic process.

3. **Immunoperoxidase techniques:** Immunohistochemical stains use specific labeled antibodies to identify marker antigens in cells and tissues (Table 19–5).

4. **Electron microscopy:**

■ Special fixation (in glutaraldehyde) and processing are required for optimal results.
■ Ultrastructural features in recognizing many types of neoplasms, eg, anaplastic squamous carcinoma, melanoma, endocrine tumors, and muscle cell tumors.

B. **Information provided by pathologic diagnosis.**

1. **Type of neoplasm:** The name of the neoplasm will be given in the pathology report.

2. **Biologic behavior:** Whenever possible the pathology report will state whether the neoplasm is benign or malignant if that information is not implicit in the name of the neoplasm.

3. Histologic grade:

■ This describes the degree of differentiation of the neoplasm, expressed either in words (eg, well or poorly differentiated) or in numbers (grade I being the least and III or IV the most malignant).
■ Highly specific criteria exist for histologic grading of different tumors.
■ The histologic grade has significant implications for prognosis, metastasis, and survival.

4. Degree of invasion and spread:
This information is vital in planning treatment of some neoplasms; eg, in malignant melanoma of the skin, the treatment is based on the depth of infiltration (see Chapter 61).

5. Pathologic stage:

■ This describes the extent of spread of a neoplasm, including the depth of invasion of the wall of a viscus, lymph-node involvement, etc.
■ Criteria for pathologic staging vary with different neoplasms and different organs:
  ● The system may be numerical (eg, stages I, II, III or IV).
  ● The TNM system may be used [size of the primary tumor (T), lymph node involvement (N), and distant metastases (M)].

Serologic Diagnosis
No general serologic screening methods exist for cancer, but several tests are of value for certain tumors (Table 19–6).

Radiologic Diagnosis
X-rays, plus CT and MRI scans, are invaluable for localizing masses as part of the primary diagnosis or for staging tumors.

TABLE 19–6. SEROLOGIC ASSAYS FOR CANCER DIAGNOSIS OR FOLLOW-UP

Substance in Serum	Cancer Type
Carcinoembryonic antigen (CEA)	Gastrointestinal tract cancer (especially colon), breast and lung cancer; elevated levels in some noncancerous states.
α-Fetoprotein (AFP)	Hepatoma, yolk sac tumors.
Human chorionic gonadotropin (hCG)	Greatly elevated in choriocarcinoma; rarely elevated in other neoplasms.
Prostatic acid phosphatase; prostate-specific epithelial antigen	Two separate molecules; levels of both are elevated in metastatic prostatic cancer.
Monoclonal immunoglobulin	Myeloma, some B cell lymphomas.
Specific hormones	Endocrine neoplasms and "ectopic" hormone-producing tumors.
CA 125	Ovarian carcinoma; other neoplasms.

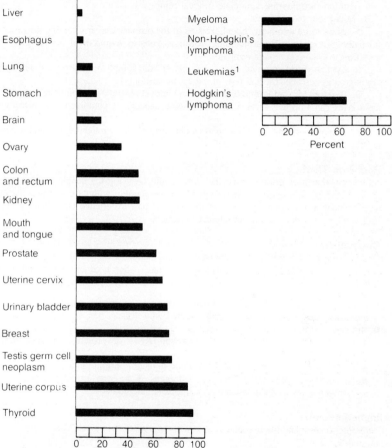

Five-year survival rates by site
(both sexes, all ages combined)

Figure 19–2. Five-year survival rates by site (both sexes, all ages combined). The rates given are the overall rates for the site and have been adjusted to include only deaths caused by the cancer. Within each site, there are different types of cancer that have greatly different survival rates. **Note:** Survival rates differ greatly for different types of leukemia (see Chapter 26).

TREATMENT OF NEOPLASMS

The purpose of accurate diagnosis of the specific tumor type is to enable the clinician to select an appropriate mode of therapy. Even with the best treatment, survival rates vary greatly for different types of neoplasms (Fig 19–2).

Surgery
  A. Benign neoplasms: Complete surgical removal is curative.
  B. Malignant Neoplasms.
    1. Wide local excision: Local excision of the primary cancer often requires careful pathologic examination (including frozen sections as required) of the margins of resection to ensure complete removal.
    2. Lymph node removal: For some cancers the lymph node group of primary drainage may also be resected (eg, in radical mastectomy).
    3. Surgery for metastatic disease: The removal of solitary or limited numbers of metastases can improve survival rates for some cancers, if combined with effective chemotherapy.
    4. Palliative surgery: Surgery plays an important role by relieving pain and restoring function in patients with incurable cancer.

Radiation Therapy

In general, the more primitive and the more rapidly growing the neoplasm, the more likely it is to be radiosensitive. Sensitivity is not synonymous with cure; the response of a given neoplasm can be predicted on the basis of past experience (see Chapter 11). Radiotherapy is often used as an adjunct to surgery.

Chemotherapy

Chemotherapy is the treatment of choice for many neoplasms, such as malignant lymphoma and leukemia. It also improves survival rates when used in conjunction with surgery in breast and lung carcinoma.

- Choriocarcinoma and testicular germ-cell neoplasms—formerly associated with high mortality rates—are now successfully treated with drugs.
- Anticancer drugs act in one of several ways:
  - By interfering with cell metabolism and RNA or protein synthesis (antimetabolites).
  - By blocking DNA replication and mitotic division (antimitotic agents).
  - By exerting hormonal effects, eg, estrogens in prostate carcinoma and antiestrogenic agents such as tamoxifen in breast carcinoma.

Immunotherapy

Attempts to stimulate the immune system with adjuvants such as BCG have met with limited success.

- Interferon and interleukin-2 (see Chapter 4) are still under investigation as treatments for such cancers as Kaposi's sarcoma, malignant melanoma, and lymphoma.
- Specific immunotherapy using monoclonal antibodies against tumor-associated antigens has been used in the treatment of malignant melanoma, lymphoma, and some carcinomas, but is still largely experimental.

Section V. The Cardiovascular System

Diseases of the Blood Vessels **20**

CONGENITAL DISORDERS

COARCTATION OF THE AORTA
Coarctation is a congenital malformation characterized by narrowing of the lumen of the aorta.

Infantile (Preductal) Coarctation
Infantile coarctation is a rare anomaly characterized by extreme narrowing of a segment of aorta proximal to the ductus arteriosus.

- The upper half of the body is supplied by the aorta proximal to the coarctation.
- The lower half is supplied from the pulmonary artery through a patent ductus arteriosus, producing cyanosis of the lower part of the body.
- Infantile coarctation is often fatal early in life unless corrected.

Adult Coarctation
Adult coarctation is more common than the infantile type, and it is more common in males than in females.

- It is characterized by localized narrowing of the aorta immediately distal to the closed ductus arteriosus.
- It is common in patients with Turner's syndrome.
- Symptoms and signs in severe adult coarctation are
  - Ischemia in the leg muscles during exercise (intermittent claudication).
  - Hypertension.
  - Presence of collateral arteries, mainly around the shoulder girdle.
  - Delay of the femoral pulse.
  - Lower blood pressure in the legs than the arms.
- Coarctation is frequently associated with bicuspid aortic valve.
- An important complication is infective endocarditis (Chapter 22) involving the abnormal aortic valve.

MARFAN'S SYNDROME
Marfan's syndrome is inherited as an autosomal dominant trait with a variable degree of expression. The exact biochemical defect is not known.

207

- Increased urinary excretion of hydroxyproline indicates high collagen turnover.
- The media of the aorta shows patchy placement of muscle by myxomatous material, resulting in
  - Dilatation of the aortic root, leading to aortic valvular incompetence.
  - A tendency to aortic dissection.
  - A tendency to spontaneous aortic rupture, with sudden death.
- Accumulation of myxomatous material also occurs in the mitral valve, leading to mitral valve prolapse syndrome and mitral incompetence.
- Marfan's syndrome is also associated with
  - Skeletal and ocular abnormalities.
  - Increased height.
  - Arachnodactyly (thin, long, "spiderlike" fingers).
  - High-arched palate.
  - Dislocation of the lens.
  - Hypermobile joints.

OTHER INHERITED DISORDERS OF CONNECTIVE TISSUE
Other rare inherited diseases in which there is defective connective tissue formation include Ehlers-Danlos syndrome, pseudoxanthoma elasticum, osteogenesis imperfecta, and the mucopolysaccharidoses. All are associated with aortic medial degeneration and weakening, predisposing to aortic root dilatation and aortic dissection and rupture.

CONGENITAL (BERRY) ANEURYSMS
Congenital aneurysms occur in small muscular arteries, such as the cerebral, renal, and splenic arteries.

- They are most commonly found in the circle of Willis, where their rupture causes subarachnoid hemorrhage.
- The aneurysm is not present at birth, but there is a congenital defect in the arterial media that causes the aneurysm to appear in adult life.

DEGENERATIVE VASCULAR DISORDERS

ATHEROSCLEROSIS

Incidence
Atherosclerosis is the main cause of both ischemic heart disease and cerebrovascular disease, and the primary cause of death in most developed countries. Deaths due to atherosclerotic arterial disease increased in the United States until about 1970, when the incidence leveled off. Since 1975 it has declined.

Etiology
Atherosclerosis is a degenerative arterial disease characterized by deposition of complex lipids in the intima.

- Its cause is uncertain.
- It occurs in older patients. (Significant atherosclerosis is uncommon under age 30.)
- Males are affected more than females. Female incidence increases after menopause, and incidence by sex is equal after age 75.

Risk Factors
A. Hypertension is the strongest risk factor for atherosclerosis in patients older than 45 years.

- Ischemic heart disease is five times more common in a hypertensive than a normotensive individual.
- Diastolic hypertension imposes a greater risk than systolic hypertension.

B. Hyperlipidemia is the strongest risk factor for atherosclerotic arterial disease in patients under age 45.

- Risk exists with both hypercholesterolemia and hypertriglyceridemia (types II, III, and IV hyperlipidemias) (Table 20–1):
  - In a patient under 45 years of age, a serum cholesterol level over 265 mg/dL is associated with a fivefold increased risk of ischemic heart disease compared to a level under 220 mg/dL.
- Low density lipoproteins (LDLs) and cholesterol levels correlate directly with the severity of atherosclerosis.
- High serum HDL cholesterol level has a protective effect; low HDL cholesterol levels increase the risk.
- Low HDL cholesterol levels are seen more commonly in:
  - Males than in females at all ages.
  - Cigarette smokers.
  - Patients with diabetes mellitus.
  - Inactive individuals.

C. Cigarette Smoking.
D. Diabetes Mellitus.

Pathology
A. The atheromatous plaque:

- The characteristic pathologic lesion consists of a mass of lipid and collagen in the intima.
- The earliest recognizable change is the accumulation of complex lipids within intimal smooth-muscle cells.
- The lipid is composed mainly of cholesterol, with smaller amounts of triglyceride and phospholipid.
- Fibroblasts enter the plaque at an early stage and lay down collagen.
- Grossly, the plaque appears as a flat yellow-white elevation on the intimal surface, covered by endothelium and containing semisolid yellow lipid material.
- Microscopically, it appears as a mass of pale eosinophilic debris in the intima in which needle-shaped cholesterol crystals are seen.

B. Distribution of atherosclerosis:

- The aorta is affected in most cases, with maximal change in the abdominal aorta.
- Involvement of muscular arteries—such as the coronary, carotid, vertebrobasilar, mesenteric, renal, and iliofemoral—is common and is responsible for many of the clinical manifestations.
- Plaques tend to be most prominent at branching of the major arteries.

TABLE 20-1. HYPERLIPIDEMIC DISORDERS

Type	Elevated Lipoprotein	Serum		Plasma on Standing[1]	Familial Disease (Inherited)	Secondary
		Cholesterol	Triglyceride			
I	Chylomicrons	N	↑	Creamy	Lipoprotein lipase deficiency (autosomal recessive)	...
IIa	LDL	↑	N	Clear	Familial hypercholesterolemia (autosomal dominant; varies)	Hypothyroidism, nephrotic syndrome, dietary, diabetes mellitus
IIb	LDL plus VLDL	↑	↑	Usually clear	Familial mixed lipoproteinemia (autosomal dominant; varies)	
III	Beta-VLDL	↑	↑	Turbid	Familial dysbetalipoproteinemia (autosomal recessive)	Obstructive jaundice
IV	VLDL	N	↑	Clear or turbid	Familial triglyceridemia (variable)	Diabetes mellitus, alcoholism, dietary
V	Chylomicrons plus VLDL	N	↑	Creamy	Very rare	...

[1] On standing, the plasma normally clears. Chylomicrons are large particles and tend to stay on the surface without precipitating, producing a creamy supernatant. This is a simple test to detect lipoprotein abnormalities.
VLDL = very low density lipoproteins (high content of triglyceride).
LDL = low-density lipoproteins (high content of cholesterol).
N = normal serum level; normal levels are defined statistically for men and women, separately for different age groups.

C. Complications of atherosclerotic plaques:

- Vessel thrombosis, which may cause sudden, complete occlusion of the artery; thrombosis is caused by slowing and turbulence of blood, and ulceration of the plaque.
- Dystrophic calcification of the plaque.
- Ulceration of the overlying endothelium may precipitate thrombosis and cause the lipid contents of the plaque to be discharged as emboli.
- Hemorrhage into the plaque may expand the plaque and occlude the lumen of the artery.
- Aneurysms may develop in vessels weakened by extensive plaque formation; the abdominal aorta is a favored site.

Pathogenesis:
A. Lipid imbibition theory hypothesizes that an abnormality in the endothelium permits entry of lipoproteins and factors that stimulate smooth muscle proliferation.

- Endothelial abnormalities may be aggravated by injury from turbulence and hypertension.
- Nicotine, carbon monoxide, and other factors that cause endothelial abnormalities have been identified in the serum of cigarette smokers.

B. Thrombus encrustation theory hypothesizes that small thrombi formed in vessels become incorporated into the intima by organization, with subsequent lipid degeneration initiating plaque formation. It is unlikely that this is the primary mechanism.

C. Monoclonal hypothesis holds that monoclonal smooth muscle proliferation is the critical event in the pathogenesis of atherosclerosis. (The smooth muscle proliferation that occurs in the atheromatous plaque is monoclonal.)

- Subsequent fatty degeneration ensues and is aggravated by hyperlipidemia and endothelial injury.
- Substances in the serum known to cause smooth muscle proliferation include endogenous lipoproteins, platelet factors and exogenous substances associated with cigarette smoking.

Clinical Features (Fig 20–1)
A. Narrowing of affected arteries:

- Ischemia from arterial narrowing is responsible for most of the clinical effects of atherosclerosis.
- A decrease in blood flow usually occurs only with severe ($> 70\%$) narrowing of the vessel.
- Aortic narrowing is almost never sufficient to cause symptoms.
- Narrowing of coronary, cerebral, renal, mesenteric, and iliofemoral vessels often causes ischemic changes.
- Thrombotic occlusion of these arteries may cause infarction.

B. Embolism:

- Ulceration of the atheromatous plaque may result in embolization of the lipid contents of the plaque.

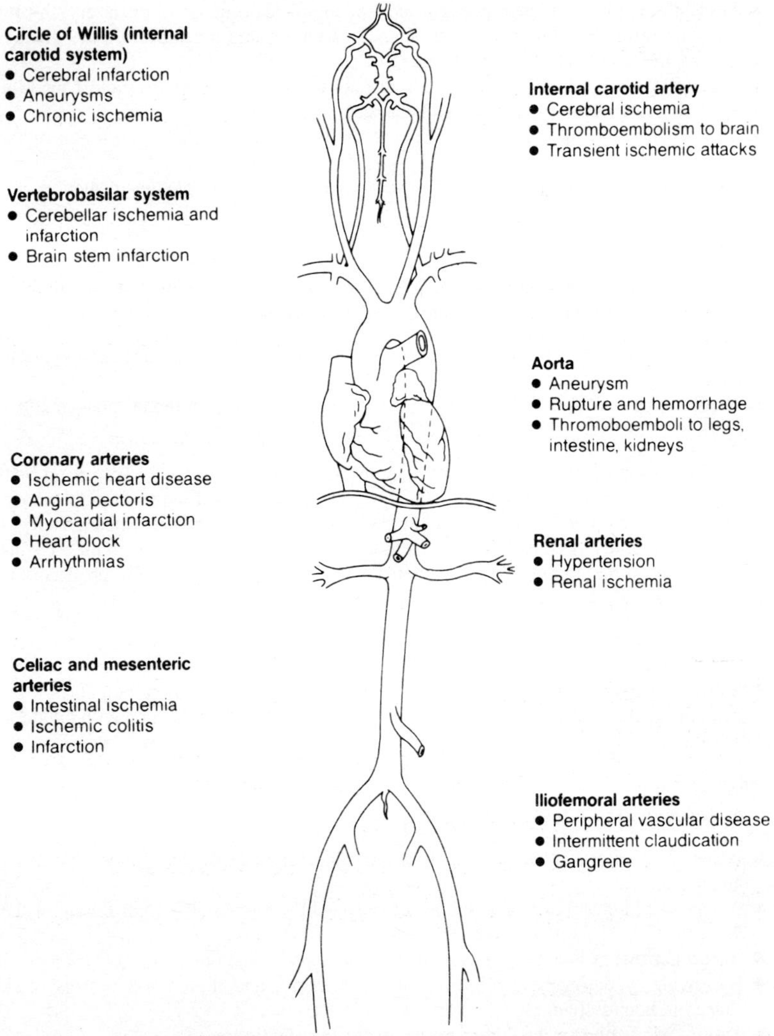

Circle of Willis (internal carotid system)
- Cerebral infarction
- Aneurysms
- Chronic ischemia

Vertebrobasilar system
- Cerebellar ischemia and infarction
- Brain stem infarction

Coronary arteries
- Ischemic heart disease
- Angina pectoris
- Myocardial infarction
- Heart block
- Arrhythmias

Celiac and mesenteric arteries
- Intestinal ischemia
- Ischemic colitis
- Infarction

Internal carotid artery
- Cerebral ischemia
- Thromboembolism to brain
- Transient ischemic attacks

Aorta
- Aneurysm
- Rupture and hemorrhage
- Thromoboemboli to legs, intestine, kidneys

Renal arteries
- Hypertension
- Renal ischemia

Iliofemoral arteries
- Peripheral vascular disease
- Intermittent claudication
- Gangrene

Figure 20–1. Clinical effects of atherosclerosis related to the major arteries involved.

- In the cerebral circulation, small emboli produce transient ischemic attacks.
- Cholesterol emboli can sometimes be visualized in the retinal arteries on funduscopic examination.

C. Aneurysm formation:

- Atherosclerotic aneurysms occur mainly in the lower abdominal aorta.
- They may appear as a fusiform dilatation of the vessel or a saccular bulge on one side of it.

SYSTEMIC HYPERTENSION
Systemic hypertension is defined as sustained elevation of systemic arterial blood pressure.

- A pressure under 140/90 mm Hg is normal, and 160/95 mm Hg is hypertensive. Pressures between these levels are regarded as borderline.
- Diastolic pressure is a more reliable indicator of significant hypertension than systolic pressure.

Incidence
Fifteen to twenty percent of adults in the United States have blood pressures over 160/95 mm Hg.

Etiology and Pathogenesis (Table 20–2)
A. Essential hypertension:

- Occurs as a primary phenomenon without known cause.
- Is the commonest type of hypertension.
- Usually occurs after age 40.
- Has a familial incidence suggestive of polygenic inheritance.
- Has uncertain pathogenesis. No constant changes in plasma levels of renin, aldosterone, catecholamines, or in the activity of the sympathetic nervous system or baroreceptors has been demonstrated.
- The currently favored theory is that essential hypertension is due to high dietary intake of sodium associated with failure of sodium excretion by the kidney.

B. Secondary hypertension (Table 20–2):

- Is defined as hypertension due to a preceding defined disease process.
- Constitutes less than 10% of cases of hypertension.
- Should be strongly suspected in a patient under age 40 who develops hypertension.

Pathology
A. Benign hypertension:

- In the earliest phase of hypertension, there are no microscopic changes in blood vessels.
- Later, there is medial muscle hypertrophy, followed by hyaline degeneration and intimal fibrosis (hyaline arteriolosclerosis).
- The tissues supplied may show changes of chronic ischemia.

TABLE 20–2. ETIOLOGY AND CLASSIFICATION OF HYPERTENSION

Essential (primary) hypertension

Secondary hypertension
 Renal diseases
  Renal vascular diseases
   Renal artery stenosis (atherosclerosis, fibromuscular hyper-
    plasia, posttransplantation)
   Arteritis, polyarteritis nodosa
   Renal artery embolism
  Renal parenchymal diseases
   Acute glomerulonephritis
   Chronic glomerulonephritis
   Chronic pyelonephritis
   Polycystic disease of the kidney
  Renal neoplasms
   Juxtaglomerular apparatus neoplasm
   Renal carcinoma
   Wilms' tumor
 Endocrine diseases
  Pheochromocytoma
  Primary aldosteronism (Conn's syndrome)
  Cushing's syndrome
  Congenital adrenal hyperplasia due to 11-hydroxylase deficiency
 Coarctation of the aorta
 Drug-induced hypertension
  Corticosteroids
  Amphetamine use
  Chronic licorice ingestion[1]
  Oral contraceptives
 Neurologic diseases
  Raised intracranial pressure
  ?Psychogenic
 Hypercalcemia

[1]Licorice has an aldosteronelike effect ("pseudoaldosteronism").

B. Malignant (accelerated) hypertension:

- Is characterized by very severe hypertension (diastolic pressure > 110 mm Hg).
- Affected vessels show fibrinoid necrosis of the media with marked intimal fibrosis and extreme narrowing.
- Tissues supplied by affected vessels show acute ischemia with microinfarcts and hemorrhages.
- Is frequently associated with elevated serum renin levels.

Clinical Features
A. Early hypertension is asymptomatic, and the diagnosis can be made only by detecting the elevation of blood pressure.

B. Hypertensive heart disease is characterized by:

- Left ventricular hypertrophy.

- Left ventricular failure, particularly in accelerated hypertension.
- An increased risk of coronary atherosclerosis and ischemic heart disease.

C. Hypertensive renal disease is characterized by:

- Decreased glomerular filtration, progressive glomerular fibrosis, and loss of nephrons.
- Renal failure with elevation of serum creatinine, usually only in patients with accelerated hypertension.
- Hematuria may occur in accelerated hypertension and be associated with acute renal failure.

D. Hypertensive cerebral disease is characterized by:

- A greatly increased incidence of cerebrovascular disease, including cerebral thrombosis (secondary to atherosclerosis) and cerebral hemorrhage.
- Hypertensive encephalopathy, which is due to transient spasm of small arteries in the brain induced by very high blood pressures; it causes headache and transient cerebral dysfunction.

E. Hypertensive retinal disease is characterized by:

- Narrow, irregular arteries with thickened walls in patients with mild to moderate hypertension.
- Retinal hemorrhages, fluffy exudates ("cotton wool spots"), and papilledema in accelerated hypertension.

MEDIAL CALCIFICATION (Monckeberg's Sclerosis)

Medial calcification, or Monckeberg's sclerosis, is a very common degenerative change seen in the elderly.

- It affects muscular arteries such as the femoral, radial, and uterine arteries, which show extensive calcification restricted to the media.
- There is no luminal narrowing or endothelial damage.
- It does not produce any clinical abnormality.

AORTIC DISSECTION (Dissecting Aneurysm of the Aorta)

Incidence & Etiology

Dissecting aneurysm of the aorta is caused by entry of blood under high pressure into the aortic media through an intimal tear.

- Dissection is usually preceded by myxomatous degeneration of the media (Erdheim's cystic medial degeneration).
- Hypertension is an important etiologic factor.
- Aortic dissection is common in patients with Marfan's syndrome and other diseases in which collagen synthesis is abnormal.

Pathology

- It is commonly associated with an intimal tear, usually just above the aortic valve or immediately distal to the ligamentum arteriosum.
- Blood dissects between layers of smooth muscle in the media.

Clinical Features

- Dissection of the media produces sudden severe pain, which is usually retrosternal and mimics the pain of myocardial infarction.
- Arteries taking origin from the aorta may become occluded.
- External rupture may occur leading to massive retroperitoneal or mediastinal hemorrhage.

VARICOSE VEINS

Varicose veins are abnormally dilated and tortuous veins. They occur in the legs, rectum (hemorrhoids), esophagus and stomach in portal hypertension, and spermatic cord (varicocele).

Etiology

In the legs, varicose veins involve the superficial saphenous venous system and result from

- Obstruction to the deep veins.
- Incompetence of the valves in the saphenous and perforating veins.

Clinical Features

- Varicose veins in the legs produce adverse cosmetic effects, chronic aching and swelling, recurrent thrombophlebitis, stasis dermatitis, and skin ulceration.
- Stasis ulcers typically occur in the region of the ankle.
- Gastroesophageal varices are a common cause of hematemesis.

INFLAMMATORY DISEASES OF BLOOD VESSELS

SYPHILITIC AORTITIS

Aortitis occurs in the tertiary stage of syphilis, often many decades after the primary infection. It has become rare because of the successful treatment of early syphilis.

- The spirochete cannot be demonstrated in the lesions.
- Immunologic hypersensitivity plays a part in pathogenesis.

Pathology

- The vasa vasorum are primarily involved by inflammation and luminal narrowing due to intimal fibrosis (endarteritis obliterans).
- This leads to degeneration and fibrosis of the outer two-thirds of the aortic media.
- Compensatory irregular fibrous thickening of the intima occurs ("tree bark appearance").

Clinical Features

Weakening of the aortic wall causes dilatation of the aortic root and aortic incompetence and aneurysms.

- Intimal fibrosis causes narrowing of the openings of the coronary arteries ("ostial stenosis"), causing myocardial ischemia.

TAKAYASU'S DISEASE

Takayasu's disease is also called occlusive thromboaortopathy, aortic arch syndrome, and pulseless disease.

- It is a disease of unknown cause that is uncommon in the United States but common in Japan.
- Females are affected more often than males by a 9:1 ratio.
- About 90% of cases occur in those under 30 years of age.

Pathology

Pathology is usually restricted to the aortic arch. In 30% of cases the whole aorta is involved, and in 10%, only the descending aorta.

- It is characterized by marked fibrosis involving all layers of the wall, causing aortic narrowing and occlusion of arteries originating from the aorta.
- Microscopic examination shows infiltration of the media and adventitia by neutrophils and chronic inflammatory cells. In a few cases, granulomas with giant cells are seen.

Clinical Features

- Occlusion of the aortic arch vessels leads to:
  - Loss of radial pulses.
  - Ischemic neurologic lesions.
  - Ocular ischemia with visual impairment.
- In cases that involve the descending aorta, involvement of renal arteries may lead to hypertension.
- The course is variable. Death may occur either in the acute phase or after many years of slowly progressive disease.

GIANT CELL ARTERITIS (Temporal Arteritis)

Temporal arteritis is an uncommon disease in individuals over age 50. The cause is uncertain. Type IV hypersensitivity against arterial wall antigens is seen in a few cases.

Pathology

Temporal arteritis is characterized by granulomatous inflammation and fibrosis of the wall with numerous multinucleated giant cells, and fragmentation of the internal elastic lamina.

- Thrombosis may occur in the acute phase.
- It affects medium-sized muscular arteries, including
  - Superficial temporal artery.
  - Intracranial arteries including the retinal artery.
  - Arteries around the scapula.

Clinical Features

Giant cell arteritis commonly presents with severe headache associated with thickening and tenderness of the superficial temporal artery. Cranial nerve palsies are less common.

- Diagnosis is by biopsy of the involved temporal artery.

- Elevation of the erythrocyte sedimentation rate, though not specific, is a useful diagnostic test.
- Treatment with corticosteroids is important to prevent permanent blindness from retinal artery involvement.

POLYARTERITIS NODOSA

Polyarteritis nodosa is an uncommon disease that occurs mainly in young adults. Males are more frequently affected than females.

- It is believed due to a type III immunologic hypersensitivity (immune complex) reaction.
- Hepatitis B surface antigen is present in the complexes in 30–40% of patients.

Pathology

Medium-sized and small arteries throughout the body are involved.

- It is characterized by segmental lesions consisting of nodular reddish swellings and multiple microaneurysms.
- Arterial rupture with tissue hemorrhages and thrombosis with tissue ischemia occurs in the acute phase. In the chronic phase, the involved artery is thickened by fibrosis.
- Microscopic examination shows fibrinoid necrosis of the media and acute inflammation involving all layers.

Clinical Features

The course is progressive, with exacerbations and remissions.

- Without treatment, the 5-year survival rate is less than 20%. With steroid therapy, 50% of patients are alive after 5 years.
- In the acute phase, patients develop fever, with variable signs and symptoms according to the pattern of organ involvement (Table 20–3).
- The diagnosis is clinical. Biopsy of acutely affected tissue may provide histologic confirmation.

WEGENER'S GRANULOMATOSIS

Wegener's granulomatosis is characterized by necrotizing vasculitis, with extensive tissue necrosis and granulomatous reaction involving the lungs, nasopharynx, and kidney. It is a rapidly progressive disease that responds somewhat to immunosuppressive therapy, but the overall prognosis is poor.

THROMBOANGIITIS OBLITERANS (Buerger's Disease)

Thromboangiitis obliterans is rare in the United States and Europe, but is common in Israel, Japan, and India.

- It occurs most often in young men in the age group from 20 to 30 years.
- It is largely restricted to heavy cigarette smokers.
- The mechanism by which smoking provokes the disease is unknown.

Pathology

It is characterized by segmental involvement of small and medium-sized arteries, mainly in the lower extremities.

TABLE 20–3. CLINICAL AND LABORATORY FINDINGS IN POLYARTERITIS NODOSA

	Percentage of Cases

Fever
Renal changes
   Microscopic hematuria
   Glomerulonephritis
Hypertension
	> 50

Skin rashes (nonspecific)
Arthritis and arthralgia
Neuropathy and mononeuritis, such as
   isolated cranial nerve palsy
Myalgia and myositis
Pulmonary changes[1]
   Hemoptysis
   Asthma
	30–50

CNS changes (nonspecific)
Cardiac changes
   Pericarditis
   Myocardial ischemia
Intestinal (ischemia)
   Abdominal pain
   Diarrhea
   Perforation
Hepatomegaly (painful)
	< 30

Hematologic abnormalities
   Anemia
   Leukocytosis and eosinophilia
   Thrombocytosis and thrombocytopenia
   Elevated erythrocyte sedimentation rate
	> 50

Serum abnormalities
   Hepatic B surface antigen
   Rheumatoid factor
   Cryoglobulins
   Decreased complement factor
	20–50

[1]Pulmonary changes do not occur in classic polyarteritis; they are seen in a variant form of the disease known as allergic granulomatosis and angiitis of Churg and Strauss.

- Frequently it involves adjacent veins and nerves.
- In the acute phase, there is marked swelling and neutrophilic infiltration of the neurovascular bundle, with extensive arterial and venous thrombosis.
- Healing by fibrosis and organization of thrombi produces thick cordlike vessels with occluded lumens.

Clinical Features

It presents with intermittent claudication, usually of the legs. As the disease progresses, the claudication distance decreases.

TABLE 20-4. DISEASES IN WHICH SMALL VESSEL IMMUNE VASCULITIS IS COMMONLY PRESENT

	Sites Involved	Antigen (Probable) in Immune Complex
Connective tissue diseases (Chapter 68) Systemic lupus erythematosus	Systemic	Nuclear antigens
Progressive systemic sclerosis	Skin, gut, lung, kidney	
Mixed connective tissue diseases	Systemic	
Mixed cryoglobulinemia	Systemic	Patient's IgG (the anti-IgG antibody is commonly IgM)
Henoch-Schönlein purpura	Skin, kidney, gut	Patient's IgA(?)
Drug hypersensitivity	Skin, other	Penicillin, sulfonamides, gold salts, antithyroid drugs, etc
Focal infective vasculitis, infective endocarditis	Skin, kidney, retina	Bacterial antigens
Erythema nodosum	Skin	Various (tuberculosis, sarcoidosis, acute rheumatic fever, fungal infections, leprosy, drugs)

- With severe disease, pain is present at rest along with trophic changes in the skin, culminating in dry gangrene.
- The disease is progressive. Abstinence from smoking frequently results in remissions.

SMALL VESSEL VASCULITIS
Necrotizing vasculitis affecting small vessels occurs in many different diseases, most of which are mediated by type III immune complex hypersensitivity (Table 20-4).

Pathology
Small arterioles are involved, and show fibrinoid necrosis accompanied by intense lymphocytic and/or neutrophil infiltration.

- Thrombosis and hemorrhage are common.
- Immunoglobulin and complement can be demonstrated in the lesions by immunologic techniques.

Clinical Features
It is characterized by involvement of multiple organs.

- Skin involvement leads to erythematous rashes and raised purpuric patches.
- Renal involvement is associated with glomerulonephritis.
- Raynaud's phenomenon—characterized by numbness and pallor or cyanosis of hands and feet in response to cold—is common.

THROMBOPHLEBITIS (See Chapter 9)
A. Phlegmasia alba dolens (painful white leg)

- This is a rare type of deep leg vein thrombophlebitis of unknown cause that occurs during the later months of pregnancy.
- It is characterized by extreme swelling of the leg, associated with severe pain and tenderness.

B. Migratory thrombophlebitis is characterized by episodic inflammation and thrombosis of superficial veins at multiple sites. It occurs in:

- Thromboangiitis obliterans.
- Patients with carcinomas of internal organs such as the pancreas, stomach, lung, or colon (Trousseau's syndrome).

LYMPHANGITIS
A. Bacterial lymphangitis commonly complicates bacterial infections of the skin.

- *Streptococcus pyogenes* is the commonest cause.
- The inflamed lymphatics appear as painful, red streaks, frequently associated with acute lymphadenitis.

B. Filarial lymphangitis is an extremely common tropical disease caused by *Wuchereria bancrofti* and *Brugia malayi*.

- Microfilariae reaching the lymphatics mature into adult worms, and death of the worms causes acute lymphangitis, followed by fibrotic occlusion of the lymphatics.
- When widespread lymphatic obstruction occurs, chronic lymphedema (elephantiasis) results.

NEOPLASMS OF VESSELS

BENIGN NEOPLASMS

Hemangioma
Hemangioma is common; 70% are present at birth.

- Skin, liver, and brain are common sites, but any organ may be involved.
- They are composed of well-formed vascular spaces lined by endothelial cells that snow no cytologic atypia.
- They are classified either as capillary hemangiomas, composed of vessels of capillary size; or cavernous hemangiomas, composed of large, thin-walled vascular spaces.

Pyogenic Granuloma
Pyogenic granuloma occurs in the skin and oral cavity, particularly during pregnancy or after trauma.

- Histologically, they are similar to capillary hemangiomas, but they often have ulcerated surfaces and are acutely inflamed.
- They present as polyps that grow rapidly to reach 1–2 cm in a few weeks, whereupon they may regress spontaneously.

Glomus Tumor (Glomangioma)
Glomangiomas are benign neoplasms arising in glomus cells, which are temperature receptor cells situated in small arterioles.

- They may occur anywhere in the skin, but are most common under the fingernails and toenails.
- They form small, firm, red-blue lesions that are extremely painful.
- Microscopically, they are composed of vascular spaces separated by nests of small, regular round cells.

Lymphangioma
Cavernous lymphangioma (also called cystic hygroma) is a benign tumor that occurs mainly in the neck in infancy, causing considerable enlargement of the neck.

- It can also occur in the mediastinum and retroperitoneum in adults.
- It can grow to large size, making complete surgical removal difficult.

MALIGNANT NEOPLASMS

Angiosarcoma (Hemangiosarcoma)
Angiosarcoma is a rare malignant neoplasm of endothelial cells, commonly occurring in skin, soft tissue, bone, liver, and breast.

- Hepatic angiosarcomas have been etiologically associated with thorium dioxide (Thorotrast), and vinyl chloride.
- They produce destructive, infiltrative mass lesions that metastasize early via the bloodstream.
- They usually present as large, hemorrhagic, rapidly growing masses.
- The prognosis is poor.

Kaposi's Sarcoma
Kaposi's sarcoma was a rare neoplasm in the United States until 1979, occurring mainly in elderly patients and involved the lower extremities as a slowly growing, localized, ulcerative skin lesion with a protracted course. Since 1979, Kaposi's sarcoma has occurred in epidemic proportions in patients with AIDS.

- Cases also occur in other immunocompromised patients, particularly after renal transplantation.
- Kaposi's sarcoma occurring in immunocompromised patients differs from that occurring in the elderly:
  - It is much more aggressive clinically.
  - It tends to disseminate and involve viscera such as intestine, lung, lymph nodes, and liver.
- The cause of Kaposi's sarcoma and how it is related to immune deficiency are unknown.

- Microscopically, it is an infiltrative lesion composed of spindle-shaped endothelial cells with slit-like spaces, erythrocyte extravasation, and hemosiderin deposition.
- Clinically it presents with purple patches, plaques, or nodules in the skin that may ulcerate; in the viscera, they appear as hemorrhagic masses.

Lymphangiosarcoma

Lymphangiosarcoma is a rare malignant neoplasm of lymphatic endothelium.

- It occurs with greatest frequency in patients who have been treated with radical mastectomy and radiation for breast carcinoma.
- The neoplasm grows rapidly and metastasizes early. Prognosis is poor.

The Heart: I. Manifestations of Cardiac Disease; Congenital Diseases

MANIFESTATIONS OF CARDIAC DISEASE

PAIN

Ischemic Pain
Myocardial ischemia is the commonest cause of cardiac pain. The pain is:

■ Caused by stimulation of nerve endings by lactic acid produced during anaerobic glycolysis.
■ Retrosternal and usually constricting.
■ May radiate to the back, to either arm (especially the left), or up the neck into the jaw.
■ Varies in severity from mild to excruciating.

Pericardial Pain
Pericardial pain is caused by inflammation of the parietal pericardium. The pain is:

■ Sharp, lower retrosternal.
■ Tends to vary with posture and respiration.
■ Often accompanied by signs of pericardial inflammation (such as pericardial rub and effusion).

CARDIAC ENLARGEMENT
Enlargement of the heart may result from dilatation of the cardiac chambers (eg, in heart failure, myocarditis) or hypertrophy of the walls (eg, in hypertension, many valvular defects). Cardiac enlargement:

■ Does not cause clinical symptoms.
■ Is a useful indication of the presence of cardiac disease.
■ May be recognized by clinical examination, radiography, or electrocardiography.

Note: Cardiac hypertrophy is assessed at autopsy by measuring the wall thickness; right ventricle thickness exceeding 0.5 cm and left ventricular thickness exceeding 1.5 cm constitutes hypertrophy.

ABNORMAL CARDIAC RHYTHM (Arrhythmia, Dysrhythmia)
Cardiac arrhythmias reflect altered activity of the SA node, ectopic foci that drive the heart at an accelerated or irregular rate, or conduction defects (Table 21–1). Clinically, arrhythmias may cause "missed beats" or palpitations.

TABLE 21–1. CLASSIFICATION OF CARDIAC ARRHYTHMIAS

Altered activity of the SA node
Sinus tachycardia
Sinus bradycardia
Sinus arrhythmia
Ectopic rhythms
Supraventricular (atrial or AV nodal)
Supraventricular extrasystoles
Paroxysmal supraventricular tachycardia
Atrial flutter
Atrial fibrillation
Ventricular
Ventricular extrasystoles
Ventricular tachycardia
Ventricular fibrillation
Heart block
Sinoatrial block (partial or complete)
Atrioventricular block (partial or complete)
Bundle branch block

Etiology

The principal cause of significant cardiac arrhythmia is ischemia. Other causes include:

- Infection (myocarditis).
- Inflammatory conditions (systemic lupus erythematosus, rheumatic fever, sarcoidosis).
- Drugs (digitalis, quinine derivatives, antidepressants, catecholamines, beta-blockers, calcium channel blockers).
- Electrolyte abnormalities (hyperkalemia).
- Endocrine disease (thyrotoxicosis).
- Congenital abnormalities of the conduction system.

Effects

- In bradyarrhythmias (slow heart rate), cardiac output falls when the reduction in heart rate cannot be compensated for by an increased stroke volume.
- In tachyarrhythmias (rapid rate), cardiac output may fall because of decreased ventricular filling resulting from shortened diastole.
- Acute heart failure is common in patients with ventricular tachyarrhythmias.
- Supraventricular tachyarrhythmias and incomplete heart block do not usually cause serious effects.
- Ventricular fibrillation and asystole result in cessation of effective ventricular ejection and causes rapid death.
- Ventricular tachycardia and complete heart block are serious arrhythmias associated with a variable decrease in cardiac output.

CARDIAC FAILURE

Cardiac failure is defined as the inability to maintain an adequate cardiac output despite normal venous return.

TABLE 21–2. COMMON CAUSES OF HEART FAILURE

Primarily left-sided
 Ischemic heart disease
 Hypertensive heart disease
 Aortic valve disease (stenosis, incompetence)
 Mitral valve disease (stenosis,[1] incompetence)
 Myocarditis
 Cardiomyopathy
 Cardiac amyloidosis
 High-output states (thyrotoxicosis, anemia, arteriovenous fistula)
Primarily right-sided
 Left-sided heart failure[2]
 Chronic pulmonary disease ("cor pulmonale")
 Pulmonary valve stenosis
 Tricuspid valve disease (stenosis, incompetence)
 Congenital heart disease (ventricular septal defect, patent ductus
  arteriosus)
 Pulmonary hypertension (primary and secondary)
 Massive pulmonary embolism

---

[1]Mitral stenosis produces functional failure of the left side of the heart; although the left ventricle itself is not in failure, the left atrium is.
[2]Left heart failure is the most common cause of right heart failure because of back pressure effects via the pulmonary circulation.

Etiology

Causes of cardiac failure are classified according to whether they produce predominantly left-sided or right-sided failure (Table 21–2).

Pathology & Clinical Effects

The effects of cardiac failure are:

- **"Forward failure,"** resulting from decreased cardiac output.
- **"Backward failure,"** due to accumulation of venous return within the heart (cardiac dilatation) or in the tissues draining to the heart (Fig 21–1).

A. Left-sided heart failure.
1. Acute cardiac arrest:

- Leads to sudden death.
- Is caused by ventricular asystole and ventricular fibrillation.

2. Acute severe decrease in output:

- May lead to cardiogenic shock.
- Causes decreased cardiac output that evokes reflex sympathetic stimulation, which results in tachycardia and vasoconstriction in skin (cold clammy extremities), muscle, intestine and kidney (pre-renal uremia).

3. Acute "backward" failure:

- Causes pulmonary edema.

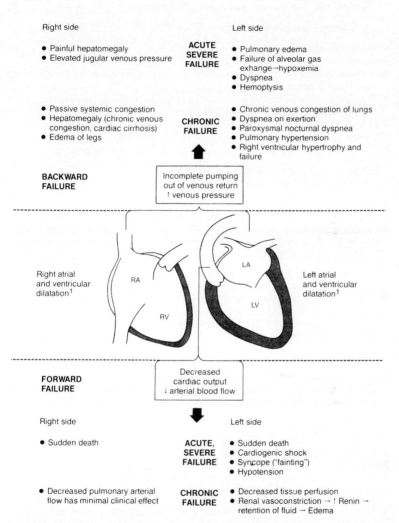

Figure 21–1. Effects of cardiac failure. **Note 1:** Dilatation partly represents a compensatory mechanism for increasing cardiac output. The stretching of myocardial fibers results in increased force of myocardial contraction.

■ Clinically, **pulmonary edema** results in dyspnea accompanied by cough productive of pink, frothy sputum, and crepitations on auscultation.

4. Chronic "backward" failure:

■ Causes **chronic pulmonary venous congestion** associated with thickening of the alveoli.
■ Produces dyspnea on exertion, orthopnea (dyspnea in the recumbent position), and paroxysmal nocturnal dyspnea.
■ Alveolar hemorrhage leads to accumulation of hemosiderin-laden macrophages in the alveoli, imparting a brown color to the lung ("brown induration of the lung").
■ Progressive fibrosis of the alveolar septa causes pulmonary hypertension which leads to right ventricular hypertrophy and right ventricular failure.
■ The commonest cause of right ventricular failure is left heart failure.

B. Right-sided heart failure.
1. Acute severe decrease in output:

■ Occurs most commonly in massive pulmonary embolism.
■ Results in circulatory arrest and **sudden death.**
■ **Cardiac tamponade** is another form of acute right heart failure caused by an increase in pericardial cavity pressure due to fluid accumulation that interferes with right ventricular diastolic filling.

2. Chronic "backward" failure:

■ Is manifested clinically by systemic venous congestion, which causes:
  ● Elevation of the jugular venous pressure.
  ● Liver enlargement due to centrizonal congestion.
  ● **Peripheral edema.**

C. Cardiac edema:

■ Occurs in both left and right heart failure.
  ● In left heart failure, edema fluid accumulates in the lungs.
  ● In right heart failure the fluid gravitates to the dependent systemic veins.
■ Is primarily the result of sodium and water retention in the kidneys.

CONGENITAL HEART DISEASE

Etiology
In most cases of congenital heart disease, there is no identifiable cause, and most congenital cardiac defects are not inherited.

■ Rubella infection of the fetus in the first trimester of pregnancy causes many cardiac anomalies.
■ Chromosomal abnormalities associated with cardiac anomalies include:
  ● **Down's syndrome** (trisomy 21)—20% of patients have defects of the atrioventricular valves or the atrial and ventricular septa.
  ● **Turner's syndrome** (45, XO) is associated with cardiac anomalies in about 20% of cases. Coarctation of the aorta is the commonest anomaly.
  ● **Trisomy 18** is associated with right ventricular origin of the aorta.

TABLE 21-3. CLASSIFICATION AND FREQUENCY[1] OF CONGENITAL HEART DISEASE

Without shunt (20%)	
Right-sided	
Pulmonary stenosis	10%
Ebstein's anomaly	Rare
Left-sided	
Coarctation of the aorta	10%
Aortic stenosis	Rare
Dextrocardia	Rare
With shunt (80%)	
Acyanotic	
Atrial septal defect	15%
Ventricular septal defect	25%
Patent ductus arteriosus	15%
Cyanotic	
Tetralogy of Fallot	10%
Transposition of great vessels	10%
Truncus arteriosus	Rare
Tricuspid atresia	Rare
Total anomalous pulmonary venous return	Rare
Hypoplastic left heart syndromes	Rare
Eisenmenger's syndrome[2]	Rare

[1] Relative frequencies of individual anomalies in children.
[2] The term "Eisenmenger's syndrome" is applied to the development of pulmonary hypertension and reversal of shunt direction in patients with atrial septal defect, ventricular septal defect, and patent ductus arteriosus. Surgery to close the defect in the presence of this degree of pulmonary hypertension has a high mortality rate.

- Drugs that cause cardiac anomalies when ingested by the mother during early pregnancy include:
  - Thalidomide.
  - Alcohol (fetal alcohol syndrome).

Classification (Table 21-3)
Congenital heart defects can occur in either side of the heart at the atrial, ventricular, or aortopulmonary level, and may or may not have a shunt.

ATRIAL SEPTAL DEFECT (ASD)

Ostium Secundum ASD
Ostium secundum ASD results from a defect in the development of the septum secundum.

- This is the most common type of ASD; it usually produces mild disease that is often not detected until adult life.
- In most cases, the defect is large enough (> 2 cm) to cause near equalization of left and right atrial pressure, with flow of blood from left to right through the ASD.
- Usually, pulmonary flow is increased to about twice that of systemic output, and the right ventricle is dilated and hypertrophied owing to the volume overload.
- Right ventricular failure is uncommon.

■ Clinically, there is:
  ● Right ventricular hypertrophy.
  ● Delayed pulmonary valve closure, causing a widely split second heart sound that does not vary with respiration ("fixed" split).
  ● Pulmonary ejection systolic murmur and loud pulmonary valve closure due to increased flow through the pulmonary valve.
■ The diagnosis is confirmed by cardiac catheterization, echocardiography, or isotope studies.
■ The main complication is the development of **pulmonary hypertension,** which may lead to:
  ● Right ventricular failure.
  ● Reversal of the shunt and cyanosis.

Ostium Primum ASD

Ostium primum ASD constitutes about 5% of all cases of ASD.

■ It is common in Down's syndrome.
■ It is characterized by a large defect in the lower part of the atrial septum, often associated with mitral valve lesions.
■ It produces severe disease in early childhood, with features of mitral incompetence superimposed on the ASD.

VENTRICULAR SEPTAL DEFECT (VSD)

VSD is the most commonly encountered cardiac anomaly in children. Most defects occur in the membranous part of the interventricular septum, just below the orifices of the semilunar valves.

Small VSD (Maladie de Roger)

Small VSDs (< 0.5 cm in diameter) produce a low-volume shunt from left to right ventricle during systole, which causes:

■ A loud pansystolic murmur heard best at the left sternal edge.
■ Slight increase in right ventricular pressure.
■ Entry of oxygenated blood into the right ventricle at cardiac catheterization.
■ Patients with small VSDs have few symptoms.
■ The defect tends to decrease in relative size as the heart grows, and may even close spontaneously.

Large VSD

A large VSD is much more serious, with clinical manifestations appearing in early childhood.

■ Initially, a large volume of blood is shunted from the left to the right ventricle during systole, producing a pansystolic murmur.
■ There is volume overload of both ventricles, leading to dilatation and hypertrophy of both ventricles.
■ Increased blood flow through the pulmonary circulation causes a loud pulmonary valve closure sound.
■ Pulmonary hypertension ensues leading to reduction in shunt volume and, finally, shunt reversal and cyanosis (Eisenmenger's syndrome).
■ Patients with both small and large VSD are at risk for infective endocarditis.

PATENT DUCTUS ARTERIOSUS (PDA)

At birth, the ductus closes normally by muscle spasm; permanent fibrotic occlusion is usually complete by 8 weeks. In premature infants, anatomic closure may be delayed several months.

- Indomethacin promotes the closure of a PDA.
- A **small PDA** leads to:
  - A small left-to-right shunt, continuous throughout the cardiac cycle, causing a typical continuous ("machinery") murmur.
  - Mild elevation of pulmonary artery pressure and minimal symptoms.
  - Entry of oxygenated blood at the pulmonary artery level during cardiac catheterization.
- A **large PDA** causes marked pulmonary hypertension and ultimately results in shunt reversal (Eisenmenger's syndrome).
- The patent ductus may be involved by a process analogous to infective endocarditis.

TETRALOGY OF FALLOT

This common cyanotic congenital cardiac anomaly is characterized by:

- A large ventricular septal defect.
- Stenosis of the pulmonary outflow tract.
- Dextroposition of the aorta, which overrides the right ventricle.
- Hypertrophy of the right ventricle.
- Right ventricular pressure is high and the shunt across the VSD is right-to-left, causing cyanosis.
- This is a severe defect that presents at birth with central cyanosis.
- The prognosis is very poor without treatment. With corrective surgery, normal survival is the rule.

The Heart: II. Endocardium & Cardiac Valves   **22**

DISEASES OF THE ENDOCARDIUM

ACUTE RHEUMATIC FEVER

Incidence
Acute rheumatic fever occurs in children, commonly between ages 5 and 15.

- It is more common among children of lower socioeconomic background and is still prevalent in underdeveloped countries.
- In the United States and Western Europe, there has been a marked decline in acute rheumatic fever in the past 2 decades.

Etiology
Rheumatic fever is believed to be an immunologic hypersensitivity reaction to streptococcal antigens.

- It occurs 2–6 weeks after streptococcal infection.
- Most serologic types of group A *Streptococcus* that cause pharyngitis have been associated with acute rheumatic fever, but less than 5% of patients with streptococcal pharyngitis develop rheumatic fever.
- Rarely, the disease follows streptococcal infections of the skin.
- Patients with histocompatibility antigen **HLA-B5** have an increased susceptibility.

Pathogenesis
The exact relationship between streptococcal infection and cardiac injury is unknown.

- Streptococcal cultures of affected heart tissue are negative.
- High levels of antistreptococcal antibodies (antistreptolysin O, anti-DNAse, antihyaluronidase) are commonly found in patients who develop rheumatic fever.
- Evidence exists for both types II and III hypersensitivity as the mechanism of injury.
- Immunoglobulin and complement can be demonstrated in myocardial fiber membrane.
- Cross-reacting antibodies with activity against both streptococcal protein and myocardial sarcolemma are present in the sera of some patients.
- Circulating immune complexes are present in some patients.

Clinical Features

- Rheumatic fever has a sudden onset with high fever and one or more of the following major features:

- **Carditis,** which is the most serious manifestation and occurs in about 30% of patients with a first attack of rheumatic fever.
- **Polyarthritis** occurs in 75% of patients; it is commonly migratory with asymmetric involvement of large joints.
- **Chorea,** which is characterized by random jerky, involuntary movements due to involvement of the basal ganglia.
- **Skin lesions,** including erythema marginatum and **erythema nodosum.**
- Subcutaneous nodules, which occur mainly over bony prominences in the extremities.

Pathology of Carditis
Cardiac involvement involves all layers of the heart (**pancarditis**).

- Endocarditis occurs in all patients with rheumatic carditis, whereas myocarditis and pericarditis are present only in severe cases.
- The **Aschoff body,** consisting of histiocyte aggregates, is diagnostic of rheumatic fever. Aschoff bodies occur in the subendocardial region and the myocardial interstitium.
- Endocarditis (*valvulitis*) is characterized by:
  - Maximal involvement of the valvular endocardium.
  - More severe and more frequent involvement of the valves of the left side, and the mitral valve more than the aortic.
  - Edema and denudation of the lining endocardium, particularly at the line of apposition of the free edge of the valve. Clinically, transient murmurs result from valve edema.
  - Formation of small, firmly adherent platelet-fibrin thrombi (**rheumatic vegetations**) in areas of endocardial damage.
- Myocarditis is characterized by:
  - Edema and the presence of numerous Aschoff bodies in the myocardium.
  - Tachycardia and dilatation of the heart.
  - Cardiac failure, which occurs in a small number of cases.
- Pericarditis is usually fibrinous, but with significant effusion in a small number of patients.

Sequelae
A. Immediate:

- The great majority of patients recover completely from the acute attack, usually within 6 weeks.
- Less than 5% die in the acute phase of severe myocarditis (heart failure and arrhythmia).

B. Recurrences:

- Are likely in a patient who has recovered from an attack of rheumatic fever.
- Greatly increase the risk of later development of chronic rheumatic heart disease.

C. Chronic rheumatic heart disease tends to follow recurrent acute episodes of
rheumatic fever by a variable interval (2–20 years).

- It may occur in patients with no history of an acute episode.
- Fibrosis of the valve with fusion of the commissures leads to **valve stenosis.**
- Severe destruction of the valve apparatus causes **valve incompetence.**
- The mitral valve is the only affected valve in 50% of cases. Combined mitral and aortic valve lesions are present in 40%, with additional involvement of the tricuspid valve in a few cases. Pulmonary valve involvement is rare.
- Fibrosis of nonvalvular endocardium is most common in the posterior left atrium (MacCallum's patch).

Prognosis

The prognosis of rheumatic fever is determined by:

- The severity of the acute illness.
- Whether or not there is cardiac involvement, since all other manifestations, including chorea, resolve completely.
- Whether or not there are recurrences.

SYSTEMIC LUPUS ERYTHEMATOSUS (SLE)

The heart is involved in 10–20% of cases of SLE. The immune complex–mediated injury may involve any layer of the heart.

- SLE is one of the most common causes of **acute pericarditis** in the United States.
- SLE **(Libman-Sacks) endocarditis** is characterized by multiple small, flat vegetations on the mitral and tricuspid valves.
- SLE valvulitis is rarely severe enough to cause valve dysfunction.

INFECTIVE ENDOCARDITIS

Classification

It is customary to classify infective endocarditis as acute or subacute; there is, however, considerable overlap. It is more important to identify the causative infectious agent (Table 22–1).

A. Acute infective endocarditis: This most severe form of infective endocarditis is less common than the subacute variety. It is caused by virulent organisms, most commonly *Staphylococcus aureus*, *Streptococcus pneumoniae*, and *Neisseria gonorrhoeae*.

- These organisms can infect healthy valves.
- It is associated with destruction of the affected valves and severe bacteremia.

B. Subacute infective endocarditis:

- Is more common than acute endocarditis.
- Is caused by organisms of low virulence such as *Streptococcus viridans*, *Streptococcus faecalis*, *Staphylococcus epidermidis*, and *Candida albicans*.
- Usually occurs in a previously damaged valve.
- Is a chronic illness characterized by low grade bacteremia, often developing over weeks to months, and commonly presenting as fever of unknown origin.
- Valvular destruction is less severe than in acute endocarditis.

TABLE 22–1. ORGANISMS MOST COMMONLY CAUSING INFECTIVE ENDOCARDITIS[1]

	Usual Clinical Picture	
	Acute	Subacute
Staphylococcus aureus, Streptococcus pyogenes, Neisseria gonorrhoeae, Proteus, Pseudomonas	███████████	██
Bacteroides, Escherichia coli, Klebsiella	████	███
Staphylococcus epidermidis, Streptococcus viridans, Streptococcus pneumoniae, Streptococcus faecalis, Haemophilus, Listeria, Candida albicans, Histoplasma, Aspergillus, Rickettsia		██████████

[1]S aureus causes more than 50% of acute cases, S viridans more than 50% of subacute cases. Many other organisms are occasionally causative.

Pathogenesis

Bacteremia (or fungemia) is the first requirement for the onset of infective endocarditis, and commonly occurs in the following circumstances:

- Following oral surgical procedures, including dentistry (usually S viridans).
- Following urologic procedures such as bladder catheterization (commonly S faecalis and gram-negative enteric bacilli).
- With intravenous drug abuse (commonly S aureus).

Endocardial injury is necessary for less virulent organisms, which can only infect previously abnormal endocardium. Precursor diseases are:

- **Chronic rheumatic heart disease,** most commonly mitral incompetence and aortic valve disease. Most cases of subacute endocarditis occur in patients with chronic rheumatic heart disease.
- **Congenital heart disease,** most often a small ventricular septal defect or bicuspid aortic valve.
- **Degenerative valvular disease,** such as calcific valves and mitral valve prolapse syndrome, are rarely complicated by infective endocarditis.
- Prosthetic cardiac valves frequently become infected. C albicans and staphylococci are common causes of prosthetic valve endocarditis.

Pathology

Infected thrombi (vegetations) on the endocardial surface, often on valves, are the characteristic findings in infective endocarditis.

- Vegetations of infective endocarditis are multiple, large, friable, and loosely attached. They commonly become detached from the valve as emboli.

VEGETATION

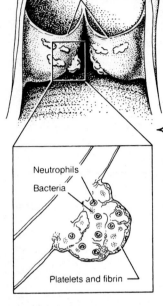

EFFECTS

Valve distortion
- Changing murmurs

Valve perforation
- Acute valvular incompetence

Bacteremia
- Splenomegaly
- Fever, malaise, weight loss
- Microabscesses (with virulent organisms)
- Involvement of viscera
- Pustular skin rashes

Immune complexes
- Osler's nodes (tender red nodules)
- Janeway lesions (red papules in palms and soles)
- Proliferative glomerulonephritis
- Vasculitis, arthritis

Emboli
- Focal embolic glomerulonephritis
- Petechial hemorrhages
  - In nail bed (splinter hemorrhages)
  - In retina (Roth's spots)
  - Cutaneous
- Mycotic aneurysms
- Microinfarcts
  - CNS dysfunction
  - Intestinal pain
  - Myocardial ischemia
  - Lung: hemoptysis

Laboratory tests
- Positive blood culture (95%)
- Leukocytosis, chronic anemia
- ↑ ESR
- Hyperglobulinemia
- ↓ Complement levels

Figure 22–1. Clinical effects of infective endocarditis resulting from infection and formation of vegetations on the valve.

■ Vegetations occur principally on the valves of the left side of the heart, mitral > aortic > tricuspid > pulmonary.

Right-sided endocarditis is uncommon but may occur in:

■ Intravenous drug abusers.
■ Patients with indwelling venous catheters extending into the right atrium.
■ Gonococcal endocarditis.
■ Endocarditis complicating ventricular septal defect.

Clinical Features (Fig 22–1)
A. Bacteremia (or fungemia):

■ Blood culture is positive in over 95% of cases and is the most important diagnostic test.

- Most patients have constant bacteremia; a few have intermittent bacteremia.
- Multiple blood cultures must be drawn at intervals before antibiotics are given.
- Fever is the most common symptom. It is low-grade and persistent in subacute endocarditis and high with rigors in acute disease.
- Bacteremia also causes **splenomegaly, petechial hemorrhages** in the skin, retina (Roth spots), and nails ("splinter hemorrhages").
- Weight loss, finger clubbing and chronic anemia also occur in subacute disease.
- With virulent pyogenic organisms, **miliary abscesses** occur in all organs of the body.

B. Circulating immune complexes formed by combination of antibodies and bacterial antigens lead to:

- Focal or diffuse proliferative glomerulonephritis. Microscopic hematuria and proteinuria occur in over 50% of patients.
- Erythematous papules on the palms and soles (Janeway lesions) and tender red nodules on the fingers or toes (Osler's nodes).

C. Valvular dysfunction resulting from the presence of vegetations and valve destruction manifests as:

- **Cardiac murmurs** that change in character as the vegetations enlarge and fragment.
- **Valve perforation,** causing acute mitral and aortic incompetence.

D. Emboli due to detachment of the friable vegetations are common, and lead to:

- Infarction in the brain, kidney, heart, intestine, spleen, and extremities when systemic with left-sided lesions.
- Pulmonary involvement when right sided.
- **Mycotic aneurysms** in the artery at the site of lodgement, due to infection.

Differential Diagnosis (Table 22–2)
Infective endocarditis must be distinguished from other noninfective causes of endocarditis in which vegetations occur, including:

- Acute rheumatic fever.
- Collagen diseases such as systemic lupus erythematosus.
- Noninfective thrombotic endocarditis.

NONINFECTIVE ENDOCARDITIS
Noninfective endocarditis was originally described as occurring in terminally ill patients (**marantic endocarditis**).

- It may occur early in the course of many diseases, notably cancer.
- The vegetations occur mainly on the mitral and aortic valves and are commonly large and friable, and may become detached as systemic emboli.

NEOPLASMS OF THE ENDOCARDIUM

CARDIAC MYXOMA
Cardiac myxoma is a benign neoplasm of endocardial mesenchymal cells.

TABLE 22–2. DIFFERENTIAL FEATURES OF DISEASES IN WHICH VALVE VEGETATIONS AND PLAQUES OCCUR

	Infective Endocarditis	Rheumatic Fever	Systemic Lupus Erythematosus	Noninfective Endocarditis	Carcinoid Syndrome
Vegetation size	Large	Small	Small	Medium	Plaques
Valves affected	Mitral, aortic	Mitral, aortic	Mitral	Mitral, aortic	Pulmonary, tricuspid
Site	Leaflet	Free edge	Atrial and ventricular surfaces	Leaflet	Both surfaces
Embolism	+++	–	–	+	–
Acute inflammatory cells	+	–	–	+	–
Organisms	+++	–	–	–	–
Valve destruction	++	–	–	–	–
Valve fibrosis	–	+++	–	–	+

- Although rare, it is by far the commonest primary neoplasm of the heart.
- It occurs almost exclusively in the atria, particularly the left atrium.
- Grossly, it appears as a firm, gelatinous polypoid mass that protrudes into the lumen of the heart.
- Microscopically, it is composed of small stellate cells embedded in an abundant mucopolysaccharide stroma.
- Clinical features include:
  - Irregular, prolonged fever, weight loss, anemia, and increased plasma globulin levels.
  - Systemic embolism, resulting from detachment of fragments of the neoplasm.
  - Mitral orifice obstruction, causing sudden death.
  - Mid-diastolic murmur that resembles mitral stenosis.

DISORDERS OF CARDIAC VALVES

MITRAL STENOSIS

Etiology
Mitral stenosis is almost always the result of chronic rheumatic heart disease. Females are affected more than males in a ratio of 9:1.

Pathophysiology
There is resistance to blood flow through the stenotic mitral valve during diastole, which causes a mid-diastolic murmur with presystolic accentuation.

- Closure of the abnormal mitral valve produces a loud first sound.
- The abnormal valve opens after aortic valve closure with an abnormal clicking sound (opening snap).
- Severity is directly proportional to the length of the diastolic murmur and inversely related to the interval between the second heart sound and the opening snap.
- There is left atrial dilatation and hypertrophy.
- Blood tends to stagnate in the left atrium, predisposing to thrombus formation which may lead to:
  - Systemic embolism.
  - Obstruction of the narrowed mitral orifice, causing sudden death ("ball-valve thrombus").
- Pulmonary venous pressure is increased and may cause:
  - Acute pulmonary edema.
  - Pulmonary hemorrhage with hemoptysis.
  - Interstitial fibrosis, pulmonary arterial hypertension, and right ventricular hypertrophy.
- With severe stenosis, left ventricular end-diastolic volume and cardiac output are decreased.

MITRAL INCOMPETENCE

Etiology
Rheumatic heart disease accounts for about 50% of cases of mitral incompetence, usually associated with mitral stenosis.

- **Mitral valve prolapse ("floppy valve") syndrome:**
  - Is a degenerative change that is present in about 1% of the population (especially young women).
  - Results from accumulation of mucopolysaccharides in the valve leaflet, causing ballooning of the valve.
  - Causes mitral incompetence in a small percentage of patients.
- Chronic left ventricular failure with dilatation of the mitral valve ring may cause functional mitral incompetence.
- Acute mitral incompetence may occur with rupture of chordae tendineae due to:
  - **Infective endocarditis.**
  - Trauma.
  - Rupture of papillary muscles due to **myocardial infarction.**

Pathophysiology

Regurgitation of blood from the left ventricle to the atrium occurs throughout systole, producing a typical pansystolic murmur.

- Flow across the mitral valve during diastole is increased, producing a third heart sound and a diastolic flow murmur.
- The left ventricle is dilated and hypertrophied.
- The left atrium is also dilated, and left atrial pressure and pulmonary venous pressure are increased.
- Acute mitral valve incompetence produces pulmonary edema and acute left heart failure.
- Chronic mitral incompetence causes pulmonary fibrosis, pulmonary arterial hypertension, and right ventricular hypertrophy followed by failure.

AORTIC STENOSIS

Etiology

Rheumatic aortic stenosis is commonly accompanied by mitral valve defects.

- **Congenital bicuspid aortic valves** may undergo progressive fibrosis and calcification, which is the cause of more than 50% of isolated aortic stenosis.
- **Calcification of the valve in the elderly** is a rare cause.
- **Congenital narrowing of the left ventricular outflow tract** above or below the aortic valve produces the same defect as aortic stenosis.
- **Hypertrophic cardiomyopathy** may also obstruct the left ventricular outflow tract (subvalvular stenosis).

Pathophysiology

Turbulent flow through the stenotic valve produces a rough ejection systolic murmur.

- Decreased flow of blood through the aortic valve causes:
  - Hypotension and syncopal attacks.
  - Soft aortic valve closure.
  - A low-volume pulse.
- Decreased coronary perfusion may cause myocardial ischemia with angina pectoris and myocardial infarction.
- Left ventricular hypertrophy and **left ventricular failure** are common.

AORTIC INCOMPETENCE

Etiology
Rheumatic heart disease accounts for about 50% of cases of aortic incompetence. In most of these cases, there is associated mitral valve disease.

- **Syphilis,** once a common cause of isolated aortic incompetence, now accounts for less than 10% of cases.
- **Ankylosing spondylitis** causes about 5% of cases of isolated aortic incompetence.
- **Rupture of the aortic valve** with blunt chest trauma and infective endocarditis causes acute aortic incompetence.
- **Myxomatous degeneration** of the aortic valve is being recognized as a possible cause.

Pathophysiology
Regurgitation of blood across the incompetent aortic valve occurs in diastole, producing a decrescendo early diastolic murmur.

- The systolic blood pressure is elevated as a result of increased left ventricular output.
- The diastolic blood pressure is markedly decreased, sometimes to zero.
- The increased pulse pressure causes the typical bounding ("water-hammer") pulse and capillary pulsations.
- The left ventricle undergoes massive dilatation and hypertrophy. Left ventricular failure is common.

PULMONARY VALVE LESIONS

Etiology
Congenital pulmonary valve stenosis is the commonest cause of isolated pulmonary stenosis. Pulmonary stenosis also occurs in Fallot's tetralogy.

- **Carcinoid syndrome** is associated with both pulmonary and tricuspid valve stenosis in about 50% of cases.
- **Pulmonary incompetence** is rare, and most often due to valve ring dilatation in right heart failure.

Pathophysiology
Pulmonary stenosis causes:

- A rough **ejection systolic murmur** over the pulmonary valve.
- Delayed closure of the pulmonary valve.
- Very soft pulmonary valve closure.

Note: Right ventricular hypertrophy and failure occur in both pulmonary stenosis and incompetence.

TRICUSPID VALVE LESIONS
Tricuspid incompetence is usually due to right ventricular dilatation in right heart failure.

- It causes a pulsatile jugular venous pulse and pulsatile enlargement of the liver.
- Tricuspid valve lesions rarely occur in chronic rheumatic heart disease, almost always with mitral and aortic valve lesions.
- Tricuspid stenosis may occur in carcinoid syndrome.

The Heart: III. Myocardium & Pericardium

23

I. DISEASES OF THE MYOCARDIUM

ISCHEMIC HEART DISEASE

Incidence
Ischemic heart disease is responsible for 500,000 deaths a year in the United States (25–30% of all deaths) and is the leading cause of death in most developed countries.

Etiology
Ischemic heart disease is caused by narrowing of one or more of the three major coronary artery branches (Fig 23–1).

- **Atherosclerosis** accounts for 98% of cases. The risk factors for ischemic heart disease are those for atherosclerosis (Chapter 20).
- Other rare causes of coronary artery narrowing include:
  - Spasm (Prinzmetal angina).
  - Embolism, most commonly in infective endocarditis.
  - Ostial narrowing in syphilis and Takayasu's aortitis.
  - Ostial occlusion in aortic dissection.
  - Arteritis involving the coronary arteries, including polyarteritis nodosa, thromboangiitis obliterans, and giant cell arteritis.

Clinical Features (Fig 23–2)

MYOCARDIAL INFARCTION

Incidence

- Approximately 1.25 million people in the United States suffer a myocardial infarction every year. Of these, 35–40% die.
- Most patients are over 45 years of age, and men are affected three times more frequently than women.

Etiology
Most patients have severe atherosclerotic narrowing of one or more coronary arteries.

- A fresh thrombus overlying an atherosclerotic plaque is found in 40–90% of cases.
- In cases where no thrombosis occurs, infarction may be precipitated by:
  - Increased myocardial demand for oxygen (during exercise and excitement).

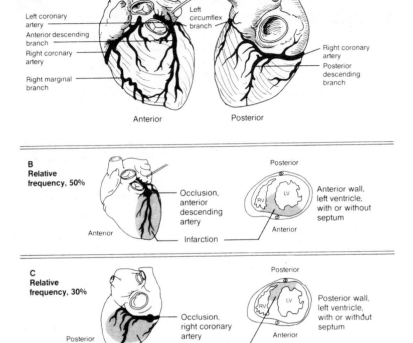

A
Normal blood supply

Left coronary artery

Anterior descending branch

Right coronary artery

Right marginal branch

Left circumflex branch

Right coronary artery

Posterior descending branch

Anterior   Posterior

B
Relative frequency, 50%

Anterior

Occlusion, anterior descending artery

Infarction

Posterior

RV   LV

Anterior

Anterior wall, left ventricle, with or without septum

C
Relative frequency, 30%

Posterior

Occlusion, right coronary artery

Infarction

Posterior

RV   LV

Anterior

Posterior wall, left ventricle, with or without septum

D
Relative frequency, 20%

Anterior

Occlusion, left circumflex artery

Infarction

Posterior

RV   LV

Anterior

Lateral wall, left ventricle

Figure 23–1. Blood supply to the myocardium (**A**) and areas of infarction resulting from the most frequent sites of coronary artery occlusion (relative frequency expressed as a percentage). The exact area of myocardium affected will vary depending on normal anatomic variation in blood supply and the extent of collateral circulation that exists at the time of coronary occlusion.

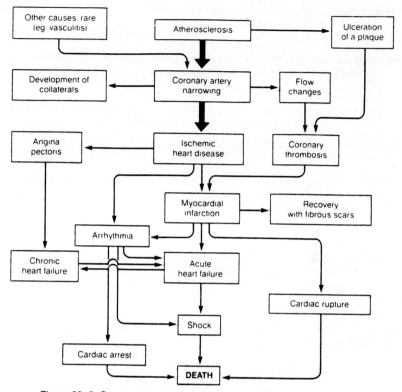

Figure 23–2. Causes and clinical consequences of ischemic heart disease.

- Reduction of coronary blood flow due to cardiac slowing during sleep.
- Segmental muscular spasm of coronary arteries.

Distribution of Infarction (Fig 23–1)

Infarction involves principally the left ventricle, interventricular septum, and conducting system.

- The atria and right ventricle are rarely involved.
- The distribution of infarction depends on which vessel is occluded. However, because collaterals develop in a chronically narrowed coronary circulation, infarction may occur in unexpected sites.
- Infarcts may be transmural, or subendocardial.

Pathology

For 2 hours after the onset of myocardial infarction there are no morphologic changes.

- At 2–4 hours, electron microscopic changes appear (swelling of mitochondria, endoplasmic reticulum, fragmentation of myofibrils).
- Light microscopic changes may appear in 4–6 hours, but are rarely detectable with certainty before 12–24 hours.
- **Coagulative necrosis** of the necrotic fibers is recognized by nuclear pyknosis, dark pink staining and loss of striations in the cytoplasm.

Clinical Features

Ischemic pain is the dominant symptom of myocardial infarction. It is a tightening, retrosternal pain that is not relieved by rest or vasodilators.

- Rarely, myocardial infarction may occur without pain ("silent infarction").
- The onset of pain is sudden and may occur during exercise, excitement, rest, or even sleep.
- Pain is often accompanied by sweating, changes in heart rate (due to autonomic stimulation), and hypotension.
- Fever and neutrophil leukocytosis are common.
- The diagnosis of myocardial infarction is made by:
  - Electrocardiography, which shows elevation of the ST segment, T wave inversion and, in transmural infarction, an abnormal Q wave.
  - Serum enzyme changes (Fig 23–3). Creatine kinase (CK)-MB isoenzyme and lactic acid dehydrogenase-isoenzyme 1 (LDH-1) levels are elevated.

Complications
A. Tachyrrhythmias:

- Occur in about 70% of cases, mainly during the first few hours after infarction.
- Ventricular extrasystoles are common.

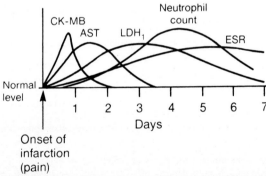

Figure 23–3. Changes in serum enzymes, neutrophil count, and erythrocyte sedimentation rates (ESR) following acute myocardial infarction. The serum level of MB isoenzyme of creatine kinase (CK-MB) rises rapidly, and CK-MB elevation is the test of choice in the first 24 hours. Since CK-MB levels return to baseline rapidly, isoenzyme 1 of lactate dehydrogenase (LDH$_1$) is the test of choice from 2 to 7 days. A test combination that includes CK-MB and LDH$_1$ is extremely effective in the diagnosis of acute myocardial infarction. Aspartate aminotransferase (AST) is of limited usefulness because of its lack of specificity, AST being present also in high concentration in liver and skeletal muscle.

- Ventricular tachycardia is less common, but can lead to acute left ventricular failure.
- Ventricular fibrillation is the most serious symptom, as it causes cardiac arrest and sudden death.
- The occurrence of tachyarrhythmias bears no relationship to the size of the infarct.

B. Heart block:

- Occurs more commonly with posterior infarcts.
- Is usually temporary, due to involvement of the conducting fibers by edema around an infarct.
- When permanent, is due to necrosis of the conducting fibers (less common).

C. Acute left ventricular failure:

- Results from arrhythmia or massive necrosis of myocardium.
- May cause sudden death, cardiogenic shock, and acute pulmonary edema.

D. Progressive infarction:

- Extension of infarction to adjacent muscle is uncommon, but may be precipitated by exercise, emotional stress, extension of the thrombus, or decreased cardiac output.
- Progression of an infarct can be diagnosed by following the serum CK-MB levels.

E. Pericarditis:

- Fibrinous or hemorrhagic pericarditis occurs in about 30% of cases.
- Usually occurs within the first few days after infarction.
- Rarely, may occur later in the recovery phase.

F. Systemic embolism from mural thrombi:

- Involvement of the endocardium leads to the formation of mural thrombi over the area of infarction.
- Mural thrombi may produce systemic embolism.

G. Myocardial rupture:

- Rupture of the necrotic muscle may involve:
  - The surface, producing hemopericardium and death from cardiac tamponade.
  - The interventricular septum, producing an acute ventricular septal defect, with a left-to-right shunt and acute right ventricular failure.
  - The papillary muscles producing acute mitral incompetence and left ventricular failure.

H. Ventricular aneurysm:

- Is a paradoxical outward bulging of the area of infarction during systole.
- May develop either in the first 2 weeks or after several months in the healed infarct.
- May cause left ventricular failure.
- Mural thrombi forming in an aneurysm may become detached as systemic emboli.

ANGINA PECTORIS

Angina pectoris is defined as episodic ischemic cardiac pain not associated with myocardial infarction.

Angina of Effort

This is a common disorder usually caused by severe atherosclerotic narrowing of the coronary arterial system.

- Pain is precipitated by exercise, stress, or excitement, and is relieved by resting or by vasodilators.
- Pathologic changes associated with angina are variable. Diffuse myocardial fibrosis is common.
- Serum enzyme levels are not elevated.
- ECG does not show changes of acute injury. Nonspecific ST depression and T wave inversion are common.
- Electrocardiography during carefully graded exercise (treadmill test) is a sensitive method for detecting ischemic heart disease.
- Patients with angina of effort have an increased risk of myocardial infarction.

Variant Angina (Prinzmetal's angina)

Prinzmetal's angina is uncommon and occurs independently of atherosclerosis.

- Pain occurs at rest and is not related to myocardial work.
- It is believed to be caused by coronary artery muscle spasm.
- Myocardial infarction is very rare.

SUDDEN DEATH

Sudden death is a well-recognized occurrence in patients whose only abnormality is severe coronary atherosclerosis.

- It has been attributed to **ventricular fibrillation.**
- Many patients who die suddenly are heavy smokers.

CARDIAC ARRHYTHMIAS

Ventricular arrhythmias commonly occur in ischemic heart disease. Ventricular fibrillation, ventricular tachycardia, and complete heart block may lead to cardiac failure or sudden death.

CARDIAC FAILURE

Chronic left ventricular failure may occur with or without a history of infarction or angina.

- Electrocardiography commonly shows nonspecific T wave inversion.
- Pathologic examination shows atherosclerotic narrowing of the coronary arteries and diffuse myocardial fibrosis.

MYOCARDITIS & CARDIOMYOPATHY

These are a group of diseases that involve the myocardium in the absence of hypertensive, congenital, ischemic, or valvular heart disease.

- **Myocarditis** denotes an acute myocardial disease characterized by inflammation.
- **Cardiomyopathy** is a more chronic condition in which inflammatory features are not conspicuous.

MYOCARDITIS

Incidence
Myocarditis is rare. Its exact incidence is difficult to establish. It is recorded as the cause of death in autopsy studies in less than 1% of cases.

Etiology
A. Infectious myocarditis:

- **Viruses** are believed to be the most common cause of myocarditis in developed countries. Coxsackie B virus is most common. Others include mumps, influenza, echo, polio, varicella, and measles.
- Myocarditis may be seen in **rickettsial diseases** such as Q fever, typhus, and Rocky Mountain spotted fever.
- **Diphtheritic** myocarditis is caused by an exotoxin.
- **American trypanosomiasis** (Chagas' disease) is endemic in South America, where it is a common cause of myocarditis.
- Myocarditis occurs in the acute phase of trichinosis and disseminated toxoplasmosis.

B. Autoimmune (hypersensitivity) myocarditis occurs in autoimmune diseases such as rheumatic fever, rheumatoid arthritis, systemic lupus erythematosus, progressive systemic sclerosis, and polyarteritis nodosa.
C. Toxic myocarditis includes:

- Alcoholic myocarditis.
- Drug-induced myocarditis caused by doxorubicin, rubidomycin, cyclophosphamide, hydralazine, phenytoin, procainamide, and the tricyclic antidepressants.

D. Sarcoidosis and radiation may be complicated by myocarditis.
E. Idiopathic myocarditis:

- Occurs without known cause.
- Is sometimes characterized by diffuse inflammation with numerous multinucleated giant cells (Fiedler's myocarditis).

Pathology
In acute myocarditis, the heart is dilated and flabby, and pale.

- Microscopically, there is edema, hyperemia, and infiltration by lymphocytes, plasma cells, and eosinophils.
- Chronic myocarditis is a controversial entity characterized by cardiac failure, ventricular hypertrophy, and the presence of lymphocytes and plasma cells in the interstitium.

Clinical Features
The onset is acute, with fever, chest pain, leukocytosis, and elevation of the erythrocyte sedimentation rate. It is commonly complicated by:

- Acute left ventricular failure.

- Arrhythmias that include extrasystoles, atrial and ventricular tachycardia, and atrial and ventricular fibrillation.
- Partial and complete heart block.
- Electrocardiography shows injury potentials in the ST segment.
- Serum creatine kinase, lactate dehydrogenase, and aspartate transaminase levels are increased.

CARDIOMYOPATHIES

Cardiomyopathies are primary myocardial diseases characterized by a chronic course and minimal features of inflammation. They should be suspected in a young, normotensive patient who develops cardiac failure in the absence of congenital, valvular, or ischemic heart disease.

Incidence & Etiology

Cardiomyopathies are rare. They may be familial or sporadic. In most cases, no cause can be found (**idiopathic**). They may occur in:

- Chronic alcoholism.
- Cardiac amyloidosis.
- Hemochromatosis.
- Endocrine disorders like hypothyroidism and thyrotoxicosis.
- Beriberi (thiamine deficiency).
- Storage diseases (glycogen storage diseases, mucopolysaccharidoses).
- Neuromuscular disorders (Friedreich's ataxas, muscular dystrophies).

Classification

A. Congestive cardiomyopathy is characterized by failure of the ventricle to empty in systole.

- Ventricular end-systolic and diastolic volumes are increased, causing bilateral ventricular dilatation and failure.
- Arrhythmias are common and sometimes cause sudden death.
- Histologic features are nonspecific, having irregular atrophy and hypertrophy of myocardial fibers with progressive fibrosis.
- Most cases are sporadic (10% are familial) and most have no detectable cause (**idiopathic congestive cardiomyopathy**).
- A few cases are associated with hypothyroidism, hyperthyroidism, hemochromatosis, thiamine deficiency, alcoholism, neuromuscular diseases, and late pregnancy (**peripartal cardiomyopathy**).

B. Hypertrophic cardiomyopathy is characterized by marked hypertrophy of the ventricular muscle with resistance to diastolic filling.

- **Asymmetric septal hypertrophy** (also called hypertrophic obstructive cardiomyopathy, or HOCM) is characterized by hypertrophy of the left ventricular outflow tract, causing subvalvular aortic stenosis.
- Twenty to thirty percent of cases of hypertrophic cardiomyopathy are familial; in some of these there is an autosomal dominant inheritance pattern.

C. Restrictive cardiomyopathy is characterized by decreased compliance of the ventricular muscle, increased resistance to filling, and cardiac failure. Many cases are due to cardiac amyloidosis.

D. Obliterative cardiomyopathy is characterized by

- Marked subendocardial fibrosis, resulting in encroachment of the lumen, decreased ventricular filling, and cardiac failure.
- Endocardial fibroelastosis, in which collagen and elastic tissue is laid down beneath the endocardium occurs in infancy.
- Endomyocardial fibrosis is an acquired disease common in Africa in which there is fibrosis of the endocardium and inner myocardium.

II. DISEASES OF THE PERICARDIUM

ACUTE PERICARDITIS

Etiology

A. Infectious acute pericarditis:

- Viral pericarditis is caused by coxsackievirus B, echovirus, and the agents of mumps, infectious mononucleosis (Epstein-Barr virus), and influenza.
- Acute idiopathic pericarditis:
  - Is very similar clinically to viral pericarditis.
  - Occurs in young adults and commonly follows a respiratory viral infection by 2–3 weeks.
  - Is self-limited, with recovery in 1–2 weeks.
- Tuberculosis pericarditis is due to direct spread of infection from a caseous mediastinal lymph node.
- Pyogenic pericarditis is usually caused by direct spread from a suppurative focus in the lung or pleura. *Streptococcus pneumoniae,* staphylococci, and gram-negative bacilli are the common causes.

B. Noninfectious acute pericarditis frequently complicates:

- Acute rheumatic fever.
- Myocardial infarction.
- Chronic renal failure (uremia).
- Connective tissue diseases such as systemic lupus erythematosus and rheumatoid arthritis.
- Malignant neoplasms.
- After radiation, cardiac trauma and cardiac surgery.
- Pericarditis occurring 2–3 weeks after myocardial infarction (Dressler's syndrome) probably has a hypersensitivity basis.

Pathology
The pericardial surface is reddened and roughened by adherent clumps of fibrin and neutrophils ("bread and butter appearance").

- Effusion varies from minimal ("dry," or fibrinous, pericarditis) to significant.
- Hemorrhagic effusions commonly occur in renal failure, malignant neoplasms, and tuberculosis.

Clinical Features

- It presents with pericardial pain and a pericardial rub.
- Effusion causes cardiac enlargement, dullness to percussion, and muffled heart sounds.
- With large effusions, diastolic filling is imparied (cardiac tamponade).

Diagnosis
Pericarditis can be diagnosed clinically by the presence of a pericardial rub or effusion.

- An effusion can be confirmed by chest X-ray and echocardiography.
- The etiology is diagnosed by examination of aspirated pericardial fluid (culture and cytologic examination).

CHRONIC ADHESIVE PERICARDITIS
Recovery from acute pericarditis frequently produces fibrous plaques ("milk spots") in the visceral pericardium or adhesions between the two pericardial layers. It is of no clinical significance.

CHRONIC CONSTRICTIVE PERICARDITIS
Chronic constrictive pericarditis is an uncommon disease.

- In most cases the cause is not known; immunologic mechanisms may account for most idiopathic cases.
- Tuberculosis and pyogenic infections were common causes in the past.
- It is characterized by encasement of the heart in a greatly thickened fibrotic pericardium. Chronic inflammatory cells and dystrophic calcification are common.
- The fibrous pericardium constricts the cardiac chambers, reducing right atrial filling and causing:
  - Elevation of jugular venous pressure.
  - Decreased cardiac output.
- Ascites and hepatic enlargement are common.
- Surgical removal of the thickened pericardial sac (pericardiectomy) is effective treatment.

NEOPLASMS OF THE MYOCARDIUM & PERICARDIUM
The myocardium and pericardium are occasionally invaded by metastatic tumor, or there may be local invasion by lung carcinoma or malignant lymphoma.

- Rhabdomyoma is a very rare hamartomatous proliferation of cardiac muscle that occurs in patients with tuberous sclerosis.
- Primary cardiac malignant neoplasms include pericardial malignant mesothelioma and angiosarcoma. They are very rare.

Section VI. The Blood & Lymph System

Blood: I. Anemias Due to Decreased Erythropoiesis

24

ANEMIAS

Anemia is defined as a reduction in the hemoglobin concentration of the blood as compared with the normal range for age and sex (Table 24–1). It is usually associated with a reduction of total circulating red cell mass. The incidence of anemia in the United States varies between 2 and 15% in various studies.

Clinical Features of Anemia

The clinical features of anemia include:

- Pallor of the skin and mucous membranes.
- Manifestations of hypoxia—most commonly weakness, fatigue, lethargy, dizziness, or syncope.
- Myocardial hypoxia, which may result in anginal pain.
- Frequently a hyperdynamic circulation, with an increase in heart rate and stroke volume. Ejection-type flow murmurs are common.
- When severe, cardiac failure may ensue.

Classification

A. Etiologic classification (Table 24–2):

- Decreased production of erythrocytes by the marrow.
- Blood loss too extensive for replacement by the marrow.
- Increased rate of destruction of erythrocytes (hemolytic anemias).

    B. Morphologic classification (Table 24–3) is according to changes in size and hemoglobin content of erythrocytes in the peripheral blood (Fig 24–1).

Anemias Due to Decreased Red Cell Production

APLASTIC ANEMIA

Aplastic anemia is the result of failure of production, suppression, or destruction of stem cells in the bone marrow.

- It leads to decreased generation of erythrocytes, leukocytes, and platelets (pancytopenia).

TABLE 24–1. NORMAL VALUES FOR PERIPHERAL BLOOD ELEMENTS[1]

	Male	Female
Hemoglobin (g/dL)	14–18	12–16
Erythrocytes (per μL)	4.6–6. × 10⁶	4.2–5.4 × 10⁶
Hematocrit (packed cell volume; PCV)	42–50%	37–47%
Mean corpuscular volume (MCV)[2]	76–96 fL	
Mean corpuscular hemoglobin concentration (MCHC)[3]	32–35%	
Total white blood cells (per μL)	4000–11,000	
Neutrophils	2500–7500[4]	
Lymphocytes	1500–3500	
Monocytes	200–800	
Eosinophils	60–600	
Basophils	0–100	
Platelets (per μL)	150,000–400,000	

[1]Normal values vary with age; adult values are given here.

[2]$MCV = \dfrac{PCV}{Red\ cell\ count}$. It is a measure of the size of individual red cells.

[3]$MCHC = \dfrac{PCV}{Hemoglobin}$. It is a measure of the hemoglobinization of individual red cells in relation to size.

[4]Recognize that absolute counts of the different types of leukocytes are more valuable than percentages.

- Drugs are the commonest cause of aplastic anemia in clinical practice.
- The bone marrow is markedly hypocellular with a reduction of all cell lines.
- The peripheral blood smear shows:
  - Normocytic and normochromic anemia, often severe, with an absence of reticulocytes in the peripheral blood.
  - Granulocytopenia, which is severe and occurs rapidly. Infections and oral ulcers may result.
  - Thrombocytopenia, which results in a bleeding tendency.
- Treatment is symptomatic; corticosteroids may help in some cases.
- Prognosis is poor.

RED CELL APLASIA
Pure red cell aplasia occurs rarely.

TABLE 24–2. ETIOLOGIC CLASSIFICATION OF ANEMIA

I. Decreased erythropoiesis
  A. Erythroid stem cell failure.
    1. Aplastic anemia
    2. Pure red cell aplasia
  B. Replacement of the bone marrow
    1. Malignant neoplasms: leukemias, plasma cell myeloma, malignant lymphoma, metastatic carcinoma
    2. Myelofibrosis
  C. Inadequate erythropoietin stimulation: chronic renal disease
  D. Defective DNA synthesis (megaloblastic anemias)
    1. Vitamin B_{12} deficiency
    2. Folic acid deficiency
  E. Defective hemoglobin synthesis
    1. Iron deficiency
    2. Anemia of chronic disease
    3. Sideroblastic anemias
  F. Other nutritional and toxic factors
    1. Scurvy
    2. Protein malnutrition
    3. Chronic liver disease
    4. Hypothyroidism
    5. "Chronic" disease, including infection and cancer
II. Blood loss
  A. Acute
  B. Chronic
III. Hemolytic anemias (see Chapter 25)
  A. Due to intrinsic red cell defects
  B. Due to extrinsic factors

■ It may be a congenital disorder (Blackfan-Diamond disease).
■ Acquired red cell aplasia is usually a transient complication of sickle cell anemia.
■ Acquired red cell aplasia may also occur as a complication of thymoma.

MARROW REPLACEMENT (LEUKOERYTHROBLASTIC) ANEMIAS

Leukoerythroblastic anemias occur when the bone marrow is invaded by metastatic neoplasms, lymphoma or leukemia, disseminated granulomatous diseases (such as tuberculosis), fibrosis, or multiple abscesses.

■ Marrow involvement of sufficient degree may result in anemia, leukopenia, or thrombocytopenia.
■ This may lead to extramedullary hematopoiesis (**myeloid metaplasia**), especially in spleen and liver.
■ It may result in the release of cells from the marrow before maturation is complete. Myelocytes and normoblasts appear in the peripheral blood (**leukoerythroblastic anemia**).

MEGALOBLASTIC ANEMIAS

Megaloblastic anemias are characterized by erythroid precursors in the marrow that are enlarged and show failure of nuclear maturation (megaloblasts).

TABLE 24–3. MORPHOLOGIC CLASSIFICATION OF ANEMIA (SEE ALSO FIG 24–1)

Type	MCV	MCHC	Common Causes
Macrocytic anemia[1]	Increased	Normal	Folic acid deficiency Vitamin B_{12} deficiency Liver disease Hypothyroidism Posthemorrhagic[2]
Microcytic anemia Hypochromic	Decreased	Decreased	Iron deficiency Thalassemia Sideroblastic anemias
Normochromic	Decreased or normal[3]	Normal	Spherocytosis
Normocytic anemia Normochromic	Normal	Normal	Aplastic anemia Anemia of chronic disease Chronic renal failure Posthemorrhagic[2] Some hemolytic anemias
Leukoerythroblastic anemia[4]	Normal	Normal	Replacement or infiltration of bone marrow

[1]A subset of macrocytic anemias shows abnormal maturation in the marrow; these are the "megaloblastic" anemias. Macrocytic anemias are normochromic.
[2]Becomes macrocytic as a result of increased numbers of reticulocytes as erythropoiesis increases.
[3]Spherocytes are erythrocytes that have lost their disk shape and are usually smaller than normal (microspherocytes). They are commonly associated with hemolysis and, therefore, the presence of increased numbers of reticulocytes, which may cause the MCV to be increased from low to normal levels.
[4]Leukoerythroblastic anemias are characterized by the presence of early forms of both white and red cells (including normoblasts) in the peripheral blood.

■ They result from conditions in which nucleic acid synthesis is abnormal, as in vitamin B_{12} and folic acid deficiency (Table 24–4).

Pathology
A. Red cell changes:

■ Erythropoiesis changes from normoblastic to megaloblastic.
■ Megaloblasts differ from normoblasts in that they are larger and show delayed nuclear maturation but normal cytoplasmic hemoglobinization (nuclear-cytoplasmic asynchrony).
■ The bone marrow is hypercellular and contains large numbers of early megaloblasts.
■ The peripheral blood smear shows macrocytosis (elevated MCV) and marked variation in size (anisocytosis) and shape (poikilocytosis; Fig 24–1).

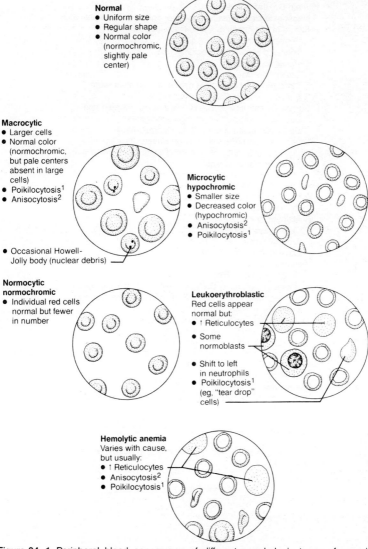

Normal
- Uniform size
- Regular shape
- Normal color (normochromic, slightly pale center)

Macrocytic
- Larger cells
- Normal color (normochromic, but pale centers absent in large cells)
- Poikilocytosis[1]
- Anisocytosis[2]
- Occasional Howell-Jolly body (nuclear debris)

Microcytic hypochromic
- Smaller size
- Decreased color (hypochromic)
- Anisocytosis[2]
- Poikilocytosis[1]

Normocytic normochromic
- Individual red cells normal but fewer in number

Leukoerythroblastic
Red cells appear normal but:
- ↑ Reticulocytes
- Some normoblasts
- Shift to left in neutrophils
- Poikilocytosis[1] (eg, "tear drop" cells)

Hemolytic anemia
Varies with cause, but usually:
- ↑ Reticulocytes
- Anisocytosis[2]
- Poikilocytosis[1]

Figure 24–1. Peripheral blood appearance of different morphologic types of anemias. **(1)** Poikilocytosis: variation in shape. **(2)** Anisocytosis: variation in size.

TABLE 24–4. CAUSES OF MEGALOBLASTIC ANEMIA

Vitamin B_{12} deficiency
  Inadequate dietary intake: very rare; only in strict vegetarians
  Failure of absorption due to intrinsic factor deficiency[1]
    Pernicious anemia
    Total and subtotal gastrectomy
  Terminal ileal disease[1]
    Crohn's disease
    Strictures and fistulas that bypass the terminal ileum
    Surgical removal of the terminal ileum
  Competition for vitamin B_{12} by intestinal microorganisms
    Bacterial overgrowth (blind loop syndromes)
    Diphyllobothrium latum (fish tapeworm) infection
  Drugs: para-aminosalicylic acid (antituberculous agent)
  Congenital deficiency of transcobalamin II (the vitamin B_{12} transport protein in blood)

Folic acid deficiency
  Inadequate intake
    Chronic alcoholism
    Malnutrition
  Failure of absorption[2]
    Tropical sprue
    Other malabsorptive states
  Increased demand
    Pregnancy and infancy
    States of increased DNA synthesis (malignant neoplasms with high rate of cell turnover, erythroid hyperplasia in congenital hemolytic anemias)
  Drugs with folic acid antagonistic activity
    Anticancer drugs such as methotrexate
    Anticonvulsants such as hydantoins

Other causes
  Arsenic poisoning
  Nitrous oxide inhalation
  Some forms of chemotherapy (in addition to folic acid antagonists)
  Orotic aciduria (a rare condition with abnormal synthesis of purines and pyrimidines)

[1]Vitamin B_{12} absorption depends on formation of a complex with intrinsic factor and absorption of this complex in the terminal ileum.
[2]Folate is absorbed throughout the small intestine; it does not require an "intrinsic factor."

B. Neutrophil changes:

■ Neutrophil precursors in the bone marrow show marked enlargement. Giant metamyelocytes are characteristic.
■ In the peripheral blood, neutrophils show **hypersegmented nuclei,** with many cells showing more than five nuclear lobes.

C. Changes in other cells in the body: The abnormality in DNA synthesis affects many other cells, notably in the intestinal mucosa, where there is cell enlargement and nuclear abnormalities.

Clinical Features & Diagnosis
Patients with megaloblastic anemia present with symptoms of severe anemia.

- It should be suspected upon finding macrocytic anemia with hypersegmented neutrophils in the peripheral blood.
- The bone marrow shows megaloblastic erythropoiesis.
- Establishment of the cause requires serum vitamin B_{12}, serum folate, vitamin B_{12} absorption studies, etc.
- Megaloblastic anemia of folate deficiency is identical to that of vitamin B_{12} deficiency except for the absence of subacute combined degeneration of the spinal cord.

PERNICIOUS (ADDISONIAN) ANEMIA
Pernicious anemia is a form of megaloblastic anemia due to vitamin B_{12} deficiency. It is common in Western Europe and among Caucasians of northern European descent in the United States. It is rare in Asia and Africa.

- It occurs predominantly after age 50.
- There is an increased familial incidence.

Pathogenesis:
Pernicious anemia is an autoimmune disease caused by immunologic destruction of the mucosa of the body and the fundus of the stomach.
- It is associated with failure to secrete acid and intrinsic factor.
  - Three autoantibodies may be found in serum and gastric juice:
  - Seventy-five percent of patients have an antibody that blocks vitamin B_{12} binding to intrinsic factor (blocking antibody).
  - Fifty percent have an antibody that binds with the intrinsic factor-vitamin B_{12} complex.
  - Ninety percent of patients have antibodies against gastric parietal cells.
- The serum autoantibodies are frequently IgG, and gastric juice antibodies are IgA.

Pathology & Clinical Features
Chronic atrophic gastritis with achlorhydria is present in all patients.

- Failure of intrinsic factor secretion leads to vitamin B_{12} deficiency and megaloblastic anemia.
- Neurologic changes due to demyelination include:
  - Peripheral neuropathy.
  - Subacute combined degeneration of the cord, which is characterized by involvement of the posterior and lateral columns of the cord.

Treatment & Prognosis
Adequate replacement therapy with injected vitamin B_{12} causes rapid reversal of anemia. Neurologic changes improve slowly and often incompletely. Patients remain at increased risk for development of gastric carcinoma in the atrophic gastric mucosa.

TABLE 24–5. CAUSES OF IRON DEFICIENCY ANEMIA

Infancy and childhood
Dietary
Chronic blood loss
Chronic infection
Prematurity
Adult female (reproductive years)
Dietary
Excessive menstrual loss
Pregnancies and miscarriages
Gastrointestinal blood loss
Hematuria, other blood loss
Adult male (and postmenopausal female)
Gastrointestinal blood loss
Drugs (eg, aspirin)
Dietary (rare)
Epistaxis, hematuria, other blood loss
Hereditary hemorrhagic telangiectasia[1]

[1] Osler-Weber-Rendu disease: Hereditary hemorrhagic telangiectasia produces multiple pinpoint bleeding foci in the gastrointestinal tract, mouth, lips, and skin.

IRON DEFICIENCY ANEMIA

Iron deficiency is the commonest cause of anemia worldwide. In underdeveloped countries, hookworm infections and malnutrition account for most cases.

■ In the United States, pregnancy and chronic blood loss due to gastrointestinal ulcers or neoplasms are the commonest causes.
■ In the USA, 50% of pregnant women, 20% of all women, 20% of preschool children, and 3% of men suffer from iron deficiency.

Causes of Iron Deficiency (Table 24–5)
A. Dietary deficiency:

■ The daily dietary iron requirement is 5–10 mg/d (equivalent to 0.5–1 mg of absorbed iron) for men and 7–20 mg/d for women.
■ The normal diet in the United States contains about 15 mg of iron, marginally adequate for women.
■ Dietary deficiency is common in underdeveloped countries.

B. Increased demand for iron is an important factor in iron deficiency anemia:

■ In the growth phase of early childhood.
■ During pregnancy and lactation.
■ In premature infants especially.

C. Malabsorption of iron may occur in severe generalized malabsorptive states such as celiac disease and tropical sprue. It occurs after total gastrectomy because gastric acid is necessary for optimal iron absorption.

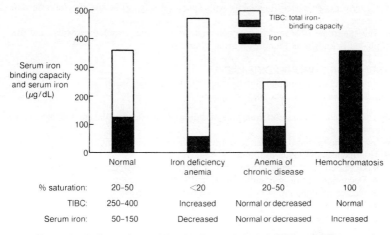

Figure 24–2. Serum iron and iron binding capacity in health and disease.

D. Chronic blood loss is a major cause of iron deficiency throughout the world.

- Common causes of chronic blood loss include:
  - Excessive menstrual blood loss from any cause.
  - Occult gastrointestinal blood loss (due to hookworm infection, peptic ulcer disease, chronic aspirin ingestion, esophageal varices, hemorrhoids, and neoplasms).
- Chronic loss of as little as 5 mL of blood per day will tip most people into negative iron balance.

Pathology and Clinical Features
Iron deficiency is first reflected in a decrease in iron stores, demonstrated by decreased serum ferritin and absence of iron in bone marrow.

- When iron stores are exhausted, the serum iron level falls, the plasma transferrin level (also called total iron binding capacity, or TIBC) increases, and the saturation of the TIBC decreases (Fig 24–2).
- Anemia is hypochromic and microcytic (Fig 24–1).
- The poorly hemoglobinized erythrocytes appear as pale cells with an expanded central clear zone and a thin ring of pink cytoplasm.
- Free erythrocytic protoporphyrin is increased because of reduced availability of iron for chelation.
- The bone marrow shows variable normoblastic hyperplasia. Stored iron is absent and the number of sideroblasts is decreased.
- Iron deficiency also results in atrophy of the mucous membranes of the mouth, tongue, pharynx, esophagus, and stomach.
- Esophageal mucosal webs may occur, causing dysphagia.
- Gastric changes may result in hypochlorhydria.

- Koilonychia (concave fingernails with abnormal ridging) is specific for iron deficiency.
- The syndrome of iron deficiency anemia, koilonychia, atrophic glossitis, and dysphagia is known as Plummer-Vinson syndrome.

ANEMIA OF CHRONIC DISEASE

Anemia occurs as a complication of many chronic diseases, such as chronic infections, collagen diseases, and malignant neoplasms.

- It is caused by failure of transport of storage iron into the plasma and developing erythrocytes.
- In most cases, the red cells are normocytic and normochromic.
- The diagnosis is made by finding:
  - Increased iron stores in the bone marrow, and elevated plasma ferritin levels.
  - Decreased serum iron and TIBC (Fig 24–2).
  - Decreased numbers of sideroblasts in the bone marrow.
  - Increased free erythrocytic protoporphyrin.
- This anemia is usually mild to moderate, but difficult to treat.

ANEMIA OF CHRONIC RENAL FAILURE

Chronic renal failure results in a normochromic, normocytic anemia due to failure of normal erythropoietin secretion by the kidney. The bone marrow may show mild hypoplasia of the erythroid series.

SIDEROBLASTIC ANEMIA

Sideroblastic anemia is an uncommon type of anemia characterized by the presence in the bone marrow of increased numbers of sideroblasts. It may be hereditary. Most acquired cases are idiopathic.

- Known causes include
  - Chronic alcoholism.
  - Pyridoxine deficiency.
  - Lead poisoning.
  - Drugs (antituberculous drugs, chloramphenicol).
- Peripheral blood shows either a hypochromic microcytic or dimorphic appearance.
- Serum iron, TIBC, and saturation are increased.
- The bone marrow shows erythroid hyperplasia, markedly increased storage iron, and an increased number of sideroblasts, including ring sideroblasts.
- In some refractory cases, increased numbers of myeloblasts are present. This is a premalignant change (dysmyelopoiesis), with 10% of these patients developing acute leukemia.

Anemia Due to Blood Loss

ACUTE BLOOD LOSS

Acute loss of whole blood leads to hypovolemia and compensatory mechanisms that maintain perfusion to vital organs.

- In the acute bleeding phase, red cell count, hemoglobin, and hematocrit are normal.

- Hypovolemia leads to retention of water and electrolytes by the kidneys. This begins immediately and causes dilution of the blood.
- Within hours, there is a decrease in red cell count, hemoglobin, and hematocrit in the peripheral blood.
- Regeneration of erythrocytes lost occurs over the next several weeks, slowly restoring the red cell count, hemoglobin, and hematocrit levels.
- During this regenerative phase, the bone marrow shows erythroid hyperplasia and depletion of iron stores, and the peripheral blood shows a reticulocytosis.
- The body's iron stores are replenished over the next few months.
- In patients who have depleted iron stores and a marginal dietary intake of iron, an episode of acute hemorrhage may precipitate iron deficiency anemia.

CHRONIC BLOOD LOSS

Chronic bleeding is compensated for initially by erythroid hyperplasia of the bone marrow and increased production of erythrocytes. This persists until iron stores have been depleted, at which time iron deficiency anemia results.

Blood: II. Hemolytic Anemias; Polycythemia

25

I. HEMOLYTIC ANEMIAS (Table 25–1)

Hemolytic anemias are diseases characterized by shortened survival of red blood cells in the circulation.

Extravascular Hemolysis (Fig 25–1)
Red cell destruction occurs in the reticuloendothelial cells, mainly in spleen. Extravascular hemolysis is characterized by:

- Hemolytic jaundice (unconjugated hyperbilirubinemia).
- Absence of bilirubin in the urine (acholuric jaundice).
- Increased bilirubin excretion in bile with increased incidence of pigment gallstones.
- Increased excretion of fecal and urinary urobilinogen.
- Erythroid hyperplasia in the bone marrow.
- Reticulocytosis in the peripheral blood.
- Systemic hemosiderosis, aggravated by increased intestinal absorption of iron and use of blood transfusions.

Intravascular Hemolysis (Fig 25–1)
With intravascular hemolysis, red cell destruction occurs in the blood stream. It is characterized by:

- Hemolytic jaundice.
- Decreased plasma haptoglobin.
- Hemoglobinemia.
- Hemoglobinuria.
- Methemalbuminemia (part of the released hemoglobin is oxidized to methemoglobin, which binds to albumin).
- Increased serum levels of lactate dehydrogenase due to its release from red cells.

INTRINSIC ERYTHROCYTE DEFECTS

Erythrocyte Membrane Defects

HEREDITARY SPHEROCYTOSIS

Etiology & Pathogenesis
Hereditary spherocytosis is a congenital autosomal-dominant disease with variable penetrance.

TABLE 25–1. CLASSIFICATION OF HEMOLYTIC ANEMIAS

Intrinsic defect of erythrocytes
  Congenital hemolytic anemias
    Membrane defects
      Hereditary spherocytosis
      Hereditary elliptocytosis
    Enzyme deficiency
      Glucose-6-phosphatase deficiency
      Pyruvate kinase deficiency
    Abnormal hemoglobin synthesis (hemoglobinopathies)
      Sickle cell disease
      Thalassemia
      Unstable hemoglobins
  Acquired hemolytic anemias
    Paroxysmal nocturnal hemoglobinuria
Hemolysis due to extrinsic factors
  Immune hemolytic anemias
    Autoimmune hemolytic anemias
      Associated with warm antibodies
      Associated with cold antibodies
    Isoimmune hemolytic anemias
      Hemolytic blood transfusion reactions
      Hemolytic disease of the newborn
    Drug-induced immune hemolytic anemias
  Direct-acting external agents
    Infections: malaria
    Snake venom
    Physical trauma: microangiopathy, hypersplenism

- It may present with severe hemolysis in childhood or with mild hemolysis manifested first during adult life.
- The exact expression of the abnormal gene is not known. Abnormal polymerization of spectrin and defective membrane autophosphorylation have been demonstrated.
- It is characterized by a change in the shape of the red cell from its normal biconcave to spherical.
- Spherocytes are less pliable than normal erythrocytes and tend to lose membrane substance in the spleen, becoming progressively smaller (microspherocytes).
- Spherocyte life span is shortened, with destruction occurring in the spleen.

Clinical Features

- Patients present with hemolytic anemia and jaundice.
- Splenic enlargement is usually present as a result of reticuloendothelial hyperplasia.
- Life-threatening aplastic crises may occur in association with infections.
- The diagnosis is confirmed by the osmotic fragility test (spherocytes are more susceptible to lysis by hypotonic saline solution).
- The red cells also show increased susceptibility to autohemolysis, which is reduced by incubating with glucose.

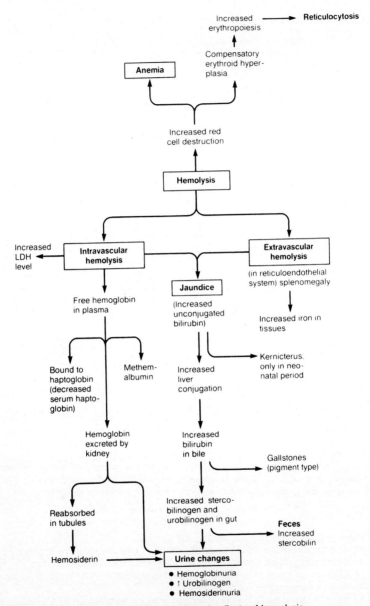

Figure 25–1. Clinicopathologic effects of hemolysis.

Treatment

- The membrane defect cannot be reversed by any known therapy.
- Splenectomy, which removes the site of maximum erythrocyte destruction, is effective treatment.

HEREDITARY ELLIPTOCYTOSIS

Hereditary elliptocytosis resembles spherocytosis except that the red cells are oval and the disease is usually less severe.

PAROXYSMAL NOCTURNAL HEMOGLOBINURIA (PNH)

This is a rare, acquired disease of red cells characterized by increased sensitivity of the membrane to complement.

- Erythrocyte lysis in the circulation results in hemoglobinemia and hemoglobinuria.
- Complement activation occurs mainly through the alternative pathway and is precipitated by:
  - Decreased pH in vivo during sleep.
  - Acidification of serum in vitro (Ham's test).
  - Addition of sucrose to serum in vitro (sucrose lysis test).
- Patients are usually young adults, and the anemia may be severe.
- PNH is associated with aplastic anemia, either preceding or following an episode. It may be caused by a clone of abnormal erythrocytes developing in an aplastic bone marrow.

Erythrocyte Enzyme Deficiency

GLUCOSE-6-PHOSPHATE DEHYDROGENASE (G6PD) DEFICIENCY

This is the most common erythrocyte enzyme abnormality. Several variants are recognized:

- G6PD-A–variant is inherited as an X-linked trait. It is present in about 10% of blacks in the United States and has a worldwide distribution. It is caused by two point mutations with full expression of the enzyme deficiency in males.
- The Mediterranean variant occurs in Middle Eastern populations and produces more severe disease.
- G6PD-deficient red cells are more vulnerable to oxidants, which cause oxidative denaturation of hemoglobin and lead to formation of Heinz bodies and hemolysis.
- Most patients with G6PD deficiency are asymptomatic.
- Acute intravascular hemolysis may occur after exposure to an oxidant drug, most commonly primaquine, sulfonamides, or nitrofurantoin.
- Rarely, patients develop a mild chronic hemolytic anemia.

OTHER ERYTHROCYTE ENZYME DEFICIENCIES

Pyruvate kinase deficiency is less common than G6PD deficiency.

- It is inherited as an autosomal recessive trait and occurs with equal frequency in both sexes.
- It is present with acute or chronic hemolytic anemia. Diagnosis is by enzyme assay.
- Deficiencies of **glutathione reductase** and **triosephosphate isomerase** are rare.

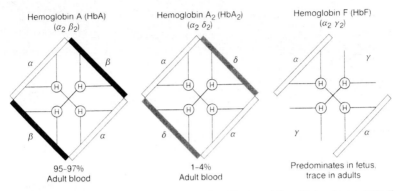

Figure 25–2. Types of hemoglobins normally found in the adult and fetus. Hemoglobin F levels rapidly decrease in the blood after birth.

Hemoglobinopathies

Several different types of hemoglobin occur in humans. All have four polypeptide chains per molecule of hemoglobin, each chain linked with one heme group (Fig 25–2). Hemoglobinopathies are diseases in which hemoglobin synthesis is abnormal. Three broad types are recognized:

■ Qualitative hemoglobinopathies are characterized by synthesis of an abnormal hemoglobin molecule, commonly due to a single gene abnormality.
■ Quantitative hemoglobinopathies (thalassemias), are characterized by failure of secretion of one chain type.
■ Combined qualitative and quantitative hemoglobinopathies also occur.

SICKLE CELL DISEASE

The abnormal HbS gene is common in Africa, India, and among blacks in the United States. It is rare in the Caucasian and Oriental races.

■ Sickle cell trait:
  ● Affects 9% of American blacks.
  ● Occurs in individuals that are heterozygous for the abnormal gene (A/S).
  ● Usually causes no symptoms.
  ● Confers some protection on the erythrocyte against infection with *Plasmodium falciparum*.
■ Sickle Cell Disease:
  ● Represents the homozygous (S/S) state.
  ● Occurs in 0.1–0.2% of blacks born in the United States; about 50,000 black Americans suffer from sickle cell disease.

Pathology

A single point mutation (codon beta-6 GAG ($\rightarrow$ GTG) dictates replacement of the normal glutamic acid with valine at position 6 in the beta chain.

- The result of this amino acid substitution is HbS.
- HbS has a tendency to polymerization, yielding semisolid crystalline structures called tactoids, under conditions of hypoxia.
- Tactoid formation causes:
  - Decreased solubility of hemoglobin.
  - Change in shape of the erythrocyte to a sickle cell.
  - Decreased deformability of the erythrocyte, which leads to phagocytosis and destruction in the spleen and liver.

Clinical Features

The onset of sickle cell disease is in childhood, and death often occurs during early adult life.

- It presents with evidence of chronic extravascular hemolysis and severe anemia, mild hemolytic jaundice with absent urinary bilirubin, and increased fecal and urinary urobilinogen.
- The bone marrow shows marked normoblastic hyperplasia, often leading to expansion of the marrow cavity causing bony deformities ("tower skull" and "hair-on-end" appearance on skull X-rays).
- Growth retardation and heart failure are common.
- Chronic leg ulcers that fail to heal are common.

Diagnosis

Sickle cells in peripheral blood smears are diagnostic but not always present. Addition of metabisulfite to the blood smears induces sickling (metabisulfite sickle preparation).

- The dithionine solubility test detects decreased solubility of hemoglobin, and is positive.
- Hemoglobin electrophoresis permits identification and quantifying of HbS in the blood.
- Patients with sickle cell disease have over 80% HbS in the blood, with absent HbA.
- Patients with sickle cell trait have HbA (50–70%) and smaller amounts of HbS (30–35%).

Complications

Aplastic crisis is a sudden, usually transient, failure of hematopoiesis in the bone marrow, which may be precipitated by infections, drugs, or other causes.

- Hemolytic crisis is characterized by a sudden increase in the level of hemolysis of erythrocytes. The cause is unknown.
- Hemochromatosis is common in long-term survivors. A positive iron balance results from stimulation of iron absorption in the intestine and multiple blood transfusions.
- Vaso-occlusive crisis is due to plugging of the microcirculation by aggregates of sickle cells. It is characterized by fever and ischemic pain and microinfarcts in heart, muscles, bone (aseptic necrosis of the femoral head), and kidneys (renal papillary necrosis).
- Autosplenectomy is caused by repeated ischemic episodes. In adults, the spleen is shrunken and shows multiple brown scars containing hemosiderin (Gamna-Gandy bodies).

TABLE 25–2. SELECTED[1] AMINO ACID SUBSTITUTION HEMOGLOBIN VARIANTS

Anemias in Homozygous state HbS–beta 6 val	Severe hemolytic anemia (sickle cell)
HbC–beta 6 lys	Mild hemolytic anemia
HbD (Punjab)–beta 121 Gln	Minimal anemia
HbE–beta 26 Lys	Mild anemia
Disease in heterozygous state *Methemoglobinemia with cyanosis* HbM (Boston)–alpha 58 Tyr HbM (Hyde Park)–beta 92 Tyr	Forms stable oxidized heme group (methemoglobin); reversible O_2 binding is prevented, and patients appear cyanosed.
Increased O_2 affinity Hb Chesapeake–alpha 92 Leu Hb Malmö–beta 97 Gln	The oxygen dissociation curve is shifted to the left; release of O_2 in tissues is reduced, leading to compensatory polycythemia.
Decreased O_2 affinity Hb Kansas–alpha 102 Thr Hb Beth Israel–beta 102 Ser	The oxygen dissociation curve is shifted to the right; increased amounts of reduced hemoglobin are present (cyanosis), but erythropoietin levels are low (anemia).
Unstable hemoglobins Hb Torino–alpha 42 Val Hb–Köln–beta 98 Met Hb Bristol–beta 67 Asp Hb Hammersmith–beta 42 Ser	Unstable hemoglobin precipitates as Heinz bodies, decreasing erythrocyte survival with varying degrees of hemolysis that is improved by splenectomy in some cases (eg, Köln, Torino).

[1]In all these conditions, substitution of a single amino acid results in a configurational change in the hemoglobin molecule.

■ The functionally asplenic state predisposes to systemic infections with encapsulated bacteria. Pneumococcal bacteremia and *Salmonella* osteomyelitis occur.

OTHER ABNORMAL HEMOGLOBINS

Many other amino acid substitution hemoglobinopathies occur (Table 25–2), and they may alter hemoglobin function.

■ Hemoglobin electrophoresis is of value in diagnosis.
■ Abnormal hemoglobins may have the following consequences:
   ● Hemolytic anemia (in general, the severity of hemolysis is less than in sickle cell disease.)
   ● Instability of the hemoglobin molecule, causing precipitation of Heinz bodies and decreased red cell survival.
   ● Increased affinity of the hemoglobin molecule for oxygen, leading to hypoxia and compensatory polycythemia.

TABLE 25–3. THALASSEMIAS

	Genotype[1]	Severity of Disease	Hemoglobins Present
Beta[2]			
Beta thalassemia major	Homozygous β^0/β^0	Severe anemia	HbA absent or reduced $\uparrow$ HbA$_2$ $\uparrow$ HbF
Beta thalassemia minor	Heterozygous β^0/β	Mild to moderate anemia	HbA present; slight $\uparrow$ HbA$_2$, HbF
Alpha			
Hydrops fetalis (deletion of all 4 α genes)	--/--	Stillborn	Hb Barts (γ^4) HbH (β^4) Hb Portland (zeta$_2$, gamma$_2$-embryonic)
HbH disease (deletion of 3 α genes)	--/-- α	Hemolytic anemia	HbA HbH Hb Barts
Alpha thalassemia minor (deletion of 2 genes)	-α/-α --/$\alpha\alpha$	Mild hemolysis	HbA; trace Hb Barts
Carrier (deletion of 1 gene)	$\alpha\alpha$/-α	No abnormality	Normal

[1]Only the β gene status is shown in beta thalassemias. β^0 = abnormal gene. Only the α gene status is shown in alpha thalassemias. Note that there are 2 alpha genes per haplotype.
[2]Other variants exist depending upon the exact effect of the defective beta gene.

- Decreased affinity for oxygen leading to anemia due to decreased erythropoietin secretion, and cyanosis.

THALASSEMIAS (Table 25–3)

Thalassemias are characterized by decreased synthesis of hemoglobin chains that are structurally normal.

■ Beta thalassemia is due to decreased synthesis of beta chains and is the most common form.
■ Alpha thalassemia is due to decreased synthesis of alpha chains.
■ Delta-beta thalassemia is due to decreased synthesis of both delta and beta chains.
  A. Homozygous beta thalassemia (Cooley's anemia) is common in persons of Mediterranean, African, and Asian ancestry. Three percent of the world's population carry the beta-thalassemia gene, which is inherited as an autosomal recessive trait.

■ Homozygous beta thalassemia is characterized by total or near-total absence of synthesis of beta chains, with a marked decrease in the amount of HbA.
■ Gamma chain production persists into adult life, resulting in persistently elevated HbF levels (to about 40–60%, but sometimes as high as 90%).

- Delta chain synthesis is also increased to compensate for the absent beta chains, causing an increase in HbA_2 levels.
- Excess free alpha chains precipitate in the cytoplasm of affected erythrocytes and are visible as inclusions.
- Clinically, homozygous beta thalassemia presents in early childhood with severe anemia, hemolytic jaundice, and splenomegaly. Growth retardation and delayed puberty are common. Extreme erythroid hyperplasia causes bony abnormalities.
- The peripheral blood picture shows hypochromic microcytic anemia with marked anisocytosis, reticulocytosis, and numerous target forms.
- Hemoglobin electrophoresis shows elevation of HbF and HbA_2 with greatly decreased or absent HbA.
- The main complication of thalassemia is secondary hemochromatosis, which affects many organs and is the most common cause of death, usually from myocardial or liver failure.

B. Heterozygous beta thalassemia (Cooley's trait):

- May be asymptomatic.
- May present clinically with a mild hemolytic process characterized by mild anemia, jaundice, splenomegaly, and a hypochromic microcytic blood picture.
- Hemoglobin electrophoresis shows sight elevation of HbA_2 (4–7%) and HbF (2–6%). Most of the hemoglobin is HbA.

C. Sickle cell-beta thalassemia:

- Is caused by heterozygosity for both the sickle cell gene and the thalassemia gene.
- Produces a hemolytic process that is intermediate in severity between sickle cell disease and sickle cell trait.
- The diagnosis is made by a combination of:
  - Positive dithionite solubility or metabisulfite sickle tests.
  - Hemoglobin electrophoresis, which shows the presence of both HbS and HbA, with the former in greater concentration. HbF and HbA_2 are increased.

D. Alpha thalassemia (Table 25–3):

- There are two alpha genes per haplotype, for a total of four in the normal situation.
- Deletion of all four leads to complete absence of alpha chain, severe fetal anemia with edema, erythroblastosis, and stillbirth.
- Absence of three or two alpha genes leads to progressively less severe disease, with varying levels of tetramer hemoglobins (β 4 and γ 4).
- Deletion of a single alpha gene has no clinical effect.

IMMUNE-MEDIATED HEMOLYTIC ANEMIAS

Autoimmune Hemolytic Anemias
These are a group of diseases in which hemolysis occurs as a result of autoantibodies.

- Binding of the autoantibody to the erythrocyte membrane may occur maximally at body temperature (37°C, warm antibodies) or at 4°C (cold antibodies).
- The antibodies may be IgG (usually warm), IgM (usually cold) or, rarely, IgA.
- Antibody acts as a lysin, opsonin, or agglutinin.

IDIOPATHIC WARM AUTOIMMUNE HEMOLYTIC ANEMIA

This anemia occurs mainly in patients over age 40 and in women more frequently than in men. It is caused by an IgG autoantibody, occurring:

- In isolation (idiopathic).
- As a complication of drugs (eg, methyldopa).
- In other diseases, such as systemic lupus erythematosus and B lymphocytic neoplasms.

Pathology & Clinical Features

This anemia has an insidious onset and a chronic course.

- It presents with hemolytic anemia or jaundice with splenomegaly.
- The peripheral blood shows a normochromic normocytic anemia with microspherocytes, fragmented forms, and poikilocytes.
- Red cell osmotic fragility and autohemolysis are increased.
- The diagnosis is established by demonstrating the autoantibody in serum using the antiglobulin (Coombs) test.

Treatment & Course

Corticosteroids represent the mainstay of treatment and are very effective.

- Splenectomy and immunosuppressive agents such as azathioprine may be used if steroids are not effective.
- Most patients have a chronic course, with relapses and remissions occurring at variable intervals.

IDIOPATHIC COLD HEMAGLUTININ DISEASE

This is a rare cause of hemolysis that occurs mainly in older patients, more commonly in women.

- It is caused by an IgM autoantibody that binds to erythrocytes at low temperatures, fixes complement, and results in hemolysis.
- Patients present with cold-induced hemolysis or Raynaud's phenomenon, in which blanching and numbness of the hands occur on exposure to cold, followed successively by cyanosis, redness, throbbing pain and tingling.
- The diagnosis is made by a positive Coombs test, with anti-IgM antibodies showing maximum reactivity at 4°C.
- Cold hemagglutinin disease also occurs in association with malignant lymphoma and as a complication of infection with *Mycoplasma pneumoniae*.

PAROXYSMAL COLD HEMOGLOBINURIA

This is a rare disorder caused by a cold antibody of the IgG class.

- The antibody is directed against the P antigen on the erythrocyte membrane.
- Complement fixation is initiated by cold but does not proceed to lysis until the blood temperature rises to 37°C.
- Patients suffer chills, fever, muscle pain, and hemoglobinuria following exposure to cold.
- Diagnosis is by the Donath Landsteiner test, demonstrating hemolysis of a blood sample following cooling to 4°C and warming to 37°C.

Isoimmune Hemolytic Anemia

These are hemolytic anemias in which the red cells of one individual are lysed as a result of the action of antibodies of another individual.

HEMOLYTIC BLOOD TRANSFUSION REACTIONS

These reactions follow transfusion of incompatible blood.

- The more severe forms produce intravascular hemolysis, occur within minutes to hours, and result in hemoglobinemia and shock.
- More rarely, hemolytic reactions are delayed several days and are associated with extravascular hemolysis.
- The transfused (donor) red cells are destroyed by antibody present in the recipient's plasma.
- ABO incompatibility is the commonest cause of serious hemolytic reactions.
- Hemolytic transfusion reactions are prevented by blood grouping and cross-matching.
- In practice, hemolytic transfusion reactions are almost all due to human (clerical) error.

HEMOLYTIC DISEASE OF THE NEWBORN

This is usually caused by Rh incompatibility between mother and fetus. More rarely, ABO or other group incompatibility is responsible.

- An Rh-negative individual does not have natural anti-Rh antibodies, but may develop immune anti-Rh antibodies (IgG):
  - When Rh-positive blood is transfused.
  - During pregnancy, when fetal Rh-positive erythrocytes enter the maternal circulation from an Rh-positive fetus. Fetomaternal passage of cells occurs mainly during delivery.
- If a sensitized Rh-negative woman becomes pregnant, the anti-Rh IgG crosses the placenta, producing hemolysis of the fetal erythrocytes in utero if the fetus is Rh-positive. This may cause:
  - Intrauterine death.
  - Hemolytic disease of the newborn.
- Hemolytic disease of the newborn is prevented by avoiding sensitization of Rh-negative women by:
  - Accurate Rh typing during blood transfusions.
  - Administration of high doses of Rh antibody (Rhogam) to an Rh-negative woman after childbirth or abortion.
- Hemolytic disease of the newborn occurs less often with ABO incompatibility, because anti-A and anti-B natural antibodies in the mother's plasma are usually IgM and do not cross the placenta.

DRUG- & CHEMICAL-INDUCED HEMOLYSIS

Immune Drug-Induced Hemolysis

Induction of autoantibody occurs with the antihypertensive agent methyldopa, which leads to a clinical syndrome resembling idiopathic autoimmune hemolytic anemia.

- A **hapten effect** occurs, where the drug combines with an erythrocyte membrane protein to form an antigenic complex that stimulates production of antibody, with penicillin and cephalosporins.

- **Immune complex** formation between a drug and induced antibody, followed by adsorption of the immune complex to the erythrocyte membrane, activating complement and causing hemolysis, is the mechanism with quinidine, phenacetin, and the antituberculous drug aminosalicylic acid.
- **Direct alterations** in the erythrocyte membrane (cephalosporins) lead to the adsorption of immunoglobulins and macrophage-mediated hemolysis.

Nonimmune Drug-Induced Hemolysis
Certain chemicals and toxins cause hemolysis by direct action on red cell membranes (amphotericin B, mushroom toxin, snake venoms, lipid solvents).

- Some chemicals affect red cell enzymes (lead, saponin), leading to hemolysis.
- Drug-induced hemolysis in G6PD deficiency was discussed earlier in this chapter.

HEMOLYSIS CAUSED BY INFECTIOUS AGENTS
Development of autoimmune hemolysis occurs in infectious mononucleosis and mycoplasma pneumonia.

- Toxins cause hemolysis in clostridial infections and in severe streptococcal septicemia.
- Direct infection of red cells results in hemolysis in bartonellosis and malaria.
- In **malaria:**
  - Red cell lysis occurs episodically upon release of proliferating merozoites from infected red cells.
  - There is intermittent fever, which coincides with hemolysis every 48 hours (tertian fever—*Plasmodium vivax, Plasmodium falciparum*) or every 72 hours (quartan fever—*Plasmodium malariae*).
- Diagnosis is by identifying the malarial parasite in peripheral blood smears.

MICROANGIOPATHIC HEMOLYTIC ANEMIA
This anemia is caused by fragmentation of erythrocytes as they traverse an abnormal microcirculation.

Etiology
It most commonly arises from disseminated intravascular coagulation (DIC) in which the fibrin strands in the microcirculation cause fragmentation of erythrocytes.

- DIC and fragmentation hemolysis are a major factor in:
  - Hemolytic uremic syndrome, which affects young children and is characterized by renal failure and microangiopathic hemolytic anemia.
  - Thrombotic thrombocytopenic purpura, a disease of young adults characterized by fever, microangiopathic hemolytic anemia, marked central nervous system changes, and renal failure.
- Other abnormalities in blood vessels associated with microangiopathic hemolytic anemia include:
  - Vasculitides of all types.
  - Malignant hypertension.

- Giant capillary hemangioma (Kassabach-Merritt syndrome).
- Arteriovenous malformations.
- Prosthetic cardiac valves or aortic prostheses.

Pathology & Diagnosis
Microangiopathic hemolytic anemia is diagnosed by the finding of abnormal fragmented erythrocytes (schistocytes, "helmet cells") in the peripheral blood smear.

- Microspherocytes and reticulocytes are also present.
- Evidence of intravascular hemolysis, including hemoglobinemia, may be present.

II. POLYCYTHEMIA

Polycythemia is defined as an increased number of red cells in the peripheral blood. It may result from:

- An increase in the total red cell mass (absolute polycythemia).
- Decreased plasma volume without an increase in total red cell mass (relative polycythemia), as in dehydration.

SECONDARY ABSOLUTE POLYCYTHEMIA
This is a normal compensatory increase in the red cell volume resulting from chronic hypoxemia, mediated by increased production of erythropoietin. It occurs in:

- Patients with chronic lung disease or congenital cyanotic heart disease.
- Individuals acclimatized to living at high altitudes.
- Cigarette smokers, who have increased carbon monoxide levels in the blood that bind hemoglobin and lead to hypoxia.
- Patients with abnormal hemoglobins that have an increased affinity for oxygen.
- Inappropriate erythropoietin secretion very rarely causes secondary absolute polycythemia. Common causes are:
  - Neoplastic diseases, most commonly renal adenocarcinoma, cerebellar hemangioblastoma, and hepatocellular carcinoma.
  - Nonneoplastic renal conditions such as renal cysts and hydronephrosis.

POLYCYTHEMIA RUBRA VERA ("Primary" Polycythemia)
This is a neoplastic myeloproliferative disorder that affects chiefly the erythroid series.

- Granulocytes and platelet numbers are also commonly increased.
- The bone marrow is hypercellular, with proliferation of all three cell lines.
- Megakaryocyte clustering is characteristic.
- Patients are usually over age 40.
- They commonly present with ruddy cyanosis of the face and plethora due to the polycythemia.
- The increased viscosity of the blood caused by the increased hematocrit often results in vascular thrombosis. Portal vein thrombosis is common.

- The diagnosis is made by demonstrating an increased total red cell mass in the absence of hypoxemia.
- Neutrophils have markedly elevated levels of the enzyme alkaline phosphatase, a feature that permits differentiation from chronic granulocytic leukemia, in which neutrophil alkaline phosphatase is greatly reduced.
- Treatment is by reducing red cell mass by repeated venesection.
- Survival for 10–15 years is usual.

Blood: III. The White Blood Cells

26

NORMAL WHITE BLOOD COUNT & DIFFERENTIAL

Normal values for the United States are given in Table 24–1. Abnormalities in the total number of individual cell types are more significant than percentage variations.

Common Abnormalities in Leukocyte Count

LYMPHOCYTOSIS (Table 26–1)

Lymphocytosis may occur in:

- Acute immune responses, with many activated or transformed lymphocytes in the blood.
- Chronic immune responses, in which most of the circulating lymphocytes resemble resting small lymphocytes.
- Neoplastic proliferations of lymphocytes.

MONOCYTOSIS

Monocytosis commonly occurs in chronic inflammatory processes such as tuberculosis, infective endocarditis, sarcoidosis, collagen diseases, and inflammatory bowel diseases. It also occurs in neoplasms of monocytes.

NEUTROPHILIA (Neutrophil Leukocytosis; Table 26–2)

Neutrophilia is defined as an increase in the absolute neutrophil count over 7500/μL.

- The term *leukemoid reaction* is used for a very severe reactive neutrophil leukocytosis, sometimes in excess of 50,000/μL, with a leftward shift owing to early release of storage pool granulocytes.
- Leukemoid reaction may be distinguished from chronic myelocytic leukemia by the neutrophil alkaline phosphatase level, which is elevated in the leukemoid reaction and decreased in chronic myelocytic leukemia.
- When the neutrophil count exceeds 100,000/μL—usually only in chronic myelocytic leukemia—vascular occlusion may occur.

EOSINOPHILIA

Eosinophilia is defined as an absolute eosinophil count in the peripheral blood that exceeds 600/μL.

- It is a common manifestation of parasitic infections, especially with metazoan parasites.

TABLE 26–1. CAUSES OF LYMPHOCYTOSIS

	Major Conditions	Immunology
With features of lymphocyte transformation, ie, medium and large lymphocytes and plasmacytoid cells[1]	Active immune responses, especially in children. Immunizations; bacterial infections (pertussis); viral infections (infectious mononucleosis, mumps, measles, viral hepatitis, rubella, influenza); toxoplasmosis.	Mixed T and B cell (polyclonal)
	Primary neoplasms—some variants of chronic lymphocytic leukemia (CLL), lymphoma	T or B cell (monoclonal)[2]
Majority resemble resting small lymphocytes	Chronic infections (tuberculosis, syphilis, brucellosis); autoimmune diseases (myasthenia gravis); metabolic diseases (thyrotoxicosis, Addison's disease).	Mixed T and B cell (polyclonal)
	Primary neoplasms—CLL, some small cell lymphomas	T or B cell (monoclonal)[2]
Lymphocytes resemble fetal lymphoblasts	Primary neoplasms—acute lymphoblastic leukemia, lymphoblastic lymphoma	Nonmarking or T cell or B cell (monoclonal)[2]
Admixture of abnormal lymphoid cells (rare)	Primary neoplasms—involvement of blood by lymphoma or myeloma	Abnormal cells are T or B cells (monoclonal)[2] often admixed with residual normal cells

[1]These medium-sized and large lymphocytes represent circulating partly transformed lymphocytes involved in disseminating the immune response (see Chapter 4). Previously they were often termed "atypical" lymphocytes, and on morphology alone they may be difficult to distinguish from neoplastic lymphocytes.
[2]Clonality as defined in Chapter 29.

■ It also occurs in:
   ● Type I hypersensitivity, eg, allergic rhinitis, bronchial asthma, urticaria, and eczema.
   ● Immunologic diseases, eg, pemphigus vulgaris, polyarteritis nodosa, and eosinophilic gastroenteritis.
   ● Patients with malignant neoplasms, most commonly Hodgkin's disease and mycosis fungoides.
   ■ Eosinophilic leukemia is extremely rare.

NEUTROPENIA (Table 26–2)
Neutropenia is defined as a decrease in the absolute neutrophil count below 1500/µL.

■ It is clinically significant when the neutrophil count drops below 1000/µL and infections, usually with pyogenic bacteria, occur frequently.

TABLE 26-2. VARIATIONS IN NEUTROPHIL PARAMETERS

	Peripheral Blood Morphology	Conditions	Comments
Normal numbers of neutrophils With shift to the left		Leukoerythroblastic anemia	Physical replacement of normal marrow by fibrosis, neoplasms
		Primary neoplasms: early "preleukemic" myeloid leukemia	Leukemic marrow
With shift to the right		Megaloblastic anemias; folate antagonists.	Vitamin B_{12} or folate levels decreased in blood; may also produce neutropenia
With abnormal giant granulocytes or inclusions		Mucopolysaccharidosis (Alder-Reilly; rare)	See Chapter 15
		Chédiak-Higashi syndrome (rare)	See Chapter 7
		Toxic granules in severe infection (more common)	
Neutrophil leukocytosis Mainly mature segmented forms; mild left shift		Metabolic diseases (uremia, gout); drugs (phenacetin, digitalis); postnecrosis (myocardial infarction, burns); post-surgery; acute infections (pyogenic cocci, *Escherichia coli*, *Proteus*, *Pseudomonas*, less often typhus, cholera, diphtheria)	Toxic granulation Giant toxic granules (Döhle bodies)

With high proportion of less mature cells (bands and metamyelocytes); marked left shift		Leukemoid reaction (very severe acute infections, especially in child)	High leukocyte alkaline phosphatase level
		Primary neoplasms: chronic myelocytic leukemia; less often, polycythemia rubra vera or myelosclerosis	Low leukocyte alkaline phosphatase level
With high proportion of "blasts"; extreme left shift		Primary neoplasms; acute myelocytic leukemia and variants	Auer rods in blast cells
Neutropenia May occur alone or may accompany lymphopenia, thrombocytopenia, anemia	Variable	Infections: Many viral infections (hepatitis, measles); some rickettsial infections; rare bacterial infections (typhoid fever, brucellosis); malaria; any very severe infection (septicemia, milliary tuberculosis)	
		Acute leukemia in early phase of marrow involvement	
		Marrow aplasia	
		Vitamin B_{12}, folate deficiency	
		Autoimmune diseases: Felty's syndrome	Antileukocyte antibodies
		Familial cyclic neutropenia	Cyclic stem cell failure (?)

TABLE 26–3. NEUTROPHIL DYSFUNCTION SYNDROMES

Disease	Inheritance	Age at Onset	Defect
Chédiak-Higashi syndrome	Autosomal recessive	Variable	Increased fusion of cytoplasmic granules in many cell types: a. Melanosomes → albinism b. Defective neutrophil degranulation → infections c. Abnormal giant granules in cytoplasm of monocytes, neutrophils, lymphocytes
Lazy leukocyte syndrome	Very rare; uncertain	Birth	Defective movement of neutrophils to chemotaxis
Chronic granulomatous disease of childhood	X-linked recessive	Childhood	Failure to produce peroxide by neutrophils, monocytes, leading to recurrent infections with catalase-producing organisms (*Staphylococcus aureus, Candida* spp, gram-negative enteric bacilli, *Aspergillus* spp)
Myeloperoxidase deficiency	Autosomal recessive	Asymptomatic	Myeloperoxidase deficiency in neutrophils, monocytes; usually no clinical effect
Corticosteroid therapy	—	—	Inhibits neutrophil movement and phagocytosis

■ When the level falls below 500/μL, such infections are inevitable.

■ Oral infections with ulceration of the throat, skin infections, and fever are the commonest manifestations.

Neutrophil Dysfunction Syndromes
This is a rare group of diseases in which patients manifest clinical complications similar to those seen in severe neutropenia, but without a decrease in the neutrophil count in the peripheral blood. Diseases in which different functions of the neutrophil are affected have been described (Table 26–3).

NEOPLASMS OF HEMATOPOIETIC CELLS

Leukemias
Leukemias are malignant neoplastic proliferations of hematopoietic cells in the bone marrow.

TABLE 26–4. TRADITIONAL CLASSIFICATION OF LEUKEMIAS BY CELL TYPE

Cell	Acute	Chronic
Lymphocyte	Acute lymphoblastic (ALL)	Chronic lymphocytic (CLL)
		Sézary syndrome
Granulocyte Neutrophil	Acute myeloblastic (AML)	Chronic myelocytic (CML)
Eosinophil		Eosinophilic[1] (rare)
Basophil		Basophilic[1] (very rare)
Monocyte	Acute monocytic	Chronic monocytic (rare)
Erythroid	Acute erythroblastic (erythro- leukemia)	Chronic erythroleukemia[1]
		Polycythemia rubra vera
Megakaryocyte	Megakaryocytic	Thrombocythemia[1]
Plasma cell	—	Plasma cell leukemia[2] (rare)
Unknown cell[3]	—	Hairy cell leukemia (rare)
Mixed cell types	Acute myelomonocytic (AMML)	Chronic myelomonocytic (rare)

[1]Often regarded as variants of CML (chronic myelocytic leukemia) with predominant differentiation to the various cell types.
[2]Leukemic dissemination of multiple myeloma.
[3]The progenitor cell of hairy cell leukemia is now known to be a B lymphocyte, but the relationship of this cell to other B lymphocytes is still unclear.

- In most cases, the neoplastic cells are also present in increased numbers in the peripheral blood.
- They may be acute or chronic and involve any one or more of the hematopoietic cell lines (Table 26–4).

Incidence
There are 25,000 new cases of leukemia in the United States per year, with 15,000–20,000 deaths.

- Death rates have fallen in the past decade because of increasing effectiveness of treatment.
- Acute leukemias account for 50–60% of all leukemias, with acute myeloblastic leukemia (AML) being slightly more common than acute lymphoblastic leukemia (ALL).
- ALL occurs predominantly in young children (peak age incidence 3–4 years).
- AML occurs at any age but is most common in young adults (peak 15–20 years).
- Chronic leukemias account for 40–50% of leukemias, with chronic lymphocytic leukemia (CLL) being slightly more common than chronic myelocytic leukemia (CML).

■ CLL occurs mainly in patients over age 60.

■ CML occurs at all ages, with a peak incidence in the age group from 40 to 50 years.

Etiology
The cause of most kinds of leukemia is unknown.

■ **Viruses:**
  ● Are known to cause animal leukemias and are highly suspect in humans.
  ● A retrovirus (human T lymphotropic virus type I; HTLV-I) is the causative agent in one type of acute T lymphocytic leukemia first described in Japan.
  ● A related virus, HTLV-II, causes chronic T cell leukemia.

■ **Radiation:**
  ● There was an increased incidence of leukemia in the first generation of radiologists.
  ● Leukemia occurred with increased frequency among survivors of the Hiroshima and Nagasaki bombs.
  ● Fetal exposure to radiation in utero and patients who receive radiation for treatment of ankylosing spondylitis and Hodgkin's disease have an increased incidence.

■ **Chemical agents:**
  ● Cytotoxic drugs used in the treatment of other cancers have an increased incidence of leukemia.
  ● Arsenic, benzene, phenylbutazone, and chloramphenicol have been implicated in some cases.

■ **Marrow aplasia** due to any cause has an increased incidence of subsequent leukemia.

■ **Immune deficiency states** are associated with an increased incidence of leukemia.

■ **Genetic factors:**
  ● Chromosomal abnormalities are present in a high proportion of patients with leukemia (Table 26–5).
  ● The Philadelphia chromosome is a small chromosome 22 resulting from the reciprocal translocation of genetic material from chromosome 22 to chromosome 9. It is typically seen in chronic myelocytic leukemia.
  ● There is an increased incidence (20 times normal) of leukemia in patients with Down's syndrome (trisomy 21).
  ● Chromosome fragility syndromes (Bloom's syndrome, Fanconi's anemia) carry a high risk of acute leukemia.

Classification
A. According to onset and clinical course:

■ Acute leukemias:
  ● Have a sudden onset with a rapidly progressive course leading to death within months if untreated.
  ● Are characterized by primitive cells ("blasts") that are morphologically poorly differentiated.

■ Chronic leukemias:
  ● Have an insidious onset and a slow clinical course, patients often surviving several years even if untreated.
  ● Are usually characterized by more mature type cells.

TABLE 26–5. CHROMOSOMAL ABNORMALITIES ASSOCIATED WITH LEUKEMIAS

Type of Leukemia	Chromosomal Abnormality
Chronic myelocytic leukemia (CML)	Philadelphia chromosome t(9;22)[1]
CML in blast crisis	t(9;22)(X2) +8,[2] isochromosome of 17 or 4
Acute myeloblastic leukemia (AML)	t(8;21), t(15;17), t(9;22) +8, 7−, 5−, 7q−, 5q−
Erythroleukemia	7q−, 5q−
Acute monocytic leukemia	t(9;11)
Acute myelomonocytic leukemia	11q−
Polycythemia rubra vera	20q−
Acute lymphoblastic leukemia (ALL)	6q−, t(4;11), t(9;22), t(8;14)
Chronic lymphocytic leukemia (CLL)	+12

[1]Note that Phi chromosome t(9;22), while typical of CML, also is seen in CML blast crisis (multiple copies), AML, and some cases of ALL (25% of adult cases).
[2]Deletions are signified by a − suffix (eg, 7q−), trisomy by a + prefix (eg, +12).

B. According to the peripheral blood picture:

- **Leukemic,** characterized by elevation of the white blood cell count and numerous leukemic cells in peripheral blood. This is the common form.
- **Subleukemic,** in which the total white count is normal or low but leukemic cells are present in the peripheral blood.
- **Aleukemic,** in which the total white count is normal or low and no leukemic cells are present in the peripheral blood.

C. According to cell type (Fig 26–1).
1. Lymphocytic leukemias.
a. Acute lymphoblastic leukemia (ALL) is characterized by the presence in the bone marrow and peripheral blood of uniform large cells that resemble the proliferating lymphoblast of fetal development. It is further classified by its morphologic features using the French-American-British (FAB) system. See Table 26–6.

b. Chronic lymphocytic leukemia (CLL) is characterized by proliferation of small "mature" lymphocytes. In 95% of cases, the lymphocytes are B cells; in the rest, they are T cells.

2. Myeloid (granulocytic) leukemias.
a. Acute myeloblastic leukemia (AML) is characterized by proliferation of myeloblasts, which are differentiated from lymphoblasts by:

- The presence of Auer rods in the cytoplasm.
- The presence of maturation into promyelocytes.
- Cytochemical or immunologic markers (Table 26–7).

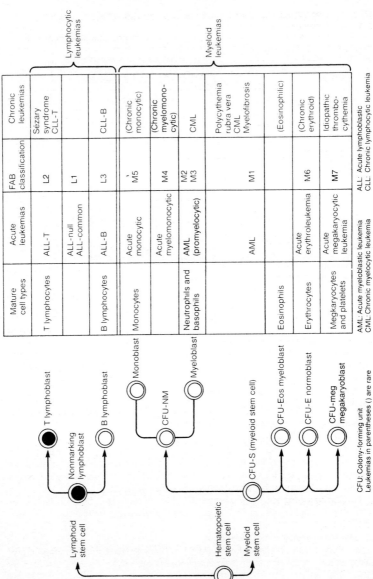

Figure 26–1. Classification of leukemias according to cell type and lineage.

CFU: Colony-forming unit
Leukemias in parentheses ( ) are rare

AML: Acute myeloblastic leukemia
CML: Chronic myelocytic leukemia

ALL: Acute lymphoblastic
CLL: Chronic lymphocytic leukemia

TABLE 26–6. THE FRENCH-AMERICAN-BRITISH (FAB) CLASSIFICATION
OF ACUTE LEUKEMIAS

Acute lymphoblastic leukemia (ALL)	
L1	Morphology medium-sized "homogeneous" blasts; immunologically non-marking but embraces several types, including common ALL and pre-B ALL; common in childhood; has the best prognosis.
L2	Heterogeneous blast cells; again a mixed group, some nonmarking, most T cell type; usual type seen in adults and has a bad prognosis.
L3	Homogeneous basophilic Burkitt-type blast cells, mark as B cells; bad prognosis
Acute myeloblastic leukemia	
M1	Consists of only myeloblasts without maturation.
M2	Myeloblasts with evidence of maturation.
M3	Acute promyelocytic leukemia; promelocytes have numerous darkly staining azurophilic cytoplasmic granules.
M4	Acute myelomonocytic leukemia is believed to arise from a cell that is the common precursor for monocytes and granulocytes (see Fig 26–1).
M5	Acute monocytic leukemia
M6	Erythroleukemia (Di Guglielmo's syndrome); predominance of erythroblasts along with myeloblasts.
M7	Megakaryoblastic leukemia

- It is further classified by the FAB system (Table 26–6) into myelomonocytic leukemia (M4), monocytic leukemia (M5), erythroleukemia (M6), and megakaryoblastic leukemia (M7), within acute myeloblastic leukemia.

    b. Chronic myelocytic leukemia (CML) is characterized by proliferation of cells of the granulocyte series that have matured beyond the myeloblast stage.

- Less than 5% of cells in the marrow are myeloblasts.
- When a patient with CML has more than 5% blasts in the bone marrow, the accelerated phase (blast crisis) is diagnosed.

3. Monocytic leukemia.

- Traditionally this included two types: acute myelomonocytic leukemia (Naegeli type, M4) and acute monocytic leukemia (Schilling type, M5), but they are now included with acute myeloblastic leukemia.
- The chronic forms of monocytic or myelomonocytic leukemia are very rare.
- Other types, such as erythroleukemia (Di Guglielmo's disease), plasma cell leukemia, eosinophilic leukemia, and megakaryocytic leukemia, are all rare.

TABLE 26–7. CYTOCHEMICAL IDENTIFICATION OF ACUTE LEUKEMIAS

Type	Peroxidase	Sudan Black	Chloroacetate Esterase	Nonspecific Esterase	Periodic Acid-Schiff	Morphologic Features
Lymphoblastic (ALL)[1]	–	–	–	–	+	Single nucleolus
Myeloblastic (AML)	+	+	+	–	–	Multiple nucleoli, Auer rods
Monocytic	–	–	–	+	–	–
Myelomonocytic	+	+	+	+	–	–
Unclassified[2]	–	–	–	–	–	–

[1]Note the subtypes of ALL may be distinguished from other acute leukemias by positivity for TdT (terminal deoxynucleotide transferase), presence of CALLA (common ALL antigen or other lymphocytic antigens), immunoglobulin or T-cell receptor gene rearrangement (see Chapter 4).
[2]Cannot be characterized cytochemically, may be identifiable by other techniques.

Clinical Features
A. Acute leukemias:

- They are characterized by an acute clinical onset and rapid progression.
- Anemia, often severe and rapidly developing, causes pallor and hypoxic symptoms.
- Thrombocytopenia may produce abnormal bleeding or purpura.
- Neutropenia results in infections, fever, and ulceration of mucous membranes.
- Patients with acute promyelocytic leukemia (M3) frequently present with disseminated intravascular coagulation.
- Enlargement of lymph nodes is common in ALL and acute monocytic leukemia but usually absent in AML.
- Involvement of tissue other than lymph nodes occurs rarely in all types of acute leukemia.
- Rarely, a local tissue mass (chloroma or granulocytic sarcoma) is the first manifestation of AML.

B. Chronic leukemias:

- They are characterized by insidious onset and a slow rate of progression.
- There is slowly developing anemia.
- Generalized lymph node enlargement is present in CLL. The histologic features are indistinguishable from those of well-differentiated lymphocytic lymphoma.
- Splenomegaly, often massive, and hepatomegaly are usually present in chronic leukemias.
- Pain in the left lower chest in CML is evidence of splenic infarction due to vascular occlusion by aggregates of granulocytes.

C. The accelerated phase (blast crisis) of CML:

- Is characterized by the appearance of myeloblasts in the bone marrow and peripheral blood.
- Occurs after a median period of 3–4 years after diagnosis of CML.
- Progresses rapidly to death if not treated.
- Is associated with the appearance of new karyotypic abnormalities (Table 26–5). Cytogenetic studies may be used to predict imminent blast crisis in patients with CML.

Diagnosis
A. Acute leukemias:

- In both AML and ALL, the peripheral blood usually shows an increased total white cell count with increased numbers of blasts.
- The bone marrow is abnormal in all cases. It is diffusely hypercellular, with proliferation of the cell type involved at the expense of the normal hematopoietic elements.
- The diagnosis of the type of acute leukemia and subclassification according to the FAB system depends on morphologic, histochemical, karyotypic and immunologic features (Tables 26–5, 26–6, and 26–7).

B. Chronic leukemias:

- Are characterized by very high peripheral white blood cell counts. The cells are mature cells.

- Neutrophil alkaline phosphatase determination is useful in distinguishing leukemoid reaction (high levels) from CML (low levels).
- The bone marrow is always abnormal.
- CML is dominated by cells of the neutrophil series (metamyelocytes and band forms dominate). Erythroid and megakaryocyte proliferation is also present.
- Myelofibrosis commonly complicates CML.
- The Philadelphia chromosome is present in 90% of cases of CML.

Treatment & Prognosis
Combination chemotherapy has dramatically improved the prognosis of patients with acute leukemias.

- Childhood ALL is now considered to be curable (over 70% five-year survival).
- The rate of cure in other types of ALL (T and B cell, 10% five-year survival), AML and acute monocytic leukemia (both with near-zero five-year survival) is much worse.
- Treatment has little effect on the survival rate of chronic leukemias. Many of these patients survive many years after diagnosis without treatment.
- Bone marrow transplantation has provided an added dimension to the treatment of leukemias.
- Hemorrhage and infection are the major causes of death of patients with leukemia, occurring as a direct effect of the leukemia or as a complication of cytotoxic therapy.

Other Related Neoplastic Processes

HAIRY CELL LEUKEMIA (Leukemic Reticuloendotheliosis)
This is a rare neoplasm of the hematopoietic system that chiefly affects individuals over age 50.

- The neoplastic cell is medium-sized, with an ovoid nucleus, a fine chromatin pattern, inconspicuous nucleoli, and abundant cytoplasm with a frayed cell membrane.
- On electron microscopy, the cell membrane shows hairy processes and a specific cytoplasmic spiral organelle (lamellar ribosomal complex).
- The cytoplasm contains tartrate-resistant acid phosphatase.
- The neoplastic cell has been demonstrated to be a B lymphocyte on the basis of the presence of immunoglobulin gene arrangement.
- Patients present with anemia, neutropenia and thrombocytopenia, and massive splenomegaly.
- They respond poorly to chemotherapy and have a median survival of 2–3 years after diagnosis.

MYELOPROLIFERATIVE DISEASES
This is a group of disorders characterized by proliferation of granulocytic, monocytic, erythroid, and megakaryocytic cell lines in the marrow.

- It includes CML, polycythemia rubra vera, idiopathic thrombocythemia, and myelofibrosis.
- The primary abnormality probably resides in the myeloid stem cell (Fig 26–1).
- A monoclonal origin is shown by the presence of one type of G6PD isoenzyme in all the proliferating cells.

- Chromosomal abnormalities are present in 50% or more of cases, including translocations involving the long arm of chromosome 1, complete or partial deletions of chromosomes 5, 7, and 20, and the appearance of the Philadelphia chromosome.
- Aspiration of marrow is often unsuccessful because of extensive fibrosis of the bone marrow (myelofibrosis).
- Residual marrow is markedly hypercellular, with proliferation of all cell lines; one cell line may evolve to dominance.
- Clusters of dysplastic megakaryocytes are typical.
- The spleen, liver, and lymph nodes commonly show extramedullary hematopoiesis.
- The peripheral blood tyically shows leukoerythroblastic anemia (except in polycythemic cases) with neutrophil leukocytosis and a marked shift to the left.

MYELODYSPLASTIC DISORDERS (Refractory Sideroblastic Anemias)

Although uncommon, these conditions are important because they may progress to AML.

- Several variants, all characterized by dyshematopoiesis, are particularly evident in erythroid cells, with increased numbers of sideroblasts.
- Primary sideroblastic anemia may occur with or without excess blasts and pancytopenia.
- Approximately 10% of patients develop AML.

Bleeding Disorders

VASCULAR DEFECTS

Vascular defects constitute the most common general cause of bleeding diathesis. The underlying defect may be production of abnormal collagen or elastin (Table 27–1) or vasculitis.

HENOCH-SCHÖNLEIN (ANAPHYLACTOID) PURPURA

This disease occurs mainly in childhood, commonly 1–3 weeks after streptococcal infection.

- It is mediated by deposition of cross-reactive IgA or immune complexes plus complement on the endothelium.
- Occasional cases have been reported with apparent hypersensitivity to other bacteria, insect bites, or food (milk, eggs, crab, strawberries).
- It presents with purpura, abdominal pain with melena, arthritis, and glomerulonephritis. Fever is common.
- Prognosis is determined by the severity of the renal lesion (focal glomerulonephritis with deposition of IgA and complement; see Chapter 48).

HEREDITARY HEMORRHAGIC TELANGIECTASIA
(Osler-Weber-Rendu Disease)

Hemorrhagic telangiectasia is inherited as an autosomal dominant trait.

- It is manifested by multiple capillary microaneurysms in the skin and mucous membranes, commonly gastrointestinal.
- Lesions tend to become more conspicuous with age and are exceedingly fragile, leading to episodes of acute severe bleeding.
- Slow occult gastrointestinal blood loss commonly causes iron deficiency anemia.

PLATELETS

Abnormalities of blood platelets that are associated with bleeding (Table 27–2) include:

- Decreased numbers (thrombocytopenia).
- Abnormal function.

IDIOPATHIC THROMBOCYTOPENIC PURPURA (ITP)

Incidence & Etiology

ITP is a common disease in which severe reduction of platelet numbers in the blood is caused by immune destruction of platelets.

- Acute ITP:
  - Is seen mainly in children.
  - Is associated with a history of viral infection 2–3 weeks before onset in 50% of cases.

TABLE 27–1. HEMORRHAGIC DISORDERS: PRINCIPAL CAUSES

Vascular defects
  Simple and senile purpura (increased capillary fragility, especially in the elderly)
  Hypersensitivity vasculitis; many autoimmune disorders (inflammation)
  Vitamin C deficiency (scurvy, defective collagen)
  Amyloidosis (affected vessels fail to constrict)
  Excess adrenocorticosteroids (therapeutic or Cushing's disease)
  Hereditary hemorrhagic telangiectasia (Osler-Weber-Rendu syndrome)
  Ehlers-Danlos disease (defective collagen)
  Henoch-Schönlein purpura (IgA and complement damage endothelium)
Disorders of platelets
  Decrease (thrombocytopenia)
  Abnormal platelet function
Disorders of coagulation
  Deficiency of coagulation factors
  Presence of anticoagulant factors
Excessive fibrinolysis
  Disseminated intravascular coagulation
  Primary fibrinolysis

- The probable mechanism is binding of immune complexes to the surface of platelets, resulting in phagocytosis by splenic macrophages.
- Spontaneous recovery is the rule; 80% are normal after 6 months, and many recover within 6 weeks.
■ Chronic ITP:
  - Occurs mainly in adults, with a predilection for females and tendency to relapse during pregnancy.
  - The probable mechanism is the presence of IgG antiplatelet autoantibody.
  - Rarely resolves spontaneously; is usually a long-standing disorder characterized by multiple relapses and remissions.
■ Neonatal thrombocytopenic purpura:
  - Occurs in children born to mothers with chronic ITP.
  - Results from transfer of the IgG antibodies across the placenta.

Pathology
The peripheral platelet survival is impaired.

■ The platelet count is markedly decreased, often to the 10,000–50,000/μL range.
■ The bone marrow typically shows increased numbers of megakaryocytes.
■ The spleen is the major site of destruction of antibody– or immune complex–coated platelets.
■ The spleen is usually either normal in size or slightly enlarged and shows sinusoidal congestion and hyperplasia of macrophages.
■ The bleeding time is prolonged and capillary fragility (tourniquet test) increased.
■ Tests of coagulation (clotting time, partial thromboplastin time, and prothrombin time) are normal. Clot retraction is defective.

Clinical Features & Treatment
Patients present with a bleeding tendency, usually purpura. Less commonly, bleeding occurs from mucosal surfaces or into brain.

TABLE 27–2. PLATELET ABNORMALITIES THAT CAUSE BLEEDING

Thrombocytopenia
  Decreased production in the bone marrow
    Aplastic anemia: any of numerous causes, including idiopathic
    Radiation
    Marrow infiltration by leukemia, metastatic neoplasms, infections
    Vitamin B_{12} and folate deficiency
    Hereditary, autosomal dominant form: Wiskott-Aldrich syndrome, May-Hegglin syndrome
  Pooling (sequestration) of platelets in an enlarged spleen
  Increased peripheral destruction of platelets
    Immune mechanisms
      Idiopathic thrombocytopenic purpura
      Systemic lupus erythematosus
      Drug-induced thrombocytopenia (gold salts, quinine, sulfonamides)
      Neonatal thrombocytopenia: transfer of maternal IgG antibodies with activity against fetal
        platelets
      Posttransfusion: due to alloantibodies to platelet antigen $P1^{A1}$ (rare but severe)
    Hypersplenism
    Increased platelet consumption
      Disseminated intravascular coagulation
      Thrombotic thrombocytopenic purpura
      Hemolytic uremic syndrome
      Valve prosthesis, artificial vascular grafts
  Dilution of platelets: massive transfusions
Qualitative platelet disorders (abnormal function)
  Congenital
    Defects of adhesion: Bernard-Soulier disease
    Defects of aggregation: thrombasthenia (Glanzmann's disease)
    Abnormal granule release: storage pool disease
    Wiskott-Aldrich syndrome
    Von Willebrand's disease
    Albinism
  Acquired
    Uremia
    Dysproteinemias
    Chronic liver disease, especially alcoholic
    Drug-induced: aspirin, phenylbutazone
    Myeloproliferative diseases
    Vascular disorders: many diseases producing vascular damage also affect platelet function

- Clinical bleeding occurs when the platelet count falls to very low levels ($< 40,000/\mu L$).
- The diagnosis of ITP is one of exclusion, reached by ruling out all other causes of thrombocytopenia (Table 27–2).
- The peripheral blood and bone marrow findings are suggestive but not specific, and there is no laboratory test to confirm the diagnosis.
- High dosage corticosteroids prolongs the life span of the antibody-coated platelets.
- Splenectomy is effective in treatment by removing the main site of platelet destruction but does nothing to correct the basic abnormality.

TABLE 27–3. ABNORMALITIES OF PLATELET FUNCTION

Disease	Inheritance	Platelet Adhesion[1]	Platelet Aggregation			Other Features
			Collagen[2]	ADP[2]	Ristocetin[2]	
Congenital						
Bernard-Soulier disease	AR	↓	N	N	↓	Giant platelets
Glanzmann's thrombasthenia	AR	N	↓	↓	N	Absent clot retraction
Storage pool disease	Variable	N	↓	↓	N	Absent dense bodies
von Willebrand's disease	AD	↓	N	N	↓	Corrected by factor VIII.vWF
Acquired						
Aspirin	—	N	↓	↓	N	Decreased cyclooxygenase
Uremia	—	↓	↓	↓	N	Pathogenesis not known
Myeloproliferative diseases	—	↓	↓	↓	N	Pathogenesis not known

AR = autosomal recessive; AD = autosomal dominant; N = normal.
[1]Tests of adhesiveness are difficult to standardize.
[2]Aggregation induced by collagen, adenosine diphosphate (ADP), or ristocetin in vitro. Other inducers of aggregation include arachidonic acid and epinephrine; the normal range is 60–100% of control.

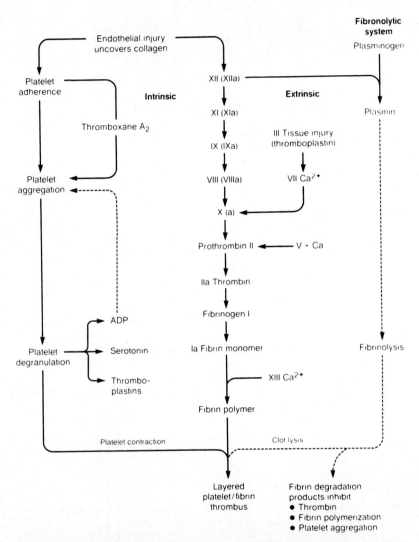

Figure 27–1. Coagulation and fibrinolytic systems. The balance between these 2 systems is very finely tuned. If this balance is disturbed, pathologic thrombosis or excessive bleeding may result.

ABNORMALITIES OF PLATELET FUNCTION

Platelet function abnormalities are characterized by symptoms and signs of platelet deficiency (ie, abnormal bleeding) but with a normal platelet count. Tests of platelet function, such as clot retraction, platelet adhesion, and aggregation in response to different agents, are abnormal and are valuable in differential diagnosis (Table 27–3).

BLOOD COAGULATION

NORMAL BLOOD COAGULATION

Coagulation is the method of permanent healing of a vascular injury; it follows vasoconstriction and formation of the platelet plug. It is achieved by the sequential interaction of several plasma factors that results in formation of fibrin (Fig 27–1).

DISORDERS OF BLOOD COAGULATION

Etiology

A. Deficiencies of coagulation factors:

- Commonly occur as inherited diseases (Table 27–4).
- Most commonly manifest as factor VIII deficiency (hemophilia A and von Willebrand's disease) and factor IX deficiency (Christmas disease).
- Acquired deficiencies of coagulation factors occur in:
  - Severe liver diseases (multiple factors).
  - Vitamin K deficiency (prothrombin and factors VII, IX, and X).

B. Presence of circulating anticoagulants:

- Anticoagulant therapy with coumarin derivatives interferes with vitamin K, thereby inhibiting synthesis of prothrombin and factors VII, IX, and X.
- Directly acting anticoagulants include:
  - Drugs such as heparin (an antithrombin).
  - Antibodies (factor VIII inhibitor and lupus anticoagulant, an antibody in systemic lupus erythematosus).
  - Natural anticoagulants (antithrombin and fibrin degradation products).

C. Increased fibrinolytic activity results from increased activation of plasmin.

Clinical Features

Patients tend to bleed excessively following minor trauma such as dentistry; bleeding is typically slow but persistent.

- In severe cases, spontaneous bleeding occurs (ie, bleeding without evident trauma), commonly into joints (hemarthrosis) and muscles.
- Determination of the cause of the abnormality requires bleeding and coagulation testing (Table 27–5).

FACTOR VIII DEFICIENCY

Factor VIII is a complex molecule composed of:

TABLE 27-4. DISEASES RESULTING FROM AN INHERITED COAGULATION
FACTOR DEFICIENCY

Deficient Factor	Disease	Inheritance	Frequency[1]	Disease Severity
Fibrinogen	Afibrinogenemia	AR	Rare	Variable
	Congenital dys-fibrinogenemia	AD	Rare	Variable
Prothrombin	. . .	. . .	Very rare	Variable
Factor V	Parahemophilia	AR	Very rare	Moderate to severe
Factor VII	. . .	AR	Very rare	Moderate to severe
Factor VIII	Hemophilia A	XR	Common	Mild to severe
	von Willebrand's disease	AD	Common	Mild to moderate
Factor IX	Hemophilia B	XR	Uncommon	Mild to severe
Factor X	. . .	AR	Rare	Variable
Factor XI	Rosenthal's syndrome	AR	Uncommon	Mild
Factor XII	Hageman trait	AR/AD	Rare	Asymptomatic
Factor XIII	. . .	AR	Rare	Severe

AR = autosomal recessive; AD = autosomal dominant; XR = X-linked recessive.
[1]Frequency: very rare = fewer than 100 reported cases; compare to hemophilia A with a frequency of 1/10,000 males.

- Factor VIII-related antigen (VIII:RAg), which is the largest part of the molecule. It is detected by immunologic methods and has no function in coagulation.
- Factor VIII coagulant (VIII:C) is the functional part of the molecule (antihemophilic globulin). Deficiency produces hemophilia A.
- Factor VIII-von Willebrand factor (VIII:VWF) is required in platelet aggregation. Deficiency produces von Willebrand's disease.

1. HEMOPHILIA A

Incidence & Etiology
Hemophilia A is inherited as an X-linked recessive trait, occurring mainly in males.

TABLE 27–5. MAJOR BLEEDING DISORDERS: DIFFERENTIAL LABORATORY FEATURES

	Tourniquet Test	Bleeding Time	Whole Blood Clotting Time	Platelet Count	Partial Thromboplastin Time (PTT)	Prothrombin Time (PT)	Comments
Vascular defects	+	↑ or N	N	N	N	N	
Platelet defects Thrombocytopenia	+	↑	N	↓	N	N	Abnormal clot retraction.
Platelet function defects	+	↑	N	N	N	N	See Table 27–3.
Coagulation defects Hemophilia A	N	N	↑	N	↑	N	VIII.C ↓ VIII.RAg and VIII.vWF normal.
von Willebrand's disease	+ or N	↑	↑ or N	N	↑	N	VIII.C ↓ VIII.RAg ↓ VIII.vWF ↓ abnormal ristocetin test.
Christmas disease (hemophilia B)	N	N	↑	N	↑	N	IX ↓
Deficiency of vitamin K-dependent factors (II, VII, IX, X)	N	N	↑ or N	N	↑	↑	Corrected by vitamin K therapy.
Liver diseases	N	N	↑ or N	N	↑	↑	Not corrected by vitamin K.
Disorders of fibrinolysis Disseminated intravascular coagulation	+ or N	↑	↑	↓	↑	↑	Presence of fibrin degradation products; positive protamine sulfate test.
Primary fibrinolysis	N	N	↑	N	↑	↑	

N = normal

- Females develop hemophilia only when they are homozygous for the abnormal gene—a rare event that occurs when a hemophiliac male mates with a carrier female.
- The incidence in the United States is 1:10,000 males.
- It occurs throughout the world.
- The presence of the abnormal gene results in deficient synthesis of the coagulant subunit of the factor VIII molecule.
- Factor VIII-related antigen and factor VIII–von Willebrand factor are present in normal amounts.
- The heterozygous female carrier shows a mild decrease in plasma level of the coagulant subunit of factor VIII (VIII:C). The ratio of VIII:C to VIII:RAg is less than 0.75 (normal is 1.0) and is a reliable means of detecting heterozygous carrier females.

Pathology & Clinical Features
Patients with severe hemophilia have less than 1% of factor VIII coagulant activity and bleed spontaneously.

- Moderately affected patients (1–5% activity) bleed excessively after minor trauma.
- Mild cases (5–25% activity) are usually asymptomatic.
- Bleeding after dental surgery is typical. Bleeding consists of a slow and persistent ooze beginning several hours after surgery and lasting many days.
- Spontaneous bleeding occurs into subcutaneous tissues, skeletal muscle, joints, and mucous membranes. This is followed by organization leading to:
  - Contractures in muscles.
  - Fibrous ankylosis and stiffness of joints.
- Intracranial hemorrhage is rare but is a major cause of death.

Diagnosis & Treatment
The partial thromboplastin time is prolonged in almost all patients.

- There is a significant decrease in factor VIII coagulant activity (to less than 20% of normal). Factor VIII-related antigen is normal, and the VIII:C to VIII:RAg ratio is markedly decreased.
- Prothrombin time and bleeding time are normal.
- Treatment consists of maintaining plasma factor VIII coagulant activity at a level that permits normal physical activity without bleeding.
- Factor VIII:C is provided in fresh plasma, cryoprecipitate, or lyophilized factor VIII concentrate.
- Cryoprecipitate and factor VIII concentrate increases the risk of hepatitis B and C, cytomegalovirus infection, and AIDS. Hemophiliacs represent a high-risk group for AIDS.

2. VON WILLEBRAND'S DISEASE
Von Willebrand's disease is inherited as an autosomal dominant trait.

- It is characterized by deficiency of the entire factor VIII molecule.
- Factor VIII coagulant activity and factor VIII-related antigen are decreased to the same extent, so that the ratio of these two components is normal.
- Clinically, patients show bleeding after minor trauma.
- The onset of symptoms is in childhood and may decrease with age.

- The commonest sites of bleeding are the skin (easy bruising) and mucous membranes (epistaxis).
- Hemarthrosis, muscle hemorrhage, and intracranial hemorrhage are uncommon.
- The diagnosis is made by demonstrating:
  - Prolonged partial thromboplastin time with normal prothrombin time.
  - Decreased factor VIII coagulant activity and factor VIII-related antigen.
  - Prolonged bleeding time due to platelet dysfunction (Table 27–5).
  - Decreased platelet aggregation by the antibiotic ristocetin.
- Von Willebrand factor is present in cryoprecipitate, which can be used in treatment.

FACTOR IX DEFICIENCY (Christmas Disease; Hemophilia B)

Factor IX deficiency is uncommon, with an incidence of 1:50,000 population.

- It results from a deficiency of factor IX.
- It is characterized by X-linked recessive inheritance, greater prevalence in males, and a clinical picture identical to that of hemophilia A.
- The diagnosis is considered when factor VIII coagulant activity is normal in a patient with symptoms of hemophilia.
- Plasma factor IX assay shows greatly decreased levels.
- Treatment is with fresh plasma or factor IX concentrate. Factor IX is not present in cryoprecipitate.

The Lymphoid System:
I. Manifestations of Disease;
Infections & Reactive
Proliferations

28

MANIFESTATIONS OF DISEASES OF THE LYMPHOID SYSTEM

IMMUNE DEFICIENCY (See Chapter 7)

- Lymphopenia, which may occur after radiotherapy, cytotoxic drugs, or corticosteroids, is associated with immunodeficiency.
- Decreased T helper cells and increased T suppressor cells occur in AIDS and some postinfectious immunodeficiency states.
- Selective atrophy of lymphoid tissues occurs in the congenital immune deficiency syndromes (Chapter 7).

PERVERTED IMMUNE FUNCTION
Abnormal immune responses include immunologic hypersensitivity and autoimmunity (Chapter 8).

- It may be associated with some proliferation of lymphoid tissue.
- The primary pathologic features and clinical effects occur in the organs that are the target of the abnormal immune response.

LYMPHADENOPATHY (Table 28–1)
Lymphadenopathy may be localized to one lymph node group in the body or may be generalized. It may be associated with enlargement of other lymphoid tissues (eg, splenomegaly; see Chapter 30).

LYMPHOCYTOSIS (See Chapter 26)
Lymphocytosis may occur either as a function of the immune response or as a result of neoplastic proliferation of lymphoid cells in lymphocytic leukemia and lymphoma.

- In leukemia, the bone marrow is always involved.
- Malignant lymphoma may or may not involve the marrow and usually involves lymph nodes and tissues.

MONOCLONAL GAMMOPATHY
Monoclonal gammopathy manifests as a discrete "spike" in serum electrophoresis, usually consisting of one immunoglobulin (M protein). It is commonly seen with neo-

TABLE 28–1. CAUSES OF LYMPHADENOPATHY[1]

Reactive hyperplasia (the immune response)
Nonspecifc
  Usually a local response to introduction of antigen, most commonly bacterial (eg, strep throat, syphilis, plague), or postvaccination, or draining a cancer site

  Occasionally generalized, as a response to viremia (eg, rubella) or drug hypersensitivity

With specific features
  Dermatopathic lymphadenitis
  Lymphangiography reaction
  Persistent generalized lymphadenopathy (AIDS-related complex)

Reactive hyperplasia (associated with specific infections)
  Pyogenic lymphadenitis
  Measles
  Infectious mononucleosis
  Toxoplasmosis
  Granulomatous (eg, tuberculosis, histoplasmosis, coccidiodomycosis)
  Granulomatous and suppurative (lymphogranuloma venereum, cat scratch disease)

Lymphadenopathy of uncertain cause
  Sarcoidosis
  With autoimmune diseases and hypersensitivity states (eg, rheumatoid arthritis, systemic lupus erythematosus, polyarteritis nodosa, serum sickness)
  Sinus histiocytosis with massive lymphadenopathy
  Giant lymph node hyperplasia
  Abnormal immune response and immunoblastic lymphadenopathy

Primary neoplastic proliferations: the lymphomas
  Non-Hodgkin's lymphomas and lymphocytic leukemias
  Hodgkin's disease
  Neoplasms of histiocytes

Secondary neoplasms: metastases
  Carcinoma
  Melanoma

[1]Most of the conditions listed may also affect lymphoid tissue elsewhere (eg, spleen, gut-associated lymphoid tissue).

plasms of B cell derivation that show evidence of plasmacytoid differentiation (myeloma, plasmacytoid lymphocytic lymphoma, heavy chain disease (see Chapter 30).

REACTIVE LYMPHOID HYPERPLASIAS

NONSPECIFIC REACTIVE HYPERPLASIA
Relative hyperplasia within lymphoid tissue represents the tissue manifestation of the immune response.

- It consists of three interrelated elements:
  - Follicular hyperplasia (the B cell response).

- Paracortical hyperplasia (the T cell response).
- Sinus histiocytosis (the histiocyte response).
- Any one of the above may predominate, but most responses represent an admixture of all three.
■ Most cases are localized to the site of antigen entry, eg, cervical lymphadenopathy in pharyngitis.
■ Generalized reactive hyperplasia may occur with an antigen that is distributed throughout the body, eg, in viral infections.

SPECIFIC REACTIVE HYPERPLASIAS

1. DERMATOPATHIC LYMPHADENITIS

■ It occurs in lymph nodes draining skin that is chronically inflamed or ulcerated, such as chronic radiation dermatitis, psoriasis, and exfoliative dermatitis.
■ Its most conspicuous feature is the presence of numerous pale histiocytes containing lipid material and melanin released by the damaged epidermis.

2. LYMPHANGIOGRAPHY-ALTERED LYMPH NODES

■ Florid hyperplasia of histiocytes occurs following lymphangiography.
■ The histiocyte cytoplasm contain globules of the oily dye.
■ It is of no clinical significance.

3. PERSISTENT GENERALIZED LYMPHADENOPATHY (PGL)

■ Patients who are at risk for AIDS commonly show persistent enlargement of lymph nodes, often generalized and often associated with fever.
■ These patients do not have AIDS as defined by the clinical criteria for the disease.
  - They have serum antibodies for the human immunodeficiency virus (HIV), and the virus can often be isolated from involved lymph nodes.
  - PGL is one of the manifestations of AIDS-related complex (ARC).
■ Ten percent of the estimated 2 million people in the United States who have contracted the virus and give a positive test for HIV antibody have evidence of persistent generalized lymphadenopathy.
■ The lymph nodes show follicular and paracortical hyperplasia, with very large conspicuous follicles, and irregular loss of the mantle zone.

SPECIFIC INFECTIONS OF LYMPH NODES

ACUTE PYOGENIC (BACTERIAL) LYMPHADENITIS
This is usually secondary to the spread of bacteria via lymphatics from a focus of infection in the area drained by the node.

■ It is characterized by acute inflammation with neutrophil infiltration of the node.
■ Clinically, there is lymph node enlargement with pain and tenderness, fever and neutrophil leukocytosis.
■ Abscess formation is common.

MEASLES

Measles is associated with a marked T cell response with expansion of the paracortical zone, and characterized by the presence of large multinucleated cells called Warthin-Finkeldey giant cells.

INFECTIOUS MONONUCLEOSIS

It is caused by the Epstein-Barr virus, which infects B cells.

- More common in children and young adults, it is transmitted via the upper respiratory tract, commonly through kissing ("kissing disease").
- Patients present with acute onset of fever, sore throat, lymphadenopathy, and hepatosplenomegaly. Mild liver dysfunction may be present.
- The peripheral blood shows lymphocytosis with atypical transformed lymphocytes (Downey cells).
- The diagnosis is confirmed serologically by:
  - Detection of heterophil antibodies by the Paul-Bunnell test (Monospot test). This is not specific for infectious mononucleosis.
  - Detection of specific antibodies against EB virus antigens (capsid, membrane and nuclear antigens).
- Lymph nodes show a florid T cell hyperplasia with numerous transformed T immunoblasts.

TOXOPLASMOSIS

Toxoplasmosis is an infection by the protozoon *Toxoplasma gondii*, which commonly infects cats, rodents, and livestock. Human infection is usually acquired by ingestion of oocysts from soil contaminated by cat feces. Less often, infection may be by ingestion of tissue cysts from undercooked pork.

A. Acquired toxoplasmosis:

- Occurs in the adult.
- Presents as an acute febrile illness with generalized lymphadenopathy.
- Lymph node biopsy shows extensive follicular hyperplasia and proliferation of histiocytes in clusters in the paracortex and within reactive centers.
- Pseudocysts of *Toxoplasma* may be seen occasionally. Tachyzoites are almost never seen.
- Immunohistologic techniques using specific antibodies are helpful in detecting the organisms.

B. Congenital toxoplasmosis:

- Is a much more serious condition in which infection is transmitted transplacentally from mother to fetus.
- Is characterized by necrosis in the brain, often severe, and retinal involvement.
- Organisms are seen in large numbers in both brain and retina.
- It may cause:
  - Stillbirth.
  - Microcephaly, hydrocephalus, and blindness in the neonatal period.
  - Delayed neurologic and learning defects.

- The diagnosis is by serologic techniques or isolation of the organism by animal inoculation.
- Serologic tests include:
  - The Sabin-Feldman dye test.
  - The more sensitive fluorescence or enzyme-linked immunoassay (ELISA).

GRANULOMATOUS LYMPHADENITIS

This represents a T cell lymphokine–mediated immune response with delayed hypersensitivity, leading to caseous epithelioid cell granulomas.

- It is caused by facultative intracellular organisms:
  - *Mycobacterium tuberculosis,* the most common.
  - Atypical mycobacteria.
  - Fungi, commonly *Histoplasma capsulatum,* and *Coccidioides immitis.*
- It usually effects only one or two lymph node groups, representing those nodes draining the sites of primary infection. Cervical nodes are most commonly affected.
- Histologically, the paracortical T cell response is admixed with caseating epithelioid cell granulomas, which may be small, or large and coalescent.
- Diagnosis is by culture.
- Organisms may be demonstrated in histologic sections using special stains:
  - Acid fast (Ziehl-Neelsen) stain for mycobacteria.
  - Periodic acid Schiff and methenamine silver stains for fungi.

SUPPURATIVE GRANULOMATOUS LYMPHADENITIS

- It is characterized by suppuration with neutrophils in the center of the epithelioid cell granulomas.
- The fully formed suppurative granuloma tends to be stellate (star-shaped).
- It is caused by several different infectious agents, including chlamydiae (lymphogranuloma venereum), cat-scratch bacillus, and others (see following).

1. LYMPHOGRANULOMA VENEREUM

This is a sexually transmitted disease, most common in the tropics, caused by *Chlamydia trachomatis.*

- It is characterized by a local papule on the external genitalia with regional lymphadenopathy, with suppuration and discharge of pus through multiple sinuses.
- Diagnosis may be suspected by finding stellate suppurative granulomas in biopsied lymph nodes, and confirmed serologically with a complement fixation test.

2. CAT-SCRATCH DISEASE

Cat-scratch disease is caused by a small gram-negative bacterium that stains positively with silver stains.

- It presents with acute onset of fever with lymphadenopathy.
- A history of a wound and exposure to cats is common.
- The diagnosis is clinical, confirmed by the presence of suppurative granulomas on lymph node biopsy and demonstration of the organism by Warthin-Starry silver stain and culture.
- The disease is self-limited.

3. OTHER CAUSES
Other rare causes of suppurative granulomas include:

- Mesenteric lymphadenitis in young children due to *Yersinia enterocolitica* and *Yersinia pseudotuberculosis.*
- Brucellosis, caused by Brucella species.
- Tularemia, due to *Pasteurella tularensis.*
- Bubonic plague, due to *Yersinia pestis.*
- Glanders and melioidosis, caused by *Pseudomonas mallei* and *Pseudomonas pseudomallei.*

LYMPHADENOPATHY OF UNCERTAIN CAUSE

SARCOIDOSIS
Sarcoidosis is a systemic disease characterized by the presence of noninfectious epithelioid cell granulomas in many tissues, particularly lung, liver, lymph nodes, and skin.

- Clinically, it ranges from asymptomatic to a severe febrile debilitating illness with cough and dyspnea, characterized by a chronic course with remissions and relapses.
- It is more common in men than in women, in blacks than in whites, and in the age group from 20 to 30 years.
- The incidence is high in Scandinavia, Western Europe, and North America.
- Histologically, there are epithelioid cell granulomas without caseation.
- Sarcoid granulomas frequently contain calcified bodies called Schaumann bodies; not specific for sarcoidosis.
- No etiologic agent has been identified.
- Serum levels of angiotensin converting enzyme are often elevated.
- Patients show depressed cell-mediated immunity (anergy), excessive B cell activity (hyperglobulinemia), and sometimes an excess of helper T cells.
- The **Kveim test** (a skin test utilizing an extract of known sarcoid tissue) is usually positive.

LYMPHADENOPTHY OF AUTOIMMUNE DISEASE
Significant lymph node enlargement may be seen in systemic lupus erythematosus, rheumatoid arthritis—particularly the juvenile form (Still's disease; Chapter 68), and Sjögren's syndrome (Chapter 33).

- Affected lymph nodes show nonspecific follicular hyperplasia, with occasional evidence of vasculitis.
- Hypersensitivity states such as serum sickness and chronic drug reactions (eg, reactions to aminosalicylic acid [PAS], an antituberculous drug) may also produce lymphadenopathy, with mixed B and T cell response.

SINUS HISTIOCYTOSIS WITH MASSIVE LYMPHADENOPATHY
This is an uncommon disease outside North Africa. In the United States, it occurs mainly in blacks.

- The cause is unknown.
- Children are mainly affected.

- Clinical presentation is with massive cervical lymphadenopathy, often bilateral, which may be associated with fever and mild anemia.
- Affected lymph nodes contain large numbers of histiocytes filling the sinuses. The histiocytes contain normal lymphocytes within their cytoplasm (**emperipolesis**).
- The disease is self-limited.

GIANT LYMPH NODE HYPERPLASIA (Castleman-Iverson Disease)

This is an uncommon condition characterized by benign nonprogressive lymphadenopathy, usually in the mediastinum or retroperitoneum.

A. Plasmacellular form:

- The lymph node shows large follicles with numerous plasma cells. The plasma cells are polyclonal.
- There is often an associated polyclonal hyperglobulinemia and low-grade fever.
- A significant number of cases progress to malignant lymphoma.

B. Angiofollicular form:

- Lymph nodes contain numerous small follicles associated with excessive numbers of peculiar hyalinized vessels.
- It is not believed to be associated with an increased incidence of malignant lymphoma.

ANGIOIMMUNOBLASTIC LYMPHADENOPATHY

This is a relatively uncommon condition, primarily affecting patients over age 50.

- It presents with weight loss, fever, hepatosplenomegaly, skin rashes, and generalized lymphadenopathy.
- Fifty percent of patients die within three years, either of infection or an aggressive malignant lymphoma (15–20%).
- The cause is unknown.
- Lymph nodes show progressive depletion of lymphoid cells, obliteration of normal architecture, loss of follicles, and numerous immunoblasts (both B and T).

The Lymphoid System: II. Malignant Lymphomas

29

THE MALIGNANT LYMPHOMAS

Malignant lymphomas are primary neoplasms of lymphoid tissue. They occur as solid tumors, usually within lymph nodes and less often in extranodal lymphoid tissues such as the tonsil, gastrointestinal tract, and spleen. They are classified as non-Hodgkin's and Hodgkin's lymphomas.

Non-Hodgkin's Lymphomas

Incidence

Leukemias and lymphomas, including Hodgkin's lymphoma, account for approximately 8% of all malignant neoplasms and together represent the sixth most common type of cancer.

- Twenty-five thousand cases of non-Hodgkin's lymphoma occur annually in the United States.
- The relative incidence of the subtypes of lymphoma varies greatly with age (Table 29–1).

Etiology

- Many animal lymphomas have a viral etiology. In humans, the viral relationship is less clearcut.
- Autoimmune and immunodeficiency diseases are associated with an increased incidence of lymphoma, eg, in AIDS and transplant patients.
- Epstein-Barr virus infection has a strong association with Burkitt's lymphoma in Africa.
- HTLV-I (Human T Leukemia Virus I) shows a strong association with T cell lymphoma-leukemia in Japan.
- HTLV-II, a related retrovirus, causes some forms of chronic T cell leukemia, and HTLV-V has been implicated in cutaneous T cell lymphomas.
- Many lymphomas show distinctive chromosomal markers (eg, Burkitt's lymphoma shows an 8;14 translocation). In many cases the breakpoint for the translocation has been shown to be at the insertion point of an oncogene (*C-MYC* oncogene in Burkitt's lymphoma).

Diagnosis

Lymphomas must be distinguished from the proliferation that occurs normally as part of the immune response (reactive hyperplasia). The usual cytologic criteria for distinguishing malignant neoplasms are not reliable in identifying a lymphoid proliferation as

TABLE 29-1. RELATIVE INCIDENCE OF LYMPHOMAS IN ADULTS AND CHILDREN

	Adult	Child
Hodgkin's lymphoma	15%	Rare
Follicular center cell[1]	35% (mostly small cleaved)	50% (all small noncleaved including Burkitt's)
Lymphocytic[1]	10%	Rare
Immunoblastic[1]	10%	Rare
Plasmacytoid[1]	10%	Rare
Convoluted[1] (lymphoblastic)	10%	40%
Others	Rare	Rare

[1]Subtypes of non-Hodgkin's lymphoma.

neoplastic. Evidence of spread in the body is not a useful criterion because both normal and neoplastic lymphocytes circulate extensively.

- Cytologic criteria are not very helpful.
  - Pleomorphism and nuclear abnormalities occur both in neoplastic and reactive immunoblasts.
  - The number of mitotic figures is often high in reactive lymph nodes. Malignant lymphomas may or may not have a high mitotic rate.
- Loss of normal lymph node architecture, particularly if coupled with a lack of the normal admixture of cell types, favors malignant lymphoma.
- Monoclonality is demonstrated by the vast majority of lymphomas, as opposed to immune responses which are polyclonal. Monoclonality can be established by:
  - Presence of monoclonal light or heavy chain immunoglobulin in a B cell population.
  - Clonal immunoglobulin gene rearrangement (B cell).
  - Clonal T receptor gene rearrangement (T cell).
  - Presence of a clonal chromosomal marker (eg, the 8;14 translocation in Burkitt's lymphoma).

NOMENCLATURE & CLASSIFICATION
Malignant lymphomas show enormous variation in clinical behavior and response to therapy. The aim of classification is to identify homogeneous subgroups that behave in a predictable way. They are named according to the normal cell they most closely resemble (Fig 29-1). Many different classifications are used.

A. Morphologic classification (Rappaport):

- The Rappaport classification (1956) of non-Hodgkin's lymphomas is shown in Table 29-2.

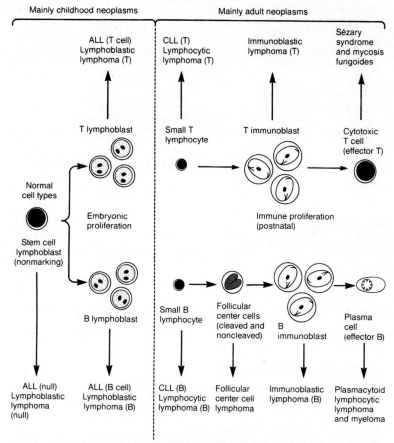

Figure 29–1. Lymphomas and leukemias derived from lymphocytes, showing relationships of the neoplastic lymphoid cells to normal lymphocyte counterparts. The cells drawn in the central area represent normal embryonic and adult lymphoid cells. Neoplasms derived from these cells are shown at top (T cell neoplasms) and bottom (B cell neoplasms). ALL = acute lymphoblastic leukemia; CLL = chronic lymphocytic leukemia.

■ Though it is scientifically inaccurate and will eventually be replaced, it is of clinical value in separating some of the lymphomas into more and less aggressive types.
■ Most "histiocytic" lymphomas are derived from transformed lymphocytes.

TABLE 29-2. THE RAPPAPORT CLASSIFICATION (MORPHOLOGIC)
OF NON-HODGKIN'S LYMPHOMA

Type of Lymphoma[1]	Cells of Origin[2]
Well-differentiated lymphocytic lymphoma	Small T lymphocyte Small B lymphocyte Effector T lymphocyte
Poorly differentiated lymphocytic lymphoma	Stem cell (nonmarking lymphoblast) Embryonic T lymphoblast Embryonic B lymphoblast Follicular center B cells
Mixed	Follicular center B cells
Histiocytic lymphoma[3]	T immunoblast B immunoblast Follicular center B cell True histiocyte

[1]Any of these types could occur in a follicular or a diffuse pattern, the former having a more favorable prognosis.
[2]As currently understood; see Fig 29–1.
[3]Note that "histiocytic" lymphomas, as the term is used here, are mainly derived from activated lymphocytes. True histiocytic lymphomas are extremely rare.

B. Immune-based classifications:

- The Lukes and Collins classification (1974) is widely used in the United States (Table 29–3).
- It has not gained widespread acceptance because of its complexity and the need for ancillary tests to reach precise diagnoses.

C. The working formulation classification:

- In 1975, a classification system called "The Working Formulation of Non-Hodgkin's Lymphoma for Clinical Usage" was proposed in a multi-institutional study. This classification is currently in use in the United States (Table 29–4).
- It divides non-Hodgkin's lymphomas into:
  - Low-grade lymphomas, which are clinically indolent diseases with long median survival times, but are rarely cured by therapy.
  - Intermediate-grade lymphomas.
  - High-grade lymphomas, which have an aggressive natural history but are responsive to chemotherapy.

SPECIFIC TYPES OF NON-HODGKIN'S LYMPHOMAS

1. B CELL LYMPHOMAS
A. Small lymphocytic lymphomas:

- Are characterized by a diffuse proliferation of uniform, small lymphocytes.
- Represent the tissue equivalent of chronic lymphocytic leukemia.

TABLE 29–3. THE LUKES-COLLINS (IMMUNE-BASED) CLASSIFICATION OF NON-HODGKIN'S LYMPHOMA (MODIFIED)

Neoplasm	Corresponding Normal Cell
Nonmarking cells[1] Acute lymphoblastic leukemia (ALL; null cell) Lymphoblastic lymphoma (null)	Stem cell (nonmarking lymphoblast)
T cells Convoluted T cell lymphoma T cell ALL	T cell lymphoblast
T-cell chronic lymphocytic leukemia (CLL)/lymphocytic lymphoma	Small T cell lymphocyte
T-cell immunoblastic lymphoma[2]	T cell immunoblast
Mycosis fungoides/Sézary syndrome	Effector T cell
B cells B cell ALL B-cell lymphoblastic lymphoma	B lymphoblast
B cell CLL/lymphocytic lymphoma	Small B lymphocyte
Follicular center cell lymphoma	Follicular center B cell[3]
B-cell immunoblastic lymphoma[2]	B immunoblast
Plasmacytoid lymphocytic lymphoma	Effector B cell
Histiocyte True histiocytic lymphoma	Histiocyte

[1]Nonmarking category was designated as U (or undefined) in original classification.

[2]Immunoblastic lymphoma is sometimes called immunoblastic sarcoma.

[3]The follicular center contains several morphologic variants of the B lymphocyte, including small cleaved, large cleaved, small noncleaved, and large noncleaved cells. Follicular center cell lymphomas corresponding to these cell types have been recognized. Burkitt's lymphoma is usually included in this category; others would place it under B lymphoblastic. These are closely related categories (see Fig 29–1), and the decision is somewhat arbitrary.

- Are low-grade.
- Rarely transform to an aggressive lymphoma (Richter's syndrome).

B. Plasmacytoid lymphocytic lymphomas:

- Are similar to small lymphocytic lymphomas, but show plasmacytoid differentiation.
- Are commonly associated with an IgM monoclonal spike (Waldenstroms macroglobulinemia).
- Are low-grade.

TABLE 29–4. THE WORKING FORMULATION OF NON-HODGKIN'S LYMPHOMAS FOR CLINICAL USE[1]

Low-grade
 Small lymphocytic lymphoma; includes chronic lymphocytic leukemia and plasmacytoid lymphocytic lymphoma.
 Follicular, small, cleaved cell lymphoma.
 Follicular, mixed small cleaved and large cell lymphoma.
Intermediate-grade
 Follicular, large cell lymphoma.
 Diffuse, small cleaved cell lymphoma.
 Diffuse, mixed small and large cell lymphoma.
 Diffuse, large cell (cleaved and noncleaved) lymphoma.
High-grade
 Large cell, immunoblastic lymphoma.
 Lymphoblastic (convoluted and nonconvoluted cell) lymphoma.
 Small noncleaved cell (Burkitt's) lymphoma.
Miscellaneous
 Composite, mycosis fungoides, histiocytic lymphoma; extramedullary plasmacytoma, unclassifiable, others.

[1]Assignment to grades is based on overall pattern (follicular or diffuse) and cell type.

C. Small cleaved cell lymphomas:

- Are characterized by small lymphocytes with hyperchromatic nuclei showing deep cleaves and scanty cytoplasm.
- May have a minority of larger cells, but few transformed cells and a low mitotic rate.
- Seventy-five percent have a follicular pattern. 25% are diffuse.
- Present with marrow involvement in over 70%.
- Tumors with a follicular pattern are low grade; those with a diffuse pattern are intermediate grade.

D. Large cell follicular center cell lymphomas:

- Mostly have large cells, but there are few transformed cells.
- Nuclei may be cleaved or noncleaved.
- May have a follicular or diffuse pattern.
- Are intermediate grade.

E. Small noncleaved cell lymphomas:

- Include Burkitt's and Burkitt-like lymphoma.
- Are composed of small cells with round nuclei containing nucleoli that resemble fetal lymphoblasts.
- Have a high mitotic rate.
- Are the tissue equivalent of acute lymphoblastic leukemia, B cell type (L3).
- Are high grade.

F. B immunoblastic sarcomas:

- Are composed of large cells with round nuclei containing prominent nucleoli and abundant cytoplasm.

- Have a high mitotic rate.
- Are high grade.

2. *T CELL LYMPHOMAS*
A. T Lymphoblastic lymphomas:

- Tend to occur in children and young adults.
- Commonly present as mediastinal mass.
- Are characterized by a diffuse proliferation of primitive cells resembling fetal T lymphoblasts.
- Have a high mitotic rate.
- Are related to T cell acute lymphoblastic leukemia (L2).

B. T Immunoblastic sarcomas:

- Resemble B immunoblastic sarcomas, from which they must be distinguished by immunologic methods.
- Are high grade.

C. Cutaneous T cell lymphomas (mycosis fungoides):

- Are characterized by small cells with convoluted ("cerebriform") nuclei (Sezary cells).
- Primarily involve skin, with or without involvement of blood, lymph nodes, bone marrow.
- Frequently composed of cells with a T helper cell phenotype.
- Have a variable rate of progression.

3. *HISTIOCYTIC LYMPHOMA*
True histiocytic lymphomas are very rare. They are distinguished from other large cell lymphomas by immunologic methods.

FACTORS DETERMINING PROGNOSIS IN NON-HODGKIN'S LYMPHOMAS
The Working Formulation grades correlate well with survival. Five-year survival rates with treatment are:

- 60% for low grade lymphomas.
- 40% for intermediate-grade lymphomas.
- 25% for high-grade lymphomas.
- **Note:** Effective treatment for high-grade lymphomas has obscured the importance of histologic type in prognosis.

Stage of Disease
The staging procedure (Table 29–5) was developed for Hodgkin's lymphoma and has been extended for non-Hodgkin's lymphomas. The stage applies only at the time of presentation and before definitive therapy is started. Staging may be:

- Clinical (physical examination, radiologic studies).
- Pathological (tissue sampling, eg, at staging laparotomy).

TREATMENT
Combined chemotherapy regimens have improved survival. Treatment has the greatest impact in high-grade lymphomas. Low-grade lymphomas are resistant.

TABLE 29–5. STAGING OF HODGKIN'S AND NON-HODGKIN'S LYMPHOMAS[1]

Stage I:	Involvement of a single lymph node region (I) or of a single extralymphoid site (I_E).
Stage II:	Involvement of 2 or more lymph node regions on the same side of the diaphragm.
Stage III:	Involvement on both sides of the diaphragm (III), which may also be accompanied by localized involvement of a single extralymphoid site (III_E) or the spleen (III_S).
Stage IV:	Diffuse or disseminated involvement of one or more extralymphoid organs or tissues with or without associated lymph node involvement.

[1] Each of these stages is divided into A and B categories—B for those with defined general symptoms and A for those without. The B classification is given those patients with unexplained weight loss, unexplained fever, and night sweats; it has a worse prognosis.

Hodgkin's Lymphoma

This is a malignant lymphoma characterized by the presence of Reed-Sternberg cells.

- It accounts for 30–40% of all lymphomas.
- Eight thousand cases occur annually in the United States.
- It shows a bimodal age incidence, with a peak in early adulthood and another in old age.

Etiology

- The cause is not known. Clusters of Hodgkin's lymphoma in restricted geographic areas have suggested some infective or other environmental agent, but no such agent has been identified.
- The origin of the Reed-Sternberg cell is uncertain. Suggested cells of origin include the lymphocyte, the histiocyte, and the interdigitating reticulum cell.

Pathologic Features

The diagnosis of Hodgkin's lymphoma depends upon the finding of Reed-Sternberg cells. Classic Reed-Sternberg cells are binucleated with round nuclei containing prominent, inclusion-like nucleoli (Fig 29–2).

- Reed-Sternberg cells show little evidence of nucleic acid synthesis or proliferative activity.
- Large mononuclear cells (called Hodgkin's cells) that resemble Reed-Sternberg cells are the proliferative cells in Hodgkin's lymphoma.
- The Reed-Sternberg cells are admixed with variable numbers of lymphocytes, plasma cells, histiocytes, eosinophils, neutrophils, and fibroblasts, all of which are reactive.
- The lymph node architecture is often totally destroyed.
- Staging, both clinical and pathologic, is similar to that for non-Hodgkin's lymphoma (Table 29–5).

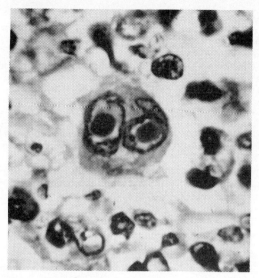

Figure 29–2. Hodgkin's lymphoma. High magnification of a classical Reed-Sternberg cell with 2 nuclei containing the typical large nucleoli.

Classification

Classification as Hodgkin's lymphoma is based on the relative proportions of Reed-Sternberg cells (and mononuclear variant cells), lymphocytes, histiocytes, and areas of fibrosis.

A. Lymphocyte-predominant Hodgkin's lymphoma:

- Is characterized by the presence of numerous lymphocytes and few classic Reed-Sternberg cells.
- May occur in nodular or diffuse form and may have numerous histiocytes (the L&H—lymphocytic and histiocytic—form of Hodgkin's lymphoma).
- Contains large polyploid variants of the Reed-Sternberg cell with lobulated nuclei ("popcorn" cells).
- Typically presents as stage I disease and progresses slowly. It is associated with prolonged survival.

B. Lymphocyte-depleted Hodgkin's lymphoma:

- Has the worst prognosis and typically presents as stage III or stage IV disease.
- Lymph nodes are replaced by a destructive process containing numerous pleomorphic mononuclear and classic Reed-Sternberg cells, variable amounts of diffuse fibrosis, and very few lymphocytes.

C. Mixed-cellularity Hodgkin's lymphoma:

- Has an intermediate histologic appearance with numerous lymphocytes, plasma cells, eosinophils, and Reed-Sternberg cells.
- Prognosis is intermediate between that of lymphocyte-predominant and lymphocyte-depleted subtypes.
- Response to therapy is usually good.

D. Nodular sclerosing Hodgkin's lymphoma:

- Usually presents as early stage disease and has a slow progression with long survival.
- Young women are particularly affected, and mediastinal involvement is common.
- Is characterized by:
  - Broad bands of collagen circumscribing nodules of neoplastic tissue.
  - Large Reed-Sternberg cell variants that have multilobated nuclei and abundant pale cytoplasm (lacunar cells).

Diagnosis & Treatment

Diagnosis is based entirely on histologic examination. Classic Reed-Sternberg cells are essential.

- Athough Reed-Sternberg cells are characteristic of Hodgkin's lymphoma, morphologically similar cells may be seen occasionally in other conditions, notably infectious mononucleosis.
- Selection of therapy depends on the histologic type, stage, and other clinical parameters.
- Localized forms of Hodgkin's lymphoma may be treated with either radiation or chemotherapy.
- Combination chemotherapy is highly effective and may lead to complete remission even in patients with late stage disease.

Neoplasms of Histiocytes

TRUE HISTIOCYTIC "LYMPHOMA"

This is rare, accounting for less than 5% of primary neoplasms of lymph nodes.

- It resembles high-grade lymphomas clinically.
- The neoplastic cells are large and pleomorphic, typically with granular pink cytoplasm. Phagocytosis may be present.
- Distinction from large cell lymphomas is difficult without immunologic tests. Malignant histiocytes show reactivity with anti-monocyte/histiocyte antibodies such as Leu M1, and Mo 1.
- It is usually aggressive and refractory to treatment.

MALIGNANT HISTIOCYTOSIS & HISTIOCYTIC MEDULLARY RETICULOSIS

These two terms are used interchangeably to denote a highly malignant systemic neoplasm of histiocytes, involving lymph nodes and soft tissue.

- They present with hepatosplenomegaly, lymphadenopathy, and pancytopenia.
- Typically there is extensive erythrophagocytosis by the neoplastic cells.
- The prognosis is poor.

HISTIOCYTOSIS X

This is a group of diseases characterized by a neoplastic histiocyte that shows a resemblance to the Langerhans cells of the skin.

- The cells are large, with large multilobated and folded nuclei.
- The cell reacts with monoclonal antibody OKT6 and contain tennis racket-shaped Birbeck granules on electron microscopy.
- The term *histiocytosis X* includes the following.

1. EOSINOPHILIC GRANULOMA

This is a relatively benign disease that involves bone, particularly the skull and ribs of children and young adults.

- It appears radiologically as a well-demarcated lytic lesion.
- Histologically, it is a diffuse infiltrate composed of histiocytes, giant cells, and eosinophils.

2. HAND-SCHÜLLER-CHRISTIAN DISEASE

This is morphologically similar to eosinophilic granuloma.

- It is multifocal, occurs in younger children, and has a less favorable prognosis.
- The base of the skull is characteristically involved, producing the triad of proptosis, lytic bone lesions in skull, and diabetes insipidus.

3. LETTERER-SIWE DISEASE

This represents the aggressive end of the spectrum of histiocytosis X.

- It presents with widespread lesions of bone and lymphoid tissue.
- Lymphadenopathy and skin nodules occur due to infiltration by large pale neoplastic histiocytes.
- It is uncommon and occurs only in young children.
- It has a rapid progression and poor prognosis.

METASTATIC NEOPLASMS

Metastatic neoplasms in lymph nodes are most commonly carcinomas and malignant melanoma.

- They are a common cause of lymph node enlargement.
- Not infrequently, an enlarged lymph node is the method of clinical presentation of a carcinoma, the primary tumor being occult, eg, cervical lymphadenopathy in nasopharyngeal carcinoma.
- The histologic diagnosis of metastatic neoplasms is easy when the neoplasm is well differentiated.
- In poorly differentiated carcinomas, the distinction from large-cell lymphoma and amelanotic malignant melanoma is often difficult to make on histologic examination.
- Immunohistochemical demonstration of specific markers (common leukocyte antigen for lymphomas; keratin for carcinomas; and S100 protein and HMB-45 for melanomas) is essential for accurate diagnosis of poorly differentiated neoplasms.

The Lymphoid System: III. Plasma Cell Neoplasms; Spleen & Thymus

30

PLASMA CELL NEOPLASMS

MONOCLONAL GAMMOPATHY

Monoclonal gammopathy is a "spike" on serum protein electrophoresis caused by accumulation of a monoclonal immunoglobulin. It commonly signifies a plasma cell neoplasm. Rarely, it occurs without a neoplasm (Table 30–1).

Diagnosis

Diagnosis is made by the presence of serum protein electrophoresis, which shows the typical sharp band ("spike") in the immunoglobulin region. It can be differentiated from the broad elevation in globulins seen in a polyclonal immunoglobulin increase (Fig 30–1).

- Serum immunoelectrophoresis permits characterization of the precipitated proteins.
- Urine electrophoresis may show a monoclonal spike if the glomeruli are permeable to the protein.
- Bence Jones protein represents free immunoglobulin light chains that are excreted in urine.

MULTIPLE MYELOMA

Incidence & Etiology

Multiple myeloma is characterized by the presence of multiple small tumors composed of plasma cells within the bone marrow.

- It is the most common form of plasma cell neoplasm, accounting for about one-sixth of all hematopoietic neoplasms.
- The peak incidence is in the eighth decade, and the disease is very rare in persons under age 40.
- Alternative names include multiple plasmacytoma, plasma cell myeloma, and Kahler's disease.
- The etiology is unknown.

Clinical Features

Presentation is usually due to symptoms of anemia, bone pain, and fractures due to bone marrow involvement, infection, renal disease, hypercalcemia, or hyperviscosity.

TABLE 30-1. CAUSES OF MONOCLONAL GAMMOPATHY
(IE, THE PRESENCE OF A MONOCLONAL OR M SPIKE IN SERUM)

		Monoclonal "Spike"
Neoplastic Multiple myeloma	Multiple plasma cell neoplasms in bone	IgG, IgA, IgM, IgD, or free light chains
Plasmacytoid lymphocytic lymphoma[1]	Lymph node or tissue mass containing neoplastic plasmacytoid lymphocytes	Usually IgM (macroglobulinemia)
Alpha heavy chain disease[2]	Plasmacytoid cell neoplasm especially involving gut wall	Alpha chain only
Amyloidosis	Usually associated with an underlying plasmacytic neoplasm	IgG or light chain
Nonneoplastic Benign monoclonal gammopathy	Mild reactive plasmacytosis in marrow: by definition not malignant[3]	Usually low-level stable IgG
Transient gammopathies	Probably a phase of florid immune response when one clonal product (antibody type) dominates; seen in some infections and with some cancers	Usually IgG, low-level
"Autoimmune" gammopathy	Monoclonal immunoglobulins are found as part of mixed cryoglobulinemia and cold agglutinin disease (see text); rare	Usually IgM, low-level

[1]Other B cell neoplasms (chronic lymphocytic leukemia, follicular center cell lymphomas, and immunoblastic sarcoma of B cell type) may also produce detectable "spikes" if very sensitive techniques are utilized.
[2]Gamma and mu chain diseases also occur but are very rare (see text).
[3]It is not known whether the condition represents a benign neoplasm or a reactive clone that becomes predominant and persists.

- Release of an osteoclast-activating factor contributes to bone lysis in myeloma.
- Diagnosis is based upon:
  - Radiologic findings, including multiple lytic lesions, especially in ribs, long bones and skull.
  - Bone marrow biopsy showing large numbers of abnormal plasma cells.
  - The presence of a monoclonal spike in serum or urine (Fig 30–1).
- The monoclonal immunoglobulin in the serum can be composed of light chain only, heavy chain only, or whole immunoglobulin.
- In classic myeloma, IgG is most commonly present, followed by free light chains and then IgA. IgD and IgM are much less common, and IgE is very rare.
- It is treated with chemotherapy, which rarely produces long-term remission.
- The median survival is three years.

Cellulose acetate pattern　　　**Densitometer tracing**

Normal serum

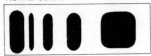
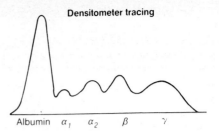

Albumin　α_1　α_2　β　γ

IgG myeloma with γ spike
(monoclonal)

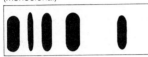
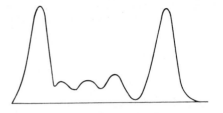

Waldenström's macroglobulinemia
with IgM spike (monoclonal)

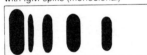
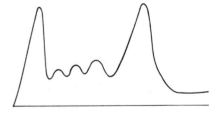

Polyclonal hypergammaglobulinemia
(polyclonal)

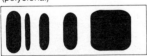
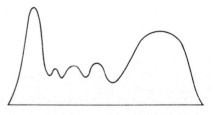

Hypogammaglobulinemia

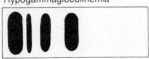
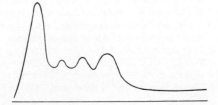

PLASMACYTOID LYMPHOCYTIC LYMPHOMA

Plasmacytoid lymphocytic lymphoma is characterized by numerous plasmacytoid lymphocytes having condensed lymphocytelike nuclei and plasma cell–like cytoplasm.

- It is almost exclusively a disease of the elderly (age 50 or older).
- It usually presents with anemia and manifestations of bleeding or hyperviscosity syndrome (Waldenström's disease).
- High levels of monoclonal IgM are present in the serum, producing hyperviscosity. IgG and IgA monoclonal proteins are present much less frequently.
- Hyperviscosity produces sludging and slowing of blood in capillaries, which may produce transient neurologic symptoms and visual impairment.
- IgM may also act as a cryoglobulin, producing Raynaud's phenomenon, characterized by cold sensitivity, pain, and focal gangrene.
- Diagnosis is by:
  - Biopsy of involved lymph nodes or tissue masses.
  - Plasma protein electrophoresis that shows an IgM monoclonal protein (Fig 30–1).
  - Detection of urinary Bence Jones protein in about 30% of cases.
  - Bone marrow biopsy, which frequently shows focal small collections of plasmacytoid lymphocytes.
- Lytic bone lesions are rare. Treatment includes:
  - Plasmapheresis to remove IgM from the patient's serum to decrease blood viscosity.
  - Chemotherapy, which is of limited efficacy.

LIGHT & HEAVY CHAIN DISEASES

1. LIGHT CHAIN DISEASE (BENCE JONES MYELOMA):

This is a type of multiple myeloma in which only light chains are secreted. It is characterized by clinical and pathologic changes identical to other forms of plasma cell myeloma.

2. HEAVY CHAIN DISEASE:

Production of heavy chains alone by plasma cell neoplasms is much less common (Table 30–2).

- Alpha heavy chain disease:
  - Is the most common form of heavy chain disease.
  - Typically presents as a lymphomatous infiltration of the gut (immunoproliferative small intestinal disease—IPSID; Mediterranean lymphoma).
  - May be diagnosed by demonstration of the monoclonal heavy chain in serum using immunoelectrophoresis or in tissue sections using immunohistologic techniques.
- Gamma and mu heavy chain disease are very rare (Table 30–2).

Figure 30–1. Serum protein electrophoresis, showing patterns seen in normal serum, monoclonal gammopathies, polyclonal hypergammaglobulinemia, and hypogammaglobulinemia.

TABLE 30–2. HEAVY CHAIN DISEASES

	Alpha Chain Disease	Gamma Chain Disease	Mu Chain Diseae
Approximate number of reported cases	150	50	15
Age at onset	10–30 years	10–40 years	> 50 years
Morphologic features	IPSID:[1] Plasma cell hyperplasia, Mediterranean lymphoma, immunoblastic sarcoma (B cell)	Usually resembles plasmacytoid lymphocytic lymphoma	Usually resembles chronic lymphocytic leukemia
Tissue site	Most often gut (IPSID);[1] rarely respiratory tract	Lymph node, spleen	Lymph nodes, marrow
Associated with amyloid	No	Yes	Yes

[1]IPSID = Immunoproliferative small intestinal disease spectrum with 3 phases.

PRIMARY AMYLOIDOSIS

Primary amyloidosis is the diffuse deposition of amyloid in the tissues without an underlying disease.

- Most cases are due to a plasma cell neoplasm closely related to multiple myeloma.
- The chief distinguishing criterion is the presence of multiple plasmacellular lytic lesions within bone marrow in myeloma and their absence in primary amyloidosis.
- It has a peak incidence in the elderly.
- It tends to have an insidious onset, presenting with evidence of peripheral neuropathy, malabsorption syndrome, renal or cardiac insufficiency.
- The diagnosis is by:
  - The presence of a monoclonal gammopathy.
  - Tissue biopsy showing amyloid deposition.
  - The absence of multiple myeloma or B cell lymphoma.
- It is slowly progressive with a high mortality rate.

THE SPLEEN

SPLENOMEGALY

Splenomegaly is a common abnormality and occurs in many diseases (Table 30–3).

- The malpighian bodies are enlarged, with reactive centers in acute and chronic infections and in autoimmune and hypersensitivity diseases.
- Epithelioid cell granulomas occur in sarcoidosis and infectious diseases, most commonly tuberculosis.
- Storage diseases typically show proliferation of histiocytes.

TABLE 30–3. CAUSES OF SPLENOMEGALY

Nonneoplastic Acute infections	Various (eg, infectious mononucleosis, typhoid fever, malaria)
Chronic infections	Various (eg, brucellosis, infective endocarditis, malaria, leishmaniasis)
Autoimmune diseases	Rheumatoid arthritis (especially Still's disease),[1] systemic lupus erythematosus, idiopathic thrombocytopenic purpura
Hypersensitivity reactions	To drugs; serum sickness
Sarcoidosis	
Amyloidosis	
Storage diseases	Gaucher's disease; Neimann-Pick disease, ceroid histiocytosis
Portal venous hypertension	Cirrhosis, portal vein thrombosis
Hematologic disorders	Hemolytic anemias (thalassemia, autoimmune); extramedullary erythropoiesis, myelofibrosis
Splenic cysts and hamartomas	
Neoplastic Lymphocytic leukemias	Especially large in chronic lymphocytic leukemia and hairy cell leukemia
Non-Hodgkin's lymphomas	
Hodgkin's disease	
Polycythemia rubra vera	
Monocytoid leukemias	
Myeloid leukemias	Especially chronic myelocytic leukemia
Histiocytosis X	Hand-Schüller-Christian disease; Letterer-Siwe disease; histocytic medullary reticulosis
Secondary neoplasms	Relatively rare

[1]Still's disease = juvenile rheumatoid arthritis.

- In portal hypertension, there is passive venous congestion.
- Splenic changes in autoimmune hemolytic anemia and idiopathic thrombocytopenic purpura consist of hyperplasia of histiocytes.
- Of the neoplasms involving the spleen, chronic lymphocytic and myeloid leukemia and hairy cell leukemia almost always produce massive splenomegaly.

- Malignant lymphomas, including Hodgkin's disease typically appears multifocally in the spleen, but may produce massive diffuse involvement.
- Myeloproliferative diseases commonly cause massive splenomegaly, associated with extramedullary hematopoiesis.
- Marked splenomegaly also occurs in histiocytic medullary reticulosis due to extensive replacement of red pulp by atypical histiocytes.
- While small foci of metastatic carcinoma are common at autopsy, metastatic carcinoma is a rare cause of clinical splenomegaly.

HYPERSPLENISM
Regardless of its cause, splenic enlargement may, rarely, result in anemia, leukopenia, and thrombocytopenia. It is caused by increased destruction of these cells in the spleen. Splenectomy is curative.

THE THYMUS

THYMIC HYPERPLASIA & MYASTHENIA GRAVIS
Thymic follicular hyperplasia is the presence of reactive follicles in the medulla of the adult thymus.

- It is very rarely seen in normal individuals, but occurs in myasthenia gravis and to a lesser extent in other autoimmune diseases.
- Eighty percent of patients with myasthenia gravis show thymic follicular hyperplasia.
- Ten percent of patients with myasthenia gravis have thymomas.
- Thymectomy leads to improvement in symptoms in many myasthenia patients, particularly young women with disease of short duration.

THYMIC NEOPLASMS

1. MALIGNANT LYMPHOMAS
Nodular sclerosing Hodgkin's disease commonly involves the mediastinum and thymus. Acute lymphoblastic leukemia (ALL) of T cell type and its tissue counterpart, T lymphoblastic (convoluted) lymphoma, commonly involve the thymus.

2. THYMOMA
Thymomas are neoplasms derived from the thymic epithelial cells. They typically contain large numbers of nonneoplastic T lymphocytes admixed with the epithelial cells (lymphoepithelial thymoma).

- Benign thymomas are usually encapsulated.
- Malignant thymomas:
  - Show capsular invasion and involvement of mediastinal structures.
  - Rarely produce distant metastases.
- May produce several different paraneoplastic syndromes (Table 30–4).

3. SEMINOMA & TERATOMA
The thymus is a site for development of primary germ cell neoplasms such as seminoma, teratoma, yolk sac carcinoma and embryonal carcinoma. Morphologically and behaviorally, they resemble the corresponding tumors of ovary or testis.

TABLE 30–4. THYMOMA AND ASSOCIATED "PARANEOPLASTIC" SYNDROMES[1]

Myasthenia gravis: 10% of myasthenia patients have thymoma.
Pure red cell aplasia: 50% of aplastic patients have thymoma.
Neutropenia with or without thrombocytopenia.
Hypogammaglobulinemia
Polymyositis
Myocarditis
Systemic lupus erythematosus
IgA deficiency and multiple neoplasms
Other (nonthymic) cancers
Other autoimmune diseases

[1]Overall, approximately 40% of patients with thymoma have one of these conditions.

Section VII. Diseases of the Head and Neck

The Oral Cavity & Salivary Glands

31

DISEASES OF THE TEETH

DENTAL CARIES

Etiology
Dental caries is a progressive decomposition of tooth substances caused by a wide variety of bacteria and fungi, most commonly *Streptococcus mutans*.

- The microorganisms proliferate in food residue on the teeth to form a hard, adherent mass of calcified debris containing bacteria and desquamated epithelial cells (plaque, tartar, calculus).
- Enzymes and acids produced by the microorganisms cause proteolysis, decalcification, and decay, first of the enamel covering of the tooth, then the dentin, finally the tooth pulp.
- There is individual variation in susceptibility of enamel to decay.
- Several factors influence the risk of dental caries:
  - Microorganisms are essential.
  - Regular brushing prevents accumulation of food residue and reduces incidence.
  - Sugar promotes bacterial growth.
- Once plaque has formed, it cannot be removed by brushing. Removal of plaque by use of dental floss or by scaling decreases the incidence.
- Fluoride has a protective effect.
- Saliva has a mechanical cleansing action and contains microbicidal substances (lysozyme, IgA). Any cause of decreased salivary secretion, such as Sjögren's syndrome or radiation, increases the risk.

Clinicopathologic Effects
A. Early caries:

- Does not cause symptoms.
- Can be recognized by clinical dental examination.

B. Pulp infection:

- Deep caries that extends through the enamel and dentin layers into the tooth pulp leads to acute pulpitis, formation of a localized abscess, or destruction of the entire pulp.
- Pulp infection is associated with severe pain and swelling.

C. Periapical infection:

- Extension of pulp infection to the apical periodontium results in an apical abscess, which may enlarge and drain through the gingiva (parulis, gum boil).
- Rarely, the infection spreads in the floor of the mouth and neck and is associated with tissue necrosis (Ludwig's angina).
- It may become chronic, leading to a periapical granuloma around the apex of the tooth. This is characterized by:
  - Bone resorption.
  - Infiltration by lymphocytes, plasma cells, and histiocytes.
  - A well-demarcated radiologically lucent area in the bone at the apex of the tooth.
- Periapical granulomas tend to undergo epithelialization and form a cystic structure lined by squamous epithelium (radicular cyst).

PERIODONTAL DISEASE
Periodontal disease is a complication of plaque formation.

- Accumulation of plaque in the crevice between the gingiva and the tooth causes gingivitis, which may progress to periodontitis.
- May cause instability of the tooth, resorption of the gingiva, purulent discharge from the gingival crevice (pyorrhea), and eventual tooth loss.

CYSTS OF THE JAW
Cysts of the jaw are very common. Many—eg, radicular cysts, follicular cysts, and odontogenic keratocysts—occur in relation to the teeth. Others, such as fissural and inclusion cysts, are not related to the teeth.

- **Radicular cyst** is the most common and is the result of epithelialization of a periapical granuloma.
- **Follicular cysts** arise from the epithelium of the tooth follicle and may be associated with failure of eruption of the involved tooth. If the unerupted tooth is present in the cyst wall, the term *dentigerous cyst* may be used.
- **Odontogenic keratocysts** are lined by a keratinized squamous epithelium and occur at the root of the tooth. They may be multiple and associated with basal cell carcinomas of the skin.
- **Fissural or inclusion cysts** are derived from epithelial inclusions along lines of fusion of the embryologic facial processes. They are classified according to their site, eg, median palatine cyst, globulomaxillary cyst.

NEOPLASMS OF TOOTH-FORMING (ODONTOGENIC) TISSUES
The commonest neoplasms in this region are those derived from bone (osteoma, osteosarcoma, etc) and soft tissues (neurofibroma, vascular neoplasms, etc).

- **Ameloblastoma** is the most common odontogenic tumor.
  - It is rare, comprising 1% of cysts and tumors of the jaw.
  - It occurs mainly between ages 20 and 50.
  - It occurs most often in the molar region of the mandible.
  - It commonly has cystic and solid areas.
  - It is a locally invasive neoplasm that does not metastasize.

DISEASES OF THE ORAL CAVITY

INFLAMMATORY LESIONS

1. HERPES SIMPLEX STOMATITIS

Herpes simplex type 1 is a common viral infection of the oral mucosa; about 20% of the population is affected.

- The primary infection occurs in children or young adults as a febrile gingivostomatitis, characterized by multiple vesicles that rupture to form ulcers.
- It is self-limited.
- The virus infects the ganglia in the acute phase, where it remains dormant for long periods.
- Reactivation of the infection may occur, causing isolated oral vesicular lesions and ulcers (herpes labialis).
- Reactivation is often precipitated by a concurrent illness or by exposure to sunlight.

2. HERPANGINA

This is an uncommon infection of the oral mucosa with coxsackievirus A. Vesicular lesions occur on the palate and posterior oral cavity and may be accompanied by skin lesions in the extremities (hand, foot, and mouth disease).

3. CANDIDIASIS (Thrush)

Candida albicans is a normal commensal of the mouth.

- Infection of the oral mucosa usually represents an opportunistic infection.
- Persons at risk include:
  - Immunocompromised patients, eg, AIDS patients or those receiving cancer chemotherapy.
  - Newborn infants.
  - Diabetics.
  - Chronically sick patients on long-term antibiotic therapy.
- *Candida* is a surface infection, forming white patches that leave raw ulcerated lesions when they are rubbed off.
- Budding yeasts and pseudohyphae of *Candida* can be identified in smears, cultures, or biopsy specimens from the lesion.

4. APHTHOUS STOMATITIS

This is a common disorder characterized by recurrent episodes of painful shallow ulcers on the oral mucosa.

- The cause is unknown; psychosomatic and allergic mechanisms have been suggested. No infectious agent has been identified.
- It is usually self-limited.
- Rarely, associated with genital and conjunctival ulcers and neurologic abnormalities (Behçet's syndrome).

5. ACTINOMYCOSIS

This is caused by *Actinomyces israelii* and *Actinomyces bovis*, gram positive filamentous bacteria.

- Infection commonly follows dental extraction.
- It presents with an indurated jaw mass that has multiple sinuses opening to the skin surface that drain pus.
- The pus contains small colonies of the organism (sulfur granules).
- Microscopy and culture are diagnostic.

6. VINCENT'S ANGINA

This is caused by a wide variety of spirochetes and fusiform bacilli that inhabit the mouth. It occurs in debilitated or malnourished individuals and is characterized by a severe ulcerative gingivitis (trench mouth).

7. SYPHILIS

In syphilis, the primary chancre may, rarely, be on the lips or tongue.

- In secondary syphilis, superficial mucous patches and "snail track" ulcers may be present.
- In tertiary syphilis, tongue ulcers and gummas may occur.
- Congenital syphilis may produce scarring at the angles of the mouth (rhagades) and abnormalities in the permanent teeth (Hutchinson's incisors and Moon's molars).

BENIGN "TUMORS" OF THE ORAL CAVITY

1. MUCOCELE (Mucus Escape Reaction)

Mucocele is a localized inflammatory reaction to the escape of mucus from a ruptured minor salivary gland or duct. It usually presents as small white cystic structures; rarely, they become large and stretch the overlying mucosa (ranula).

2. PYOGENIC GRANULOMA

This is a common oral lesion that is the result of a reactive inflammatory proliferation of granulation tissue.

- It presents as a small, bright red nodule with ulceration of the overlying mucosa.
- It occurs commonly during pregnancy (pregnancy tumor).
- The cause is unknown; it resolves spontaneously.

3. EPULIS

Epulis is a local reactive inflammatory lesion of the gum that presents as a mass.

- It may be composed of multinucleated giant cells (giant cell epulis).

- Congenital epulis is characterized by the proliferation of large cells with abundant granular cytoplasm (granular cell epulis).

4. LINGUAL THYROID

Thyroid tissue at the root of the tongue is a rare condition that represents incomplete descent of thyroid tissue in the embryo. It usually coexists with a normal thyroid but in rare cases represents the individual's only thyroid tissue.

BENIGN NEOPLASMS OF THE ORAL CAVITY

These arise from the squamous epithelium (squamous papilloma) mesenchymal cells (fibroma, lipoma, neurofibroma), or from minor salivary glands (adenomas). Granular cell tumor, a variant of a schwannoma in which the cells have abundant granular cytoplasm, occurs commonly in the tongue.

SQUAMOUS CARCINOMA OF THE ORAL CAVITY

Incidence & Etiology

Squamous carcinoma accounts for over 95% of malignant neoplasms in the oral cavity and 5% of all cancers in the United States.

- The lower lip (40%), the tongue (20%), and the floor of the mouth (15%) are the common sites. The upper lip, palate, gingiva, and tonsillar area (5% each) are less common.
- They are much more common in men than in women, and whites are affected more commonly than blacks.
- Etiologic factors include cigarette and pipe smoking, tobacco chewing, and alcohol.
- Oral cancer is extremely common in Sri Lanka and parts of India, where chewing betel is common (betel is a green leaf that is chewed with areca nut, limestone, and tobacco).
- It is also common in parts of Italy, where it is customary to smoke cigars with the lighted end inside the mouth.

Clinical Features

It begins as a painless indurated plaque on the tongue or oral mucosa that commonly forms a malignant ulcer.

- Diagnosis is made by biopsy.
- A significant number of patients with oral cancer present first with involved cervical lymph nodes.
- In very advanced local disease, there may be fixation of the tongue, interfering with speech and swallowing.

Pathology

The earliest lesion is squamous epithelial dysplasia, the most severe form of which is carcinoma in situ. This may sometimes produce a white plaque (leukoplakia).

- Most lesions are invasive to a variable depth at the time of diagnosis.
- Most tumors are well differentiated with keratinization.
- They spread primarily by lymphatics. Cervical lymph nodes are involved early. Bloodstream metastasis occurs late.

Treatment & Prognosis

Treatment is by radical surgery, radiotherapy, and chemotherapy.

- Lesions are moderately sensitive to radiation therapy.
- Prognosis depends on the stage of the disease and is relatively good in the absence of cervical lymph node involvement.

DISEASES OF THE SALIVARY GLANDS

INFLAMMATORY LESIONS

1. SALIVARY DUCT CALCULI (Sialolithiasis)

Sialolithiasis occurs mainly in the duct of the submandibular gland. Obstruction of a salivary gland duct produces acute inflammation (acute sialadenitis) followed by chronic inflammation, glandular atrophy, and fibrosis (chronic sialadenitis).

2. SJÖGREN'S SYNDROME

This is an autoimmune disease in which there is immune-mediated destruction of the lacrimal and salivary glands.

- It is manifested clinically as dry eyes (keratoconjunctivitis sicca) and dry mouth (xerostomia).
- It is commonly associated with other autoimmune diseases, notably rheumatoid arthritis.
- Seventy-five percent of patients have rheumatoid factor in the blood, and 70% have antinuclear antibodies.
- Specific autoantibodies designated SS-A and SS-B have been identified in the serum of 60% of patients with Sjögren's syndrome.
- There is an increased incidence of malignant lymphomas in the salivary gland.
- Histologically, the lacrimal and salivary glands show marked lymphocytic and plasma cell infiltration with destruction of the glandular epithelium and fibrosis.
- Diagnosis can be made by:
  - Clinical tests to demonstrate absence of secretion of tears.
  - Lip biopsy, which shows the typical histologic changes in the mucus glands of the lip.

3. INFECTIONS OF THE SALIVARY GLANDS

The parotid gland is the commonest site of involvement in **mumps virus** infection. **Bacterial parotitis** occurs in debilitated patients with dehydration and poor oral hygiene. It is frequently complicated by abscess formation.

NEOPLASMS OF THE SALIVARY GLANDS (Table 31–1)

These are common. Eighty percent occur in the parotids, 15% in the submandibular gland, and 5% in minor salivary glands.

- They present as a mass causing enlargement of the affected gland.
- Computerized tomography is helpful in assessment of the location and extent of salivary gland neoplasms.
- Diagnosis requires cytologic (fine-needle aspiration) or histologic examination.

TABLE 31-1. SALIVARY GLAND NEOPLASMS

Neoplasm	Rate of Occurrence	Degree of Malignancy
Adenomas		
Pleomorphic adenoma (mixed parotid tumor)[1]	60%	Benign but tend to recur as a result of local extension
Adenolymphoma (Warthin's tumor)	10%	Benign
Monomorphic adenomas (various subtypes)	3%	Benign
Carcinomas		
Adenocarcinoma	5%	Variable degree of malignancy
Mucoepidermoid tumor	5%	Combined squamous and mucous cells, variable malignancy
Adenoid cystic carcinoma	3%	Malignant; marked tendency to invade locally; metastases occur late
Acinic cell carcinoma	3%	Low-grade[2]
Carcinoma in mixed tumor	3%	Variable degree of malignancy
Undifferentiated carcinoma	3%	Highly malignant[2]
Others[3]	Rare	

[1]Most of these tumors occur most often in the parotid gland, but any salivary gland may be involved.
[2]For highly malignant tumors, the 5-year survival rate is 20% or less; low-grade cancers have a 5-year survival rate of 80%.
[3]Others include lymphomas, squamous carcinomas.

1. PLEOMORPHIC ADENOMA (Mixed Tumor)

Pleomorphic adenoma accounts for over 50% of salivary gland tumors.

- They are well-circumscribed but incompletely encapsulated.
- Simple enucleation is followed by a high rate of local recurrence due to regrowth of residual tumor.
- Wide excision is necessary for cure.
- Grossly, they appear as a firm, solid mass.
- Histologically, they are composed of uniform epithelial and myoepithelial cells arranged in cords, nests, and strands within a matrix of mucoid material which frequently resembles cartilage.

2. WARTHIN'S TUMOR (Adenolymphoma)

Most Warthin's tumors occur in the parotid gland.

- They are rarely multicentric and bilateral.

- Histologically, they are composed of cystic spaces lined by a uniform double-layered epithelium that is frequently papillary.
- Neoplastic epithelial cells are large, with abundant pink cytoplasm, and surrounded by a dense lymphocytic infiltrate.

3. MALIGNANT SALIVARY GLAND NEOPLASMS
Malignant salivary gland neoplasms are of several different pathologic types (Table 31–1).

- Most are slow-growing. Exceptions are the rare undifferentiated carcinomas and the high-grade mucoepidermoid carcinomas.
- Low-grade mucoepidermoid carcinoma is a well-circumscribed neoplasm with variable solid and cystic areas; it is cured in over 90% of cases by surgical removal.
- Adenoid cystic carcinoma is a highly infiltrative neoplasm with a tendency to invade along nerves.
  - It is rarely cured by surgery.
  - Local recurrences and metastases occur many (5–25) years after original treatment.
- Carcinomas arising in mixed tumors and acinic cell carcinoma have variable clinical courses.

The Ear, Nose, Pharynx, & Larynx

32

I. THE EAR

THE EXTERNAL EAR

Preauricular Sinus & Cyst
This is a developmental anomaly associated with abnormal fusion of the facial folds.

- It is characterized by a blind-ending epithelium-lined tract that opens as a small pit anterior to the ear.
- Obstruction of the opening may lead to the development of an epidermal cyst.
- Infection may cause abscess and discharging sinus.

Otitis Externa
This is commonly caused by saprophytic fungi, often *Aspergillus* spp.

- It causes pain and a thick discharge.
- A foreign body or excessive exposure to water (swimmer's ear) predisposes to infection.

Herpes Zoster
Herpes zoster involving the facial nerve ganglion (Ramsay Hunt syndrome) results in typical viral vesicles in the external ear, and is commonly associated with severe pain.

Chondrodermatitis Nodularis Helicis
This is a common lesion characterized clinically by the occurrence of a painful nodule in the helix.

- It is thought to result from trauma and is more common in males.
- There is ulceration of the skin and a chronic inflammatory infiltrate involving the perichondrium of the underlying cartilage.
- Surgical excision is curative.

Cauliflower Ear
Cauliflower ear is the result of trauma and is most commonly seen in professional boxers. It is caused by thickening due to multiple organized and contracted hematomas.

Neoplasms of the External Ear

The skin of the external ear is a common site for basal cell and squamous carcinoma. Nevi and malignant melanoma also occur in the skin of the ear. Neoplasms of the external auditory meatus, such as osteoma and ceruminous gland adenoma, are very rare.

THE MIDDLE EAR

OTITIS MEDIA

Incidence & Etiology

This is a common disease characterized by acute or chronic suppurative inflammation of the middle ear.

- Common causes are *Streptococcus pyogenes* and the pneumococcus. These are pharyngeal organisms that reach the middle ear via the auditory tube.
- It usually occurs in children as a complication of viral and bacterial infections of the pharynx.

Pathologic Features

- In acute otitis media:
  - The middle ear is filled with purulent exudate.
  - The reddened tympanic membrane bulges into the external auditory meatus and may rupture, leading to a purulent discharge from the ear.
- In chronic otitis media:
  - There is chronic suppuration with fibrosis of the ossicles, leading to hearing loss.
  - There may be ingrowth of keratinizing squamous epithelium from the tympanic membrane, forming a pearly-white keratinized mass called a cholesteatoma.

Clinical Features

- Acute otitis media:
  - Presents with earache and fever.
  - Diagnosis is by presence of an outward-bulging, tense, reddened tympanic membrane.
  - When the membrane ruptures, there is a purulent discharge from the ear.
  - Culture of the exudate is necessary to identify the causative bacterium.
- Chronic suppurative otitis media:
  - Presents with chronic purulent ear discharge, commonly associated with hearing loss of varying degree.
  - Systemic symptoms are usually not prominent.
  - The tympanic membrane may show evidence of rupture.
  - Granulation tissue in the middle ear may protrude from the external auditory meatus as a polypoid mass ("aural polyp").
  - A cholesteatoma may be present in the middle ear.

Complications

They usually result from spread of the infection and include:

- Mastoiditis with inflammation of the mastoid air cells, leading to bone inflammation and necrosis (osteomyelitis).
- Epidural abscess, meningitis, and brain abscess; abscesses commonly occur in the cerebellum or temporal lobes.
- Thrombophlebitis of the lateral and sigmoid venous sinuses is characterized by high fever, severe headache, and bacteremia.

OTOSCLEROSIS
This is a disease of uncertain cause characterized by sclerosis of the middle ear ossicles, often with fusion of bone; it is usually bilateral.

- Bony ankylosis impairs transmission of sound waves to the cochlea, leading to deafness.
- There is a strong familial tendency, with about 40% of patients giving a positive family history.
- Autosomal dominant inheritance with variable penetrance appears likely.
- It is characterized by progressive deafness, usually beginning in the third decade.
- Low tones are lost first, followed by failure of high tone perception.

GLOMUS JUGULARE TUMOR
This is a **paraganglioma** that arises in the jugular glomus that lies in the adventitia of the internal jugular vein at the skull base.

- It frequently erodes into the middle ear, forming a red nodular mass and causing conduction deafness.
- It is extremely vascular and bleeds profusely when handled.
- The diagnosis is established by histologic examination.
- Tumors are locally aggressive but do not usually metastasize.

THE INNER EAR

ACUTE LABYRINTHITIS
This is a common cause of sudden unilateral hearing loss and acute vertigo.

- Viral infection is the commonest cause.
  - May be part of a systemic viral infection, as occurs in mumps and measles.
  - May be an isolated infection of the inner ear.
- It is usually a self-limited illness, but a significant number of patients have permanent hearing loss.
- Bacterial labyrinthitis is rarer and due to extension of suppurative otitis media. It leads to necrosis of the inner ear and commonly results in permanent deafness.

MENIERE'S DISEASE
This is an uncommon lesion involving the cochlea.

- The cause is not known. Infection, allergy and vascular disturbance have all been suggested.
- It occurs mainly in middle age and is more common in men than in women.
- It is bilateral in 20% of cases.

- It is characterized by accumulation of endolymphatic fluid in the cochlea ("hydrops of the labyrinth").
- With repeated attacks there is degeneration of the cochlear hair cells leading to deafness.
- Clinically, it is characterized by fluctuating hearing loss and tinnitus, and episodic vertigo; after several years, permanent and progressive hearing loss develops.
- No effective treatment is available.

II. THE UPPER RESPIRATORY TRACT

THE NOSE, PARANASAL SINUSES, & PHARYNX

Inflammatory Diseases

ACUTE RHINITIS (Coryza, Common Cold)

Acute rhinitis is almost always the result of viral infection and is one of the commonest infections of humans.

- It is caused by many different viruses, commonly rhinoviruses, influenza virus, myxoviruses, paramyxoviruses, and adenoviruses.
- It is characterized by watery nasal discharge accompanied by sore throat, fever, and muscle aches.
- It is self-limited.

ALLERGIC RHINITIS

Type I hypersensitivity (atopy) is also a common cause of acute rhinitis (hay fever).

- Susceptible patients are affected by a variety of allergens, most commonly pollens and dust.
- Commonly they have a positive family history and an increased frequency of developing other atopic diseases such as bronchial asthma and atopic dermatitis.

ACUTE PHARYNGOTONSILLITIS

Over 90% of cases of pharyngotonsillitis are the result of viral infections. Influenza, parainfluenza, myxo- and paramyxoviruses, adenovirus, respiratory syncytial virus, and enteroviruses are the usual causes.

- Epstein-Barr virus (infectious mononucleosis) and cytomegalovirus produce pharyngotonsillitis as part of a distinctive systemic illness.
- Bacterial infection, most commonly with *Streptococcus pyogenes,* is responsible for less than 10% of cases.
- *Neisseria gonorrhoeae, Mycoplasma pneumoniae,* and *Corynebacterium diphtheriae* are rare causes.
- Clinically, it is characterized by erythema of the mucosa with pain and fever.
- Culture of a throat swab is essential for diagnosis of bacterial infections.

- A quick (30-minute) nonculture test is now available for the rapid diagnosis of streptococcal sore throat.
- Viral infections are usually self-limited.
- Bacterial infections may lead to peritonsillar abscess and retropharyngeal space abscess.

INFLAMMATORY & ALLERGIC NASAL POLYPS
Repeated episodes of acute rhinitis result in the development of polyps in the nose and sinuses.

- They occur mainly in young adults and are usually multiple.
- They are composed of edematous stroma in which are found numerous neutrophils, eosinophils, lymphocytes, and plasma cells.
- They may cause nasal obstruction and frequently need to be removed surgically.

CHRONIC RHINITIS
Chronic inflammation of the nasal cavity occurs in leprosy, leishmaniasis, and syphilis, with marked destruction of the nose.

- Nonspecific inflammation also occurs with cocaine sniffing, in which septal perforation may occur.
- Nonspecific chronic bacterial infection of the nose leads to mucosal atrophy, crusting and an offensive odor (ozena or chronic atrophic rhinitis).
- Rhinoscleroma:
  - Is an uncommon infection in the United States.
  - Occurs commonly in eastern Europe and Central America.
  - Is caused by *Klebsiella rhinoscleromatis*.
  - Is characterized by accumulation of foamy macrophages (Mikulicz cells) filled with bacteria.
  - Results in nodular polypoid masses and ulceration (Hebra nose).
  - Diagnosis is made by demonstration of the organism in histologic sections and culture.
- Rhinosporidiosis:
  - Occurs in South India and Sri Lanka. It is rare elsewhere.
  - Is caused by the fungus *Rhinosporidium seeberi,* which appears in the nasal submucosa as large spherules containing endospores.
  - It results in nasal polyps.
  - Diagnosis is made by demonstrating the organism in histologic sections. *Rhinosporidium* cannot be cultured.

PARANASAL SINUSITIS
Inflammation of the maxillary, ethmoid, and frontal sinuses is a common complication of acute rhinitis.

- It results from obstruction of the nasal openings of these sinuses by edema.
- Chronic suppurative inflammation may occur.
- *Haemophilus influenzae* and *Streptococcus pneumoniae* are the organisms found most commonly.

- It causes headache, sometimes accompanied by fever and cervical lymph node enlargement.
- Extension of the inflammation to adjacent structures may, rarely, lead to:
  - Osteomyelitis affecting the maxilla.
  - Orbital cellulitis.
  - Cavernous sinus thrombophlebitis.
  - Meningitis, and brain abscess.

FUNGAL INFECTIONS

Phycomycosis (mucormycosis)
Phycomycosis is caused by fungi of the class Phycomycetes, most commonly *Mucor* species.

- It occurs only in:
  - A host with increased susceptibility.
  - Patients with diabetic ketoacidotic coma.
  - Immunocompromised patients.
- It presents as an acute nasal inflammation with extensive tissue necrosis, frequently spreading to the adjacent orbit and the cranial cavity.
- Death is common unless emergent treatment is instituted.
- Diagnosis is by identifying irregularly branching nonseptate hyphae by microscopy and culture.

Aspergillosis:
Aspergillosis causes a necrotizing inflammation of the nasal cavity in immunocompromised patients.

- *Aspergillus* is distinguished from *Mucor* by culture and recognition of the thinner, dichotomously branching, septate hyphae.
- *Aspergillus* spp may also cause a noninvasive infection in the nasal sinuses, forming an intracavitary mass ("fungus ball").

WEGENER'S GRANULOMATOSIS
This is a rare disease that in its fully expressed form involves the upper and lower respiratory tract and the renal glomeruli.

- Nasal and paranasal sinus lesions occur in 60% of cases.
- It is characterized by a rapidly progressive necrotic lesion.
- Biopsies show a necrotizing granulomatous vasculitis.

Lethal Midline Granuloma
This is a clinical term applied to a group of diseases characterized by a severe acute destructive ulcerative lesion of the middle of the face, including the nasal cavity and palate.

- It may be caused by bacterial or fungal infections, Wegener's granulomatosis, or neoplasms.
- Often it represents a progressive lymphoproliferative disease called *polymorphic reticulosis,* which is a form of malignant lymphoma.

TABLE 32–1. NEOPLASMS OF THE NASAL CAVITY AND PARANASAL SINUSES

Neoplasm	Location	Behavior	Histologic Appearance	Age and Sex
Juvenile angiofibroma	Roof of nasal cavity	Benign	Large blood vessels and fibrous stroma	Mainly in young adult males
Squamous papilloma	Nasal cavity, septum, sinuses	Benign	Papillary squamous epithelium	Adults
Inverted papilloma	Nasal cavity, lateral wall	Benign but may recur	Papillary epithelial growth; infiltrative	Adults
Extramedullary plasmacytoma	Nasal cavity	Malignant[1]	Diffuse sheets of abnormal plasma cells	Elderly
Malignant lymphoma	Nasal cavity, sinuses	Malignant	Monoclonal lymphoid proliferation	All ages
Nasal "glioma" (not a true neoplasm)	Roof of nasal cavity	Represents a herniation of normal brain through the cribriform plate or ectopic glial tissue		Newborn
Neoplasms of minor salivary glands	Sinuses	See Chapter 31		
Embryonal rhabdomyosarcoma (sarcoma botryoides)	Nasal cavity	Malignant	Primitive small cells; striated muscle differentiation	Children
Olfactory neuroblastoma (esthesioneuroblastoma)	Nasal cavity	Malignant	Primitive small cells; rosettes and neurofibrils	Children, adults
Squamous carcinoma	Nasal cavity, sinuses, nasopharynx, hypopharynx	Malignant	Infiltrative proliferation of atypical squamous epithelium	Adults
Malignant melanoma	Nasal cavity	Malignant	Infiltrative melanocyte proliferation	Adults

[1]Malignant plasmacytoma may occur as a solitary lesion or as part of multiple myeloma. Distinction from plasmacytosis in chronic inflammation is best achieved by demonstrating monoclonality in plasmacytoma (see Chapter 30).

Neoplasms

NEOPLASMS OF THE NASAL CAVITY (Table 32–1)

These are uncommon but display great variety. They commonly present as polypoid masses obstructing the nasal cavity.

- Both benign and malignant tumors may ulcerate and bleed, producing epistaxis.
- The most common benign neoplasm is a squamous papilloma.
- A variant of squamous papilloma known as inverted papilloma has a locally infiltrative growth pattern with a tendency to recur locally after surgical excision.
- Malignant neoplasms, such as squamous carcinoma and embryonal rhabdomyosarcoma, infiltrate extensively and metastasize to cervical lymph nodes.
- The diagnosis of the specific type is made by biopsy.
- Neoplasms of the paranasal sinuses (Table 32–1) tend to remain silent clinically until they are large.

CARCINOMA OF THE NASOPHARYNX

This is very common in the Far East and in eastern Africa.

- It has been linked etiologically to Epstein-Barr virus (EBV).
- Affected individuals show evidence of EBV infection, and the viral genome has been identified in the tumor cells.
- Cigarette smoking is an important etiologic factor.
- Nasopharyngeal carcinoma may occur at all ages, including younger patients.
- It is a poorly differentiated, nonkeratinizing squamous carcinoma with an abundant lymphoid stroma ("lymphoepithelioma").
- It presents with:
  - Enlarged cervical lymph nodes due to metastases.
  - Cranial nerve palsies due to infiltration of the skull base.
  - Otitis media due to obstruction of the auditory tube.
- Diagnosis is by biopsy.

MALIGNANT LYMPHOMA

The ring of lymphoid tissue in the oropharynx (Waldeyer's ring) is a common site for occurrence of extranodal malignant lymphoma.

- Most are of B cell origin.
- Intermediate- and high-grade lymphomas are most common.
- They present as nodular or ulcerative masses that grossly resemble carcinoma.
- The diagnosis is made by histologic examination with immunologic confirmation.

THE LARYNX

Inflammatory Conditions

ACUTE LARYNGITIS

Acute laryngitis frequently accompanies viral and bacterial infections of the upper respiratory tract, causing pain and hoarseness. Acute epiglottitis is a common infection in very young children, caused either by *Haemophilus influenzae* or by viruses. It may cause acute respiratory obstruction.

DIPHTHERIA

Incidence and Etiology
Diphtheria is caused by the gram-positive bacillus *Corynebacterium diphtheriae*.

- It has become rare in the United States and other developed countries because of effective immunization in childhood.
- It still occurs frequently in underdeveloped countries, where it is predominantly a disease of young children.

Pathology
Nasal, faucial, and laryngeal forms of diphtheria are recognized depending on the site of maximum involvement.

- Laryngeal diphtheria is the most common form, as well as the most dangerous.
- It is characterized by acute membranous inflammation.
- Detachment of the membrane and impaction in the trachea may cause sudden death from respiratory obstruction.
- The bacterium remains localized and does not enter the bloodstream.
- Some strains produce an **exotoxin** that enters the bloodstream and causes myocardial and nerve damage.

Clinical Features & Treatment
Patients present with pain, hoarseness, high fever, and marked enlargement of cervical lymph nodes.

- Diagnosis is by clinical examination and culture.
- Treatment includes antibiotics plus antitoxin to neutralize exotoxin.
- Mortality rates are low.

LARYNGEAL NODULE
This is a common lesion that occurs in the middle third of the true vocal cord.

- It is related to excessive use of the voice and occurs in singers ("singer's nodule"), teachers, and preachers.
- It appears grossly as a firm, rounded nodule covered by mucosa.
- Microscopically, dilated vascular spaces, fibrosis, and myxomatous degeneration are present to varying degree.
- Clinically, patients present with hoarseness and loss of ability to speak.
- Surgical excision is curative.

Laryngeal Neoplasms

SQUAMOUS PAPILLOMA
Squamous papilloma occurs in two distinct forms:

- Solitary papillomas occur in adults, and are cured by local excision.
- Juvenile papillomatosis, which is due to papillomavirus infection, occurs mainly in children and is characterized by multiple lesions and a high incidence of local recurrence after surgical removal. Lesions regress after puberty.

SQUAMOUS CARCINOMA

Incidence & Etiology
It is the commonest malignant neoplasm of the larynx.

- Most cases occur after age 50, and men are affected 7 times more frequently than women.
- Cigarette smoking and exposure to asbestos have a statistical association.

Pathologic Features
Squamous carcinoma is classified anatomically as:

- Glottic, involving the vocal cord.
- Supraglottic, involving the aryepiglottic folds and epiglottis.
- Subglottic, below the vocal cords.
- It often begins as an area of squamous epithelial dysplasia that may appear as a thickened white mucosal plaque.
- Invasion is associated with nodularity and ulceration.
- Microscopically, the majority are well-differentiated squamous carcinomas.
- Verrucous carcinoma is a highly differentiated form of squamous carcinoma characterized by a wartlike exophytic growth pattern with little invasion.

Clinical Features and Treatment
It commonly presents with persistent hoarseness.

- Large masses may cause respiratory obstruction and hemoptysis.
- Metastasis to cervical lymph nodes occurs early; distant metastases occur late.
- Diagnosis is made by laryngoscopy and biopsy.
- Surgical removal is highly successful when the patient has an early neoplasm and in verrucous carcinoma.
- In tumors with subglottic or supraglottic involvement, total laryngectomy and removal of cervical lymph nodes is frequently necessary, and survival rates are much lower.
- Radiation therapy is effective.

The Eye

THE EYELIDS

STY (Hordeolum)
Sty is an acute suppurative inflammation of the hair follicle or associated glandular structures: the sebaceous glands of Zeis and the apocrine glands of Moll. It is usually caused by *Staphylococcus aureus* and produces a painful localized abscess.

CHALAZION
Chalazion is a common chronic inflammatory process involving the meibomian glands. It is caused by duct obstruction, leading to retention of secretions, infection, and chronic inflammation with macrophages, lymphocytes, and plasma cells. Clinically, it produces an indurated mass.

XANTHELASMA
Xanthelasma is a yellow plaque composed of lipid-laden foamy macrophages in the subepithelial zone. It occurs in some hyperlipidemic conditions and in diabetes.

CYSTS
Congenital dermoid cysts occur along the lines of fusion of the facial skin folds, most often at the external angle of the upper eyelid. Acquired cysts arising in ducts of glands (eg, eccrine and apocrine hydrocystomas) and epidermal inclusions (epidermal cysts) are common.

MALIGNANT NEOPLASMS

Basal Cell Carcinoma
This is the commonest malignant neoplasm of the eyelid.

- It occurs much more commonly in the lower than in the upper lid.
- It presents as nodules that grow and ulcerate, forming an ulcer with an elevated pearly margin.
- It invades locally and may extend deeply into the orbit, but does not metastasize.

Squamous Carcinoma
Squamous carcinoma is uncommon in the eyelids.

Meibomian Gland Carcinoma
This occurs chiefly in the upper eyelid, which is the predominant location of meibomian glands.

- Clinically, it appears as a slowly growing yellowish mass.

TABLE 33–1. CAUSES OF CONJUNCTIVITIS AND KERATITIS

Infections
  Bacterial
    Haemophilus aegyptius, staphylococci, pneumococci.
    Neisseria gonorrhoeae (ophthalmia neonatorum) in babies
      born to mothers with active gonococcal cervicitis.
    Treponema pallidum; interstitial keratitis in congenital syphilis.
  Viral
    Especially severe in herpes simplex keratitis; occasionally
      herpes zoster, adenoviruses.
  Chlamydial
    Trachoma.
    Inclusion conjunctivitis.
  Protozoal
    Acanthamoeba (grows in contact lens cleaning fluid).
  Filarial
    Onchocerca volvulus, Loa loa.
Allergic conjunctivitis
  Includes seasonal or vernal conjunctivitis.
Chemical conjunctivitis
  Reaction to drugs, eye washes, makeup.
Solar conjunctivitis
  Ultraviolet light (snow blindness)
Trauma, foreign bodies

- Microscopically, the tumor consists of large invasive cells with abundant lipid-containing cytoplasm.
- It has a more aggressive biologic behavior than squamous carcinoma.
- Lymph node metastasis is common.

THE CONJUNCTIVA & CORNEA

KERATOCONJUNCTIVITIS

Etiology
For etiology, see Table 33–1.

Pathology & Clinical Features
Acute bacterial conjunctivitis is characterized by pain, hyperemia (red eye), and a purulent discharge in which numerous neutrophils are present. Ulceration occurs in severe cases and, when this involves the cornea, visual impairment may occur.

- Inclusion conjunctivitis (swimming pool conjunctivitis):
  - Commonly occurs in epidemics.
  - Is characterized by pain, red eye, and discharge.
  - Is caused by chlamydiae, which may be demonstrated as cytoplasmic inclusions in infected cells in the exudate.
- Trachoma is a serious chronic chlamydial infection causing corneal destruction and blindness. It is the commonest cause of blindness in underdeveloped tropical countries.

- *Acanthamoeba* keratoconjunctivitis may occur in users of soft contact lenses due to use of contaminated lens cleaning fluids.
- Allergic conjunctivitis is typically seasonal and associated with hay fever.
- Phlyctenular conjunctivitis is characterized by an elevated, hard, red triangular plaque at the limbus, which ulcerates and then heals in about two weeks. It may be associated with tuberculosis.

Diagnosis
Diagnosis of conjunctivitis is made clinically. Fluorescein staining is necessary to identify corneal involvement. Culture and microscopic examination of conjunctival discharge and scrapings from corneal lesions are necessary for identification of the etiology.

Degenerative Conjunctival & Corneal Conditions

PINGUECULA
This is a common degenerative disease caused by ultraviolet solar radiation.

- It is characterized by epithelial atrophy, degeneration of collagen, and hyalinization of elastic tissue.
- The exposed interpalpebral part of the conjunctiva is chiefly affected.
- It appears clinically as a thickened, yellowish area in the conjunctiva. It may become secondarily infected and ulcerate.
- The risk of squamous carcinoma is small.

PTERYGIUM
Pterygium affects the sclerocorneal junction (limbus) and may extend into the cornea as a layer of vascularized connective tissue, producing corneal opacification and visual impairment.

- In the cornea, there is replacement of Bowman's layer by collagen and elastic tissue.
- It has a tendency to recur after excision.
- Incidence of secondary infection, ulceration, and epithelial dysplasia is low.

Neoplasms of the Conjunctiva

BENIGN NEOPLASMS
Squamous papilloma, melanocytic nevus, hemangioma, and neurofibroma occur rarely in the conjunctiva. Benign lymphoid hyperplasia may produce a conjunctival mass.

SQUAMOUS CARCINOMA
Squamous carcinoma is rare. Most cases are believed to be due to ultraviolet radiation, complicating pinguecula and pterygium. Usually it invades superficially and it almost never metastasizes. It is treated by limited local excision, and has an excellent prognosis.

MALIGNANT MELANOMA
Malignant melanomas are rare.

- Melanomas may occur:
  - De novo.

- In a preexistent melanocytic nevus.
- In an acquired melanocytic hyperplasia (lentigo).
■ They present as nodules that may or may not be pigmented.
■ The prognosis is related to depth of invasion.
■ The more superficial lesions can be treated by local excision and have a good prognosis.
■ With deeper invasion, lymphatic and vascular involvement commonly occurs, and the prognosis is guarded even after radical exenteration of the orbit.

THE ORBITAL SOFT TISSUES

INFLAMMATORY PSEUDOTUMOR

This is an uncommon inflammatory lesion of unknown cause.

■ Clinically it is characterized by proptosis, pain, swelling, and restriction of ocular movement.
■ Histologically, there is edema, hyperemia, and infiltration of the orbital soft tissue with neutrophils, eosinophils, lymphocytes, and plasma cells.

GRAVES' DISEASE

Graves' disease (primary hyperthyroidism) is associated with exophthalmos caused by edema and accumulation of mucopolysaccharides in the orbital soft tissues.

■ Orbital muscles show marked myxoid change and weakness.
■ It is usually bilateral.
■ It is caused by an autoantibody (exophthalmos-producing factor) that may persist even after the hyperthyroidism is treated.

Primary Neoplasms of the Orbit

MALIGNANT LYMPHOMA

This is the most common malignant neoplasm of the orbit in adults.

■ Most are low-grade B cell lymphomas.
■ An exception is Burkitt's lymphoma, which is a high grade lymphoma.
■ The diagnosis is established by histologic examination, and confirmed by immunologic methods.

EMBRYONAL RHABDOMYOSARCOMA

This is a rare orbital primary tumor, occurring mainly in children.

■ It is highly malignant, with a rapid growth rate.
■ Diagnosis is made by demonstrating an undifferentiated neoplasm containing rhabdomyoblasts or by muscle differentiation using electron microscopy or immunohistochemistry.
■ Untreated, it is rapidly fatal. With chemotherapy and radiation, orbital embryonal rhabdomyosarcomas can be controlled and sometimes cured.

OPTIC NERVE GLIOMA

This is a rare neoplasm of the optic nerve, usually affecting the intraorbital part of the nerve.

- Commonly it is a well-differentiated, very low-grade, fibrillary astrocytoma that grows slowly over several years.
- Most cases occur in children, and are often associated with neurofibromatosis (von Recklinghausen's disease).

NEOPLASMS OF BONE

Common primary neoplasms of orbital bone are **osteoma** and **Histiocytosis X** (Hand-Schüller-Christian disease and eosinophilic granuloma). Metastatic neoplasms, such as neuroblastoma in children and metastatic carcinoma in adults, may present as orbital masses.

THE EYEBALL

Inflammatory Conditions

BACTERIAL INFECTIONS

Acute bacterial endophthalmitis and panophthalmitis are caused by bacteria such as staphylococci following penetrating injuries to the eye, orbital cellulitis, or septicemia. Untreated, there may be severe destruction with softening and collapse of the eyeball (phthisis bulbi).

TOXOPLASMA CHORIORETINITIS

This occurs either as a congenital transplacental or an acquired infection. Chorioretinitis may be the only manifestation of congenital toxoplasmosis.

- The organism persists in the choroid as pseudocysts, causing symptoms in childhood and early adult life.
- In acquired toxoplasmosis in adults, ocular involvement is common.
- Pathologically, there is focal coagulative necrosis of the retina and choroid, with granulomatous inflammation and fibrosis.
- *Toxoplasma* can be identified as small crescent-shaped trophozoites and as larger pseudocysts.

OCULAR LARVA MIGRANS

This is usually caused by larvae of *Toxocara canis* (a dog nematode) that reach the interior of the eye through the uveal or retinal blood vessels.

- It causes a granulomatous endophthalmitis with large numbers of eosinophils around the larvae.
- Marked fibrosis frequently causes retinal detachment and visual loss.

NONINFECTIOUS INFLAMMATORY CONDITIONS

Sarcoidosis produces an acute iridocyclitis, with fever and pain, and a chronic granulomatous disease, with corneal opacification and visual impairment.

- Rheumatoid arthritis produces scleritis and uveitis.
- Both ulcerative colitis and Crohn's disease are associated with nonspecific chronic iritis.
- Ankylosing spondylitis is associated with anterior uveitis in 20–50% of cases.
- Sympathetic ophthalmia is an uncommon diffuse granulomatous uveitis that affects

TABLE 33–2. PRINCIPAL TYPES AND CAUSES OF CATARACT

Congenital, inherited (autosomal dominant), unilateral or bilateral.
Congenital, due to fetal infection, especially rubella.
Congenital, associated with chromosomal abnormalities: trisomy 13.
Galactosemia.
Hypoparathyroidism.
Radiation to the eye.
Trauma, including penetration and contusion.
Toxic, drug-induced: dinitrophenol, long-term steroids.
Senile (aggravated by solar radiation).
Diabetic (resembles accelerated senile cataract).

both eyes after a penetrating injury to one eye. It is believed to be the result of an immunologic reaction.

■ Behçet's syndrome (uveitis plus oral and genital lesions) and Reiter's syndrome (conjunctivitis, uveitis, arthritis, and urethritis) probably represent postinfectious autohypersensitivity responses.

Degenerative Conditions of the Eyeball

CATARACT
Cataract is defined as the opacification of the lens.

■ Most individuals develop some lens opacification in later life (senile cataract).
■ Numerous other causes exist (Table 33–2).
■ Clinically, there is progressive loss of visual acuity, and halos or spots in the visual field.
■ Treatment with extraction of the cataract and implantation of a prosthetic lens is very successful.

GLAUCOMA
Glaucoma is defined as an increase in intraocular pressure sufficient to cause degeneration of the optic disk and optic nerve fibers.

■ Normal intraocular pressure, measured by tonometry, is 10–20 mm Hg.
■ Elevation in pressure induces deformational changes in the optic disk plus decreased retinal blood flow.
■ The correlation between intraocular pressure and optic nerve damage is not exact.
■ Glaucoma is the result of an abnormality in the dynamics of aqueous humor circulation.
■ It has many causes. Obstruction to the outflow of aqueous flow from the anterior chamber is the most common (Table 33–3).
■ Glaucoma is a common disorder, with about 2% of all people over age 40 being affected.
■ It may occur as a primary disease or as a complication of other diseases affecting the eye (secondary glaucoma).

TABLE 33–3. GLAUCOMA: CLASSIFICATION AND CAUSES

Congenital (rare)
Primary: Defects in canal of Schlemm, congenital and infantile
"Secondary": In association with other congenital anomalies: aniridia, Marfan's syndrome, neurofibromatosis, pigmentary glaucoma (degeneration of iris releases pigment that blocks outflow)

Primary (most common)
Open (wide) angle glaucoma: Most common form, often familial
Due to degeneration of canal of Schlemm, age > 40 years
?Due to primary vascular changes in optic nerve
Closed (narrow) angle or angle closure glaucoma: Blockage of the narrow anterior chamber by iris, especially when dilated at night; increase in lens size, causing further narrowing of anterior chamber

Secondary (common)
Several mechanisms; usually act through obstruction outflow from anterior chamber
Adhesions from uveitis (anterior synechiae)
Adhesions from intraocular hemorrhage or trauma
Dislocation of lens
Retinal artery narrowing (or occlusion), especially in diabetes mellitus
Arteriovenous fistulas (producing a direct increase in pressure)

1. PRIMARY OPEN-ANGLE GLAUCOMA

Open-angle glaucoma is also called simple or chronic glaucoma.

- It is a slowly progressive bilateral disease of insidious onset, occurring in individuals over age 40.
- It is responsible for over 90% of cases of primary glaucoma.
- It is characterized by a slow rise in intraocular pressure with subtle microscopic abnormalities in the canal of Schlemm.
- Progressive degeneration of the optic disk causes an increase in size of the blind spot (scotoma), and peripheral visual field loss. Blindness is common.
- Examination of the optic fundus shows deepening and enlargement of the optic cup.
- Treatment with pupillary constrictors such as pilocarpine, laser trabeculoplasty, and surgery are successful in arresting visual loss.

2. PRIMARY ANGLE-CLOSURE GLAUCOMA

Angle-closure glaucoma usually presents acutely.

- Many patients have a shallow anterior chamber and a narrow anterior chamber angle.
- Acute attacks may be precipitated by dilatation of the pupil (as in preparation for funduscopy).
- It is characterized by a rapid increase of intraocular pressure associated with severe pain, vomiting and rapid visual impairment.
- This is an ophthalmologic emergency. Complete blindness can occur within days. Treatment includes:
  - Osmotic agents and pupillary constrictors, which are effective in the acute phase.

● Peripheral iridectomy by laser, which is effective both in the acute relief of symptoms and in preventing further episodes.

DISLOCATION OF THE LENS
Dislocation of the lens may be caused by severe trauma.

■ It occurs in patients with abnormal collagen (as in Marfan's syndrome and homocystinuria) who have weak zonular fibers.
■ Anterior lens dislocation often causes obstruction to aqueous flow, leading to acute secondary glaucoma.
■ Posterior dislocation of an intact lens does not cause severe symptoms except visual impairment.
■ If the lens capsule is ruptured, lens protein may enter the blood stream, and cause an immunologic endophthalmitis.

RETINITIS PIGMENTOSA
This is a group of degenerative disorders with variable inheritance, most often recessive.

■ Retinal degeneration usually begins in early life and progresses slowly to blindness at age 50–60 years.
■ Degeneration beings in the peripheral part of the retina, causing progressive loss of the peripheral visual field.
■ Pathologically, there is disappearance of the rod and cone layer and loss of ganglion cells.
■ The fundus becomes slate-gray in color due to increased pigment.
■ Clinically, loss of night vision is an early symptom.
■ There is no treatment at present.

RETROLENTAL FIBROPLASIA OF PREMATURITY
This is caused by excessive oxygen, usually given for therapy of respiratory distress syndrome in premature infants.

■ The immature retina is exquisitely sensitive to oxygen, which causes vasospasm and proliferation of small retinal vessels into the vitreous.
■ Edema and hemorrhage leads to retinal detachment and blindness.
■ Careful control of oxygen therapy in the newborn has reduced the incidence of retrolental fibroplasia.

VASCULAR DISEASES OF THE RETINA
Retinal vessels are commonly affected in diabetes mellitus (Chapter 46) and hypertension (Chapter 20).

■ Occlusion of the central artery of the retina results in retinal infarction.
■ Hemorrhagic infarction occurs when the central vein of the retina is occluded.
■ Arterial emboli, either cholesterol emboli (derived from atheromatous plaques in the carotid circulation) or septic emboli in infective endocarditis may cause microinfarcts.

RETINAL DETACHMENT
Retinal detachment is defined as the separation of the neuroepithelial layer of the retina from the pigment layer.

- It is caused by:
  - Fibrous contraction, usually secondary to organization of vitreous hemorrhage.
  - Fluid collection between the two layers, due to inflammation or venous obstruction.
  - Neoplasms.
- Detachment deprives the neuroepithelial layer of its choroidal blood supply and causes degeneration within 4–6 weeks.
- Severe myopia is associated with retinal detachment (1% of myopic patients develop retinal detachment)
- Clinically, there is a sudden loss of part of the field of vision.
- Untreated, the detachment progresses, ultimately involving the entire retina and causing blindness.
- Laser treatment is effective in stopping the progression of retinal detachment and reversing the visual loss.

OPTIC ATROPHY

Optic atrophy presents as extreme pallor of the optic disk (optic nerve head). It usually reflects degeneration of optic nerve fibers and is associated with visual loss. It is classified as:

- Primary optic atrophy resulting from diseases of the optic disk.
- Secondary optic atrophy, which is due to long-standing papilledema.

Neoplasms of the Eyeball

MALIGNANT MELANOMA

This occurs almost exclusively in white adults. It is the commonest intraocular malignant neoplasm in the Unites States and Europe. It is uncommon in Asia, Africa, and South America.

Pathology

Intraocular melanomas arise in the uveal tract (85% in the choroid, 10% in the ciliary body, 5% in the iris).

- They are composed of proliferating invasive melanocytes, with several morphologic subtypes:
  - Spindle cell type A tumor, composed of slender cells with elongated nuclei and no nucleoli. These have the best prognosis (85% 10-year survival).
  - Spindle cell type B tumors, composed of more ovoid spindle cells with nucleoli. These have a slightly worse prognosis (80% 10-year survival).
  - Epithelioid cell tumors, composed of large pleomorphic round cells with hyperchromatic nuclei, nucleoli, and a high mitotic rate. They have a bad prognosis (35% 10-year survival).

Clinical Features

- Melanomas in the iris:
  - Become visible as a black mass in the front of the eye and usually present at an early stage.
  - Are commonly spindle type A tumors.
  - Have an excellent prognosis after removal.

- Melanomas arising in the ciliary body and choroid:
  - Usually attain a large size before they are detected.
  - Produce large masses that project into the vitreous, causing retinal detachment and visual impairment.
  - Are treated by enucleation of the eye.
  - Prognosis depends mainly on the histologic type.

RETINOBLASTOMA

Retinoblastoma has a worldwide distribution. It occurs in two forms: an inherited form (30%) and a sporadic form (70%). It occurs almost exclusively in children under age 5.

Genetic Features (Chapter 18)

A pair of mutant recessive genes are required to cause neoplasia.

- In the sporadic form, both mutations are acquired.
- In the hereditary form, one recessive gene is inherited in mutant form and the other suffers an acquired mutation.
- This pattern of inheritance mimics incomplete penetrance of a dominant gene.
- Patients with inherited retinoblastoma commonly have bilateral disease.
- More than 90% of sporadic cases have unilateral disease.
- It is associated with a constant karyotypic abnormality (deletion of 13q−).

Pathology

It arises in the retina from primitive neural cells. It is an aggressive neoplasm, infiltrating the retina, extending into the vitreous and along the optic nerve into the cranial cavity.

- Seeding of the cerebrospinal fluid may result in widespread dissemination in the subarachnoid space.
- Hematogenous spread also occurs.
- Microscopically, retinoblastoma is composed of undifferentiated small cells with a high nuclear:cytoplasmic ratio, hyperchromatic nuclei and a high mitotic rate. Flexner-Wintersteiner rosettes are characteristic.

Clinical Features

Commonly a white spot in the pupil (leukocoria) of a child's eye is noticed by an adult.

- Increased size of the orbit due to the mass effect is a late feature.
- Fundal examination shows the presence of the neoplasm.
- Without treatment, retinoblastoma causes rapid death in most cases.
- Treatment with radiation and chemotherapy has improved the prognosis.
- One to two percent of retinoblastomas undergo spontaneous regression. Regression is associated with cessation of proliferation of the neoplasm followed by fibrosis.
- Patients with retinoblastomas that have regressed represent a source of transmission of the abnormal gene to the next generation.

Section VIII. The Respiratory System

The Lung: I. Manifestations of Disease; Congenital Diseases; Infections

34

MANIFESTATIONS OF RESPIRATORY DISEASE

RESPIRATORY FAILURE

Respiratory failure is defined as a condition in which arterial Po_2 is decreased below, or arterial Pco_2 is increased above, its normal level.

■ Normal Pco_2 is 40 ± 5 mm Hg and does not vary with age.
■ Mean Po_2 varies with age and is derived from the following equation: $Po_2 = 100.1 - 0.323 \times$ age in years. The normal range is this calculated value ± 5 mm Hg.
■ The diagnosis of respiratory failure is made by arterial blood gas analysis and not by clinical examination.
■ Failure may be acute or chronic and results from failure of ventilation, diffusion, or perfusion of the lungs (Table 34–1). Changes in arterial blood gases with different mechanisms are shown in Table 34–2.

CYANOSIS

Cyanosis is a dusky, bluish discoloration of the skin and mucous membranes caused by the presence in the blood of increased amounts (over 5 g/dL) of reduced hemoglobin.

■ Central cyanosis is caused by admixture of deoxygenated venous blood with oxygenated arterial blood in the heart and lungs.
■ Peripheral cyanosis is caused by increased extraction of oxygen in the tissues, resulting in excessive reduction of normally saturated hemoglobin.
■ Central cyanosis can be differentiated from peripheral cyanosis by the presence of blue discoloration of mucous membranes in addition to the skin.

HEMOPTYSIS

Hemoptysis occurs in left heart failure, necrotizing parenchymal diseases such as infarcts, tuberculosis, and pneumonia, and neoplasms, most commonly lung carcinoma.

357

TABLE 34–1. CLASSIFICATION OF CAUSES OF RESPIRATORY FAILURE

Mechanism	Acute	Chronic
Reduced ventilation Restrictive Neuromuscular diseases (failure of respiratory muscles)	Tetanus, botulism, poliomyelitis, polyneuritis, spinal cord injury	Muscular dystrophy, myasthenia gravis
Chest wall diseases (failure of chest expansion)	Pneumothorax, flail chest (trauma)	Kyphoscoliosis, obesity, pleural effusion, mesothelioma, ankylosing spondylitis
Obstructive	Foreign bodies, epiglottitis, angioedema, diphtheria, bronchiolitis, bronchial asthma	COPD,[1] bronchiectasis
Abnormal perfusion	Pulmonary embolism, fat embolism	Recurrent emboli, vasculitis
Impaired diffusion Interstitial diseases	Shock, interstitial pneumonitis	Sarcoidosis, pneumoconiosis, interstitial pneumonitis, interstitial fibrosis
Pulmonary edema	Acute left ventricular failure, toxic gases, mitral stenosis	Chronic left ventricular failure

[1]COPD = chronic obstructive pulmonary disease.

CONGENITAL DISEASES OF THE LUNG

BRONCHOPULMONARY SEQUESTRATION

The lungs normally develop from buds arising from the embryonic foregut. Occasionally, an additional segment of lung develops from an abnormal accessory lung bud. The bronchi in this sequestered segment may not communicate with the normal bronchial tree.

- Sequestration is characterized by accumulation of mucus secretion in dilated bronchi, infection with abscess formation, and parenchymal fibrosis.
- Patients usually present with a mass in the lung or, more rarely, with accessory lung tissue in the mediastinum.

BRONCHOGENIC CYST

These cysts arise from accessory bronchial buds that lose communication with the tracheobronchial tree.

- They are lined by respiratory epithelium and frequently have cartilage in their walls.

TABLE 34-2. ARTERIAL BLOOD GAS CHANGES IN RESPIRATORY FAILURE

	Po_2	Pco_2	pH	Pathophysiology
Ventilation failure	Decreased	Increased	Decreased	Nonventilated lung is effectively right-to-left shunt, allowing venous type blood (low Po_2, high Pco_2) to pass directly to the left heart. Alveolar Po_2 is low, and Pco_2 is high in underventilated areas.
Perfusion failure	Decreased	Normal	Normal	Effective dead space is increased; hyperventilation of remaining lung may correct Pco_2 level, but oxygen exchange is already maximal and hyperventilation does not correct the fall in Po_2.
Diffusion failure	Decreased	Decreased	Increased	Diffusion failure affects only exchange of oxygen, not CO_2, the resulting hypoxemia causes compensatory hyperventilation, washing out CO_2 and causing hypocapnia.

- Usually they remain attached to the trachea. Rarely, they are found elsewhere in the mediastinum or esophagus.

CONGENITAL CYSTIC ADENOMATOID MALFORMATION
This malformation commonly presents during the newborn period.

- Usually it involves one lobe, which is enlarged and composed of abnormal cystic cavities lined by bronchiolar and columnar mucinous epithelium.
- The cystic mass may compress adjacent normal lung and displace the mediastinum, interfering with normal cardiac and lung function.
- Surgical removal of the involved lobe is curative.

TRACHEOESOPHAGEAL FISTULA
Usually this fistula is manifested by cyanosis and respiratory distress at the time of the first feeding. If feeding is continued, severe aspiration pneumonia occurs, causing death. Closure of the fistula is curative.

CONGENITAL ATELECTASIS
Failure of the lungs to expand at birth is termed *atelectasis*. It may be focal or may affect all of both lungs. Causes include inadequate attempts at respiration by the newborn (due

to neurologic damage, severe anoxia), bronchial obstruction, or absence of surfactant (see Respiratory Distress Syndrome, following).

NEONATAL RESPIRATORY DISTRESS SYNDROME (RDS)

This syndrome is also called hyaline membrane disease (HMD). It is a common complication in premature infants with immature lungs. It is also seen in babies born to diabetic mothers, and occurs more frequently in children delivered by cesarian section.

- The basic defect is deficient production of surfactant by type II pneumocytes. (Surfactant normally reaches adequate levels after the 35th week of gestation.)
- RDS accounts for about 7000 neonatal deaths every year in the United States.
- RDS occurs in 60% of babies born after less than 28 weeks of gestation, 40% of those born between 28 and 32 weeks, 20% of those born between 32 and 36 weeks, and less than 5% of those born after more than 36 weeks of gestation.
- RDS has a mortality rate of about 25%. In babies with a birth weight of less than 1000 g, the mortality rate is over 50%.
- In the immediate neonatal period, surfactant is important in maintaining expansion of the lung. In surfactant deficiency, the alveoli tend to undergo collapse after initial expansion.
- Grossly, the involved lung is heavy and purple as a result of fluid exudation and hemorrhage.
- Microscopically, there is intra-alveolar hemorrhage and hyaline membranes lining the damaged alveoli and respiratory bronchioles.
- Babies that survive severe RDS—particularly if oxygen has been used in therapy— may progress to chronic lung disease with fibrosis (bronchopulmonary dysplasia).
- Amniocentesis permits evaluation of lung maturity in premature babies by testing for the lecithin:sphingomyelin (L:S) ratio in amniotic fluid. When the L:S ratio reaches 2:1, the risk of RDS is very small.

INFECTIONS OF THE LUNG PARENCHYMA

Classification
A. Acute versus chronic infections:

- Acute infections causes alveolar involvement with consolidation (pneumonia), or interstitial inflammation.
- Chronic infections produce chronic inflammatory responses associated with fibrosis and persistent suppuration or the formation of granulomas.

B. Alveolar versus interstitial inflammation:

- Alveolar acute inflammation (pneumonia) is characterized by exudation of fluid and neutrophil emigration into the alveolar spaces (consolidation).
- Alveolar inflammation is further classified as:
  - Lobar pneumonia, where consolidation affects large confluent areas of lung.
  - Bronchopneumonia, where consolidation is patchy and adjacent to inflamed bronchioles.
- Alveolar inflammatory processes are caused by bacteria and lobar pneumonia is usually caused by more virulent bacteria than bronchopneumonia.

TABLE 34–3. USUAL LABORATORY FINDINGS IN COMMON LUNG INFECTIONS[1]

	Sputum	Sputum Culture	Blood Culture	White Blood Count	Chest X-Ray
Pneumococcus	Gram-positive diplococci	Positive	Often positive	10,000+	Lobar or bronchopneumonia
Staphylococcus aureus	Gram-positive clusters of cocci	Positive	Often positive	10,000+	Bronchopneumonia, abscesses
Group A streptococci	Gram-positive cocci	Positive	Often positive	20,000+	Bronchopneumonia
Haemophilus influenzae	Gram-negative short bacilli	Positive on chocolate agar in CO_2	Usually negative	10,000+	Bronchopneumonia
Klebsiella pneumoniae	Gram-negative short fat rods	Positive	Occasionally positive	20,000+	Broncho- or lobar-pneumonia; suppurative
Other enterobacteria: Escherichia coli, Pseudomonas, Proteus	Gram-negative large rods	Positive	Often positive late in course	10,000+	Bronchopneumonia; suppurative
Bacteroides	Gram-negative rods	Positive in anaerobic culture	Usually negative	10,000+	Bronchopneumonia; suppurative
Legionella	Gram-negative; silver and fluorescence stains positive	Positive in charcoal yeast agar	Negative	20,000+	Bronchopneumonia

(continued)

TABLE 34–3. (Continued)

	Sputum	Sputum Culture	Blood Culture	White Blood Count	Chest X-Ray
Mycobacterium tuberculosis	Acid-fast bacilli	Positive but takes 6 weeks	Negative	May be normal	Bronchopneumonia; granulomas; cavities; fibrosis
Fungi: *Histoplasma, Coccidioides, Aspergillus, Cryptococcus, Candida*	Periodic acid-Schiff or silver stains show fungi	Sabouraud agar positive; growth is slow	Usually negative (except cryptococcus)	May be normal	Bronchopneumonia; granulomas; fibrosis; cavities
Viruses and *Chlamydia:* Influenza, measles, respiratory syncytial virus, adenovirus, varicella, psittacosis, Q fever	Not useful; show commensal flora	Not useful (long delay)	Negative	May be normal, or lymphocytosis	Interstitial infiltrates (pneumonitis)
Mycoplasma	Not useful	Positive on special media, but slow growth	Negative	Occasionally 10,000+	Pneumonitis or mild bronchopneumonia

[1]*Note:* Many other organisms may cause lung infections; these are the more common ones.

■ Acute interstitial pneumonitis is characterized by edema, hyperemia, and lymphocytic infiltration of the alveolar septa. It occurs in infections with viruses, chlamydiae (psittacosis), rickettsiae (Q fever), and *Mycoplasma pneumoniae.*

C. Etiologic classification (Table 34–3):

■ Identification of the causative organism is the basis of treatment of pneumonia.
■ Methods of microbiologic diagnosis include a Gram-stained smear of sputum, sputum culture, and antibiotic sensitivity assays.

INFECTIONS CAUSING ACUTE INFLAMMATION

LOBAR PNEUMONIA

Incidence & Etiology
Streptococcus pneumoniae (pneumococcus) causes 90% of cases of lobar pneumonia. Other organisms include staphylococci, *Klebsiella, Pseudomonas,* and *Proteus.* The organisms are inhaled or aspirated into the alveoli.

Pathology & Clinical Features
A. Acute congestion:

■ This is the early stage where bacteria are actively multiplying in the alveoli and spreading in the lung.
■ There is hyperemia and fluid exudation into the alveoli.
■ Clinically, there is high fever, bacteremia (positive blood culture is common), and cough productive of purulent sputum tinged with blood.
■ Involvement of the pleura is common in this stage, causing chest pain, a pleural friction rub, and accumulation of effusion fluid.

B. Red hepatization:

■ Continued exudation and neutrophil emigration into the alveolar spaces causes consolidation, with alveoli being filled with fibrinous exudate and neutrophils.
■ The involved area appears grossly like liver ("hepatization").
■ Clinically, the illness is at its most severe stage, with high fever and cough.
■ Physical signs of consolidation are present.

C. Gray hepatization:

■ This is the early recovery phase, with clinical improvement.
■ The organism has been controlled by the body defenses and antibiotic therapy.
■ The alveoli still contain the exudate, and the physical signs and radiologic evidence of consolidation are still present.

D. Resolution:

■ The process by which the alveolar exudate is removed and the lung returns to normal is termed *resolution.*
■ Complete resolution may take several weeks, during which radiologic abnormalities persist despite clinical return to normal.

Diagnosis & Treatment

Alveolar consolidation is demonstrated by clinical and radiologic examination.

- The causative agent is identified in Gram-stained smears of sputum and by culture of sputum or blood.
- Predisposing factors that may have favored establishment of the infection should be identified and controlled.
- Failure to do so may lead to failure of antibiotic therapy and recurrence of pneumonia.

Complications

Lobar pneumonia interferes with gas exchange in the involved area.

- When both lungs are massively involved by the consolidation, respiratory failure may occur.
- Pleural effusion is common in the acute phase.
- Rarely, chronic suppuration (empyema) occurs.
- Bacteremia is a serious complication which increases the likelihood of death.
- Bacteremia may also lead to pneumococcal meningitis and endocarditis.
- Suppuration with formation of lung abscess occurs in pneumonia caused by type 3 pneumococci, *Staphylococcus aureus* and gram-negative bacilli.

BRONCHOPNEUMONIA

Etiology & Pathogenesis

Bronchopneumonia is a common finding at autopsy and contributes significantly to death in many patients, especially those with chronic diseases.

- Aspiration of pharyngeal secretions plays an important role in pathogenesis.
- In most cases of bronchopneumonia, a mixed bacterial flora that includes many bacteria is cultured from sputum.
- Pneumococci are present in 80% of cases.
- In seriously ill patients, gram-negative enteric bacilli are frequently found.
- Other organisms include *H influenzae* and streptococci other than *S pneumoniae*.
- When bronchopneumonia complicates a viral pneumonitis such as influenza or measles, *S aureus* is the most common pathogen.
- *Pneumocystis carinii* pneumonia is an opportunistic bronchopneumonia occurring in patients with AIDS, in malnourished children, and in patients undergoing chemotherapy for cancer.
- Bronchopneumonias caused by virulent organisms such as *S aureus*, type 3 pneumococci, and gram-negative organisms such as *K pneumoniae* are associated with multiple abscesses, bacteremia and a high mortality.

Clinical Features

Bronchopneumonia presents an extremely varied clinical picture.

- Severe infections caused by virulent organisms present as an acute febrile illness with cough and dyspnea very similar to lobar pneumonia.
- Physical examination usually reveals rales without consolidation.
- X-rays show the patchy nature of the process.

- With less virulent organisms, bronchopneumonia may have a less acute course, and clinical diagnosis can be difficult.
- The specific etiologic diagnosis is made by identifying the organisms in sputum (Gram's stain and culture) or lung biopsy (*P carinii* pneumonia).

ACUTE NECROTIZING PNEUMONIA

This is an acute pneumonia caused by highly virulent organisms associated with extensive necrosis and intra-alveolar hemorrhage. It is characterized clinically by a sudden onset and a severe course, often with rapid progression to death.

1. PLAGUE

Plague is caused by *Yersinia pestis*. It is found in wild rodents, particularly squirrels, in many parts of the United States.

- **Bubonic plague** is transmitted from rodents to humans by the bite of an infected flea.
  - The site of the bite shows inflammation and ulceration with marked regional lymph node enlargement.
  - Bacteremia follows.
- **Pneumonic plague,** a rapidly fatal necrotizing pneumonia, is the result of airborne spread of *Y pestis* from person to person.

2. ANTHRAX

Anthrax is caused by *Bacillus anthracis*. It involves the skin in 95% of cases.; in 5% of cases, anthrax spores are inhaled and lead to a severe necrotizing pneumonia with a high mortality rate.

3. LEGIONNAIRES' DISEASE

This is caused by *Legionella pneumophila,* a gram-negative bacillus.

- It may cause epidemics or sporadic disease.
- It is also common in immunocompromised hosts.
- Infection is frequently traced to contamination of air conditioners, ventilation systems, and shower heads.
- Clinically, most patients develop a mild lobar pneumonia, with recovery within 2–3 weeks.
- In about 20% of cases, there is a severe necrotizing pneumonia with a high mortality rate.
- Diagnosis can be made by demonstrating the organism in sputum, bronchial washings, or lung biopsy using silver and acid-fast stains, and immunofluorescence.

ACUTE INTERSTITIAL PNEUMONITIS

Etiology

Pneumonitis is caused by:

- Viruses, including influenza and parainfluenza virus, respiratory syncytial virus, adenoviruses, cytomegalovirus, herpesviruses, measles virus, echovirus, and coxsackieviruses.
- Chlamydiae: *Chlamydia psittaci*.

■ Rickettsiae: *Coxiella burneti* (the agent of Q fever).
■ *Mycoplasma pneumoniae.*

Pathology

The alveolar septa are expanded by hyperemia and a cellular infiltrate composed of plasma cells, lymphocytes, and macrophages. In a few cases, there are additional changes:

■ Necrosis of pneumocytes, most commonly in influenza and adenovirus infections, leads to intra-alveolar hemorrhage, and formation of hyaline membranes.
■ Inclusion bodies may be present with cytomegalovirus infection, herpes simplex infection, varicella, adenovirus infection, measles, influenza, and psittacosis.
■ Multinucleated giant cells are found in measles and in respiratory syncytial virus infection.

Clinical Features

It is characterized by an acute onset of fever, cough, and dyspnea.

■ The illness is usually mild and self-limited.
■ Because of the absence of alveolar exudation and consolidation, there are few abnormal findings on physical examination.
■ Chest X-ray shows the pattern of interstitial inflammation.

INFLUENZA

Etiology & Epidemiology

Influenza is caused by an RNA virus related to myxoviruses.

■ Type A influenza virus is a major cause of epidemic disease, type B less so, and type C rarely.
■ The virus has an outer envelope that shows frequent antigenic changes (antigenic drift), developing into new strains that are not affected by immune responses.
■ It occurs endemically year-round with seasonal variation, peaking in the winter months.
■ Epidemics occur every 3–4 years, and pandemics usually signify emergence of an antigenic strain that most of the population have not encountered previously.

Pathology & Clinical Features

■ The incubation period is 2–3 days.
■ The virus infects and multiples in the respiratory epithelium.
■ In severe cases, there is necrosis of alveolar epithelial cells, intra-alveolar hemorrhage and exudation, and formation of hyaline membranes.
■ Clinical onset is abrupt, with fever, chills, malaise, headache, and muscle pains. Sputum is usually scanty but may be bloody.

Complications

■ Secondary bacterial infection is most important. Common secondary invaders include *H influenzae,* staphylococci, pneumococci, and other streptococci.

- Less commonly, the influenza virus causes a severe necrotizing viral pneumonitis that progresses rapidly to respiratory failure and death.
- Other less common complications include myocarditis, encephalitis, polyneuritis, and Guillain-Barré syndrome.
- Reye's syndrome (acute encephalopathy with acute fatty degeneration of liver and kidney) may rarely complicate influenza, especially when high doses of salicylates are given to dehydrated children with infection.

Prevention
Vaccination is successful against endemic influenza or in slowly developing epidemics when the antigenic characteristics of the strain are known. It is less effective in explosive pandemics that by definition represent an emergent new strain and require development of a new vaccine.

INFECTIONS CAUSING CHRONIC SUPPURATIVE INFLAMMATION

CHRONIC LUNG ABSCESS
Chronic lung abscess occurs in several situations:

- As a sequela of unresolved acute pneumonia with suppuration.
- As a common complication of bronchopneumonia following aspiration.
- Distal to a bronchus that is obstructed by neoplasms or foreign bodies.
- Following aspiration during coma from any cause.
- Clinically, patients present with low-grade fever, weight loss, clubbing of fingers, and cough productive of a large volume of foul-smelling purulent sputum.
- Leukocytosis and increased serum immunoglobulin levels are common.
- Radiologic examination shows a cavitary lesion with an air-fluid level.
- Sputum culture usually grows multiple bacteria, commonly including anaerobes such as *Bacteroides* species.

ACTINOMYCOSIS & NOCARDIOSIS
Actinomyces israelii and *Nocardia asteroides* are gram-positive filamentous bacteria that cause chronic suppuration with extensive fibrosis.

- Multiple abscesses with colonies of organisms are present.
- The infection tends to spread by local extension and may produce chest wall abscesses that drain through the skin.

INFECTIONS CAUSING CHRONIC GRANULOMATOUS INFLAMMATION
Chronic granulomatous inflammation of the lung is caused by facultative intracellular organisms:

- *Mycobacterium tuberculosis*.
- Atypical mycobacteria.
- Fungi, commonly *Histoplasma capsulatum, Coccidioides immitis, Blastomyces dermatitidis, Paracoccidioides brasiliensis,* and *Cryptococcus neoformans*.

PULMONARY TUBERCULOSIS

Pulmonary tuberculosis is caused by *Mycobacterium tuberculosis.*

■ The human strain infects only humans. Patients with pulmonary tuberculosis are the source of infection.
■ It is well controlled in most developed countries, but still common in underdeveloped countries.
■ In the United States, tuberculosis is a problem in crowded cities with a high concentration of immigrants.

1. Primary (Childhood) Tuberculosis (Fig 34–1)

Pathology

■ It occurs when a child who has not been previously exposed to tubercle bacilli inhales the organism.
■ The organism enters the alveoli and leads to the formation of the primary (Ghon) complex, which is composed of the Ghon focus and enlarged regional (hilar) lymph nodes.
■ The Ghon focus is an epithelioid-cell granulomatous inflammation at the site of parenchymal infection. It is usually small and subpleural, but may be large and located anywhere in the lung.
■ Before immunity is established, tubercle bacilli are transported via lymphatics and the bloodstream throughout the body (preallergic lymphohematogenous dissemination).
■ The immune response against the tubercle bacillus results in:
  ● Macrophage activation leading to destruction of tubercle bacilli.
  ● Inhibition of macrophage migration, which reduces further spread of bacilli in the body.
  ● Delayed (type IV) hypersensitivity, which leads to caseous necrosis of granulomas in the Ghon focus and elsewhere in the body.
  ● Hypersensitivity is responsible for "tuberculin conversion." The infected individual gives a positive reaction to intradermal injection of tuberculin.

Clinical Features

■ It is usually asymptomatic or manifested as a mild flulike illness.
■ In 95% of cases, immunity stops disease progression and healing occurs.
■ Complications occur in 5% of cases of primary pulmonary tuberculosis, including:
  ● Locally progressive pulmonary disease, causing extensive caseous consolidation of the lung (caseous pneumonia).

Figure 34–1. Pulmonary tuberculosis. Infection with *Mycobacterium tuberculosis* in the nonimmune host, usually in a child, causes primary tuberculosis. While most patients recover from this, many have subclinical lymphohematogenous dissemination of bacilli to many organs. These bacilli can remain dormant and become reactivated many years later, leading to secondary pulmonary and extrapulmonary tuberculosis. Secondary pulmonary tuberculosis may also result from reinfection in adult life. The pathologic features of reinfection and reactivation types of secondary pulmonary tuberculosis are identical. Note that extrapulmonary tuberculosis may occur in a patient without overt lung involvement.

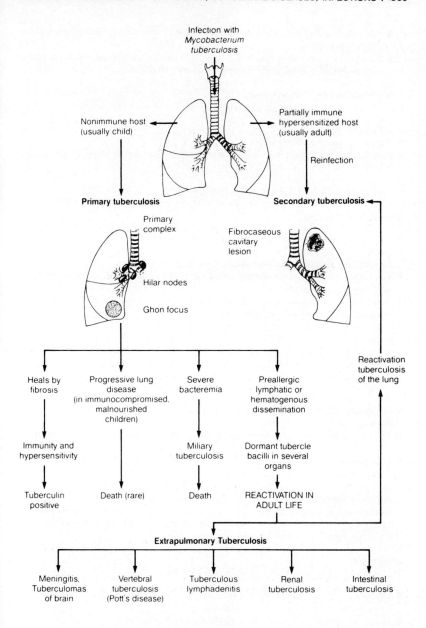

- Erosion of a caseous granuloma into a bronchus, which may result in tuberculous bronchopneumonia.
- Erosion into a blood vessel, which may cause severe bacteremia and small tuberculous granulomas all over the body (miliary tuberculosis).

Effects of Primary Tuberculosis
Patients who have had a primary infection show:

- Tuberculin positivity.
- Partial immunity to tuberculosis.
- Dormant tubercle bacilli in the lungs, brain, meninges, bone, kidneys, lymph nodes, intestines, etc. (Fig 34–1).

2. Secondary (Adult) Tuberculosis (Fig 34–1)

Definition & Etiology

- It occurs in a patient who has had a prior primary infection.
- Usually it occurs in an adult and may be due to either reinfection or reactivation. Reactivation is probably responsible for the majority of cases.
- The mechanism that keeps dormant bacilli in check is uncertain, as are the reasons why they become reactivated.
- Reactivation commonly occurs when a tuberculin-positive individual is given immunosuppressive drugs such as corticosteroids.

Pathology
Multiplication of tubercle bacilli occurs in the presence of a rapidly developing secondary immune response, which localizes the tubercle bacilli to the area.

- Enhanced delayed hypersensitivity produces a heightened local response with extensive caseous necrosis.
- Secondary tuberculosis may occur in any tissue by reactivation; the commonest site is the lung apex.
- The typical lesion is a large fibrocaseous mass (tuberculoma) that undergoes liquefaction and cavitation.
- The liquefied granuloma may open into a bronchus, leading to coughing up sputum that is infectious.

Clinical Features
Almost always symptoms include chronic cough, frequently with hemoptysis. Marked weight loss, low-grade fever, and night sweats are common. Physical examination and chest X-ray show apical fibrosis and cavitation.

Diagnosis
The diagnosis of tuberculosis must always be confirmed by microbiologic techniques.

- Demonstration of tubercle bacilli can be by acid-fast stain of smears of sputum or in tissue sections of tissue biopsies.
- Failure to demonstrate bacilli in a single specimen does not exclude a diagnosis of tuberculosis.

- Culture of *M tuberculosis* from sputum or tissue takes 4–6 weeks.
- The tuberculin test is usually strongly positive. A significant number of patients with active tuberculosis demonstrate immunologic anergy and give a false-negative tuberculin test.

Treatment & Prognosis
The most effective antituberculous drugs are isoniazid (INH) and rifampin.

- The tubercle bacillus rapidly develops resistance to antimicrobial drugs, and it is customary to start treatment of a new case with three drugs, one of which is isoniazid.
- Asymptomatic patients who have recently become tuberculin-positive are advised to undergo chemoprophylaxis.

ATYPICAL MYCOBACTERIAL INFECTION
Atypical mycobacteria are commonly found in the soil.

- They are less pathogenic for humans than *M tuberculosis* and cause disease less often.
- *Mycobacterium kansasii* may rarely infect normal individuals.
- *Mycobacterium avium-intracellulare* infection occurs in immunodeficient states and is one of the opportunistic infections commonly seen in patients with AIDS.
- Pulmonary disease caused by atypical mycobacteria is very similar to pulmonary tuberculosis and is distinguished only by culture.

FUNGAL GRANULOMAS OF THE LUNG
These granulomas produce pathologic lesions in the lung very similar to those seen in tuberculosis. One major difference is that the source of infection is not an infected patient. Infection occurs after exposure to soil containing spores of fungi.

Etiology & Epidemiology

- Histoplasmosis, caused by *Histoplasma capsulatum,* is common in the midwestern United States, and a very high incidence in the Mississippi Valley.
- Coccidioidomycosis, caused by *Coccidioides immitis,* is common in the Southwestern United States (San Joaquin Valley fever).
- Blastomycosis (*Blastomyces dermatitidis*), paracoccidioidomycosis (*Paracoccidioides brasiliensis*), and sporotrichosis (*Sporothrix schenckii*) are uncommon causes of pulmonary infection in the United States.

Pathology
The pathologic lesions are chronic granulomas with extensive caseation and fibrosis.

Clinical Features
Primary infection is characterized by a parenchymal granulomatous focus and regional lymph node enlargement. The disease is usually asymptomatic, and recovery is the rule.

- About 90% of the population in the Mississippi Valley and 80% of people in the San Joaquin Valley in California have positive skin tests for histoplasmin and coccidioidin, respectively.
- The level of immunity after a primary infection with these fungi is low, so that reinfection is relatively common.

■ Progressive primary infection with widespread dissemination of fungus in the body, is common in malnourished or immunodeficient individuals.

■ Dormant infection followed by reactivation is responsible for many cases of pulmonary and all cases of secondary extrapulmonary fungal granulomas.

■ Secondary infection is associated with large caseous granulomas that cause marked fibrosis and chronic cavitary lung disease.

Diagnosis

Precise diagnosis depends on identifying the fungus in sputum or in tissue by microscopy (Fig 34–2) or culture.

PULMONARY CRYPTOCOCCOSIS

Cryptococcus neoformans may cause pulmonary disease, both in healthy individuals (uncommon) and in immunodeficient patients (common).

■ In individuals with a normal immune system, a chronic granulomatous inflammation occurs.

■ Differentiation from tuberculosis and other fungal granulomas depends on demonstrating cryptococci microscopically or by culture.

■ In the immunodeficient host, the yeast multiplies in the alveoli with little or no inflammatory reaction and produces an area of consolidation.

■ *Cryptococcus* is identified by its variability in size (10–25 μm), thick mucoid capsule, and narrow-based single budding.

■ Disseminated cryptococcal infection with meningeal involvement is common in the immunodeficient host.

PARASITIC INFECTIONS OF THE LUNG

DIROFILARIA IMMITIS INFECTION

Dirofilaria immitis is a filarial worm whose normal site of infection is the heart and pulmonary arteries of dogs ("dog heartworm").

■ Accidental infection of humans occasionally occurs, mainly in the Southeastern United States.

◗ The worm infects the pulmonary arteries; when the worm dies, it evokes an inflammatory reaction that causes fibrous occlusion of the vessel and pulmonary infarction.

■ This causes chest pain, hemoptysis and a circumscribed opacity ("coin" lesion) on chest X-ray.

OTHER PARASITIC LUNG INFECTIONS

■ Tropical pulmonary eosinophilia is associated with filariasis and characterized by fever, wheezing, weight loss, peripheral blood eosinophilia, hyperglobulinemia, and diffuse infiltrates on chest X-ray.

Figure 34–2. Morphologic features in tissue sections of the fungi that commonly cause granulomas.

2-4 μm group

Histoplasma capsulatum

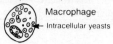

Macrophage

— Intracellular yeasts

Sporothrix schenckii

10-30 μm group

Cryptococcus neoformans

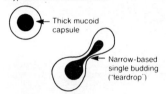

— Thick mucoid capsule

— Narrow-based single budding ("teardrop")

Blastomyces dermatitidis

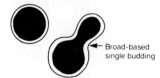

— Broad-based single budding

Paracoccidioides brasiliensis

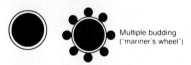

Multiple budding ("mariner's wheel")

Over 30 μm

Coccidioides immitis

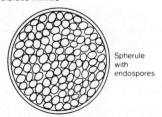

Spherule with endospores

- Hydatid cysts, cysticercosis, lung fluke (*Paragonimus westermani*) infection, and amoebic (*Entamoeba histolytica*) lung abscess are all rare.
- Larval migration of *Ascaris lumbricoides* (roundworm) and *Strongyloides stercoralis* may also produce symptoms similar to those of pulmonary eosinophilia.

The Lung: II. Toxic, Immunologic, & Vascular Diseases

35

ACUTE DISEASES OF THE AIRWAYS

Infections of the Air Passages

ACUTE TRACHEOBRONCHITIS

Acute tracheobronchitis commonly complicates a severe upper respiratory tract infection, particularly:

- *Haemophilus influenzae* infection of the larynx in young children.
- Influenza in adults and children.
- Viral tracheobronchitis may also be complicated by secondary bacterial infection, most commonly with *Staphylococcus aureus*.

ACUTE BRONCHIOLITIS

Acute bronchiolitis is a common, often epidemic, infection of the small airways that occurs mainly in children under age 2.

- Most cases are mild, but 1–2% require hospitalization, and about 1% of these children die.
- Most cases are caused by respiratory syncytial virus. More rarely, parainfluenza virus and adenoviruses are responsible.
- The bronchioles show acute epithelial damage, lymphocytic infiltration and luminal mucus plugs.
- Patients present with acute-onset tachypnea and wheezing. Fever is low-grade and may be absent.

WHOOPING COUGH (Pertussis)

Whooping cough is caused by *Bordetella pertussis*. It is an extremely serious acute respiratory tract infection in the young.

- Prior to immunization, it accounted for 40% of all deaths in the first 6 months of life.
- Clinically, it is characterized by paroxysmal coughing and an inspiratory whoop.
- Otitis media, bronchitis, and bronchiectasis are serious complications.
- Tetracycline is effective in therapy.

BRONCHIAL ASTHMA

Bronchial asthma is characterized by acute narrowing of bronchioles due to bronchospasm, which causes obstruction to air flow, maximal in expiration, and a high-pitched wheeze.

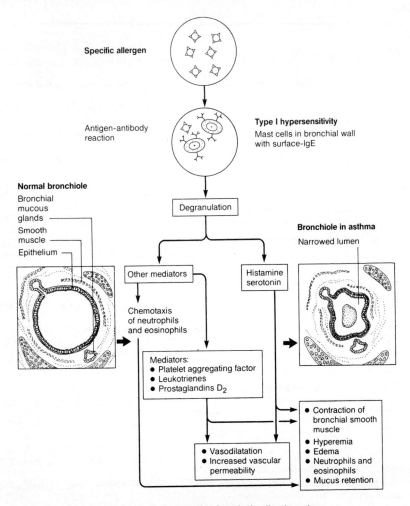

Figure 35-1. Pathogenesis of extrinsic allergic asthma.

- Attacks are usually of short duration and reverse completely.
- Rarely, they may be severe and prolonged ("status asthmaticus"), and may lead to acute ventilatory failure and even death.

Etiology & Classification
A. Extrinsic allergic asthma:

- Is a reagin-mediated type I hypersensitivity (atopic) reaction (Fig 35-1).
- Is common in childhood and has a familial tendency.

TABLE 35–1. FACTORS INVOLVED IN ASTHMA

Allergens
Household dust
 Contains waste products of house mite *Dermatophagoides pteronyssimus*
Other organic dusts
 Includes allergic *Aspergillosis* in which the response is to antigens on fungi actually growing in
  the bronchi
Pollens
 Especially grasses and trees; types vary in different geographic regions. This form of asthma
  usually is seasonal and often coexists with "hay fever" (allergic rhinitis)
Animal dander, fur
 Cats, dogs, horses, birds; allergy is usually to fur and feathers; usually only one species (eg,
  cats, not dogs)
Food products
 Ingested antigens may produce asthma after absorption and distribution in the bloodstream
Drugs
 Ingested, act as haptens

Precipitating factors
Heat, cold, aerosols, chemicals, gases, cigarette smoke
Exercise
Infection
Emotional stress
Drugs, especially aspirin, may precipitate nonallergic asthma
In nonallergic asthma, bronchi are abnormally sensitive because of decreased beta-adrenergic
 responses

- Many different antigens may be involved (Table 35–1).
- Inhaled antigens combine with specific IgE on the surface of mast cells in the respiratory mucosa.
- Serum IgE is increased, and skin tests against the offending antigens are positive.

B. Intrinsic (nonallergic) asthma:

- Is characterized by hyperreactive airways that constrict in response to a variety of nonspecific stimuli, due in part to abnormal β-adrenergic responses.
- Aspirin, cold, exercise, and respiratory infections are common precipitants of attacks.
- Serum IgE levels are normal, and skin tests are negative.
- Intrinsic asthma occurs in older patients.

Pathology

- Histologic changes are nonspecific.
- Inspissated mucus plugs obstruct bronchioles and causes focal collapse of alveoli.
- Expiratory obstruction leads to air trapping and distention of distal alveoli.
- Mild inflammation and edema with numerous eosinophils are seen in the bronchiolar wall.
- Infection may complicate prolonged attacks.

Clinical Features

- There are episodic attacks of dyspnea and wheezing.
- In severe attacks, there is frequently secondary bacterial infection.

- Allergic asthma occurs in childhood and tends to disappear as the child grows.
- Intrinsic asthma occurs in older individuals and tends to produce a more chronic disease.

Treatment & Prevention

The acute attack is treated with bronchodilator drugs such as theophylline, epinephrine, and β_2-adrenergic agents like metaproterenol.

- Corticosteroids are effective in severe cases.
- Control of secondary infection is necessary in a severe attack.
- Identification of allergens by skin testing may be followed by their avoidance or by desensitization.
- Disodium cromoglycate, which appears to stabilize mast cell membranes, is used prophylactically.

ALLERGIC BRONCHOPULMONARY ASPERGILLOSIS

This is a specific form of allergic asthma caused by inhalation of spores of *Aspergillus* species.

- The fungus grows in the bronchioles and evokes a hypersensitivity reaction (Table 35–2) that appears to be a combined type I (elevated serum IgE) and type III reaction (elevated serum levels of precipitating antibodies and an Arthus-type reaction in the lungs).
- Clinically, the asthmatic attacks tend to be more persistent, with infiltrates appearing on chest X-ray.
- Pulmonary fibrosis may ensue.

CHRONIC OBSTRUCTIVE PULMONARY DISEASE (COPD)

COPD is characterized by features of chronic obstruction to air flow in the lungs, as shown by a decreased FEV_1:FVC ratio. Normally, the FEV_1:FVC ratio is over 75%. In COPD, the degree of reduction correlates well with disease severity and survival.

Incidence

COPD is second only to ischemic heart disease as a cause of chronic disability in older individuals and the incidence is increasing.

Pathology

COPD is associated with two distinctive pathologic conditions—chronic obstructive bronchitis and emphysema—which contribute in variable degree.

A. Chronic obstructive bronchitis: Chronic obstructive bronchitis is defined clinically as the presence of a chronic cough productive of mucoid sputum.

- Pathologic examination shows hypertrophy of bronchial wall mucous glands, chronic inflammation, and fibrous replacement of bronchiolar smooth muscle.
- The Reid index—the ratio of mucous gland thickness to bronchial wall thickness—is increased above the normal value of 0.5.
- Fibrotic bronchioles collapse in expiration due to the positive intrathoracic pressure, resulting in ventilatory obstruction in expiration.

TABLE 35–2. IMMUNOLOGIC HYPERSENSITIVITY IN LUNG DISEASE

Hypersensitivity Reaction	Clinicopathologic Effect
Type I IgE-mediated	Bronchial asthma Allergic bronchopulmonary aspergillosis
Type II Antibody against basement membrane	Goodpasture's syndrome Idiopathic pulmonary hemosiderosis
Type III Immune complex	Hypersensitivity pneumonitis Connective tissue diseases Allergic bronchopulmonary aspergillosis
Type IV Cell-mediated hypersensitivity	Tuberculous and fungal granulomas Some type of interstitial pneumonitis
Uncertain	Idiopathic interstitial pneumonitis Wegener's granulomatosis

B. Emphysema in COPD:

- Is characterized by permanent dilatation of the air spaces distal to the terminal bronchiole, usually with destruction of lung parenchyma.
- To produce clinical COPD, large areas of the lung must be involved by emphysema.
- There are two principal types:
  - Centrilobular emphysema, in which dilatation and destruction primarily involve the central part of the acinus formed by the respiratory bronchioles.
  - Panacinar emphysema, in which dilatation and destruction involve the alveoli and alveolar ducts as well as the respiratory bronchioles.
- Other forms of emphysema are recognized but are not usually associated with COPD (Table 35–3).

Pathogenesis

- It is 5–10 times more common in heavy cigarette smokers. Cigarette smoking acts as a local irritant, causing hypertrophy of bronchial mucous glands and hypersecretion of mucus.
- Other inhaled irritants such as sulfur dioxide and oxides of nitrogen produce similar changes, but are not present at high enough concentration in most environments to play a significant role.
- Hypersecretion of mucus increases the susceptibility to bacterial infection. *Haemophilus influenzae,* pneumococci, and *Streptococcus viridans* are common pathogens.

Pathogenesis of Emphysema

The destruction of lung parenchyma in emphysema is due to the action of proteolytic enzymes.

TABLE 35–3. CHRONIC BRONCHITIS AND EMPHYSEMA

	Causal Factors	Clinical Effects
Destructive lung disease Chronic bronchitis, centrilobular emphysema, panacinar emphysema	Cigarettes Recurrent infection ?Pollutants Alpha$_1$-antitrypsin deficiency	Chronic obstructive pulmonary disease (COPD)
Senile emphysema	Aging	Asymptomatic
Paraseptal emphysema (paracicatricial)	Associated with any cause of collapse or fibrosis (scars [paracicatricial])	Rarely sufficient to produce symptoms
Bullous emphysema	Unknown	Asymptomatic, but rupture leads to pneumothorax
Nondestructive disease Compensatory emphysema (dilatation without destruction)	Removal or collapse of part of lung; remaining lung expands	Asymptomatic
Focal dust emphysema (dilatation without destruction)	Various dust diseases, pneumoconioses, eg, coal miners's lung	Usually insufficient to produce symptoms
Dilatation distal to obstruction; no destruction	Acute bronchial asthma: air trapping	Symptoms of asthma

■ One important source of these proteases is leukocytes associated with pulmonary inflammation.

■ Normally, antiproteolytic substances such as antitrypsins in the plasma inactivate these enzymes.

■ Lung destruction—and emphysema—occur in patients who either produce an excess of proteolytic enzymes or have too little antiproteolytic activity in the plasma (α_1-antitrypsin deficiency; see following).

■ Cigarette smoking is an important etiologic factor in emphysema. Smoking increases numbers of neutrophils, and promotes elastase release from neutrophils.

■ The lungs of heavy smokers show centrilobular emphysema beginning at a relatively young age.

■ **Alpha$_1$-antitrypsin** deficiency predisposes to emphysema because of reduced plasma antiproteolytic activity.

● The α_1-antitrypsin level in serum is determined by inheritance at a single (Pi, or protease inhibitor) locus. A normal individual is PiMM.

● The **Z gene** is the commonest of several abnormal genes that may be inherited.

● PiZZ homozygotes have severe deficiency of α_1-antitrypsin and almost invariably develop panacinar emphysema by age 40.

● PiZZ occurs with a frequency of 1:4000 and thus is a very rare cause of emphysema.

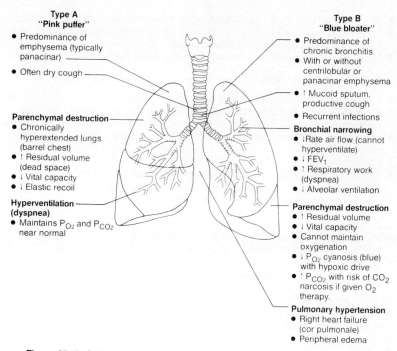

Type A
"Pink puffer"

- Predominance of emphysema (typically panacinar)
- Often dry cough

Parenchymal destruction
- Chronically hyperextended lungs (barrel chest)
- ↑ Residual volume (dead space)
- ↓ Vital capacity
- ↓ Elastic recoil

Hyperventilation (dyspnea)
- Maintains P_{O_2} and P_{CO_2} near normal

Type B
"Blue bloater"

- Predominance of chronic bronchitis
- With or without centrilobular or panacinar emphysema
- ↑ Mucoid sputum, productive cough
- Recurrent infections

Bronchial narrowing
- ↓Rate air flow (cannot hyperventilate)
- ↓ FEV_1
- ↑ Respiratory work (dyspnea)
- ↓ Alveolar ventilation

Parenchymal destruction
- ↑ Residual volume
- ↓ Vital capacity
- Cannot maintain oxygenation
- ↓ P_{O_2} cyanosis (blue) with hypoxic drive
- ↑ P_{CO_2} with risk of CO_2 narcosis if given O_2 therapy.

Pulmonary hypertension
- Right heart failure (cor pulmonale)
- Peripheral edema

Figure 35–2. Clinical effects and types of chronic obstructive pulmonary disease.

- The heterozygous PiMZ state occurs in about 5% of the population of the United States, and is associated with a moderate reduction in serum α_1-antitrypsin.
- While PiMZ has been associated with emphysema in some families, general population studies have not confirmed a causal association between emphysema and the PiMZ genotype.

Clinical Features

It is asymptomatic in the early stages of the disease because of pulmonary reserve.

■ FEV_1:FVC ratio is decreased, as is vital capacity and maximal ventilatory volume.
■ The total lung capacity and residual volume are often increased as a result of air trapping in the distended air spaces.
■ In the later symptomatic phase, COPD patients present with a spectrum of symptoms, the 2 extremes of which are designated types A and B (Fig 35–2).

A. Type A patients ("pink puffers"):

■ Present with chronic cough—either dry or productive of mucoid sputum—progressive dyspnea, and wheezing.

- Hyperventilate, and often sit hunched forward with mouth open and nostrils dilated.
- Their lungs are overinflated, with increased anteroposterior diameter of the chest ("barrel chest") and flattened diaphragm on chest X-ray.
- These patients successfully maintain oxygenation of the blood by hyperventilation.

B. Type B patients ("blue bloaters"):

- Have marked chronic bronchitis and cannot hyperventilate.
- Show decreased oxygenation of blood (cyanosis) and increased arterial carbon dioxide content.
- Have pulmonary hypertension, right ventricular hypertrophy and failure ("cor pulmonale").
- Peripheral edema is a dominant clinical feature.
- Type A patients frequently have dominant emphysematous changes, while type B patients usually have dominant chronic obstructive bronchitis.
- Changes in blood gases in patients with COPD are variable.
- Hypoxemia is a constant feature in advanced disease and is caused by decreased alveolar ventilation and imbalanced ventilation and perfusion.
- In type B patients with chronic hypercapnia (elevated Pco_2), the respiratory center becomes insensitive to the Pco_2 stimulus and is driven by the hypoxemia.
- Administration of oxygen in these patients can cause carbon dioxide retention and death ("carbon dioxide narcosis").

BRONCHIECTASIS

Bronchiectasis is defined as abnormal and irreversible dilatation of the bronchial tree proximal to the terminal bronchioles.

Etiology

- It is the result of chronic infection with resulting parenchymal destruction, fibrosis, and abnormal permanent dilatation of damaged bronchi.
- Long-standing bronchial obstruction, as occurs in bronchial tumors and stenosis, leads to bronchopneumonia and bronchiectasis in the lung distal to the obstruction.
- Mucoviscidosis (fibrocystic disease of the pancreas), where bronchial mucus is abnormally thick and plugs the smaller bronchi, causing obstruction, infection and bronchiectasis.
- Bronchopneumonia, particularly following childhood infections such as measles and whooping cough, is a common antecedent of bronchiectasis.
- **Kartagener's syndrome:**
  - Is due to a congenital defect in ciliary motion caused by absence of the dynein arms of cilia.
  - It is inherited as an autosomal recessive trait.
  - Failure of ciliary clearance of bronchial mucus predisposes to bronchopneumonia and bronchiectasis.
  - Other features of the syndrome are absent frontal sinuses, infertility, and dextrocardia.

Pathology

- It is usually patchy in distribution, with lower lobes more commonly involved.
- The dilated bronchi and bronchioles may be cylindric, fusiform, or saccular.

- The walls of the distended bronchi show inflammation and fibrosis.
- The mucosa may be ulcerated, and the lumen is commonly filled with pus.

Clinical Features

This is a chronic illness with cough, usually productive of a large volume of foul-smelling sputum, and episodic fever.

- Clubbing of fingers and hyperglobulinemia are common.
- Bacteria cultured from bronchiectatic cavities include *Staphylococcus aureus, Staphylococcus epidermidis;* streptococci of all types (pneumococci; *Haemophilus influenzae;* enteric gram-negative bacilli) and anaerobes.

CHRONIC DIFFUSE INTERSTITIAL LUNG DISEASE

Noninfectious disorders characterized by diffuse inflammation and fibrosis involving the interstitium of the alveolar septum. The end stage is associated with extensive parenchymal destruction, fibrosis, with the formation of abnormal cystic spaces (honeycomb lung).

General Clinical & Pathologic Features

- It presents with dyspnea, tachypnea, and cyanosis.
- The vital capacity is reduced but there is no airway obstruction.
- The FEV_1:FVC ratio is normal.
- Diffusion of oxygen is impaired, leading to hypoxemia, increased ventilation and low Pco_2 levels.
- Chest X-ray shows a reticulonodular pattern of interstitial involvement.

Etiology

Diffuse infiltrative lung disease has many causes (Table 35–4).

Immunologic Interstitial Pneumonitis & Fibrosis

IDIOPATHIC INTERSTITIAL PNEUMONITIS (Fibrosing Alveolitis, Hamman-Rich Syndrome)

This is a group of diseases characterized by diffuse interstitial fibrosis occurring without recognized cause.

- The presence of circulating immune complexes, immunoglobulin deposition in the interstitium, and the response of early disease to treatment with steroids strongly suggest an immunologic basis.
- Clinically, patients present with progressive dyspnea and cough, and ventilatory failure of the restrictive type.
- The rate of progression is quite variable; a rapidly progressive variant may cause death in 1–2 years.
- The following distinctive pathologic types are recognized.

A. Usual interstitial pneumonitis (UIP):

- Accounts for the majority of cases.
- In the acute phase, there is interstitial infiltration with lymphocytes, acute alveolar damage, and hyaline membranes.

TABLE 35-4. CAUSES OF CHRONIC DIFFUSE INTERSTITIAL LUNG DISEASE

Immunologic injury
"Idiopathic": Usual interstitial pneumonitis, desquamative interstitial pneumonitis, lymphocytic interstitial pneumonitis

Hypersensitivity pneumonitis

Connective tissue diseases (systemic lupus erythematosus, progressive systemic sclerosis, rheumatoid arthritis)

Goodpasture's syndrome and idiopathic pulmonary hemosiderosis

Physical and chemical agents
Inhaled mineral dusts (pneumoconioses): Silica, asbestos

Inhaled gases: Oxygen toxicity

Ingested toxins and drugs: Paraquat (a herbicide); cancer chemotherapeutic agents such as bleomycin, methotrexate, busulfan, and cyclophosphamide; nitrofurantoin (a urinary antiseptic)

Radiation

Intravenous drug (heroin) abuse

Uncertain etiology
Sarcoidosis

Eosinophilic granuloma

Wegener's granulomatosis

Lymphomatoid granulomatosis

Vascular
Chronic left heart failure: Passive venous congestion

Multiple small pulmonary emboli

Prior infections
Following recurrent pneumonitis

Following recurrent bronchopneumonia

- This is followed by proliferation of fibroblasts and the laying down of collagen in the alveolar interstitium.
- The rate of fibrosis is variable, but the occurrence of fibrosis represents irreversibility.
- The course is protracted, with respiratory failure occurring many years after onset.
- When interstitial fibrosis (honeycomb lung) is present, the clinical response to steroids is poor.

B. Desquamative interstitial pneumonitis (DIP):

■ Is similar to UIP, except for the aggregation of desquamated type II pneumocytes and macrophages in alveoli.
■ The course is similar to that of slowly progressive usual interstitial pneumonitis.

C. Lymphocytic interstitial pneumonitis (LIP):

■ Is also called pseudolymphoma.
■ Is characterized by extensive infiltration of the interstitium with lymphocytes and plasma cells.
■ It may be diffuse or may involve a single area of lung, producing a mass lesion ("pseudolymphoma").
■ It is associated with an increased incidence of primary pulmonary malignant lymphoma.
■ In some cases, the process appears to be a primary low-grade lymphoma.

HYPERSENSITIVITY PNEUMONITIS (Extrinsic Allergic Alveolitis)

Hypersensitivity pneumonitis results from inhalation by susceptible individuals of small organic particles (antigens), most commonly spores of thermophilic fungi.

■ These fungi grow best at 50–60°C in decaying vegetation such as hay and sugar cane, or in heated water in air-conditioning and heating systems.
■ A variety of occupations are at risk, and the disease frequently bears the name of these occupations:
  ● Farmer's lung (moldy hay).
  ● Bagassosis (moldy sugar cane).
  ● Mushroom worker's disease.
  ● Bird-fancier's lung.
  ● Maple bark-stripper's disease.
  ● Malt worker's lung.
■ In urban areas, the spores are most frequently found in contaminated forced air heating and air-conditioning systems.

Pathogenesis

It is caused by a combination of type III hypersensitivity and lymphocyte-mediated type IV hypersensitivity (Table 35–2).

■ It is associated with precipitating IgG antibodies, which are present in the serum of 70% of patients.
■ There is a local Arthus type immune complex reaction with complement deposition in the lung.

Pathology

This is an acute interstitial pneumonitis.

■ Poorly formed alveolar noncaseating epithelioid cell granulomas with giant cells are typically present.
■ Fibrous obliteration of bronchioles (bronchiolitis obliterans) is a characteristic change.

- If the disease is recognized early and the patient removed from the source of antigen, the disease is reversible.
- With continued exposure, diffuse interstitial fibrosis occurs, leading to end-stage honeycomb lung.

Clinical Features

- It presents with acute dyspnea, fever, and cough, 4–6 hours after exposure to the antigen.
- Initially, these symptoms subside spontaneously in 12–18 hours.
- As pulmonary fibrosis ensues, the disease goes into its chronic phase, with all the features of diffuse interstitial lung disease.

INTERSTITIAL PNEUMONITIS IN CONNECTIVE TISSUE DISEASES

Diffuse interstitial pneumonitis, with fibrosis leading to honeycomb lung indistinguishable from usual interstitial pneumonitis, occurs in progressive systemic sclerosis (scleroderma) and rheumatoid arthritis. Systemic lupus erythematosus may be complicated by immune complex vasculitis and acute alveolar damage.

GOODPASTURE'S SYNDROME

This is a rare disease characterized by a combination of hemoptysis and pulmonary infiltrates, glomerulonephritis, and the presence of circulating anti-basement membrane antibodies.

Pathology

- Circulating anti-basement membrane antibody fixes onto the basement membrane of pulmonary alveoli and renal glomeruli, causing a complement-mediated type II hypersensitivity reaction (Table 35–2).
- Immunofluorescence shows linear deposition of IgG and complement in the alveoli.
- Pulmonary hemorrhage is the dominant feature; hemosiderin-containing macrophages may be found in the sputum.
- In the acute phase, the lungs are consolidated, heavy, and hemorrhagic.
- In the chronic phase, the lung shows marked interstitial fibrosis, hemosiderin deposition and honeycomb lung.

Clinical Features

- There is a striking male predominance.
- Onset is most frequently in the second or third decade of life.
- Patients present with recurrent hemoptysis.
- Massive pulmonary hemorrhage occurs rarely.
- In the chronic phase, there is progressive dyspnea, cough, and right heart failure due to pulmonary fibrosis.
- Iron deficiency anemia may result from chronic blood loss.
- Chest X-ray shows pulmonary infiltrates due to intra-alveolar hemorrhage.
- Changes of increasing pulmonary fibrosis dominate chronic disease.
- Patients almost invariably have evidence of glomerulonephritis, and in many cases the renal disease dominates the clinical picture and determines the prognosis, which is poor.

TABLE 35–5. DIFFERENT TYPES OF PNEUMONOCONIOSES IN HUMANS

Disease	Inorganic Dust	Occupations
Anthracosis	Coal dust[1]	Coal mining, railroad work
Silicosis	Crystalline silica	Mining, sandblasting, stone masonry, foundry work; glass, tile, brick, and pottery manufacture
Silicate pneumoconiosis Asbestosis	Asbestos	Asbestos mining and milling, shipyard workers, welders, pipe fitters, boilermakers, insulators, brake lining manufacturers, "tearing-out" of old asbestos insulation
Talcosis	Talc	Often found with asbestos
Kaolin pneumoconiosis	Kaolin or porcelain clay	Ceramics manufacture
Fuller's earth pneumoconiosis	Fuller's earth	Oil refining, foundry work
Diatomaceous earth pneumoconiosis	Diatomaceous earth	Water filtration
Mica pneumoconiosis	Mica	Rare
Graphite pneumoconiosis	Graphite[1]	Graphite mining
Berylliosis	Beryllium	Fluorescent lights
Aluminum pneumoconiosis	Aluminum oxide	"Shaver's disease"
Tungsten carbide pneumoconiosis	?Cobalt	Battery manufacture
Stannosis	Tin[1]	Rare

[1] These dusts in pure form tend not to cause fibrosis (noncollagenous pneumoconioses) and have minimal clinical effects. Other dusts, especially silica and asbestos, may lead to severe fibrosis (collagenous pneumoconioses).

IDIOPATHIC PULMONARY HEMOSIDEROSIS

This is morphologically identical to Goodpasture's syndrome and considered by some to be a variant of Goodpasture's without renal involvement.

■ It differs from Goodpasture's syndrome in:
  ● A tendency to affect a younger age group.
  ● Absence of a male preponderance.
  ● Absence of anti-basement membrane antibodies in the plasma, though they are present on the alveolar membranes.

Pneumoconioses

Pneumoconioses denotes pulmonary disease secondary to inhalation of various inorganic dusts (Table 35–5).

- Some dusts, like coal dust, do not evoke a fibrous response (noncollagenous pneumoconioses), whereas others such as silica do (collagenous pneumoconioses).
- There is a variable latent period between exposure to dust and onset of clinical disease that may be as long as 20–30 years.

COAL WORKER'S PNEUMOCONIOSIS (Anthracosis)

Anthracosis results from exposure to coal (carbon) dust and is seen most extensively in coal miners and workers for old coal-burning railways.

- Lesser degrees of anthracosis occur in almost all urban dwellers.
- The basic pathologic lesion is the coal dust macule, which is a collection of carbon-laden macrophages around the respiratory bronchiole.
- It is associated with minimal fibrosis and mild dilatation of the respiratory bronchiole ("focal dust emphysema").
- There are usually no symptoms and no detectable abnormalities in lung function.
- Rarely, coal workers develop **progressive massive fibrosis** when heavy exposure is coupled with infection with *Mycobacterium tuberculosis,* or associated silicosis.
- Progressive massive fibrosis is characterized by multiple irregular firm, black fibrous masses in both lungs.
- When coal miners develop rheumatoid arthritis, they develop large rheumatoid nodules in the lung (Caplan's syndrome).

SILICOSIS

Silicosis is caused by inhalation of crystalline silicon dioxide (silica) dust particles in the 1- to 3-μm range.

- Silica exists in nature as quartz, chrystobalite, and tridymite.
- Occupations at increased risk for silicosis are hardrock, gold, tin, and copper mining; sand blasting; and iron, steel, and granite working.
- More than 1 million workers in the United States are at risk for developing silicosis.
- Significant pulmonary disease usually occurs with 10–15 years of exposure but may rarely occur after as little as 1 year.

Pathology

- It is characterized by a nodule composed of hyalinized collagen around the silica crystals, and may be found in the lungs and hilar lymph nodes.
- Grossly, the silicotic nodule is gray-black, hard, and brittle, and has concentric rings of hyalinized collagen in cross section.
- Microscopically, the nodules are composed of a solid mass of macrophages, fibroblasts, and collagen.
- Silica particles are recognized as birefringent needle-shaped crystals in the nodules when examined by polarized light.

Clinical Features

It is often asymptomatic, being found incidentally at chest X-ray or histologic examination of lungs and hilar lymph nodes removed for an unrelated reason.

- Rarely, when patients are exposed to massive amounts of dust, acute lung disease may occur, with accumulation of proteinaceous material in the alveoli (acute silicotic proteinosis).
- More often, there is chronic pulmonary fibrosis with a mild restrictive ventilatory defect, decreased compliance, slowly progressive dyspnea, and pulmonary hypertension (cor pulmonale).

Complications

- Progressive massive fibrosis, particularly when the level of exposure to dust is high. It is characterized by confluence of silicotic nodules into large fibrotic masses.
- Tuberculosis, which causes extensive necrosis in the nodules.
- Increased incidence of autoimmune disease, especially progressive systemic sclerosis.

ASBESTOSIS

Asbestos is a fibrous silicate found in nature as the minerals chrysotile, amosite, and crocidolite.

- It is present in insulation, flame retardants, flooring and roofing materials, water and sewage pipes, and vehicular brake linings.
- Low-grade exposure is almost universal among urban dwellers.
- It is estimated that up to 11 million workers in the United States have had significant asbestos exposure since 1940.
- Asbestosis is most common in those with the highest levels of exposure, ie, workers in shipyards and the construction industry.
- Approximately 40% of World War II shipyard pipe fitters now have evidence of asbestosis.
- About 10,000 deaths every year in the United States are due to asbestos-related diseases.

Pathology

- There is thickening of the parietal pleura by a plaquelike deposition of hyalinized collagen, maximal in the lateral and diaphragmatic pleura.
- Pulmonary changes are a diffuse interstitial fibrosis.
- Microscopically, asbestos fibers are visible as ferruginous bodies ("asbestos bodies") composed of a thin central asbestos fiber 5–10 μm long encased in an iron-containing glycoprotein coat which is brown in color.
- Ferruginous bodies are best seen in sections that have been stained for iron with Prussian blue. (While ferruginous bodies are most commonly seen in asbestosis, they are not specific for it.)

Clinical Features

It presents with the features of diffuse interstitial lung disease, ie, chronic cough, progressive dyspnea, a diffuse infiltrative pattern on chest X-ray, decreased vital capacity with no obstructive element, decreased compliance, and hypoxemia.

- The most significant effect of asbestos exposure is the greatly increased risk of malignant neoplasms:

- Bronchogenic carcinoma, which is the commonest neoplasm associated with asbestosis.
- Cigarette smoking has a profound additive effect to asbestos exposure in causing bronchogenic carcinoma.
- Malignant mesothelioma of the pleura, peritoneum, and pericardium. Although less common than bronchogenic carcinoma, it is the most specific neoplasm associated with asbestos exposure.

Iatrogenic Drug-, Chemical-, or Radiation-Induced Interstitial Fibrosis
A large number of drugs—notably the anticancer drugs bleomycin, busulfan, melphalan, methotrexate, and cyclophosphamide—cause a dose-related diffuse pulmonary fibrosis. Fibrosis is insidious, progressive, and may cause death.

- **Paraquat,** a commonly used herbicide, causes severe pulmonary edema, hemorrhage, and interstitial inflammation progressing rapidly to pulmonary fibrosis and death.
- **Radiation** therapy for cancer may result in acute pneumonitis (high doses) or chronic fibrosis (lower doses) if the lungs are included in the field of radiation.
- **Toxic gases** (mustard gas, 100% oxygen) produce diffuse fibrosis that may be severe.

Interstitial Diseases of Uncertain Etiology

SARCOIDOSIS
This is a systemic disorder of uncertain cause that is commonly manifested in the lungs.

- Abnormalities of the immune system are usually present, including:
  - Depressed cell mediated immunity, manifested by decreased numbers of T cells in the peripheral blood and anergy.
  - Hyperactive humoral immunity with an increased number of B lymphocytes in the peripheral blood, and hyperimmunoglobulinemia.

Pathology

- It is characterized by small, noncaseating epithelioid cell granulomas.
- Several types of nonspecific inclusions may be present, including Schaumann bodies (round, calcified, laminated bodies in the cytoplasm) and asteroid bodies.
- In the lung, granulomas are found in the alveolar septa and along the lymphatics, and are associated with interstitial inflammation and fibrosis.
- Chronic disease progresses to end-stage honeycomb lung.
- Granulomas may also be found in lymph nodes, liver, spleen, skin, and many other organs.
- The diagnosis of sarcoidosis is made on clinical grounds.
- Elevated serum level of angiotensin-converting enzyme is seen in 60% of patients, but is not specific.

Clinical Features (Fig 35–3)
In the United States, sarcoidosis occurs 10 times more frequently in blacks than in whites.

- Women are more commonly affected.

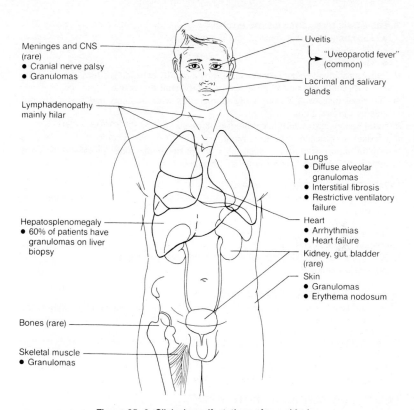

Figure 35–3. Clinical manifestations of sarcoidosis.

- The most common age at onset is between 20 and 35 years.
- An abnormality in the chest X-ray is present in over 90% of patients with sarcoidosis.
- Bilateral hilar lymphadenopathy and lung infiltrates are common.
- It has a variable course. About 65% of patients with hilar adenopathy alone undergo spontaneous remission.
- Pulmonary parenchymal involvement usually signifies progressive chronic disease.
- Steroids are effective in controlling the disease and are indicated when there is symptomatic lung involvement, ocular lesions, cardiac disease, or neurologic disease.

WEGENER'S GRANULOMATOSIS
This is a disease of unknown cause, though a hypersensitivity reaction to an unknown antigen has been postulated.

- It is characterized by necrotizing vasculitis of small arteries.
- The inflammation around the affected vessel is granulomatous.

- The classic form of the disease involves:
  - The nose, paranasal sinuses, and nasopharynx.
  - The lungs.
  - The kidneys.
- Pulmonary involvement is characterized by a rapidly expanding infiltrate, often bilateral with multiple nodular mass lesions which tend to cavitate.
- The renal disease is a necrotizing glomerulitis with crescents that frequently progresses to renal failure.
- Nasal lesions are usually ulcerating granulomas.
- Clinical progression to death is rapid.
- Immunosuppressive drugs such as cyclophosphamide have prolonged survival, though the ultimate prognosis is still very poor.

LYMPHOMATOID GRANULOMATOSIS
This is a systemic disorder affecting the lung, nervous system, kidney, skin, and many other organs.

- Histologically, there are necrotizing granulomas in the lung that are infiltrated by atypical lymphocytes.
- Patients are at high risk for pulmonary malignant lymphoma.
- Prognosis is poor.

BRONCHOCENTRIC GRANULOMATOSIS
This is a disease of uncertain cause characterized by granulomatous inflammation centered around the airways.

- The walls of the airways are destroyed, and their lumens are filled with necrotic material.
- Patients present with dyspnea, wheezing, and the consequences of bronchial obstruction, such as pneumonia, lung abscess, and bronchiectasis.

PULMONARY ALVEOLAR PROTEINOSIS
It is characterized by filling of the alveolar spaces with a homogeneous, proteinaceous, lipid-rich material thought to be composed of surfactant and cellular debris. The cause is unknown.

- Patients present with dyspnea and dry cough.
- Chest X-ray shows consolidation first affecting the lung bases.
- The infiltrates have a typical ground-glass appearance on chest X-ray.
- Hypoxemia is common and often severe.
- It is usually a benign disease, with most patients undergoing spontaneous remission.
- There is good clinical response to treatment with pulmonary lavage.

PULMONARY VASCULAR DISORDERS

ADULT RESPIRATORY DISTRESS SYNDROME (ARDS; "Shock Lung")
ARDS is an acute diffuse alveolar injury that occurs in:

- Severe hypovolemic shock, most commonly following trauma ("Viet Nam lung").
- Sepsis, particularly that associated with gram-negative organisms.

- Acute pancreatitis.
- Fat embolism.
- Following inhalation of toxic gases such as chlorine and sulfur dioxide.
- Disseminated intravascular coagulation.
- An estimated 150,000 patients in the United States develop ARDS annually.

Pathology
It is characterized by acute diffuse alveolar damage leading to necrosis and loss of type I pneumocytes.

- Exudation of protein-rich fluid into the alveoli results in pulmonary edema, hemorrhage, and formation of hyaline membranes.
- Grossly, the lungs are purple, heavy, and solid. Hemorrhagic fluid exudes from the cut surface.

Clinical Features

- Rapidly increasing dyspnea, hypoxemia, and cyanosis.
- Chest X-ray shows diffuse interstitial or alveolar edema, but may be normal in the early stages.
- ARDS is commonly the terminal event in many of these patients.

PULMONARY EMBOLISM (See also Chapter 9)
Pulmonary embolism causes over 50,000 deaths per year in the United States.

- Pulmonary emboli originate from deep leg vein thrombi in over 90% of cases.
- Thrombi in pelvic veins are second in frequency.
- Deep vein thrombosis and pulmonary embolism occur most commonly:
  - After surgery.
  - After childbirth.
  - In patients who are immobilized for any reason.
  - In patients with cardiovascular diseases.
- Effects of pulmonary embolism are:
  - Sudden death with a large embolus that obstructs the right ventricular outflow tract, causing circulatory arrest.
  - Pulmonary infarction, which occurs with a medium-sized embolus in a patient with left heart failure or pulmonary hypertension.
  - Pulmonary hypertension, which results from multiple small emboli over a long period.
- Pulmonary infarcts:
  - Are hemorrhagic (red).
  - Present with pleuritic chest pain, dyspnea, fever, and hemoptysis, and a hemorrhagic pleural effusion.

PULMONARY HYPERTENSION
Pulmonary hypertension is defined as elevation of the mean pulmonary arterial pressure.

- Most patients with pulmonary hypertension have a recognizable cause for the elevated pressure (secondary pulmonary hypertension) (Table 35–6).

TABLE 35–6. PULMONARY HYPERTENSION

Causes
Idiopathic (primary)
Secondary
  Mitral valve disease
  Left ventricular failure
  Congenital heart disease with left-to-right shunt
    Atrial septal defect
    Ventricular septal defect
    Patent duct arteriosus
  Chronic pulmonary disease (cor pulmonale)
    Emphysema
    Chronic bronchitis
    Diffuse interstitial fibrosis
  Multiple recurrent pulmonary emboli
Results
Hypertrophy of muscular pulmonary arteries
Fibrous thickening of pulmonary arteries
Pulmonary atherosclerosis
Progressive increase in pulmonary artery blood pressure
Right ventricular hypertrophy
Right heart failure

- In a small number of patients, there is no recognizable cause (primary pulmonary hypertension).
- Primary pulmonary hypertension occurs mainly in young women and is frequently associated with immunologically mediated collagen diseases such as rheumatoid arthritis.
- The pathologic features of both primary and secondary pulmonary hypertension are similar.
- Clinically, pulmonary hypertension causes right ventricular hypertrophy, a loud split pulmonary valve closure sound, and right ventricular failure.
- Primary pulmonary hypertension is irreversible and slowly progressive; few patients survive 10 years after diagnosis.

The Lung: III. Neoplasms   **36**

CARCINOMA OF THE LUNG (Bronchogenic Carcinoma)

Incidence
In the United States, lung cancer causes about 120,000 deaths annually; in England and Wales, it accounts for 40,000 deaths annually—about one-third of total cancer deaths and almost one-tenth of all deaths.

- The incidence has increased markedly since 1950 (approximately five-fold) and continues to increase.
- It is more common in males; the male:female ratio was 7:1 in 1960 but has fallen to about 2.5:1 in 1987.
- Lung cancer is the leading cause of death by cancer in both men and women.
- It affects older individuals, being rare under age 40.

Etiology
A. Cigarette smoking is the main cause of lung carcinoma.

- Heavy cigarette smokers (over 40 cigarettes a day) have a 20-fold increase in incidence compared to nonsmokers.
- Cessation of smoking decreases the risk; ten years after stopping, the risk falls to that of a nonsmoker.
- The risk is only slightly less with "low-tar" filter cigarettes; cigar and pipe smoking carry a lower risk.
- A number of potent carcinogens are present in cigarette smoke, including polycyclic hydrocarbons, aromatic amines, and heavy metals such as nickel.
- Cigarette smoking is most strongly associated with squamous carcinoma and small cell undifferentiated carcinoma and to a lesser degree with adenocarcinoma.

B. Industrial carcinogens:

- Exposure to asbestos increases the risk of lung carcinoma.
- The risk of lung cancer following asbestos exposure is compounded by cigarette smoking.
- Mining of uranium, nickel, chromate, gold is also associated with an increased risk of lung cancer.

C. Radiation: Exposure to natural radiation in Central European mines was shown to cause lung cancer.

D. Urban pollution: While there is great concern, most studies to date have failed to demonstrate a significant association between lung carcinoma and urban pollutants.

E. "Scar cancer": There is a slightly increased incidence of peripheral adenocarcinoma in areas of scarring.

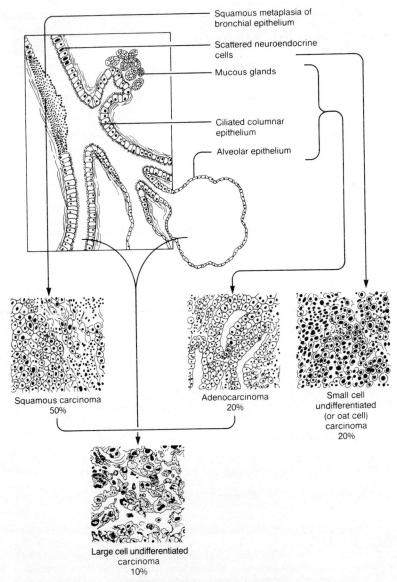

Figure 36–1. Histogenetic classification of bronchogenic lung carcinoma.

Classification (Fig 36-1)

The **International Classification of Lung Carcinoma (World Health Organization)** recognizes four major and several minor types.

A. Squamous (epidermoid) carcinoma:

- Arises in metaplastic squamous epithelium of the bronchi.
- Is characterized by marked cytologic pleomorphism, intercellular bridges between tumor cells, and keratinization of the cytoplasm.
- Is strongly associated with cigarette smoking.
- Accounts for 40–60% of all lung cancers.
- Tends to remain localized, resulting in large masses in the lung. Central cavitation is common.

B. Adenocarcinoma:

- Is characterized by formation of glands or secretion of mucin by the tumor cells. It includes:
  - Adenocarcinoma arising centrally in large bronchi.
  - Adenocarcinoma arising in peripheral scars.
  - Bronchiolo-alveolar carcinoma.
- The histologic appearance of adenocarcinoma may be mimicked by metastatic adenocarcinoma.
- It constitutes 10–25% of lung carcinomas.
- It has an equal sex incidence, and is less associated with cigarette smoking than squamous carcinoma.

C. Small-cell undifferentiated ("oat cell") carcinoma:

- Is composed of small round to oval cells with scant cytoplasm, a high nuclear:cytoplasmic ratio, and hyperchromatic nuclei that do not have prominent nucleoli.
- Arises from neuroendocrine cells in the bronchial mucosa.
- Stains positively with neuroendocrine immunologic markers such as chromogranin and neuron-specific enolase, and has neurosecretory granules in the cytoplasm on electron microscopy.
- Is highly malignant; bloodstream metastasis occurs early in the course of the neoplasm.
- Account for 10–25% of lung carcinomas and is strongly associated with smoking.
- Almost always occur in the hilum.

D. Large cell undifferentiated carcinoma is composed of large cells that show no squamous or glandular differentiation on light microscopy.

- Pleomorphic giant-cell carcinoma is a highly malignant variant with numerous multinucleated giant cells.
- It accounts for 5–20% of lung carcinomas.

Pathology

A. Central (bronchogenic) carcinoma (75%):

- Arise in the first-, second-, or third-order bronchi near the hilum of the lung.

- Tend to be hidden in chest X-rays during their early growth phase.
- Can be seen and biopsied at an early stage by bronchoscopy.
- All histologic types occur, but the majority are squamous or small-cell undifferentiated carcinomas.
- From its mucosal origin, the neoplasm grows into the bronchial lumen (causing ulceration, bleeding, or obstruction) and infiltrates the bronchial wall and adjacent lung parenchyma.

B. Peripheral lung carcinoma (25%):

- Arise in relation to small bronchi, bronchioles, or alveoli.
- Are visible on chest X-ray at an early stage as a circumscribed mass but cannot be seen by bronchoscopy.
- Tend to be adenocarcinomas. Small-cell undifferentiated carcinoma rarely occurs in the periphery.

Spread of Lung Carcinoma

Local invasion in central carcinomas may involve the superior vena cava and pericardium. Peripheral lung carcinomas tend to involve the pleura early.

- Lymphatic metastases to lymph nodes occurs early in all types of lung carcinoma.
- Involvement of the hilar lymph nodes is present in 50% of cases at presentation.
- Pleural lymphatic involvement causes multiple pleural nodules and pleural effusion.
- Bloodstream metastasis also occurs early, and patients with lung carcinoma frequently present with a distant metastasis.
- In small-cell undifferentiated carcinoma, distant metastases are almost invariably present at the time of diagnosis.
- Common sites of metastasis of lung carcinoma are the adrenals, liver, brain, bone, and kidneys.

Staging of Lung Carcinoma

- Stage I: confined to the lung and are either large (> 3 cm) without node involvement, or small (< 3 cm) with local nodal involvement only.
- Stage II: lesions are large (> 3 cm) and confined to the lung, with only local nodal involvement.
- Stage III: includes all other lesions.

Clinical Features (Fig 36–2)

Earliest symptoms are cough, hemoptysis, dyspnea, chest pain, and weight loss. Unfortunately, these occur at a relatively advanced stage.

- A minority of cases of lung carcinoma are detected at an asymptomatic stage by routine chest X-ray.
- A few patients with central lesions present with features of bronchial obstruction (unresolving pneumonia, lung abscess, and bronchiectasis).
- They may have symptoms due to local invasion such as pleural and pericardial effusion, superior vena caval obstruction, and tracheoesophageal fistula.
- Pancoast's syndrome results from an apical lung carcinoma (usually squamous) that involves the T1 intercostal nerve and the cervical sympathetic trunk.

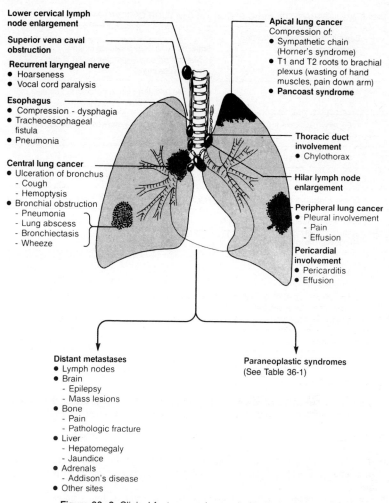

Lower cervical lymph node enlargement

Superior vena caval obstruction

Recurrent laryngeal nerve
- Hoarseness
- Vocal cord paralysis

Esophagus
- Compression - dysphagia
- Tracheoesophageal fistula
- Pneumonia

Central lung cancer
- Ulceration of bronchus
  - Cough
  - Hemoptysis
- Bronchial obstruction
  - Pneumonia
  - Lung abscess
  - Bronchiectasis
  - Wheeze

Apical lung cancer
Compression of:
- Sympathetic chain (Horner's syndrome)
- T1 and T2 roots to brachial plexus (wasting of hand muscles, pain down arm)
- **Pancoast syndrome**

Thoracic duct involvement
- Chylothorax

Hilar lymph node enlargement

Peripheral lung cancer
- Pleural involvement
  - Pain
  - Effusion

Pericardial involvement
- Pericarditis
- Effusion

Distant metastases
- Lymph nodes
- Brain
  - Epilepsy
  - Mass lesions
- Bone
  - Pain
  - Pathologic fracture
- Liver
  - Hepatomegaly
  - Jaundice
- Adrenals
  - Addison's disease
- Other sites

Paraneoplastic syndromes
(See Table 36-1)

Figure 36–2. Clinical features and spread of lung carcinoma.

- A significant number of patients with lung carcinoma present with evidence of lymph node or hematogenous metastases.
- A minority of patients present with symptoms that cannot be attributed to the direct effects of destruction by primary or metastatic tumors (paraneoplastic syndromes; Table 36–1).

TABLE 36–1. PARANEOPLASTIC SYNDROMES IN LUNG CARCINOMA

Ectopic hormone syndromes	
Adrenocorticotropic hormone	Small-cell undifferentiated carcinoma; causes bilateral adrenal hyperplasia and Cushing's syndrome
Antidiuretic hormone	Small-cell undifferentiated carcinoma; causes hyponatremia
Parathyroid hormone (PTH)	Squamous carcinoma; causes hypercalcemia
5-Hydroxytryptamine	Carcinoid syndrome
Gonadotropins	Gynecomastia
Finger clubbing and pulmonary hypertrophic osteoarthropathy	
Dermatomyositis and polymyositis	
Migratory thrombophlebitis	
Neuromuscular syndromes Peripheral neuropathy Myopathy Myasthenic syndrome (Eaton-Lambert syndrome) Cerebellar degeneration Leukoencephalopathy	
Skin rashes	

Diagnosis

Chest X-ray and computerized tomography are effective for demonstrating the presence of a mass in the lung. (They have a significant failure rate in small hilar lesions.)

- Cytologic examination of sputum or pleural effusions for malignant cells is a good technique.
- Bronchoscopy permits visualization, biopsy, recovery of brush cytology specimens from endobronchial lesions, and transbronchial needle biopsies from parenchymal masses.
- Percutaneous needle aspiration biopsy may be done under radiologic guidance when a mass lesion is visible on chest X-ray or CT scan.
- Open lung biopsy may, rarely, be necessary.
- With all these techniques, both cytologic and histologic examinations provide the diagnosis and the classification of lung carcinoma.

Treatment & Prognosis

The overall 5-year survival rate of patients with lung cancer is a dismal 10–20%.

- Recent chemotherapeutic regimens combined with aggressive surgery have shown an improving trend.

- Small-cell undifferentiated carcinoma is treated primarily by chemotherapy, which has improved median survival from less than 6 months to about 2 years. Few patients survive 5 years.
- Non-small–cell carcinoma is treated primarily by surgical resection, which is possible only in about 30% of cases.
- Five-year survival rates are as follows: Patients with surgically resected stage I tumors, 50%; patients with surgically resected stage II tumors, 20–30%; patients with stage III tumors, 5–10%.
- Overall 5-year survival rates of squamous carcinoma, adenocarcinoma, and large-cell undifferentiated carcinoma are 20–30%.
- Solitary well-differentiated bronchiolo-alveolar carcinoma has a 60% survival rate at 5 years.

OTHER "TUMORS" OF THE LUNG

Many other benign or malignant neoplasms, as well as inflammatory lesions, may present as a mass in the lung.

- The term *bronchial adenoma* was used in the past to include bronchial carcinoid tumor, mucoepidermoid tumor, and adenoid cystic carcinoma. These are low-grade malignant neoplasms.
- Other neoplasms of the lung include sclerosing hemangioma (benign), chondroid hamartoma (benign), pulmonary blastoma and carcinosarcoma (malignant).
- Inflammatory lesions such as infectious granulomas, plasma cell granuloma, and inflammatory pseudotumor may present with mass lesions in the lung.

METASTATIC NEOPLASMS TO THE LUNG

Metastatic neoplasms occur commonly in the lung from a variety of primary sites. It is often difficult to distinguish metastatic from primary lung neoplasms on the basis of histologic examination alone. Carcinomas, sarcomas, melanomas, and almost any other malignant neoplasm may give rise to lung metastases.

DISEASES OF THE PLEURA

PLEURAL EFFUSION

Pleural effusion is a collection of fluid in the pleural cavity. The presence of a pleural effusion can be detected clinically and by chest X-ray.

- Aspiration of pleural fluid is helpful in identifying the cause of an effusion.
- A transudate can be differentiated from exudates by the low specific gravity and protein content and absence of inflammatory cells.
- Bacterial infection commonly produces a frankly purulent exudate (empyema).
- Hemorrhagic exudates occur in malignant effusions, tuberculosis, uremia, and pulmonary infarction.
- Cytologic examination of effusion sediment for malignant cells is frequently positive when malignant neoplasia is the cause of the effusion.
- Pleural biopsy is useful in the diagnosis of tuberculosis or cancer.

CHYLOTHORAX

Chylothorax is a specific kind of pleural effusion characterized by accumulation of chyle in the pleural cavity.

- Chylothorax may be differentiated from other turbid pleural effusions by the presence of chylomicrons and a high triglyceride content.
- Chylothorax may result from injuries to the thoracic duct by trauma and surgery or by infiltration of the thoracic duct by malignant neoplasms.

PNEUMOTHORAX

Pneumothorax is the presence of air in the pleural cavity. It may be caused by:

- Trauma, due to a chest wall defect or lung laceration.
- Spontaneous rupture into the pleural cavity of a bulla on the lung surface.
- Spontaneous pneumothorax may complicate many lung diseases such as bronchial asthma, emphysema, and tuberculosis.
- It presents with acute onset of chest pain and dyspnea.
- Physical examination reveals an absence of chest expansion, mediastinal shift, decreased breath sounds, and a tympanic sound on percussion. The diagnosis may be confirmed by chest X-ray.
- In most cases, the air is slowly reabsorbed with reexpansion of the lung.
- Rarely, a valvelike effect develops, producing a tension pneumothorax and increasing respiratory difficulty. Insertion of a chest tube is essential.

NEOPLASMS OF THE PLEURA

BENIGN FIBROUS MESOTHELIOMA

This is a rare benign neoplasm of the pleura, usually discovered incidentally on routine chest X-ray.

- It appears grossly as a localized growth of firm, dense fibrous tissue on the visceral pleura, often attached to the lung surface by a pedicle.
- Most are small; rarely, they may become large.
- Microscopically, it is composed of fibroblastlike spindle cells and collagen.
- It does not invade, and the prognosis after surgical excision is excellent.

MALIGNANT MESOTHELIOMA

This is a rare neoplasm strongly related etiologically to asbestos exposure. Many cases have occurred in World War II shipyard workers.

- There is a long lag period (as long as 40 years) between asbestos exposure and tumor development.
- Commonly it occurs over age 50.
- Clinical presentation is with dyspnea and pleural effusion.
- Grossly, the tumor diffusely involves the pleura, encasing large areas of lung as a firm, grayish, gelatinous mass.
- Invasion of both lung parenchyma and chest wall occurs frequently.
- Microscopically, the tumor is biphasic, with a sarcomatoid spindle cell component and epithelial elements that form tubular and papillary structures.
- The prognosis is very poor, with 50% of patients dead within 1 year and a few 2-year survivals.

SECONDARY PLEURAL NEOPLASMS

Secondary involvement of the pleura by malignant neoplasms is much more common than mesothelioma.

- Direct involvement of the pleura by lung carcinoma is the commonest.
- Metastases from distant sites such as the breast, colon, kidney, and thyroid also occur.
- Involvement of the pleura by malignant lymphoma is uncommon.
- It causes dyspnea and effusion. On X-rays, nodular pleural masses may be identified.
- The diagnosis may be established by identifying malignant cells in aspirated pleural fluid.
- The differentiation of secondary pleural neoplasms from malignant mesothelioma may be difficult.

Section IX. The Gastrointestinal System

The Esophagus

37

CLINICAL EFFECTS OF ESOPHAGEAL DISEASE

- **Dysphagia** refers to any difficulty in swallowing.
- **Odynophagia** refers to pain during deglutition.
- **Retrosternal pain** ("heartburn") unassociated with deglutition occurs when acidic gastric juice refluxes into the esophagus.
- **Hematemesis** is due to acute hemorrhage into the lumen of the esophagus or stomach. Peptic ulcer disease and rupture of esophageal varices are the most common causes (Table 37–1).
- Slower, more sustained bleeding produces melena (tarry black stools containing blood altered by the action of gastric acid).

METHODS OF EVALUATING THE ESOPHAGUS

The esophagus is inaccessible for physical examination, because most of its course is in the posterior mediastinum.

- **Barium swallow** permits visualization of peristalsis, the presence of any obstructive lesions, and mucosal abnormalities.
- **Computerized tomography** permits evaluation of lesions in the wall of the esophagus and is a good technique for evaluating spread of esophageal neoplasms.
- **Esophagoscopy** permits direct visualization and biopsy of mucosal lesions.
- **Manometry, motility studies, and pH measurement** are useful in the evaluation of esophageal peristalsis and competence of the lower esophageal sphincter.

CONGENITAL ESOPHAGEAL ANOMALIES

TRACHEOESOPHAGEAL FISTULA

Tracheoesophageal fistula is the commonest congenital anomaly of the esophagus.

- Several clinical types exist (Fig 37–1,B–D), some associated with varying degrees of esophageal atresia.
- The most dangerous fistulas are those in which swallowed material enters the trachea, causing cyanosis and aspiration pneumonia.

OTHER ANOMALIES

Other congenital anomalies are rare.

TABLE 37–1. CAUSES OF HEMATEMESIS[1,2]

Esophageal causes
 *Esophageal varices in portal hypertension
 *Carcinoma of the esophagus
 *Mallory-Weiss syndrome
 Peptic ulcer and reflux esophagitis
 Esophageal perforation
  Traumatic, postendoscopic
 Other neoplasms of the esophagus
  Leiomyosarcoma, malignant lymphoma

Gastric causes
 *Chronic gastric ulcer
 Postgastrectomy marginal ulcer
 *Acute gastric ulcer and acute gastritis
  Stress ulcers (burns, postsurgical)
  Drug-induced gastritis
   Aspirin (salicylates), indomethacin, phenylbuta-
    zone, ibuprofen, corticosteroids
  Alcoholic gastritis
 Benign polyps of the stomach
  Inflammatory, adenomatous, hyperplastic
 *Gastric malignant neoplasms
  Carcinoma, lymphoma, leiomyosarcoma
 Pancreatic pseudocyst perforating into the stomach

Duodenal causes
 *Chronic duodenal ulcer
 *Acute duodenal ulcer
  Stress ulcers
 Duodenal neoplasms
  Periampullary carcinoma
  Benign neoplasms
   Brunner's gland adenoma, adenomas (Gardner's
    syndrome), paraganglioma

Generalized diseases
 *Hereditary hemorrhagic telangiectasia
 Scurvy
 Congenital diseases of collagen synthesis
  Pseudoxanthoma elasticum, Ehlers-Danlos syndrome,
   blue rubber bleb nevus syndrome
 Henoch-Schönlein purpura
 Polyarteritis nodosa
 Amyloidosis
 Kaposi's sarcoma (in AIDS)

[1]More common causes are marked with asterisk.
[2]Hematemesis usually occurs when there is rapid bleeding into the gastrointestinal tract above the duodenojejunal junction. Exceptions to this rule are uncommon.

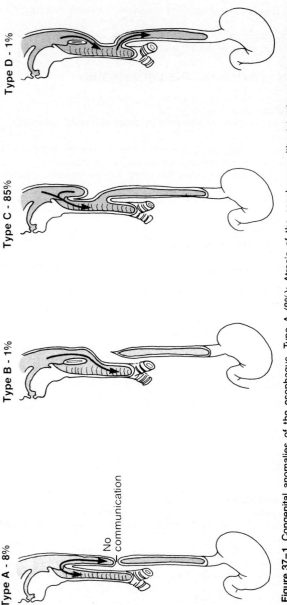

Figure 37–1. Congenital anomalies of the esophagus. Type A (8%): Atresia of the esophagus without tracheoesophageal fistula. Collection of food and fluid in the upper esophagus may result in aspiration into the larynx. Type B (1%): Atresia of the esophagus with fistula between the blind upper segment and the trachea. Type C (85%): Atresia of the esophagus with fistula between the trachea and distal segment. Type D (1%): Esophageal atresia with fistulous communication between both segments and the trachea. In type E (5%, not shown), there is a fistula between a normal esophagus and the trachea. Those children in whom the defect causes milk to enter the trachea, either directly (**B**, **D**, and **E**) or by reflux (**A** and **C**), present with coughing and cyanosis during feeding; aspiration broncho-pneumonia may follow. Those anomalies in which the trachea communicates with the lower esophagus (**C**, **D**, and **E**) are associated with gastric dilatation due to "swallowed" air.

Type A - 8%

No communication

Type B - 1%

Type C - 85%

Type D - 1%

- Esophageal atresia (Fig 37–1A) is a marked congenital narrowing of a part of the esophagus.
- Congenital short esophagus and congenital ectopic gastric mucosa in the esophagus are uncommon, but important in the differential diagnosis of Barrett's esophagus.

INFLAMMATORY LESIONS OF THE ESOPHAGUS

REFLUX ESOPHAGITIS

Reflux of acid gastric juice into the lower esophagus occurs in normal individuals.

- Symptomatic esophagitis is believed to occur when there is excessive reflux or when the normal mechanisms for clearing the lower esophagus are impaired.
- The refluxed fluid is usually acid; when bile reflux into the stomach is present, alkaline reflux may occur.
- Reflux occurs in sliding-type hiatal hernias because obliteration of the cardioesophageal angle renders the lower esophageal sphincter incompetent.

Pathology

- Reflux is recognized endoscopically as reddening and superficial erosion of the lower esophagus.
- Histologically, there is hyperplasia of the basal cells, elongation of submucosal papillae, and the presence of neutrophils in the epithelium.

Clinical Features

- Reflux causes low retrosternal burning pain (heartburn), typically when the patient lies flat.
- In chronic cases, pain may be constant, and dysphagia may occur as a result of fibrous stricture.

Complications
A. Barrett's esophagus:

- Is defined as metaplasia of the epithelium of the esophagus from squamous to glandular type.
- Three types of glandular epithelium occur:
  - Cardiac type, resembling gastric cardiac mucosa.
  - Fundic type, resembling gastric fundus with acid-secreting cells.
  - Intestinal type, with villi and goblet cells (also called specialized Barrett's epithelium; Fig 37–2).
- It is caused by prolonged reflux.
- It is a precancerous lesion. Epithelial dysplasia precedes invasive cancer.
- Most primary adenocarcinomas of the lower end of the esophagus arise in Barrett's esophagus.

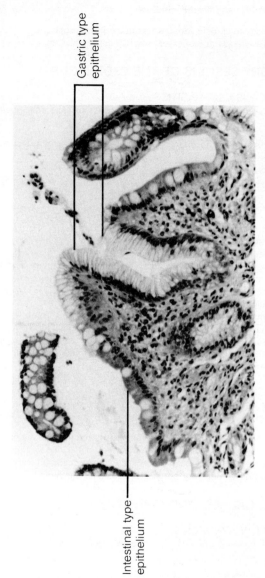

Gastric type epithelium

Intestinal type epithelium

Figure 37–2. Barrett's esophagus, showing the characteristic specialized columnar epithelium composed of a mixture of gastric and intestinal type epithelial cells.

B. Peptic ulceration and fibrous strictures:

■ Severe reflux leads to chronic peptic ulcers in the lower esophagus.
■ Subsequent fibrosis leads to esophageal stricture and dysphagia.

INFLAMMATORY LESIONS OF THE ESOPHAGUS

CANDIDA ALBICANS ESOPHAGITIS
This is a common opportunistic infection in patients receiving cancer chemotherapy and those with AIDS.

■ The yeast infects the superficial layers of the squamous epithelium, forming grossly visible adherent white plaques.
■ The main symptom is odynophagia.
■ Diagnosis is by identifying the fungus in smears, cultures, or biopsy specimens.

VIRAL ESOPHAGITIS

■ Herpes simplex esophagitis:
  ● Is common in AIDS.
  ● Infects squamous epithelial cells.
  ● Can be recognized in biopsies by the presence of Cowdry type A intranuclear inclusions and herpetic giant cells and by the immunologic demonstration of herpes simplex antigen.
■ Cytomegalovirus:
  ● Is also a common cause of esophagitis in AIDS.
  ● Infects submucosal endothelial cells, causing focal ischemia, hemorrhage, inflammation, and ulceration.
  ● Enlarged cells with large intranuclear inclusions and granular cytoplasmic inclusions are present.

TRAUMATIC & CHEMICAL ESOPHAGITIS
Prolonged feeding through a nasogastric tube frequently causes mucosal inflammation, often with ulceration.

■ Ingestion of corrosives such as phenol, strong acids, and mercuric chloride leads to chemical esophagitis followed by fibrous strictures.
■ Strictures caused by lye ingestion are associated with a greatly increased risk (1000 times normal) of development of esophageal squamous carcinoma.

FUNCTIONAL CAUSES OF DYSPHAGIA

PLUMMER-VINSON SYNDROME
Plummer-Vinson syndrome consists of severe iron deficiency anemia, koilonychia, atrophic glossitis, and dysphagia.

■ It has a marked female preponderance owing to the frequency of negative iron balance in women as a result of menstrual blood loss.

- Dysphagia results from:
  - Atrophy of the pharyngeal mucosa, causing failure of the deglutition reflex.
  - Weblike mucosal folds in the upper esophagus.
- There is a greater than normal risk of developing squamous carcinoma of the upper esophagus, oropharynx, and posterior tongue.

PROGRESSIVE SYSTEMIC SCLEROSIS

The esophagus is commonly involved in systemic sclerosis, and dysphagia is a common symptom. Vasculitis with muscle wall degeneration and fibrosis leads to failure of peristalsis.

ACHALASIA OF THE CARDIA

This is a common disease resulting from loss of ganglion cells in the myenteric plexus of the esophagus. Ganglion cell loss is present throughout the body of the esophagus.

- The cause is unknown in most cases; a few cases are caused by *Trypanosoma cruzi* (Chagas' disease).
- Failure of propulsive peristalsis leads to failure of relaxation of the lower esophageal sphincter, and obstruction.
- The esophagus dilates massively above the cardia.
- Patients present with dysphagia.
- An important complication is aspiration pneumonia.
- Treatment is by intraluminal dilatation or surgical myotomy.
- It imposes a slight increased risk of carcinoma.

ESOPHAGEAL VARICES

Gastroesophageal varices are found in the lower esophagus and fundus of the stomach in portal hypertension. The dilated veins are submucosal, and their rupture causes severe hemorrhage (hematemesis and melena).

MALLORY-WEISS SYNDROME

This is common in alcoholics and pregnant women who have severe vomiting associated with violent retching. It is characterized by a longitudinal tear in the mucosa of the lowest part of the esophagus. Severe hemorrhage with hematemesis occurs.

NEOPLASMS OF THE ESOPHAGUS

CARCINOMA OF THE ESOPHAGUS

Incidence

- Accounts for over 95% of neoplasms of the esophagus and about 1% of cancers involving the gastrointestinal tract.
- Causes about 2% of all cancer deaths in the United States (about 9000 per year).
- Occurs mainly in people over age 50.
- Is more common in males and blacks.
- Exhibits very high incidence in the Far East (notably China) and in certain parts of Africa and Iran.

Etiology

- Chronic alcoholism increases the risk 20- to 30-fold.
- Cigarette smoking increases the risk 10- to 20-fold.
- The cause of esophageal cancer in the high-incidence areas of the world is unknown.
- Hot rice and tea, nitrosamines and aflatoxins in food, contaminants in locally brewed beer, and smoked fish have been suggested as causative factors.
- Premalignant conditions associated with an increased risk of esophageal carcinoma include lye strictures (squamous carcinoma), Plummer-Vinson syndrome (squamous carcinoma), and Barrett's esophagus (adenocarcinoma).

Pathology

In the United States, 50% of esophageal cancers arise in the middle third, 30% in the lower third, and 20% in the upper third of the organ.

- The early lesion is a plaquelike thickening of the mucosa.
- Late lesions may be a polypoid, fungating mass, a malignant ulcer, or a malignant stricture.
- Ninety percent of esophageal carcinomas are squamous carcinomas.
- Most adenocarcinomas arise in Barrett's esophagus, and occur in the lower third of the esophagus.

Spread

- Local invasion through the esophageal wall to involve adjacent cervical and mediastinal structures occurs early.
- Invasion of the bronchial wall may rarely result in tracheoesophageal fistula.
- Invasion of the aorta may lead to massive hemorrhage.
- Recurrent laryngeal nerve involvement leads to vocal cord paralysis (hoarseness).
- Lymphatic spread occurs early, and lymph node metastases are usually present at the time of diagnosis.
- Bloodstream spread with metastases to liver and lung also occurs early.

Clinical Features & Diagnosis

- Most patients present with dysphagia and severe weight loss, and most have large unresectable tumors.
- Less often, presentation is with anemia, hematemesis, or melena.
- The diagnosis is best established by endoscopic visualization of the tumor followed by biopsy.

Treatment & Prognosis

- Surgery followed by radiation is the primary treatment.
- Chemotherapy has not been very effective until recently.
- The overall prognosis is very poor, 70% of patients being dead within 1 year after diagnosis and fewer than 10% surviving 5 years.

OTHER NEOPLASMS OF THE ESOPHAGUS

Neoplasms other than carcinomas are rare in the esophagus. Leiomyoma is the commonest benign neoplasm, but it rarely causes symptoms. Leiomyosarcoma, malignant lymphoma, malignant melanoma, and carcinoid tumors have been reported.

The Stomach

38

CLINICAL MANIFESTATIONS OF GASTRIC DISEASE

Pain is a feature in acute gastritis and peptic ulcer disease. It is epigastric, burning in nature, and is related to intake of food.

- **Dyspepsia** may include pain, but is also manifested by nausea, bloating, distention, and eructation.
- **Anorexia** (loss of appetite) occurs in gastritis and gastric carcinoma.
- **Early satiety** occurs in conditions where gastric volume is decreased (commonly neoplasms).
- **Bleeding** occurs in any disease where the mucosal surface becomes eroded.
  - When bleeding is severe hematemesis and melena occur.
  - With chronic slow bleeding, iron deficiency anemia results.
- **Gastric outlet obstruction** (pyloric stenosis):
  - May be congenital, or associated with peptic ulcer disease and neoplasms.
  - Leads to dilatation of the stomach and active peristalsis, which may be visible.
  - Causes vomiting, often profuse and sometimes projectile.
  - Results in hypokalemic alkalosis.

METHODS OF EVALUATING THE STOMACH

Barium meal and gastric endoscopy permits study of the mucosal structure. Endoscopy also permits photography and biopsy of suspicious areas. Abdominal ultrasound and computerized tomography are useful in the detection of mass lesions.

- **Gastric outlet obstruction** (pyloric stenosis):
  - May be congenital, or associated with peptic ulcer disease and neoplasms. stimulation.
  - Schilling's test for absorption of vitamin B_{12}, which assesses intrinsic factor.
  - Serum gastrin assay.
  - Serum assay for antibodies against parietal cell components and intrinsic factor.

CONGENITAL PYLORIC STENOSIS

Pyloric stenosis is one of the most common congenital disorders of the gastrointestinal tract, occurring in 1:500 live births.

- It is four times more common in males than in females and tends to affect the firstborn.
- There is a familial tendency, but no clear inheritance pattern has been demonstrated.
- Marked hypertrophy of the muscle at the pyloric sphincter results in obstruction to gastric emptying.
- Symptoms of gastric outlet obstruction typically appear 1–2 weeks after birth, and include projectile vomiting, visible enlargement of the stomach, and visible peristalsis.

- In most cases the hypertrophied pylorus can be palpated as a firm, ovoid mass.
- Treatment consists of surgical myotomy of the pylorus.

INFLAMMATORY LESIONS OF THE STOMACH

ACUTE GASTRITIS

This is a common pathologic finding in autopsies and in gastric biopsies.

- It is characterized by hyperemia, edema, and neutrophilic infiltration of the lamina propria.
- Affected areas show diffuse reddening of the mucosa with multiple small erosions and ulcers.
- In severe cases there are multiple ulcers, and acute hemorrhage may occur.

Etiology & Pathogenesis

The etiology is often obscure. It may result from:

- Direct infection with viruses, *Salmonella* and *Helicobacter pylori* cause acute gastritis.
- Direct toxicity by ethyl alcohol and bile reflux, which are responsible for a few cases.
- Decreased mucosal resistance to acid, which is believed responsible for most other cases of gastritis, and may be caused by:
  - Inhibition of prostaglandin secretion by aspirin, other anti-inflammatory agents, and smoking.
  - Interference with mucosal epithelial regeneration by antimitotic drugs.
  - Ischemia of the mucosa, which is believed to play a role in the gastritis associated with shock.

Clinical Features

Mild acute gastritis causes no symptoms. Epigastric pain, nausea, vomiting, and anorexia occur in moderate and severe gastritis.

- The correlation between symptoms, endoscopic changes, and histologic changes is poor.
- Acute gastric hemorrhage causing hematemesis and melena occurs mainly with drug-induced (usually aspirin) and stress-induced gastritis.

CHRONIC GASTRITIS

Chronic gastritis is defined as an increase in the number of lymphocytes and plasma cells in the gastric mucosa. The correlation between these changes and endoscopic and clinical features is poor.

Etiology & Classification

A. Chronic atrophic gastritis of pernicious anemia is an autoimmune disease.

- Three different autoantibodies may be present in the serum:
  - Anti-parietal cell antibody (also called parietal canalicular antibody), present in 90%.
  - Intrinsic factor–blocking antibody in 75%.
  - Intrinsic factor–binding antibody in 50%.

- The antibodies against intrinsic factor are also found in gastric juice.
- The immune reaction manifests as a lymphoplasmacytic infiltrate around parietal cells, which progressively decrease in number.
- Mucosal atrophy results and the glands become lined by mucous cells.
- Results in failure of secretion of acid (achlorhydria) and intrinsic factor, the latter causing failure of absorption of vitamin B_{12}.
- Failure of vitamin B_{12} absorption causes megaloblastic anemia (See Chapter 24).
- Patients with pernicious anemia have an increased incidence of developing gastric carcinoma.
- The epithelial cells pass through increasing degrees of dysplasia before cancer develops. Recognition of these changes in biopsies is an indication for gastrectomy.

B. Chronic antral gastritis is characterized by infiltration of the pyloric antrum by lymphocytes and plasma cells, commonly associated with intestinal metaplasia.

- The fundus and body mucosa is normal, and there is no parietal cell loss or decreased secretion of intrinsic factor.
- Acid secretion may be reduced, owing to loss of antral gastrin-producing G cells.
- Multiple etiologic factors are involved:
  - Bile acids and lysolecithin are likely injurious agents in cases with bile reflux.
  - *Helicobacter pylori* is commonly present in biopsies and cultures in antral gastritis and is believed to be causally related.

Clinical Features
Most patients with chronic gastritis are asymptomatic.

- Mild epigastric discomfort and pain, nausea, and anorexia may occur, particularly when acute gastritis is superimposed.
- The diagnosis is made by biopsy.

MENETRIER'S DISEASE (Hypertrophic Gastritis; Rugal Hypertrophy)
This is a rare condition of unknown cause that occurs mainly in males over age 40.

- It is characterized by greatly thickened gastric rugal folds that are visible both radiologically and by endoscopy.
- There is hyperplasia and cystic dilatation of mucous glands, and proliferation of the smooth muscle of the muscularis mucosae.
- Most patients have reduced or normal acid secretion.
- Overproduction of gastric mucus leads to increased protein loss (protein-losing enteropathy).
- Note that enlarged gastric mucosal folds may also occur in malignant lymphoma, gastric carcinoma, Zollinger-Ellison syndrome, and eosinophilic gastroenteritis.

EOSINOPHILIC GASTROENTERITIS
This is a rare disease believed to be due to immunologic hypersensitivity.

- The gastric and intestinal mucosa is infiltrated by chronic inflammatory cells and numerous eosinophils.
- The deeper parts of the intestinal wall may be affected, causing thickening of the intestine and intestinal obstruction.

PEPTIC ULCER DISEASE

Peptic ulcer disease is defined as ulcers occurring in any part of the gastrointestinal tract exposed to the action of acid gastric juice.

- Seventy-five percent occur in the first part of the duodenum (duodenal ulcer) and 25% in the stomach (gastric ulcer).
- Other rare sites include:
  - Lower esophagus.
  - The stoma of a gastroenterostomy.
  - Meckel's diverticulum.
  - Distal duodenum and jejunum in Zollinger-Ellison syndrome.
- Peptic ulcer disease is common all over the world.
- In the United States, 5–10% of individuals suffer from peptic ulcers during their lifetime. Duodenal ulcer is 2–3 times more frequent in males, particularly those under age 50.
- Peptic ulcers occur at all ages; most commonly onset is between ages 20 and 40.
- A familial tendency exists for duodenal ulcers but not gastric ulcers.
- Duodenal ulcers are associated with blood group O, absence of blood group antigens in saliva ("nonsecretors"), and HLA-B5 histocompatibility antigen.

Pathogenesis
A. Hypersecretion of acid:

- Acid is necessary for peptic ulcers to form, and ulcers do not occur in achlorhydric states.
- The exact role played by the acid is uncertain.
- Patients with duodenal ulcers have increased acid secretion with heightened responses to normal stimuli, but patients with gastric ulcers frequently have normal or low acid production.
- Severe, intractable peptic ulcers affecting the stomach, duodenum, and jejunum occur in Zollinger-Ellison syndrome.
  - It is caused by a gastrin-producing neoplasm of the pancreas.
  - The high gastrin levels stimulate continuous maximal acid secretion by parietal cells.
  - High acid output is the primary cause of peptic ulceration.

B. Decreased mucosal resistance to acid is believed to be the primary cause of most gastric ulcers.

- Prostaglandin E_2:
  - In gastric juice are consistently decreased in patients with peptic ulcer.
  - Rise during the healing phase and remain low in patients whose ulcers do not heal.
  - Inhibitors such as aspirin, ibuprofen, and indomethacin—and cigarette smoking—have an adverse effect on peptic ulcer healing.
  - Analogues like misoprostol accelerate healing in experimental studies.

C. Abnormal gastric motility with an increased rate of gastric emptying is common in patients with duodenal ulcer.
D. Pepsinogen:

- Increased levels of pepsinogen occur in some ulcer-prone families.

A
Peptic ulcer

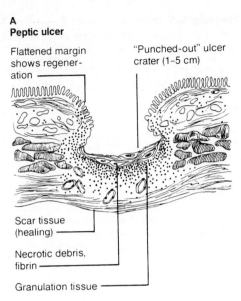

Flattened margin shows regeneration

"Punched-out" ulcer crater (1–5 cm)

Scar tissue (healing)

Necrotic debris, fibrin

Granulation tissue

B
Malignant ulcer

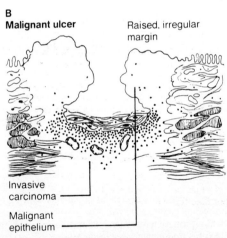

Raised, irregular margin

Invasive carcinoma

Malignant epithelium

Figure 38–1. Comparative features of benign versus malignant gastric ulcers. A: Chronic peptic ulcer, showing the flat, punched-out ulcer with regenerating epithelium at the edges. B: Carcinomatous ulcer with raised edges composed of malignant epithelial cells. The shaded gray areas in the base and at the edges of the ulcer represent malignant epithelial cells.

■ In the majority of patients with peptic ulcer disease, pepsinogen secretion is unchanged.

Pathology

Chronic peptic ulcers are usually solitary, often large (over 1 cm, rarely larger than 5 cm), and round-to-oval with a punched-out appearance.

■ Microscopically, the base of a chronic peptic ulcer is composed of necrotic, acutely inflamed debris below which is granulation tissue and collagen.
■ The epithelium at the edge of the ulcer shows regenerative hyperplasia, which frequently demonstrates marked cytologic atypia, mimicking neoplastic change.
■ Differentiation from ulcerating gastric carcinoma (Fig 38–1) may be difficult without biopsy.

Clinical Features

It has a chronic course, with remissions and relapses of symptoms associated with healing and activation of the ulcer disease.

■ Relapses may be precipitated by emotional stress, by drugs such as aspirin, ibuprofen, or steroids, and by cigarette smoking.
■ Burning or gnawing epigastric pain related to meals is the characteristic symptom of chronic peptic ulcer. Pain is relieved by food and antacids.
■ The diagnosis is best established by endoscopy, including biopsy to rule out carcinoma in gastric ulcers.

Complications

A. Bleeding is the result of erosion of a blood vessel by the ulcer and occurs in about 30% of patients with peptic ulcer.

■ If slow, it causes occult blood loss in feces, leading to iron deficiency anemia.
■ When rapid, hematemesis and melena occur.
■ Peptic ulcer disease is the commonest cause of hematemesis.
■ Hemorrhage is responsible for 10% of deaths from peptic ulcer disease.

B. Perforation occurs in about 5% of peptic ulcer patients, being most common with anterior duodenal ulcers.

■ The entry of gastric juice into the peritoneal cavity results in chemical peritonitis, with sudden onset of abdominal pain and boardlike rigidity of the abdominal muscles.
■ Perforation is responsible for over 70% of deaths due to peptic ulcer.

C. Pyloric obstruction may result from the fibrosis associated with an ulcer in the pyloric canal or first part of the duodenum. Severe vomiting with hypochloremic alkalosis results.

D. Penetration refers to extension of the ulcerative process through the full thickness of the wall into adjacent organs.

■ The fibrotic base of the ulcer is intact in penetration, and there is no perforation.
■ Penetration into the pancreas may lead to constant back pain.

E. Malignant transformation:

- Patients with gastric ulcers are at increased risk—probably small (1–3%)—to develop gastric carcinoma.
- Duodenal and prepyloric ulcers are not associated with an increased risk of malignant transformation.

Treatment

Symptomatic treatment includes frequent small meals, avoidance of cigarette smoking, coffee, and alcohol, and the use of antacids.

- Cimetidine (and other histamine H_2 receptor antagonists) is the most effective form of treatment.
- Surgical treatment includes removal of the ulcer and procedures to decrease gastric acid secretion such as vagotomy and pyloric antrectomy.

NEOPLASMS OF THE STOMACH

Benign Neoplasms

MUCOSAL POLYPS

Epithelial polyps are rare in the stomach. There are two types: adenomatous (10%) and hyperplastic (90%). Both types are usually pedunculated and may be multiple.

- They are associated with an increased risk of carcinoma—smaller with hyperplastic than with adenomatous polyps. The cancer frequently occurs in the adjacent mucosa, not in the polyp itself, and removal of the polyp does not remove the risk.
- Though adenomatous polyps are to be regarded as premalignant lesions, only a very small number of gastric carcinomas arise in adenomatous polyps.

MESENCHYMAL NEOPLASMS

Mesenchymal neoplasms, most commonly leiomyomas and neurofibroma, are uncommon.

- Also presenting as a mass in the submucosa of the stomach is heterotopic pancreas (also called choristoma).

Malignant Neoplasms

GASTRIC ADENOCARCINOMA

Incidence & Etiology

Gastric adenocarcinoma accounts for over 90% of malignant neoplasms of the stomach.

- In the United States, it accounts for approximately 14,000 deaths per year.
  - This represents a decline since 1950.
  - The decline has been attributed to better refrigeration of meat and decreased use of preservatives, mainly nitrites.
- Incidence of gastric carcinoma is 5–10 times higher in Japan than in the United States. Incidence is also high in Iceland and Chile.

- Japanese immigrants to the United States show a decreased incidence from generation to generation, suggesting an environmental carcinogen.
- It has been postulated that polycyclic hydrocarbons in smoked fish may be responsible.
- It is commoner in individuals with blood group A.
- There is no significant familial tendency.

Precancerous Lesions

- Gastric carcinoma occurs with increased frequency:
  - In chronic atrophic gastritis associated with pernicious anemia (high risk).
  - In chronic atrophic gastritis not associated with pernicious anemia, particularly when there is intestinal metaplasia (uncertain risk).
  - In adenomatous and hyperplastic polyps (low risk).
  - In chronic gastric ulcer (very low risk).
- Following subtotal gastrectomy, the residual gastric stump is believed to be at increased risk, though a recent study casts serious doubt on this.

Pathology
A. Gross appearance:

- Early gastric cancer:
  - Is defined as a carcinoma restricted to the mucosa and submucosa.
  - Appears as a small, flat mucosal thickening that may have a minimal polypoid and ulcerative component.
  - In the United States, less than 5% of gastric carcinomas are detected at this early stage.
- Late gastric cancer:
  - Is defined as a carcinoma that has invaded the muscle wall.
  - Is the stage at which the tumor is commonly diagnosed in the United States.
  - May present as a fungating mass that protrudes into the lumen, as a malignant ulcer with raised, everted edges (Fig 38–1), as an excavated ulcer resembling a chronic peptic ulcer, or as a diffuse thickening of the stomach wall (linitis plastica).

B. Microscopic appearance:

- Gastric carcinomas are adenocarcinomas.
- The most common form is poorly differentiated, with cells distended by intracellular mucin ("signet ring cell carcinoma").
- Well-differentiated adenocarcinoma is less common.

C. Spread:

- Gastric carcinoma infiltrates the submucosa and invades through the muscle wall into the omental fat.
- Involvement of the serosa leads to spread of tumor cells in the peritoneal fluid (transcoelomic spread) to the ovary (Krukenberg tumor) and rectovesical pouch.
- Lymphatic involvement also leads to metastasis to lymph nodes around the stomach and up the thoracic duct with involvement of the left supraclavicular node (Virchow's node).
- Bloodstream spread to the liver and lungs also occurs early.

Clinical Features

Gastric carcinoma is asymptomatic in its early stages.

- A few patients with early gastric cancer have symptoms resembling chronic peptic ulcer.
- All nonhealing gastric ulcers must be biopsied.
- Late gastric cancer presents with anorexia, anemia, and weight loss.
- Early satiety may occur with a large mass or a contracted (linitis plastica) stomach.
- Hematemesis, melena, and gastric outlet obstruction are common complications.
- Diagnosis is established by endoscopy and biopsy.

Prognosis

The likelihood of metastatic disease depends almost entirely on the depth of invasion of the neoplasm.

- Early gastric cancer has a 5-year survival rate of about 85%.
- Late gastric cancer with negative lymph nodes has a 30% 5-year survival rate.
- When there is extension of tumor through the entire gastric wall or when lymph node involvement is present, the 5-year survival rate drops to about 5%.
- Histologic features and degree of differentiation are of little prognostic importance.

MALIGNANT LYMPHOMA

Lymphoma accounts for about 3% of malignant tumors of the stomach.

- Most are aggressive B cell non-Hodgkin's lymphomas, B-immunoblastic sarcoma being the commonest histologic type.
- They present as polypoid masses, ulcers, thickened mucosal folds, and large intramural masses.
- Histologic examination shows a proliferation of large transformed lymphoid cells.
- Immunohistochemical demonstration of lymphoid markers is confirmatory.
- They respond well to chemotherapy. The 5-year survival rate is around 50–60% for disease localized to the stomach.

GASTRIC LEIOMYOSARCOMA

Malignant smooth muscle neoplasms, although they are the commonest mesenchymal neoplasm in the stomach, account for only 2% of gastric malignancies.

- They present as large masses that originate in and involve the wall, usually protruding both into the mucosa and out as an extragastric mass.
- Mucosal ulceration and cavitation of the central part of the tumor occur commonly.
- Microscopically, they are composed of a cellular mass of smooth muscle cells showing increased mitotic activity and areas of necrosis and hemorrhage.
- They present with bleeding, blood-loss anemia, or a palpable mass.
- Diagnosis is by radiologic studies followed by biopsy.
- With surgical resection, over 50% of patients survive for 5 years.

The Intestines: I. Malabsorption Syndrome; Intestinal Obstruction

39

CLINICAL MANIFESTATIONS OF INTESTINAL DISEASE

INTESTINAL OBSTRUCTION

Causes
A. Mechanical obstruction may result from:

- Lesions outside the intestine that compress or constrict the intestine, eg, fibrous adhesions in the peritoneal cavity and hernial sacs.
- Intramural lesions such as fibrous strictures and neoplasms.
- Volvulus and intussusception.
- Intraluminal foreign bodies.

B. Functional obstruction due to failure of peristalsis may due to:

- Paralytic ileus, which occurs after surgery, in acute peritonitis, and in severe inflammation (eg, toxic megacolon).
- Abnormalities of the myenteric plexus, eg, Hirschsprung's disease, Chagas' disease.
- Intestinal smooth muscle diseases, eg, familial visceral myopathy.

Effects

- Vomiting, constipation and absence of flatus.
- Abdominal distension due to dilatation of the intestine proximal to the obstruction. The dilated bowel loops are filled with fluid, food, and gas.
- Hypovolemia and electrolyte imbalance due to fluid accumulation in the bowel.
- Increased peristalsis when the obstruction is mechanical, resulting in colicky abdominal pain and increased bowel sounds on abdominal auscultation.
- In cases where intestinal obstruction is due to muscle paralysis, pain and bowel sounds are absent.

INTESTINAL PERFORATION
Complete disruption of the bowel wall permits leakage of luminal contents into the peritoneal cavity.

- When perforation occurs in a part of the intestine whose wall is not covered by serosa, eg, the posterior wall of the descending colon, the contents leak into the pericolic fat, causing pericolic abscess.

- The effect of intestinal perforation depends on its site.
- Perforation of a duodenal ulcer produces chemical peritonitis due to the acid content.
- Perforation of the intestine distal to the first part of the duodenum leads to bacterial infection.
- In all cases of perforation, gas enters the peritoneal cavity and can be detected under the diaphragm on X-ray.

INTESTINAL HEMORRHAGE
Bleeding into the lumen of the intestines may be manifested in several ways:

- Bright red blood per rectum occurs with rapid bleeding and when the source of bleeding is near the rectum.
- Passage of dark stools containing altered blood admixed with stools occurs with bleeding originating in the proximal colon and small intestine.
- Passage of tarry black stools occurs when bleeding is in the stomach and duodenum and the blood is altered by the action of acid.
- Iron deficiency anemia may develop with chronic slow bleeding and is associated with occult blood in stools.

PROTEIN-LOSING ENTEROPATHY
Increased loss of protein in the intestine resulting in hypoproteinemia and edema is called *protein-losing enteropathy*.

DIARRHEA
Diarrhea is the passage of fluid feces; it occurs when the rate of movement of intestinal contents is increased, so that complete digestion and absorption of fluid in the intestine fails to occur.

- The volume of feces is usually greatly increased in diarrhea, leading to increased frequency of evacuation and increased loss of water and electrolytes.
- The mechanisms in the production of diarrhea are summarized in Table 39–1.
- Diarrhea may result from:
  - Increased fluid secretion into the intestine (secretory diarrhea).
  - Presence of increased amounts of osmotically active substances in the intestinal lumen.
  - Inflammation of the intestine.
  - Increased peristalsis, eg, in carcinoid syndrome and in irritable bowel syndrome.
  - Failure of colonic water absorption, eg, after surgical removal of the colon.
- **Steatorrhea:**
  - Is a specific form of diarrhea defined by the presence of excessive fat (> 6 g/d) in the feces.
  - Is a typical clinical manifestation of maldigestion or malabsorption of fat.
- **Dysentery:**
  - Is a specific type of diarrhea characterized by passage of liquid feces admixed with bright red blood and mucus at frequent intervals.
  - Is a characteristic symptom of acute colonic inflammation.
  - When the rectum is inflamed, dysentery is accompanied by a constant and painful desire to defecate (tenesmus).

TABLE 39–1. MECHANISMS IN THE PRODUCTION OF DIARRHEA

Secretory diarrhea
  Associated with cAMP increase
    Enterotoxin of *Vibrio cholerae*
    Enterotoxin of *Escherichia coli*
    Vasoactive intestinal polypeptide (from pancreatic islet cell neoplasms)
    Bile acids
  Not associated with cAMP
    Enterotoxin of *Staphylococcus aureus*
    Enterotoxin of *Clostridium perfringens*
    Some laxatives (bisacodyl, phenolphthalein)
    AIDS (unknown mechanism)
  Mucosal injury
    Infections: Viral and *Salmonella* gastroenteritis, *Shigella, E coli, Campylobacter* colitis
    Inflammatory bowel disease
  Neoplasms
    Gastrinoma (gastrin)
    Carcinoid syndrome (serotonin, prostaglandins)
    Villous adenoma

Osmotic diarrhea
  Disaccharidase deficiency (lactose or sucrose intolerance)
  Postgastrectomy
  Postvagotomy
  Laxatives (lactulose, magnesium salts)

Motility disorders
  Irritable bowel syndrome
  Autonomic neuropathy (diabetes mellitus)
  Laxatives

MALABSORPTION SYNDROME

NORMAL ABSORPTION IN THE SMALL INTESTINE

Absorption of Fat
A. Luminal phase:

- Pancreatic lipase hydrolyzes triglycerides to fatty acids and monoglycerides.
- The fatty acids and monoglycerides, along with fat-soluble vitamins, are complexed with bile acids to form a globular structure called a *micelle*.

B. Cellular phase:

- The micelles dissociate at the surface of the intestinal mucosal cell, and the fatty acids, monoglycerides, and fat-soluble vitamins move into the cell while the bile acids remain in the lumen.

- The bile acids are reabsorbed in the terminal ileum and pass to the liver for reexcretion (the enterohepatic circulation of bile acids).
- Fat absorption occurs mainly in the upper jejunum, and about 100 cm are required for normal fat absorption.
- In the intestinal cells, monoglycerides are further hydrolyzed by mucosal cell lipase.
- The fatty acids are then reconverted to triglycerides in the endoplasmic reticulum and complexed with protein, phospholipid, and some cholesterol to form chylomicrons.
- Chylomicrons exit the cell at the antiluminal border of the mucosal cell and enter intestinal lymphatics.
- Medium-chain triglycerides (containing 6–10 fatty acids) are capable of limited direct absorption without micelle formation, and can pass directly into the portal circulation, bypassing lymphatics.

Absorption of Protein & Carbohydrate

Proteins and carbohydrates are hydrolyzed by enzymes in saliva (amylase), gastric juice (pepsin), pancreatic juice (amylase, trypsin, and chymotrypsin), and intestinal juice (disaccharidases, carboxypeptidases) into amino acids and monosaccharides. These hydrophilic substances are absorbed into the mucosal cells and pass into the portal venous radicals.

DEFINITION OF MALABSORPTION SYNDROME

This is a clinical syndrome characterized by increased fecal excretion of fat (steatorrhea) and the systemic effects of deficiency of vitamins, minerals, protein, and carbohydrates (Table 39–2). The presence of steatorrhea is established when fat excretion exceeding 6 g/d is demonstrated in a 72-hour stool sample.

PATHOPHYSIOLOGY OF MALABSORPTION (TABLE 39–3)

Deficiency of Pancreatic Enzymes

Absence of pancreatic lipase leads to steatorrhea.

- Pancreatic amylase and trypsin are important for carbohydrate and protein digestion, but their function can be taken over by other enzymes in intestinal juice.
- Absence of pancreatic lipase is usually the result of chronic pancreatitis.
- In the rare Zollinger-Ellison syndrome, lipase activity is decreased because of increased acidity.

Deficiency of Bile Acids

- Bile acid deficiency occurs:
  - In biliary obstruction.
  - When bile acids are deconjugated in the lumen of the small intestine. This results from bacterial overgrowth, which occurs when there is stasis of luminal contents from any cause.
  - When normal reabsorption of bile acids in the terminal ileum does not occur, due either to absence or disease of that segment of intestine.
- Deficiency of bile acids results in failure of micelle formation, interfering with absorption of fat and fat-soluble vitamins.
- Medium-chain triglycerides, proteins, and carbohydrates are absorbed normally.

TABLE 39-2. SYSTEMIC EFFECTS OF MALABSORPTION

Dietary Substance	Clinical Effect
Total calories (fat, carbohydrate)	Weight loss, general weakness
Protein	Muscle wasting (increased gluconeogenesis) Osteoporosis Decreased pituitary hormone output (causes amenorrhea) Hypoproteinemia, edema
Calcium	Hypocalcemia Tetany, paresthesias Secondary hyperparathyroidism Osteomalacia, osteitis fibrosa cystica Bone pain
Magnesium	Hypomagnesemia, tetany
Iron	Hypochromic microcytic anemia Glossitis, koilonychia
Folic acid	Macrocytic megaloblastic anemia
Vitamin B_{12}	Macrocytic megaloblastic anemia Peripheral neuropathy Subacute combined degeneration of the spinal cord
Vitamin B complex	Cheilosis, angular stomatitis, glossitis
Vitamin K	Hypoprothrombinemia Hemorrhagic diathesis
Vitamin D	Hypocalcemia Osteomalacia
Vitamin A	Night blindness Bitot's spots, xerophthalmia

Abnormalities in the Absorptive Mucosa

Quantitative abnormalities include:

- Reduction in the length of small intestine due to extensive surgical resection.
- Decreased available surface area of absorptive mucosa, as occurs in villous atrophy and giardiasis.
- Changes in the villi such as—amyloidosis and Whipple's disease.

Decreased Intestinal Transit Time

Malabsorption may occur in conditions where there is increased intestinal motility, such as carcinoid syndrome and post gastrectomy.

TABLE 39–3. MECHANISMS AND CAUSES OF MALABSORPTION SYNDROME

Inadequate digestion
  Postgastrectomy
  Deficiency of pancreatic lipase
    Chronic pancreatitis
    Cystic fibrosis
    Pancreatic resection
    Zollinger-Ellison syndrome (high acid inhibits lipase)

Deficient bile salt concentration
  Obstructive jaundice
  Bacterial overgrowth (leading to bile salt deconjugation)
    Stasis in blind loops, diverticula
    Fistulas
    Hypomotility states (diabetes, scleroderma, visceral myopathy)
  Interrupted enterohepatic circulation of bile salts
    Terminal ileal resection
    Crohn's disease
  Precipitation of bile salts
    Neomycin, cholestyramine

Primary mucosal abnormalities
  Celiac disease
  Tropical sprue
  Whipple's disease
  Amyloidosis
  Radiation enteritis

Inadequate small intestine
  Intestinal resection
    Crohn's disease
    Mesenteric vascular disease with infarction
  Jejunoileal bypass

Lymphatic obstruction
  Intestinal lymphangiectasia
  Malignant lymphoma

Failure of Removal of Intestinal Triglyceride

Triglycerides formed in the mucosal cell must be complexed with a carrier protein to form chylomicrons before they can enter the intestinal lymphatics.

- Failure of synthesis of proteins necessary for formation of chylomicrons occurs in abetalipoproteinemia, a rare autosomal-recessive inherited disease characterized by decreased serum betalipoprotein levels and abnormal erythrocytes. The triglyceride accumulates in the intestinal mucosal cell.
- Obstruction of lymphatics, as in intestinal lymphangiectasia and extensive intestinal lymphomas, leads to malabsorption.

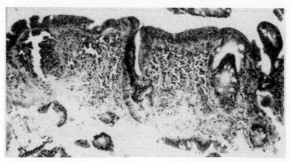

Figure 39–1. Total villous atrophy in a case of celiac disease. Note the flat surface epithelium without villi. The surface epithelium also appears more cuboidal, with less cytoplasmic mucin than is normal. The hypercellular appearance of the surface epithelium is due to the presence of numerous intraepethelial lymphocytes (visible only at higher magnification).

Diseases Causing Malabsorption

CELIAC DISEASE (Nontropical Sprue; Gluten-Induced Enteropathy)

Celiac disease is caused by the action of acidic peptides contained in the gliadin fraction of the wheat protein gluten on the intestinal mucosa.

- Serum contains IgA antibodies to gliadin in most patients, and antibody titers fall when these patients are maintained on a gluten-free diet.
- Susceptibility to gluten-induced intestinal damage is rare and has a familial tendency; 80–90% of patients have the histocompatibility antigen HLA-B8 or HLA-DR3.

Pathology

The changes of celiac disease are restricted to the small intestinal mucosa.

- It is characterized by total villous atrophy, surface epithelial cell damage manifested by decreased cell height and decreased cytoplasmic mucus, and lymphocytic infiltration of the epithelium (Fig 39–1).
- Immunologic studies show the presence of anti-gliadin IgA antibodies in the mucosa.

Clinical Features & Diagnosis

Celiac disease presents with severe malabsorption syndrome, most commonly in childhood.

- Small bowel follow-through shows an abnormal mucosal pattern.
- Jejunal biopsy shows total villous atrophy and epithelial abnormalities.
- Withdrawal of gluten from the diet produces dramatic improvement in both clinical symptoms and histologic changes in the small intestine.
- Confirmation of diagnosis is by demonstrating reversal of histologic changes after the patient has been on a gluten-free diet for 6 months.

Complications
Celiac disease is regarded a premalignant condition with an increased risk of malignant lymphoma of the intestine.

TROPICAL SPRUE
This is an acquired disease that is commonly seen in the Caribbean, Far East, and India. It is thought to result from chronic bacterial infection of the small intestine, because treatment with broad-spectrum antibiotics is often successful.

- It occurs in adults and is characterized by a severe malabsorption syndrome in which folic acid deficiency is often a dominant feature.
- Jejunal biopsy shows partial villous atrophy.

WHIPPLE'S DISEASE (Intestinal Lipodystrophy)
This is a rare disease characterized pathologically by distention of the lamina propria of the small intestine by macrophages with abundant pale foamy cytoplasm.

- The macrophages contain large numbers of bacilli (seen on electron microscopy) that produce a positive staining with periodic acid-Schiff (PAS) stain.
- The villi are increased in size, giving the mucosal surface a coarse appearance resembling the pile of a shaggy rug.
- Treatment with antibiotics causes improvement of symptoms as well as disappearance of the bacillary bodies, suggesting that this is also a form of bacterial infection.
- No specific organism or organisms responsible has been identified.
- Presentation is with severe malabsorption syndrome, commonly in males over age 30.
- Diagnosis may be made by demonstration of the typical macrophages on jejunal biopsy.
- Forty percent of patients have extraintestinal manifestations, including:
  - Lymph node enlargement, commonly mesenteric.
  - Fever, present in 30% of patients, commonly with polyarthritis and polyserositis (pleural effusion and ascites).
  - Rarely, the spleen, liver, kidney, lungs, heart, and brain may be affected.
- It may sometimes be intestinally asymptomic. Diagnosis is made by finding the abnormal macrophages in affected tissues.

CONGENITAL DISEASES OF THE INTESTINE

INTESTINAL ATRESIA
This is a rare disorder consisting of failure of development of the lumen in one part of the intestine.

- The jejunum and ileum are most commonly affected, and multiple bowel segments may be affected.
- Atresia presents with intestinal obstruction in the first week of life.
- Surgical correction is curative.

IMPERFORATE ANUS
This is a common congenital abnormality that results from failure of the entodermal hindgut to open at the anal dimple. Varying degrees of abnormality result, sometimes associated with fistulous communications with the bladder, urethra, and vagina.

MALROTATION
Malrotation is characterized by failure of the cecum to reach its normal position in the right lower quadrant. The abnormal mobility of the cecum predisposes to twisting (volvulus) and intestinal obstruction.

MECKEL'S DIVERTICULUM
Meckel's diverticulum represents persistence of the intestinal end of the omphalomes-enteric duct.

- It is present in 2% of the population (the commonest congenital anomaly of the gastrointestinal tract).
- It is located within 2 feet (1 m) of the ileocecal valve, and is usually 2 inches (5 cm) long.
- The diverticulum is usually lined by small intestinal mucosa. About 40% of cases have heterotopic gastric mucosa or pancreatic tissue.
- Complications include:
  - Peptic ulceration, which may occur when there is gastric mucosa.
  - Bleeding from an ulcerated Meckel diverticulum, which may result in iron deficiency anemia.
  - Meckel's diverticulitis, which presents a clinical picture very similar to that of acute appendicitis.
  - Perforation secondary to inflammation or peptic ulcer.
  - Volvulus, especially when it is attached to the umbilicus by the obliterated omphalomesenteric duct.
  - Inversion of the diverticulum into the ileum, followed by intussusception.

CONGENITAL MEGACOLON (Hirschsprung's Disease)
This is caused by failure of development of ganglion cells in the myenteric and sub-mucosal plexuses of the colon.

- The aganglionic segment usually starts at the anorectal junction and extends proximally for a variable distance.
- In 90% of cases, aganglionosis is restricted to the rectum. Rarely, the aganglionic segment is longer, and in exceptional cases the entire colon is aganglionic.
- The aganglionic segment remains narrow and spastic and represents a zone of functional intestinal obstruction.
- The colon proximal to the aganglionic segment dilates, often massively, leading to abdominal distention.
- Most affected children present soon after birth with failure to pass meconium followed by distention and vomiting. In a few cases, the onset is delayed.
- Without treatment, death occurs from fluid and electrolyte imbalance or from perforation of a massively dilated cecum.

- Diagnosis may be made by demonstrating absence of ganglion cells in the submucosa of an adequate rectal biopsy.
- Treatment is surgical removal of the aganglionic segment.

VASCULAR DISEASES OF THE INTESTINES

ACUTE SMALL INTESTINAL INFARCTION

Etiology

A. Sudden occlusion of the superior mesenteric artery is responsible for 50% of cases of small bowel infarction. It is caused by:

- Atherosclerosis in over 90% of cases.
- Vasculitis—most commonly polyarteritis nodosa.
- Aortic dissection.
- Embolism from mural cardiac thrombi and valvular vegetations in patients with cardiac disease.
- Fibromuscular dysplasia of mesenteric arteries.

B. Nonocclusive infarction:

- In 25% of cases, intestinal infarction occurs without occlusion of the mesenteric arteries.
- Usually it occurs in severe shock, where there is prolonged vasoconstriction in the intestinal circulation.

C. Mesenteric vein occlusion:

- In 25% of cases intestinal infarction is due to mesenteric venous occlusion.
- Mesenteric vein occlusion may be caused by:
  - Thrombosis, commonly in hypercoagulable states such as polycythemia vera and with oral contraceptive use.
  - Infiltration by malignant neoplasms.

Pathology

- Affected small bowel loops are hemorrhagic, appearing purple to black.
- The demarcation of viable and nonviable bowel on gross examination at surgery may not be clear.
- Microscopically, there is transmural necrosis of the intestinal wall, rapidly followed by bacterial infection from the lumen and acute inflammation, leading to wet gangrene.
- The distinction between arterial and venous infarction cannot be made on examination of the bowel; it is necessary to dissect the vessels at the root of the mesentery or to have angiographic evidence of arterial occlusion.
- Intestinal infarction associated with vasculitis and nonocclusive infarction characteristically causes multiple discontinuous areas of intestinal necrosis, maximally affecting the mucosa.

Clinical Features

- Intestinal infarction occurs most often in elderly individuals with severe atherosclerosis.
- Embolism occurs in patients with cardiac diseases (infective endocarditis, myocardial infarction, mitral stenosis, atrial fibrillation).
- In a few patients, infarction may be preceded by "abdominal angina," which is characterized by abdominal pain 15–30 minutes after a meal.
- Infarction is characterized by a sudden onset of severe abdominal pain accompanied by fever, vomiting, abdominal distention, absent bowel sounds, and bloody diarrhea.
- The disease progresses very rapidly, with shock and peritonitis due to gangrene within 1–2 days after onset.
- Without treatment, there is a 100% mortality rate. Even with emergency intestinal resection, the mortality rate is 50–75%.

ISCHEMIC COLITIS

This is caused by extensive atherosclerotic narrowing of the arteries that supply the colon.

- The splenic flexure and rectosigmoid area are most commonly involved.
- It is characterized by patchy mucosal necrosis in the affected region, accompanied by acute inflammation and ulceration.
- The condition is usually self-limited, with healing by fibrosis and epithelial regeneration.
- Rarely, fibrosis may be so extensive as to cause narrowing (stricture) of the colon.
- Patients present with an acute onset of fever, left-sided abdominal pain, and bloody diarrhea.
- Colonoscopy and histologic examination of biopsies show nonspecific necrosis, inflammation, and ulceration.
- Differentiation from other inflammatory lesions of the colon (infections, idiopathic inflammatory bowel disease) is difficult.

ANGIODYSPLASIA OF THE COLON

This is a common and important cause of intestinal bleeding, mainly affecting elderly patients.

- It commonly involves the right side of the colon, but may occur anywhere in the gastrointestinal tract.
- It is characterized by the presence of numerous dilated, tortuous, thin-walled blood vessels in the mucosa and submucosa of the colon. Rupture of these vessels causes painless bleeding, which can be sudden and severe.
- The diagnosis is best made by angiography, which shows the vascular malformation bleeding into the lumen.
- Surgical resection of the involved segment of intestine is usually necessary to control the bleeding.

MISCELLANEOUS DISEASES OF THE INTESTINE

ABDOMINAL HERNIA

An abdominal hernia is the protrusion of a sac of peritoneum through a defect or weakness in the abdominal wall.

- Anatomic types of hernia include:
  - Indirect inguinal hernia, through the internal inguinal ring.
  - Direct inguinal hernia, through the posterior wall of the inguinal canal.
  - Femoral hernia, into the femoral canal.
  - Periumbilical hernia, around the umbilicus.
  - Incisional hernia, through areas weakened by surgical scars.
  - Lumbar hernia, through the posterior abdominal wall.
  - Diaphragmatic hernia, through the diaphragm.
- Inguinal, umbilical, diaphragmatic and incisional hernias are very common.
- The peritoneal sac of a hernia may contain a variety of abdominal tissues, commonly omentum and intestine and, more rarely, bladder.
- When intestine constitutes part of the contents:
  - Intestinal obstruction may occur.
  - Strangulation due to constriction of venous drainage and arterial supply at the neck may occur, causing infarction and gangrene.

INTUSSUSCEPTION

Intussusception is telescoping of one segment of bowel into another. Once the intussusception begins, peristalsis pushes the intussusceptum farther distally.

- The common location for an intussusception is the terminal ileum.
- Intussusception occurs in:
  - Weaning infants, due probably to hyperplastic lymphoid tissue.
  - Adults with polypoid tumors, commonly lipomas or leiomyomas. It is the tumor that acts as the apex.
- Intussusception causes intestinal obstruction, with abdominal distension, pain, and vomiting.
- The intussusceptum commonly undergoes hemorrhagic infarction and gangrene, leading to passage of blood per rectum.
- The intussuscepted bowel may be palpable as a sausage-shaped mass in the abdomen.
- Treatment is surgical reduction or resection.

VOLVULUS

Volvulus is a twisting of the intestine about the axis of its mesentery or around an abnormal fibrous band.

- Abnormal fibrous bands usually result from previous local peritonitis followed by fibrous adhesions.
- Complete twisting leads to intestinal obstruction and often strangulation of the vascular supply, causing infarction.
- Volvulus commonly occurs in the sigmoid colon in elderly individuals.
- Cecal volvulus occurs in younger people who have developmental malrotation of the bowel.

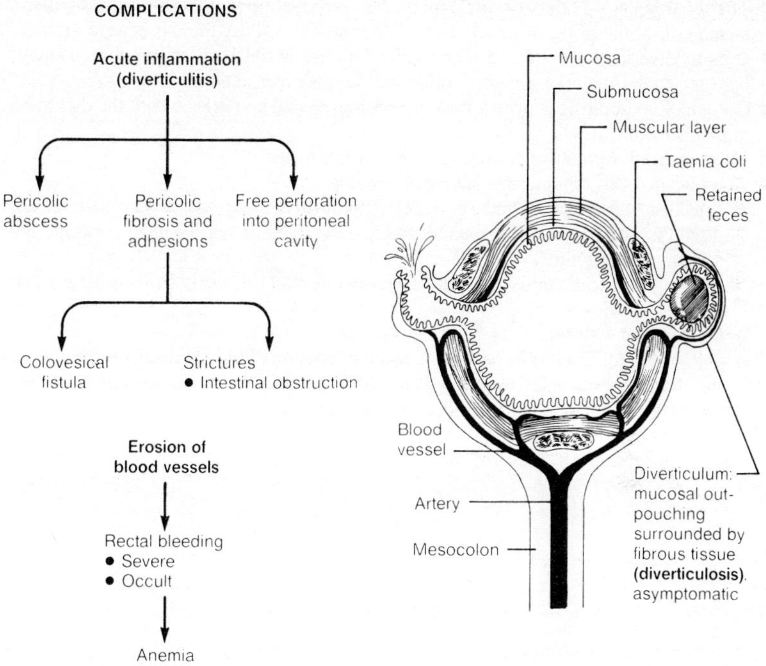

COMPLICATIONS

Figure 39–2. Cross section of sigmoid colon, showing diverticulosis. Complications associated with diverticulosis are shown on the left side.

DIVERTICULOSIS

A diverticulum is an outpouching of the mucosa of the intestine.

- True diverticula have all the layers of the intestine in their wall (congenital ones such as Meckel's diverticula are true diverticula.)
- False diverticula, which are mucosal herniations through a weak point in the muscle wall, are lined by mucosa and fibrous tissue only. Most acquired diverticula are false diverticula.

1. JEJUNAL DIVERTICULOSIS

This is relatively uncommon and is characterized by the presence of multiple diverticula in the jejunum. Bacterial overgrowth in the static contents of the diverticula causes bile acid deconjugation and malabsorption.

2. COLONIC DIVERTICULOSIS (FIG 39–2)

This is common in developed countries, being present in over 50% of patients over age 60.

- The sigmoid colon is most commonly involved.

- The diverticula are false, occuring in a double vertical row along the antimesenteric taenia coli at the point of penetration of the muscle wall by the mesenteric arteries.
- Colonic diverticulosis is the result of a diet deficient in fiber, which promotes a small, hard stool that requires a high luminal pressure for evacuation.
- Colonic diverticulosis is uncommon in underdeveloped countries where the diet has a high fiber content.
- Most cases of sigmoid diverticulosis are asymptomatic.
- Complications of colonic diverticulosis include:
  - Infection (diverticulitis) causes fever, leukocytosis, and left lower quadrant abdominal pain ("left-sided appendicitis"). Diverticulitis may lead to pericolic abscesses or peritonitis.
  - Intestinal obstruction as a result of marked pericolic fibrosis from healed diverticulitis.
  - Colovesical fistulas.
  - Hemorrhage, which may occur as a result of erosion of blood vessels in the wall of the diverticulum, causing the passage of bright red blood per rectum or slower occult bleeding, leading to iron deficiency anemia.

Intestines: II. Infections; Inflammatory Bowel Diseases

40

I. INFECTIONS OF THE INTESTINE

Most intestinal infections are transmitted by fecal contamination of food or drinking water. They are common in parts of the world where public health sanitary measures such as disposal of feces and purification of water supplies are not adequate. Clinically, infections that involve the small intestine result in profuse watery diarrhea, while those that involve the colon produce dysentery.

Classification (Table 40–1)
A. Enterotoxin-mediated:

- The disease is caused by a bacterial exotoxin (enterotoxin).
- The toxin-producing bacterium does not invade the tissues and in some cases does not even enter the body (staphylococcal toxin, botulism).
- Fever is usually absent.

B. Invasive infections:

- The organism invades the intestinal mucosa evoking an inflammation.
- Fever is usually present.

C. Noninvasive infections: The organism exists in the intestinal lumen and does not invade the tissues.

Diagnosis

- Stool culture for Shigella, Salmonella, Campylobacter, Escherichia coli.
- Identification of organisms in smear preparations of stool (eg, Entamoeba, Giardia, Cryptosporidium, Isospora).
- Serologic diagnosis is of value in certain instances (eg, typhoid fever).
- In diseases produced by toxins, identification of the toxin is often the only means of diagnosis (eg, Clostridium difficile enterocolitis).
- With intestinal worm infections, stool specimens may reveal whole worms, body segments, larvae, or eggs, depending upon the species.

TABLE 40–1. INFECTIONS OF INTESTINES

Organism	Source of Toxin or Infectious Agent	Clinical Illness
Toxin-mediated *Vibrio cholerae*	Contaminated water	Severe diarrhea
Escherichia coli, toxigenic	Food, water	Traveler's diarrhea
Staphylococcus aureus toxin	Toxin in food	Food poisoning
Clostridium perfringens	Reheated foods	Food poisoning
Bacillus cereus	Reheated foods	Food poisoning
Vibrio parahaemolyticus	Shellfish	Food poisoning
Clostridium botulinum	Neurotoxin in food	Botulism

Invasive infections
Viral
  Rotaviruses and adeno-
  viruses
	Person to person	Infantile diarrhea

Parvoviruses	Person to person	"Stomach flu"
Cytomegalovirus	Person to person	Enterocolitis (mainly in immunocompromised patients)
Bacterial *Salmonella* species	Food, milk, or water	Food poisoning
Salmonella typhi	Food, water	Typhoid
Shigella species	Food, water	Dysentery
Enteropathogenic *E coli*	Mostly person to person	Diarrhea and dysentery
Campylobacter fetus	Animals, infected persons, food	Childhood diarrhea
Yersinia species	Infected persons, food	Mesenteric adenitis, diarrhea
Mycobacterium tuberculosis	Infected person or milk	Chronic disease
Atypical mycobacteria	Infected person, soil	Chronic diarrhea (mainly in immunodeficient patients)
Protozoal *Entamoeba histolytica*	Fecal contamination (cysts)	Amebic colitis

(continued)

TABLE 40–1. (*Continued*)

Organism	Source of Toxin or Infectious Agent	Clinical Illness
Invasive infections Metazoan parasites (see Table 40–3)		
Noninvasive infections *Giardia lamblia*	Contaminated water	Giardiasis
Cryptosporidium, Isospora	Contaminated food, water	Diarrhea (mainly in immuno-compromised patients)
Metazoan parasites (see Table 40–3)		

ENTEROTOXIN-MEDIATED DISEASES

CHOLERA

Cholera is caused by *Vibrio cholerae*. It is endemic in several Southeast Asian countries and occurs also in the Southeastern United States.

- Infection occurs when the organism is ingested with fecally contaminated food or water.
- The organism multiplies in the intestinal lumen and produces an exotoxin that binds irreversibly to ganglioside receptors on the surface membranes of small intestinal mucosal cells.
- Toxin binding results in increased cAMP synthesis in the cell, which stimulates secretion of fluid and electrolytes, causing secretory diarrhea.
- Pathologic examination reveals a normal small intestinal mucosa on gross, light microscopic, and electron microscopic examination, even in fatal cases.
- Clinically, there is a severe diarrhea, often without abdominal pain or fever, causing rapid dehydration and hypovolemic shock; death may occur within 24 hours.
- The diagnosis is made by demonstrating the vibrio in a stool sample.
- Correction of dehydration with fluid therapy is vital in the acute phase.
- Tetracycline is an effective antibiotic.
- The mortality rate in epidemics of cholera is high, because of the rapidity with which dehydration occurs and because epidemics commonly occur in regions where medical facilities are inadequate.

TOXIGENIC *ESCHERICHIA COLI* INFECTION

Certain strains of *E coli* produce a heat-labile enterotoxin similar to cholera toxin in its mode of action. The ability to produce toxin is plasmid-induced and may therefore be transferred to other organisms.

- Toxigenic *E coli* causes:
  - Traveler's diarrhea in adults.
  - Epidemic diarrhea in neonatal units.

- The disease is usually mild, though in neonates diarrhea may result in dangerous fluid and electrolyte depletion.
- Diagnosis is difficult to establish because *E coli* is a normal commensal in the colon; techniques using tissue culture systems for identifying the heat-labile toxin of *E coli* are necessary.

STAPHYLOCOCCAL FOOD POISONING

This is a common form of epidemic food poisoning. It is caused by enterotoxin-producing strains of *Staphylococcus aureus.*

- The organism multiplies in cooked food that has been kept without refrigeration for several hours before it is eaten, leading to accumulation of the enterotoxin.
- Heating the food before ingestion destroys staphylococci but not the heat-stable toxin.
- The toxin causes severe nausea and vomiting of short duration, usually accompanied by abdominal cramps and diarrhea.
- The disease is self-limited. Death almost never occurs.

CLOSTRIDIUM DIFFICILE PSEUDOMEMBRANOUS ENTEROCOLITIS

Pseudomembranous enterocolitis complicates treatment with certain antibiotics—most commonly clindamycin, ampicillin, or tetracycline.

- These alter the intestinal bacterial flora, permitting the overgrowth of *C difficile,* which produces a powerful exotoxin.
- The toxin has a cytotoxic effect on mucosal epithelial cells, resulting in superficial necrosis and acute inflammation of the intestinal mucosa.
- The necrotic mucosa and exudate remain adherent to the mucosal surface as yellow plaques or membranes.
- Clinically, there is an acute severe diarrhea with blood and mucus, accompanied by fever and leukocytosis.
- The disease progresses rapidly and is frequently fatal in the absence of prompt treatment.
- Diagnosis is based on:
  - Endoscopic visualization of mucosal plaques and membranes.
  - Superficial mucosal necrosis and mushroom-shaped membrane of inflammatory exudate on microscopic examination of biopsies.
  - Demonstration of *C difficile* exotoxin in blood and stool.
- Vancomycin is effective in treatment.

OTHER ENTEROTOXIC DISEASES (Table 40–2)

Clostridium perfringens, Bacillus cereus and *Vibrio parahaemolyticus* cause food poisoning similar clinically to staphylococcal food poisoning.

- **Botulism:**
  - *C botulinum* toxin may be present in inadequately processed food (commonly sausage or home-canned food).
  - The toxin is destroyed by heating for 20 minutes at 100°C, which is achieved in commercial canning.
  - Though classified as a form of "food poisoning," botulism rarely causes diarrhea.
  - It presents with neuromuscular paralysis due to the systemic action of the exotoxin (see Chapter 13).

TABLE 40–2. FOOD POISONING

Organism	Mechanism of Disease	Incubation	Illness
Staphylococcus aureus	Preformed heat-stable toxin, pies, non-refrigerated dairy products	2–4 hours	Vomiting, diarrhea
Bacillus cereus	Heat-stable toxin formed in food or gut, especially re-heated fried rice	2–14 hours	Vomiting, diarrhea
Escherichia coli (toxin)	Organisms produce toxin in gut	24–72 hours	Mild traveler's diarrhea in adults; severe diarrhea in neonates
Clostridium perfringens	Organisms ingested in poorly cooked or re-heated food; produces enterotoxin	8–14 hours	Diarrhea
Vibrio parahaemolyticus	Organism in poorly cooked shellfish; produces toxin in gut	8–96 hours	Vomiting, diarrhea, mild fever
Salmonella species (*typhimurium, enteritidis, newport,* etc)	Ingested organisms in food (especially shellfish) or water; invasive infection	8–24 hours	Fever, vomiting, diarrhea
Clostridium botulinum	Toxin in inadequately processed canned food or sausage	24–96 hours	Vomiting rare; diplopia, dysphagia, respiratory difficulty

INVASIVE VIRAL & BACTERIAL INFECTIONS

VIRAL GASTROENTERITIS

These are very common infections caused by many viruses, most commonly rotaviruses and parvoviruses (eg, the Norwalk agent).

- The viruses infect the small-intestinal epithelial cells, causing blunting of villi and infiltration of the mucosa with lymphocytes and plasma cells.
- They present with fever, acute diarrhea, vomiting, and abdominal pain.
- The illness is self-limited and mild, lasting 3–4 days.
- Diagnosis may be made by demonstrating the virus in stools or detecting a rise in antibody titer.

CYTOMEGALOVIRUS ENTEROCOLITIS

This is an important cause of intestinal infection in immunocompromised patients and is common in AIDS. The virus infects the entire intestine, producing a severe chronic diarrhea that may cause death.

- Cytomegalovirus vasculitis may result in focal ischemic necrosis of the wall.
- Rarely, perforation of the intestine results.
- The diagnosis is established by demonstrating infected cells—greatly enlarged and containing large intranuclear inclusions and granular cytoplasmic inclusions—in endoscopic biopsy specimens.

SALMONELLA GASTROENTERITIS

Salmonella species other than *Salmonella typhi* are a common cause of bacterial "food poisoning" all over the world (Table 40–2). Infection results when food, water, and dairy products are contaminated with infected human or animal feces.

- Pasteurization of milk has decreased the incidence of this disease.
- Infection causes acute inflammation of the small intestine, with diffuse mucosal hyperemia, swelling, superficial ulceration, and neutrophil infiltration.
- It presents with an acute onset of fever, abdominal pain, and diarrhea for 1–3 days after infection.
- The disease is usually mild; rarely, a more severe illness with bacteremia may occur.

TYPHOID FEVER

Typhoid fever is caused by *Salmonella typhi*. The organism infects only humans, and infection results from contamination of food and water with feces from a case or carrier of typhoid. Typhoid is uncommon in the United States but is still prevalent in Third World countries.

Pathology & Clinical Features

- The ingested bacillus invades the small intestinal lymphoid tissue where it multiplies during the 1- to 3-week incubation period.
- At the end of the incubation period, the bacilli enter the bloodstream (bacteremic phase), resulting in fever, headache, and muscle aches.
- Many tissues, including liver, heart, kidney, lungs, meninges, and bone, may be infected during this phase.
- Fever may be accompanied by splenomegaly, a petechial skin rash (rose spots), bradycardia, and neutropenia.
- Diagnosis is established in the first week by blood culture, which is positive in 95% of cases.
- In the second week, *S typhi* reenters the intestinal lumen through bile (intestinal phase), now causing acute inflammation and necrosis of lymphoid tissue in the ileum and colon with mucosal ulceration.
- The mucosal ulcers take the shape of the underlying lymphoid follicles and are typically longitudinal (i.e. parallel to the long axis of the intestine).
- Microscopic examination shows edema and acute inflammation composed of macrophages, lymphocytes, and plasma cells.
- Clinically, the intestinal phase is characterized by diarrhea and continued fever.
- In the second week, stool and urine culture are positive. Blood culture is still positive in about 60% of patients.

Complications

- Bacteremia may cause meningitis, endocarditis, chrondritis, osteomyelitis, or widespread focal necrosis of muscle (Zenker's degeneration).
- Hemorrhage and perforation commonly complicate the intestinal phase.
- After clinical recovery, 5% of patients continue to excrete bacilli in urine or feces (carrier state).

SHIGELLA COLITIS (Bacillary Dysentery)

Shigella sonnei and *Shigella flexneri* are the common species and cause a relatively mild illness.

- *Shigella boydii* is uncommon.
- *Shigella dysenteriae* type I (Shiga's bacillus) produces a severe illness and is endemic in Central America and parts of Asia.
- *Shigella* dysentery is common in the United States.
- *Shigella* affects the colon, producing an acute inflammation with diffuse hyperemia, edema, neutrophil infiltration and superficial ulceration.
- Bacillary dysentery is an acute illness characterized by high fever, severe diarrhea with blood and mucus in the stool, and neutrophilic leukocytosis.
- Diagnosis is made by stool culture. Blood culture is rarely positive.

ENTEROINVASIVE ESCHERICHIA COLI INFECTION

Some strains of *Escherichia coli* invade the intestinal mucosa and cause a disease that resembles *Salmonella* enteritis and *Shigella* colitis.

- It causes epidemics of enterocolitis in neonatal units.
- Identification of serotypes of *E coli* that are invasive is very difficult.

CAMPYLOBACTER FETUS INFECTION

C fetus is responsible for about 10% of cases of bacterial diarrhea in children. The disease is acquired from infected humans and animals.

- Both small intestine and colon are affected, causing diarrhea and dysentery, usually mild.
- Diagnosis is by stool culture.
- Treatment with antibiotics is effective.

YERSINIA ENTEROCOLITICA & YERSINIA PSEUDOTUBERCULOSIS INFECTION

These two *Yersinia* species cause fever, diarrhea, and marked painful enlargement of mesenteric lymph nodes (mesenteric adenitis).

- Patients may have right lower quadrant abdominal pain that resembles acute appendicitis.
- Diagnosis is made by stool culture.

INTESTINAL TUBERCULOSIS

Primary intestinal tuberculosis has become rare as a result of pasteurization of milk and eradication of bovine tuberculosis in dairy herds.

- Most cases of intestinal tuberculosis are secondary and occur in adults.
- Secondary tuberculosis occurs as a result of:
  - Swallowing infected sputum by patients with active pulmonary disease.
  - Reactivation of a dormant intestinal focus, usually in the terminal ileum or cecum.
- It is characterized by caseous granulomatous inflammation.
- It forms mucosal ulcers that are transverse (i.e. perpendicular to the long axis of the intestine).
- Clinically, intestinal tuberculosis is a chronic illness characterized by low-grade fever and diarrhea.
- Rarely, a mass may be palpable in the right lower quadrant (hyperplastic cecal tuberculosis).
- The diagnosis is made by culturing tubercle bacilli from the stools.
- Complications of intestinal tuberculosis include:
  - Intestinal obstruction due to strictures associated with marked fibrosis.
  - Tuberculous peritonitis.
  - Fistulas between intestinal loops due to serosal involvement and extension of infection.

ATYPICAL MYCOBACTERIOSIS

Intestinal infection with *Mycobacterium avium-intracellulare* occurs in elderly or immunocompromised patients.

- *M avium-intracellulare* enteritis is one cause of severe chronic diarrhea in patients with AIDS.
- The organisms accumulate in large numbers in macrophages in the mucosa, and there is little or no inflammation.
- The diagnosis may be established by biopsy or by identification of the organism in stools on direct examination (using acid-fast stain) or culture.

ACUTE APPENDICITIS

Acute appendicitis is the commonest surgical emergency. It occurs at all ages, with a peak incidence in young adulthood.

- In most cases, inflammation of the appendix is preceded by obstruction of the appendiceal lumen (Fig 40–1).
- Multiple enteric bacteria including *Escherichia coli, Streptococcus faecalis,* and anaerobes are involved.

Pathology

- Acute inflammation of the mucosa rapidly extends to involve the entire wall. Suppuration commonly occurs.
- Grossly, the appendix is swollen and red, with a surface that is covered by a fibrinopurulent exudate.

Clinical Features

- It presents with acute onset of fever, abdominal pain, and vomiting.
- Pain is initially periumbilical (referred pain), but becomes localized to the right lower quadrant when the parietal peritoneum is involved.

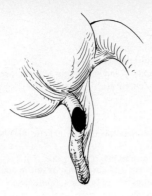

Acute appendicitis

Obstruction of lumen
- Fecalith
- Lymphoid hyper-
  plasia

Multiplication of
luminal bacteria
- Invasion of mucosa
  and wall
- Inflammation

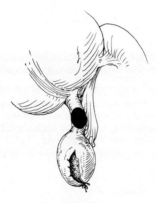

**Perforated acute
appendicitis**

- Rapid involvement
  of full thickness of
  wall
- Perforation
- Generalized
  peritonitis
- Pelvic abscess
- Subphrenic abscess

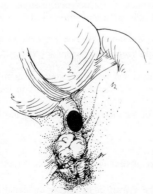

**Localized peritoneal
involvement**

- Inflammatory mass
  or "phlegmon"
- Suppuration
- Appendiceal
  abscess
- Necrosis of
  appendix
- Gangrenous
  appendicitis

Figure 40–1. Pathogenesis and complications of acute appendicitis.

- Tenderness and guarding are commonly present.
- The peripheral blood shows neutrophilic leukocytosis.
- The diagnosis is clinical, since laboratory and radiologic features are nonspecific.
- Surgical treatment (appendectomy) is curative.

Complications

- Local extension into periappendiceal tissues results in an inflammatory mass (**phlegmon**) in the right lower quadrant.
- Suppuration may cause an appendiceal abscess.
- Perforation of the appendix into the peritoneal cavity may result in acute peritonitis, and distant abscesses may form—commonly pelvic or subphrenic.
- Infection of the portal venous radicals—very rare—causes portal vein thrombophlebitis with multiple liver abscesses (pylephlebitis suppurativa).

PROTOZOAL INFECTIONS

AMOEBIASIS
Entamoeba histolytica is a common pathogen of the colon in underdeveloped countries. In the United States it occurs mainly in cities with high immigrant populations.

- Infection occurs by ingestion of cysts in food and water contaminated with feces.
- Ingested cysts release active amoebas (trophozoites) that invade the colonic mucosa and enter the submucosa, which is the site of maximum involvement.
- They cause necrosis and acute inflammation, leading to flask-shaped submucosal abscesses separated by healthy-appearing undermined mucosa.
- *E histolytica* trophozoites containing cytoplasmic erythrocytes are found in the abscess wall and necrotic material.
- In severe cases, necrosis involves the muscle, leading to intestinal perforation.
- Venous spread to the liver may occur (Chapter 42).
- Clinically, patients with amoebic colitis present with bloody and mucous diarrhea and low-grade fever.
- Diagnosis is made by finding trophozoites of *E histolytica* in stools or in a biopsy.
- Amoebicidal drugs such as metronidazole are highly effective in treatment.

GIARDIASIS
This is a common infection caused by the protozoan flagellate *Giardia lamblia*.

- Infection is by ingestion of cysts in food and water contaminated with feces.
- After ingestion, excystment and release of trophozoites occurs in the duodenum, which is maximally involved.
- *Giardia* attaches itself to the surface of the mucosal cells, causing mechanical interference and partial villous atrophy.
- Acute malabsorption results.
- The organism does not invade tissues.
- Clinically, infected individuals develop cramping abdominal pain, with diarrhea and steatorrhea.
- Diagnosis is made by identifying the organism in stools, duodenal aspirates, or duodenal biopsies.

INTESTINAL CRYPTOSPORIDIOSIS & ISOSPORIASIS IN AIDS

These two protozoa have been identified as common causes of chronic watery diarrhea in patients with AIDS.

- Diarrhea is severe and not uncommonly causes death.
- *Cryptosporidium* is present in large numbers, usually attached to the surface of the epithelial cell.
- Diagnosis is established by identifying the organism in stool smears stained with acid-fast stains.

TABLE 40–3. HELMINTHIC INFECTIONS OF THE INTESTINE

Parasite	Site	Clinical Effects
Ascaris lumbricoides (roundworm)	Small intestine	Intestinal obstruction by worm mass; migration up bile duct (cholangitis, gallstones) and pancreatic duct
	Lung (larval migration)	Cough, wheezing (Löffler's syndrome)
Enterobius vermicularis (pinworm)	Cecal region	Anal pruritus; migration up vagina, urethra (rare)
Trichuris trichiura (whipworm)	Colon	Bloody diarrhea, rectal prolapse (rare; only in heavy infestations)
Ancylostoma duodenale and *Necator americanus* (hookworm)	Small intestine	Iron deficiency anemia caused by sucking of blood by worm (common)
Strongyloides stercoralis	Small intestine	Bloody diarrhea
	Lung (larval migration)	Hyperinfection in immunodeficient patients
Trichinella spiralis	Small intestine	Abdominal pain and diarrhea
	Parasitemia	Myositis, myocarditis, encephalitis
Taenia solium	Small intestine	Asymptomatic
	Larval migration	Cysticercosis
Taenia saginata	Small intestine	Asymptomatic
Diphyllobothrium latum	Small intestine	Vitamin B_{12} deficiency
Schistosoma mansoni	Colon	Bloody diarrhea; portal hypertension
Schistosoma japonicum	Small intestine	Diarrhea; portal hypertension
Fasciolopsis buski	Small intestine	Abdominal pain, diarrhea (with heavy infestations)

INTESTINAL HELMINTHIASIS

Intestinal helminthiasis has been estimated as inflicting about 25% of the world population. In many of these diseases, the worm lives in the lumen without causing major
symptoms; in others, significant clinical manifestations occur (Table 40–3).

II. IDIOPATHIC INFLAMMATORY BOWEL DISEASE

The term *idiopathic inflammatory bowel disease* is used for two diseases—**Crohn's
disease** and **ulcerative colitis.** Though their causes are unknown, the two diseases
probably have an immunologic basis. Nevertheless, they are two distinct entities with
distinct clinical and pathologic features (Table 40–4). In 10% of patients with idiopathic
inflammatory bowel disease affecting the colon, features of both Crohn's disease and
ulcerative colitis are present (indeterminate idiopathic inflammatory bowel disease).

CROHN'S DISEASE

Most commonly, Crohn's disease affects the ileum and colon, but it has the potential to
involve any part of the gastrointestinal tract from the mouth to the anus. It is characterized by involvement of discontinuous segments of intestine ("skip areas"), noncaseating epithelioid cell granulomas, and transmural (full-thickness) inflammation of the
affected parts (Fig 40–2).

Incidence

It occurs mainly in Western Europe and the United States and is uncommon in Asia and
South America.

- In the United States, it affects chiefly whites; blacks, Native Americans, and His-
  panics are less frequently affected. The highest incidence is in Jews.
- Both sexes are affected equally. The disease can occur at any age but is commonest in
  young adults.
- There is a positive family history in 20–30% of cases.

Etiology

Despite extensive search, no infectious agent has been found.

- Evidence of an immunologic basis includes:
  - Identification of antibodies against intestinal epithelial cells in the serum and
    lymphocytes.
  - Frequent T cell dysfunction (anergy to tuberculin and mumps antigen, low pe-
    ripheral blood T cell count).

Pathology (Fig 40–2)
A. Sites of involvement:

- Combined ileal and colonic disease is most common (50%).
- The ileum alone is involved in 30% of patients and the colon alone in 20%.

TABLE 40–4. DIFFERENCES BETWEEN ULCERATIVE COLITIS AND CROHN'S COLITIS

	Ulcerative Colitis	Crohn's Colitis
Clinical features		
Rectal involvement	Over 90%	Rectum spared in > 50%
Distribution of lesions	Continuous	Skip lesions
Mucosal appearance	Friable, purulent, diffusely involved	Aphthous, linear ulcers with cobblestoning
Associated ileal disease	10%, mild, terminal ileal inflammation	50% have combined ileal and colon involvement
Perianal abscess, fistulas	Rare	Common
Intestinal strictures and obstruction	Not seen	Common
Intestinal fistulas	Not seen	Common
Fissures (radiologic)	Not seen	Common
Intestinal perforation	Rare	Rare
Intestinal hemorrhage (severe)	Common	Rare
Pathologic features		
Depth of inflammation	Mucosal (submucosal rarely)	Transmural
Creeping mesenteric fat	Not seen	Common
Fibrous thickening of wall	Not seen	Common ("lead pipe")
Crypt abscesses	Common	Common
Pseudopolyps	Common	Common
Granulomas (epithelioid, noncaseating)	Not seen	Common
Fissures (microscopic)	Not seen	Common
Dysplasia	Common	Rare
Carcinoma	10%	Rare

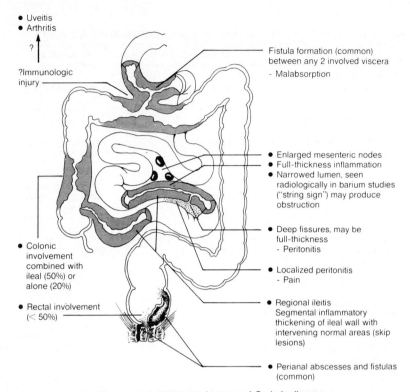

- Uveitis
- Arthritis

?

?Immunologic injury

- Colonic involvement combined with ileal (50%) or alone (20%)

- Rectal involvement (< 50%)

Fistula formation (common) between any 2 involved viscera
- Malabsorption

- Enlarged mesenteric nodes
- Full-thickness inflammation
- Narrowed lumen, seen radiologically in barium studies ("string sign") may produce obstruction

- Deep fissures, may be full-thickness
- Peritonitis

- Localized peritonitis
- Pain

- Regional ileitis Segmental inflammatory thickening of ileal wall with intervening normal areas (skip lesions)

- Perianal abscesses and fistulas (common)

Figure 40–2. Pathologic features of Crohn's disease.

- Involvement of the oral cavity, larynx, esophagus, stomach, and perineum are rare.
- Seventy-five percent of patients have perianal lesions such as abscesses, fistulas, and skin tags. Perianal disease is independent of rectal involvement.

B. Gross appearance:

- Involvement is typically segmental, with skip areas of normal intestine between areas of involved bowel.
- Normal and affected intestine are sharply demarcated from one another.
- In the acute phase, the intestine is swollen and reddened. The mucosa shows diffuse hyperemia, acute inflammation, and ulceration.
- In the chronic phase, the affected segment is greatly thickened and rigid ("lead pipe" or "garden hose" appearance).
- In involved ileal segments, the mesenteric fat creeps from the mesentery to surround the bowel wall ("creeping fat").
- The mucosal surface shows longitudinal serpiginous ulcers separated by irregular islands of edematous mucosa ("cobblestone" effect).

C. Microscopic features:

- It is characterized by distortion of mucosal crypt architecture, transmural inflammation, and epithelioid granulomas.
- Granulomas are present in about 60% of patients.
- Fissure ulcers are a typical feature.
- The regional mesenteric lymph nodes are frequently enlarged and may contain noncaseating granulomas.

Clinical Features

- In the acute phase, fever, diarrhea, and right lower quadrant pain may mimic acute appendicitis.
- Chronic disease is characterized by remissions and relapses that may last several months.
- Active disease is characterized by diarrhea, weight loss, anemia, and low-grade fever.
- Thickening of the intestine may produce an ill-defined abdominal mass.

Diagnosis

- Diagnosis is based on a combination of clinical, radiologic, and pathologic findings.
- There is no specific laboratory test.

Complications

- Intestinal obstruction is a common complication of the extensive transmural fibrosis.
- Fistula formation occurs between involved loops of bowel and adjacent viscera (bladder, vagina).
- Malabsorption syndrome may also follow disease in the terminal ileum due to failure of absorption of vitamin B_{12} and bile acids.
- Iron deficiency anemia may occur as a result of chronic occult bleeding, and protein-losing enteropathy as a result of loss of protein from the inflamed mucosa.
- Extraintestinal manifestations include arthritis and uveitis.
- Crohn's disease carries a very slightly increased risk of development of carcinoma of the colon—much less than in ulcerative colitis.

ULCERATIVE COLITIS

Incidence
In the United States, about 400,000 patients suffer from ulcerative colitis, and there are about 25,000 new cases every year.

- It is common in the 20- to 30-year age group but may occur at any age.
- It is slightly commoner in females than in males.
- In the United States, whites are more often affected than blacks, and Jews more often than non-Jews.
- Worldwide, the disease is most prevalent in North America and Western Europe and less prevalent in Asia, Africa, and South America.

Etiology
The cause is unknown; no infectious agent has been identified.

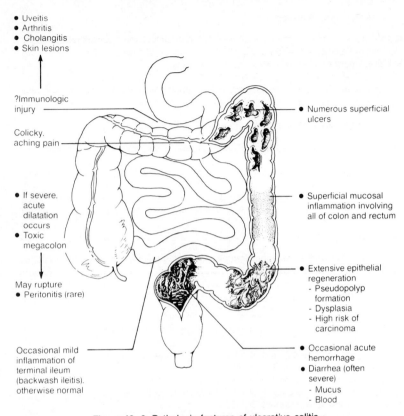

- Uveitis
- Arthritis
- Cholangitis
- Skin lesions

?Immunologic injury

Colicky. aching pain

- If severe. acute dilatation occurs
- Toxic megacolon

May rupture
- Peritonitis (rare)

Occasional mild inflammation of terminal ileum (backwash ileitis). otherwise normal

- Numerous superficial ulcers

- Superficial mucosal inflammation involving all of colon and rectum

- Extensive epithelial regeneration
  - Pseudopolyp formation
  - Dysplasia
  - High risk of carcinoma

- Occasional acute hemorrhage
- Diarrhea (often severe)
  - Mucus
  - Blood

Figure 40–3. Pathologic features of ulcerative colitis.

- Antibodies that cross-react with intestinal epithelial cells and certain serotypes of *Escherichia coli* have been demonstrated in the serum of some patients.
- Psychologic stress frequently precipitates ulcerative colitis.

Pathology (Fig 40–3)
A. Sites of involvement:

- The rectum is involved in almost all cases and in some patients remains the only site of disease.
- Involvement tends to extend proximally from the rectum in a continuous manner without skip areas.
- Total colonic involvement is not uncommon.
- The ileum is not involved as a rule; 10% of cases show mild nonspecific mucosal inflammation for a few centimeters proximal to the ileocecal valve ("backwash ileitis").

B. Gross appearance:

- Ulcerative colitis involves mainly the mucosa, which shows diffuse hyperemia with numerous superficial ulcerations in the acute phase ("velvety" appearance).
- There is rarely any thickening of the wall.
- In the chronic phase of the disease, the mucosa appears flat and atrophic.
- The regenerated or nonulcerated mucosa may appear polypoid (inflammatory "pseudopolyps") in contrast with the atrophic areas or ulcers.

C. Microscopic appearance:

- In the acute phase, the mucosa shows marked inflammation with neutrophils in lamina propria and glands (crypt abscesses).
- In the chronic phase, the crypts are decreased in number (crypt atrophy) and show distorted architecture due to abnormal branching, and there are numerous chronic inflammatory cells in the lamina propria.
- The inflammation is usually restricted to the mucosa and superficial submucosa.

Clinical Features

- In the acute phase and during relapse, the patient has fever, leukocytosis, lower abdominal pain, and diarrhea with blood and mucus.
- The disease usually has a chronic course, with remissions and exacerbations.
- Some patients have a chromic continuous disease with mild diarrhea and bleeding.

Diagnosis

Diagnosis is based on a combination of clinical, radiologic, and pathologic findings.

- In mucosal biopsies, crypt atrophy, distortion of crypt architecture, and an increased number of lymphocytes and plasma cells are diagnostic of idiopathic inflammatory bowel disease, but can be seen in both ulcerative colitis and Crohn's disease.
- The only finding on mucosal biopsy that reliably differentiates ulcerative colitis and Crohn's disease is the presence of noncaseating epithelioid granulomas in the latter.

Complications

- Severe bleeding may occur in the acute phase.
- Toxic megacolon in severe acute disease is characterized by dilatation of the colon with functional obstruction and, rarely, perforation. It carries a high mortality rate and requires emergency colectomy.
- Extraintestinal manifestations occur more commonly in ulcerative colitis than in Crohn's disease. They include:
  - Arthritis.
  - Uveitis.
  - Skin lesions, including pyoderma gangrenosum.
  - Sclerosing pericholangitis, which causes obstructive jaundice.
- Patients with chronic ulcerative colitis have an increased risk of developing colon carcinoma.
  - The overall risk is about 10%.
  - The risk increases progressively with:

o Disease duration beyond 7 years.
o Involvement of the entire colon (pancolitis).
o Onset at an early age.
o The presence of severe dysplasia in mucosal biopsies.

The Intestines: III. Neoplasms

41

I. BENIGN EPITHELIAL TUMORS

BENIGN NEOPLASMS

COLONIC ADENOMA
Adenomas of the colon are present in 20–30% of all individuals over age 50.

1. TUBULAR ADENOMA (Adenomatous Polyp)
These account for over 90% of colonic adenomas.

- They are commonly multiple, 10–20 lesions being present in some patients.
- The are pedunculated with a well-defined stalk (Fig 41–1B).
- Histologically, neoplastic glands are lined by epithelial cells which are hyperchromatic and stratified and show loss of normal mucin content ("adenomatous change").
- The proliferating epithelium is confined to the mucosa with no evidence of invasion of the stalk (Fig 41–1B).
- Tubular adenomas can be removed by colonoscopy.
- Tubular adenomas are premalignant lesions. Though the risk of cancer is 1–3%, the frequency of these polyps in the population makes them the most important precancerous colonic lesion.
- The risk of carcinoma increases with:
  - Increasing size of the polyp over 2 cm.
  - Increasing number of adenomatous polyps.
  - Increasing degrees of epithelial dysplasia.
- The only means of differentiating a tubular adenoma from a polypoid adenocarcinoma is by the presence of stalk invasion in the latter (Fig 41–1B).
- The risk of lymph node involvement in a cancerous polyp with tumor confined to the upper part of the stalk (Fig 41–1B) is only about 1–2%. Simple removal of such a malignant polyp with stalk invasion is therefore curative in 98–99% of cases.
- When the invasion by cancer cells involves the base of the polyp (Fig 41–1B), the patient needs colon resection to remove residual cancer.
- Clinically, most patients with tubular adenomas are asymptomatic. A few will present with overt rectal bleeding. Most will have occult blood in the stools if multiple samples are taken.
- Diagnosis is made by colonoscopic visualization and biopsy. Adenomatous polyps

A

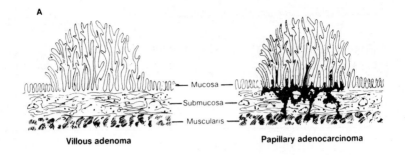

Villous adenoma   Papillary adenocarcinoma

B

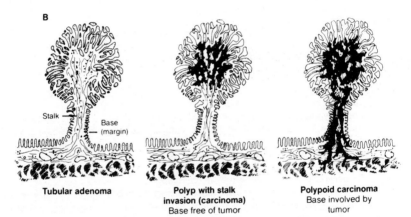

Tubular adenoma   Polyp with stalk invasion (carcinoma) Base free of tumor   Polypoid carcinoma Base involved by tumor

Figure 41–1. Villous adenoma (**A**) and tubular adenoma (**B**) of the colon, with their malignant counterparts. Dark areas represent invasive carcinoma.

must be distinguished histologically from other types of polyp (hyperplastic, juvenile retention, hamartomatous, inflammatory, lymphoid, etc.)

2. VILLOUS ADENOMA

These comprise less than 10% of colonic adenomas.

- They commonly occur in older individuals as a solitary large, sessile lesion (Fig 41–1A), most commonly in the rectum.
- They appear grossly as soft, velvety, papillary growths that project into the lumen. Even large growths may be difficult to feel on digital rectal examination.
- They are usually 1–5 cm in diameter and cause rectal bleeding or mucous discharge.
- Diagnosis may be made by colonoscopy and biopsy.

- Histologically, villous adenoma is composed of neoplastic proliferation of colonic epithelial cells organized into long fingerlike papillary or villous processes.
- They cannot be removed endoscopically.
- Villous adenoma differs from a papillary adenocarcinoma by the absence of invasion of the muscularis mucosae at the base of the lesion (Fig 41–1A).
- Villous adenomas have a 30–70% incidence of carcinoma.
- Treatment usually consists of surgical excision.

NONNEOPLASTIC EPITHELIAL TUMORS

INTESTINAL HAMARTOMAS

These are uncommon polyps of the intestinal mucosa. They can be found as isolated lesions anywhere in the intestine and as familial hamartomatous polyposis in Peutz-Jeghers syndrome (see following).

- They are composed of a disorganized proliferating mass of intestinal epithelium, various intestinal glands, and smooth muscle.
- All constituent tissues are histologically normal.
- They are not associated with an increased risk of carcinoma.

HYPERPLASTIC POLYPS

Hyperplastic polyps are very common in the colonic mucosa.

- They are commonly small (usually <5 mm in diameter) and appear as small sessile polyps in the mucosa.
- They are composed of hyperplastic colonic epithelial cells with basal nuclei and markedly increased cytoplasmic mucin. The lumens of glands are serrated.
- They do not have an increased risk of cancer.

JUVENILE RETENTION POLYPS

Juvenile retention polyps are common, occurring mainly in the rectum in children and young adults. They are characterized by cystically dilated mucous glands lined by flat epithelium surrounded by an inflamed stroma. They are not associated with an increased risk of carcinoma.

FAMILIAL POLYPOSIS SYNDROMES (Table 41–1)

FAMILIAL POLYPOSIS COLI

Polyposis coli is the commonest of the familial polyposis syndromes. It has an autosomal dominant inheritance pattern.

- It is characterized by multiple adenomatous polyps, exceeding 100 in all cases and frequently innumerable.
- Polyps are not present at birth but begin to appear at about 10–20 years of age.
- Clinically, there is rectal bleeding.
- Diagnosis is made by demonstration of numerous adenomas by colonoscopy and biopsy.
- Colon carcinoma supervenes in 100% of cases. The mean age at development of carcinoma is 35–40 years.
- Total colectomy to prevent cancer is essential.

TABLE 41-1. FAMILIAL POLYPOSIS SYNDROMES

Syndrome	Type of Polyp	Locations	Cancer Risk	Inheritance[1]	Other Features
Polyposis coli	Adenoma	Colon	100%	AD	
Gardner's syndrome	Adenoma	Colon, small intestine	100%	AD	Bone and soft tissue lesions; ampullary cancer common
Turcot's syndrome	Adenoma	Colon	100%	?AR	Nervous system neoplasms
Peutz-Jeghers syndrome	Hamartoma	Jejunum, rest of intestine	Slight increase	AD	Pigmentation in mouth; theca or granulosa cell tumors of ovary
Juvenile polyposis[2]	Retention	Colon	Slight increase	AD	

[1]AD/AR = autosomal dominant/recessive.
[2]Canada-Cronkite syndrome is a nonfamilial juvenile polyposis syndrome.

GARDNER'S SYNDROME
Gardner's syndrome is similar to polyposis coli in inheritance pattern, appearance of the colon, and risk of carcinoma.

■ It differs from polyposis coli in:
  ● The presence of adenomatous polyps elsewhere in the intestinal tract.
  ● The presence of extraintestinal lesions such as osteomas in the jaw bones, epidermal cysts, fibromas in the skin, and fibromatosis of soft tissues.
  ● An increased incidence of periampullary (duodenal) carcinoma.

TURCOT'S SYNDROME
This is an extremely rare syndrome characterized by the association of multiple colonic adenomas with central nervous system neoplasms (usually glioblastoma multiforme).

■ It is inherited as an autosomal recessive trait.
■ It has a 100% risk of colon carcinoma, which tends to occur at an earlier age.

PEUTZ-JEGHERS SYNDROME
This is characterized by hamartomatous polyps throughout the intestine, with maximum density in the jejunum. Patients have pigmented macules in the circumoral skin and buccal mucosa. There is a slightly increased risk of colon carcinoma.

JUVENILE POLYPOSIS SYNDROME

This is a very rare syndrome characterized by the presence of multiple juvenile retention polyps in the colon. There is a slightly increased risk of colon carcinoma. An acquired form of multiple juvenile polyposis is called Canada-Cronkite syndrome.

PRIMARY MALIGNANT EPITHELIAL NEOPLASMS

CARCINOMA OF THE COLON & RECTUM

Incidence

Colorectal carcinoma accounts for over 90% of malignant neoplasms of the intestine. It is second only to lung cancer as a cause of cancer deaths in the United States—over 50,000 a year—when both sexes are considered together.

- It is common in North America and Europe and uncommon in Asia, Africa, and South America.
- About 110,000 new cases occur every year in the United States.
- 90% of cases occur over age 50.
- Females show a 2 : 1 preponderance of colon cancer; rectal cancer is slightly more common in males.

Etiology

The cause of colorectal carcinoma is unknown. The high incidence in developed countries is thought to be due to a diet rich in animal fat and low in fiber.

Premalignant Lesions

Most colon carcinomas are believed to arise in premalignant lesions, only a few arising de novo in previously normal mucosa.

- Heredofamilial adenomatous polyposis syndromes have a 100% risk of colon cancer.
- Villous adenomas have 30–70% risk.
- The overall risk is 10% in chronic ulcerative colitis. Prophylactic colectomy is justified when there is total colonic involvement, disease over 10 years in duration, and epithelial dysplasia on biopsy.
- Tubular adenomas have a 1–3% risk of carcinoma, but because they are so common they are believed to be the most frequent precursor lesion for colon carcinoma.

Pathology (Fig 41–2)

The rectosigmoid region accounts for about 50% of colon carcinomas, the remainder being distributed throughout the colon. Multiple carcinomas are present in 5% of cases.

- Carcinomas in the right side of the colon tend to be large polypoid masses that project into the lumen.
- Left-sided cancers tend to involve the whole circumference and often constrict the lumen ("napkinring" or "apple core").
- Rectal carcinomas are most commonly malignant ulcers with raised everted edges.
- Microscopically, most colon carcinomas are adenocarcinomas of varying differentiation.

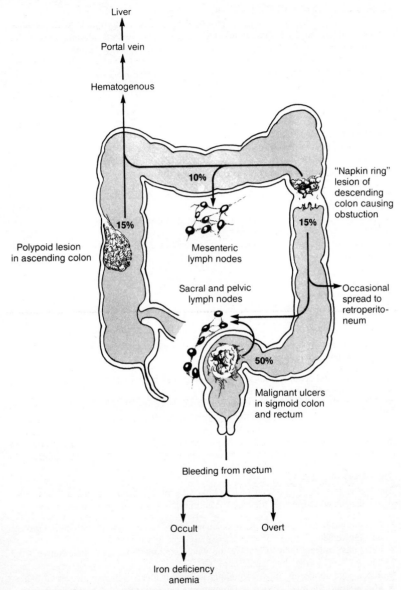

Figure 41-2. Colon carcinoma—sites, gross appearances, and spread.

Clinical Features

Colon carcinoma is asymptomatic in its early stages. Diagnosis can only be made by screening sigmoidoscopy, which is recommended after age 40.

- Asymptomatic rectal carcinomas are detected by rectal examination, which should be part of every routine physical examination.
- The earliest detectable abnormality is the presence of occult blood in the stools. Testing stools for occult blood is the only cost-effective means of detecting early colon carcinoma.
- Chronic intestinal blood loss causes iron deficiency anemia. All patients with iron deficiency anemia must be evaluated for intestinal cancer.
- Symptoms in colon carcinoma are any change in bowel habits, including constipation and diarrhea, and bleeding per rectum.
- Left-sided colon cancers commonly present with intestinal obstruction.
- Right-sided carcinomas commonly present with abdominal pain, weight loss, anemia, and a palpable mass.

Diagnosis & Treatment

Colonoscopy and barium enema examination are accurate.

- Colonoscopy permits biopsy and pathologic diagnosis.
- Surgical resection of the involved segment of colon is the primary treatment.
- Radiotherapy and chemotherapy are not very effective.

Prognostic Factors

A. Clinicopathologic stage is an expression of the degree of spread, and is determined by microscopic examination of the resected colon. This is the most important prognostic factor. The most commonly used staging system in the United States is the Astler-Coller modification of Dukes' system (Table 41–2).

B. Histologic grade is an expression of the degree of differentiation of the adenocar-

TABLE 41–2. ASTLER-COLLER MODIFICATION OF DUKES STAGING SYSTEM FOR COLON CARCINOMA

Dukes Stage	Invasion of Colonic Wall	Lymph Node Metastases	Distant Metastases	Five-Year Survival Rate
A	Mucosa and submucosa[1]	No	No	> 90%
B1	Partial muscle wall thickness	No	No	67%
B2	Full thickness of muscle wall	No	No	55%
C1	Partial muscle wall thickness	Yes	No	40%
C2	Full thickness of muscle wall	Yes	No	20%
D	Any	Yes or No	Yes	< 10%

[1] Involvement of the submucosa is not addressed in the original Astler-Coller classification, and is placed in stage A arbitrarily. Some authorities place submucosal lesions in stage B1.

cinoma. It is a minor prognostic factor. Poorly differentiated (grade III) neoplasms and those with large amounts of extracellular mucin (mucinous carcinoma) have a worse prognosis than well-differentiated (grade I) carcinoma.

C. Vascular invasion is a minor adverse prognostic factor.

CARCINOMA OF THE ANAL CANAL
Anal canal carcinoma is rare but is being seen with increasing frequency in anoreceptive male homosexuals.

- Sexual transmission of human papilloma virus is strongly suspected of causing this neoplasm.
- Pathologically, there is an infiltrative mass in the anal canal.
- Histologic types include:
  - Squamous carcinoma.
  - Basaloid (or cloacogenic) carcinoma which arises at the anorectal junction.
- Clinically, patients present with rectal discomfort, discharge, bleeding, or a mass.
- Treatment by radiation and chemotherapy in combination with surgery has improved survival rates considerably.

ADENOCARCINOMA OF THE SMALL INTESTINE
Carcinoma of the small intestine is very rare, and accounts for less than 1% of malignant gastrointestinal neoplasms. The most common location for small intestine carcinoma is the periampullary region of the duodenum. The pathologic features, staging scheme, and prognosis are similar to those of colon carcinoma.

MUCINOUS NEOPLASMS OF THE APPENDIX
Mucinous neoplasms occur rarely in the appendix.

- Most are benign mucinous cystadenomas that are differentiated from low-grade mucinous cystadenocarcinoma by the absence of invasion.
- Pathologically, the lumen of the appendix is dilated, filled with mucin and lined by the neoplastic mucinous epithelium.
- Invasion of the wall may lead to extensive seeding of the peritoneum and mucinous peritonitis, characterized by mucin lakes containing adenocarcinoma cells (pseudo-myxoma peritonei).

II. PRIMARY NONEPITHELIAL NEOPLASMS

MALIGNANT LYMPHOMA
The intestine is a common site of primary extranodal malignant lymphoma, most often non-Hodgkin's lymphomas of B cell type.

- Lymphomas may occur in any part of the intestine. The ileocecal region is a favored site for Burkitt's lymphoma.
- An increased incidence of intestinal lymphoma is seen in:
  - AIDS.

- Alpha heavy chain disease (see Chapter 30).
- Celiac disease.

SMOOTH MUSCLE NEOPLASMS

Leiomyoma and leiomyosarcoma are the commonest mesenchymal neoplasms of the intestine.

- They may form submucosal polypoid masses that precipitate intussusception or large mural masses.
- Ulceration with bleeding and intestinal obstruction are common presenting features. A mass may be palpable.
- The likelihood of malignancy in smooth muscle tumors increases with increasing size, the presence of necrosis, and mitotic rate.
- Even leiomyosarcomas tend to be well-circumscribed, and surgical removal has a 60% 5-year survival rate.

CARCINOID TUMORS

Origin & Sites of Occurrence

Carcinoid tumors arise from neuroendocrine cells present in the mucosa throughout the gastrointestinal tract.

- The tip of the appendix is the most common site for carcinoid tumor (Table 41–3). Appendiceal carcinoids are usually incidental findings at appendectomy, are almost always less than 2 cm in diameter, and are benign in over 95% of cases. Only those rare tumors that are over 2 cm in diameter have potentially malignant behavior.
- The ileum is the next most frequent site. Ileal carcinoids are malignant in about 60% of cases. Most malignant ileal carcinoids are over 1 cm in diameter.

Pathology

Grossly, carcinoid tumors are firm, yellow nodules in the submucosa, elevating and ulcerating the mucosa and locally infiltrating the wall.

- Multiple lesions are present in 25% of cases.
- They may be associated with marked fibrosis and distortion of the intestine.
- Microscopically, they are composed of nests and cords of small, uniform round cells separated by vascular channels.

TABLE 41–3. INCIDENCE AND RISK OF CANCER OF INTESTINAL CARCINOIDS

Site	Incidence	Percentage Malignant
Appendix	40%	1%
Ileum	25%	60%
Rectum	20%	15%
Stomach	5%	?High
Colon	10%	?High

- Local and blood vessel invasion is common and does not correlate with malignant behavior. Malignancy in a carcinoid tumor is certain only when metastases occur.
- Histologic diagnosis can be confirmed by:
  - Affinity for silver stains (argentaffin positive).
  - Positive staining for neuron-specific enolase or chromogranin by immunoperoxidase.
  - Presence in the cytoplasm of membrane-bound dense- core neurosecretory granules by electron microscopy.
- Carcinoid tumors commonly secrete amines—notably 5-hydroxytryptamine (serotonin) and histamine—or polypeptide hormones.

Clinical Features

The average age at presentation for carcinoid tumors is 55 years, but there is a wide age distribution.

- Most are asymptomatic and are incidental findings at appendectomy and autopsy.
- The most common clinical presentation of carcinoid tumor is intestinal obstruction.
- **Carcinoid syndrome:**
  - Is a rare presentation of a carcinoid tumor resulting from the entry of serotonin into the systemic circulation.
  - Serotonin secretion by an intestinal carcinoid does not cause carcinoid syndrome because the serotonin produced is inactivated to 5-hydroxyindole acetic acid in the liver.
  - Occurs only when a malignant intestinal carcinoid has metastasized to the liver. Serotonin produced by the hepatic metastases reaches the systemic circulation.
  - Is characterized by abdominal cramps, diarrhea, bronchospasm, episodic cutaneous flushing, and pulmonary valve stenosis.

III. METASTATIC NEOPLASMS

Metastases to the intestine occur rarely. The most common are lung carcinoma and malignant melanoma. Direct invasion of the colon by carcinomas of the urinary bladder and cervix is not rare, and may result in fistulas.

The Liver: I. Manifestations of Disease; Infections

42

MANIFESTATIONS OF LIVER DISEASE

PAIN

Pain is an uncommon symptom of liver disease. It is caused by stretching of the capsule when rapid enlargement of the liver occurs. It occurs in acute hepatitis and right heart failure.

ALTERATION IN LIVER SIZE

Most liver diseases are associated with palpable hepatomegaly.

- Enlargement may be localized in a focal lesion such as neoplasm or abscess.
- The enlarged liver of heart failure is firm, tender, and has a smooth surface.
- The enlarged liver of cirrhosis is firm and has a nodular surface.
- Shrinkage of the liver occurs in massive liver necrosis and some forms of cirrhosis.

ABNORMAL LIVER FUNCTION TESTS (Table 42-1)

An abnormality in a liver function test detected on routine blood examination is a common presentation of liver disease.

- Patients with asymptomatic chronic liver disease (eg, chronic hepatitis, cirrhosis) may show decreased serum albumin, increased enzyme levels, or an increased prothrombin time.
- Patients with mass lesions in the liver may have an elevated alkaline phosphatase level in serum.

JAUNDICE

Jaundice manifests in an increase in the plasma bilirubin above its normal upper limit of 0.8 mg/dL. The different types of jaundice can be diagnosed by laboratory testing (Table 42-2).

Etiology

    A. Hemolytic jaundice (see Chapter 25).
    B. Hepatocellular Jaundice:

- **Defective hepatic uptake of bilirubin** due to absence of intracellular transport proteins occurs in **Gilbert's syndrome.** This is an autosomal dominant trait characterized by transient episodes of mild jaundice, usually precipitated by intercurrent illness. Patients have a normal life expectancy.

465

TABLE 42-1. LIVER FUNCTION TESTS

Test[1]	Functional Significance
*Serum bilirubin levels Indirect (unconjugated)	↑ in hemolysis or defective bilirubin uptake
Direct (conjugated)	↑ in hepatocellular failure and biliary obstruction
*Urine bilirubin	↑ in biliary obstruction
*Urine urobilinogen	↓ in biliary obstruction
	↑ hemolysis, hepatocellular failure
Dye excretion tests (rose bengal, Bromsulphalein)[2]	↓ in hepatocellular damage and biliary obstruction
*Serum alkaline phosphatase	↑ in biliary obstruction, mass lesions of liver
*Serum aspartate and alanine aminotransferase[3]	↑ ↑ ↑ in liver cell necrosis
	↑ in obstruction
*Serum albumin (albumin : globulin ratio)[4]	↓ albumin in hepatocellular failure; globulin levels ↑ in chronic liver disease
Serum ammonia (NH_3)	↑ in hepatocellular failure
Serum cholesterol	↓ in hepatitis and cirrhosis
	↑ in biliary obstruction
*Prothrombin time (one stage)	prolonged in biliary obstruction and liver damage; reflects ↓ synthesis of prothrombin, coagulation factors V, VII, and X
Plasma glucose	↓ in acute liver failure
*Serum alpha-fetoprotein	↑ in hepatocellular carcinoma (also some cases of cirrhosis with active regeneration)
*Serum α_1-antitrypsin	↓ in α_1-antitrypsin deficiency
Serum ceruloplasmin	↓ in Wilson's disease
Serum free copper (or liver cell copper)	↑ in Wilson's disease (lesser increases in primary biliary cirrhosis)
Serum iron	↑ in hemochromatosis

[1] Asterisk indicates most commonly used tests.
[2] Dye excretion tests are largely obsolete; BSP (sulfobromophthalein, Bromsulphalein) is sensitive but may produce hypersensitivity reactions.
[3] Liver enzymes; aspartate aminotransferase (AST), formerly known as GOT (glutamate oxaloacetic transferase); and alanine aminotransferase (ALT), formerly known as GPT (glutamate pyruvate transferase) are most commonly used. Lactate dehydrogenase and isocitrate dehydrogenase are also used to detect liver cell necrosis.
[4] Various flocculation tests reflected these changes in serum albumin and globulin but are now obsolete.

TABLE 42–2. LABORATORY FINDINGS IN THE DIFFERENTIAL DIAGNOSIS OF JAUNDICE

Type of Jaundice	Blood						Stools Color	Urine	
	Hct	Unconjugated Bilirubin (Indirect)	Conjugated Bilirubin (Direct)	Alkaline Phosphatase	Aminotransferases	Cholesterol		Bilirubin	Urobilinogen
Hemolytic	↓	↑↑	N	N	N	N	N	0	↑
Hepatocellular									
Gilbert's syndrome	N	↑	N	N	N	N	N	0	N or ↓
Abnormal conjugation	N	↑	N	N	N	N	N	0	N or ↓
Hepatocellular damage	N	↑	↑	↑	↑↑	N	N	↑	↑
Obstructive									
Defective excretion	N	N	↑	N	N	N	N	↑	N
Intrahepatic cholestasis	N	N	↑	↑	N	N or ↑	Pale	↑	↓
Extrahepatic biliary obstruction	N	N	↑	↑↑	N or ↑	↑	Pale	↑	↓

- **Abnormal conjugation of bilirubin** due to deficiency of UDP-glucuronyl transferase occurs in:
  - **Neonates (neonatal or physiologic jaundice),** particularly in premature infants.
  - **Crigler-Najjar syndrome,** a very rare autosomal recessive disease characterized by severe jaundice and death in early life.
  - **Novobiocin therapy.**
- **Hepatocellular damage:**
  - Acute or chronic, leads to jaundice when the number of functioning liver cells is sufficiently reduced.
  - Jaundice is commonly due to intrahepatic cholestasis and failure of conjugation, producing a mixed conjugated and unconjugated hyperbilirubinemia.

C. Obstructive jaundice:

- **Defective excretion** of conjugated bilirubin from the liver cell into the biliary canaliculus occurs in the inherited **Dubin-Johnson syndrome** and **Rotor's syndrome.** The defect is usually partial; life expectancy is normal.
- Obstruction to flow of bile in the intralobular biliary canaliculi is called **intrahepatic cholestasis,** which occurs in:
  - Viral hepatitis.
  - Alcoholic liver disease.
  - Drug toxicity to androgens (methyltestosterone), anabolic steroids, oral contraceptives, and phenothiazines.
  - Benign familial cholestatic jaundice.
  - The last trimester of pregnancy (recurrent jaundice of pregnancy).
- **Extrahepatic biliary obstruction** causes jaundice when obstruction involves both main hepatic ducts, the common hepatic duct, or the common bile duct.

Effects

It causes yellow discoloration of tissues, most easily seen in the sclera. Jaundice must always be confirmed by serum bilirubin measurement because other pigments such as carotene may cause yellow discoloration of eyes.

- Deposition of bilirubin by itself does not cause symptoms.
- Patients with obstructive jaundice frequently have intense pruritus believed to be caused by bile acids, which also accumulate in serum.
- Unconjugated hyperbilirubinemia in the neonatal period causes kernicterus (see Chapter 1).

HEPATOCELLULAR FAILURE (Fig 42–1)

Acute Liver Failure
A. Causes:

- **Massive liver cell necrosis** due to:
  - Viral hepatitis (B and C).
  - Drugs (halothane, isoniazid, acetaminophen).
  - Toxic chemicals (chloroform, mushroom poisoning).
- Acute fatty change of the liver (see Chapter 1):
  - **Reye's syndrome,** a disease of children characterized by acute liver failure plus

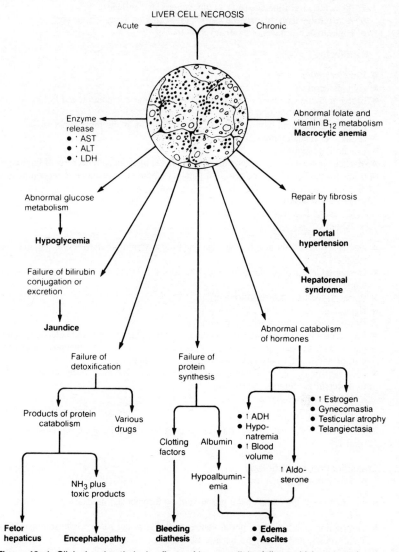

Figure 42–1. Clinical and pathologic effects of hepatocellular failure, which commonly results from conditions associated with acute or chronic necrosis of liver cells.

acute fatty change in liver, kidney, and heart, which has been linked to aspirin use for acute viral illnesses such as chickenpox and influenza.

● **Acute fatty liver of pregnancy,** which occurs in the last trimester.
● High-dosage intravenous **tetracycline** therapy.

B. Effects:

■ Jaundice, often severe.
■ Hypoglycemia.
■ Bleeding tendency, due to disseminated intravascular coagulation and failure of synthesis of clotting factors.
■ Electrolyte and acid-base disturbances (hypokalemia is the most dangerous).
■ Hepatic encephalopathy.
■ Hepatorenal syndrome.
■ Marked elevation of serum enzymes (Table 42–1) in cases with necrosis of liver cells.
■ It has a very high mortality rate, but patients who recover usually do so completely.

Chronic Liver Failure
A. Causes: It usually results from cirrhosis or chronic active hepatitis.
B. Effects:

■ Decreased synthesis of albumin, leading to low serum albumin levels, edema, and ascites.
■ Decreased levels of prothrombin and of factors VII, IX, and X, resulting in a bleeding tendency.
■ Portal hypertension (see following).
■ Hepatic encephalopathy (see following).
■ Hepatorenal syndrome (see following).
■ Endocrine changes leading to gynecomastia, testicular atrophy, and cutaneous spider angiomas (estrogen excess), secondary hyperaldosteronism, and inappropriate secretion of antidiuretic hormone, which causes hyponatremia.
■ Fetor hepaticus—a breath like that of "a freshly opened corpse"—believed to be due to deficient methionine catabolism.

PORTAL HYPERTENSION
This is defined as elevation of portal venous pressure above the upper limit of normal of 12 mm Hg.

Classification and Etiology
A. Presinusoidal, due to:

■ Obstruction of the extrahepatic portal vein by thrombosis, neoplasms, or inflammation.
■ Obstruction of intrahepatic portal venous radicals, as occurs in schistosomiasis, biliary cirrhosis, and congenital hepatic fibrosis.
■ Idiopathic portal hypertension.

B. Sinusoidal accounts for over 90% of cases and is caused by cirrhosis of the liver.

C. Postsinusoidal, due to:

- Obstruction of the hepatic venous radicles by thrombosis (Budd-Chiari syndrome) or neoplasm, commonly hepatocellular carcinoma.
- Right ventricular failure and constrictive pericarditis.

Effects of Portal Hypertension

- **Splenomegaly** due to passive venous congestion.
- **Development of portosystemic venous anastomoses,** bypassing the obstructed portal circulation. The anastomoses result in dilated, tortuous veins in:
  - The lower esophagus and fundus of the stomach (gastroesophageal varices).
  - The rectum (hemorrhoids).
  - Around the umbilicus (caput medusae).
- Entry of portal venous blood into the systemic circulation through these collateral channels may result in hepatic encephalopathy.
- **Ascites,** which is due to decreased serum albumin, sodium and water retention and portal hypertension. There is increased transudation of fluid over the surface of the liver.

HEPATIC ENCEPHALOPATHY

This is characterized by cerebral dysfunction (hypersomnia, delirium, "flapping" tremors of the hands) leading to convulsions, coma, and death.

- It occurs in both acute and chronic liver disease.
- It is caused by nitrogenous products of intestinal bacteria entering the systemic blood, having bypassed the liver through portosystemic anastomoses or having undergone deficient detoxification by the failing liver cells.
- Substances suspected of causing encephalopathy are:
  - Ammonia, which is present in high plasma and cerebrospinal fluid concentrations.
  - Octopamine, which acts as false neurotransmitter.

HEPATORENAL SYNDROME

This is defined as the occurrence of acute renal failure in a patient with liver disease.

- The mechanism by which renal failure occurs is uncertain.
- There are no pathologic changes in the kidneys, and when these kidneys are transplanted into normal individuals, they function normally.
- Renal failure has features of "prerenal" failure occurring in shock, with production of a small volume of concentrated urine.
- It has a bad prognosis.

HEPATOCELLULAR NECROSIS

Focal Necrosis

- This is randomly occurring necrosis of single cells or small clusters of cells in all areas of liver lobules.

- It is recognized in biopsies by acidophilic (Councilman) bodies, and areas of lysed liver cells surrounded by collections of Kupffer cells and inflammatory cells.
- It is commonly seen in viral hepatitis, toxic damage, and bacteremic infections.

Zonal Necrosis
This is necrosis occurring in identical regions in all liver lobules.

- Centrizonal necrosis occurs in viral hepatitis, carbon tetrachloride and chloroform toxicity, and anoxic states.
- Midzonal necrosis is uncommon and occurs in yellow fever.
- Peripheral zonal necrosis occurs in eclampsia and phosphorus poisoning.

Submassive & Massive Necrosis

- This is necrosis that extends across lobular boundaries, bridging portal areas and central veins ("bridging necrosis").
- The most severe form is massive necrosis, in which large confluent areas of liver undergo necrosis, leaving only small islands of viable liver cells.
- The liver is smaller, appears soft, yellow, and flabby, and with a wrinkled capsule ("acute yellow atrophy").
- Massive liver necrosis is caused by hepatitis viruses (B and C), drugs (halothane, acetaminophen, isoniazid, methyldopa), or toxic chemicals (*Amanita phalloides* mushrooms, chlorinated hydrocarbon insecticides, chloroform, carbon tetrachloride).

CONGENITAL DISEASES OF THE LIVER

CONGENITAL HEPATIC FIBROSIS
This is uncommon and is usually associated with polycystic renal disease.

- It is characterized by fibrosis connecting adjacent portal tracts and abnormal proliferation of bile ducts (bile duct hamartomas, Meyenberg complexes).
- Cases with larger biliary cysts are termed congenital polycystic disease of the liver.
- It usually presents as an incidental finding in a patient with polycystic renal disease.
- It rarely causes presinusoidal portal hypertension.

VASCULAR LESIONS OF THE LIVER

CHRONIC HEPATIC VENOUS CONGESTION
This occurs in right heart failure and constrictive pericarditis.

- The liver is enlarged and shows centrizonal congestion.
- Grossly, the liver has a characteristic mottled appearance ("nutmeg liver").
- Prolonged congestion leads to centrizonal fibrosis producing a finely granular liver ("cardiac sclerosis").
- Clinically, it is characterized by tender, enlarged liver. Mild abnormalities in liver function are common, but liver failure almost never occurs.

INFARCTION OF THE LIVER
Infarction is rare and usually due to sudden occlusion of the hepatic artery beyond the origin of the gastroduodenal and right gastric arteries.

- Occlusion may be caused by thrombosis, atherosclerosis, polyarteritis nodosa, or accidental ligation at surgery.
- Hepatic infarcts are hemorrhagic.

BUDD-CHIARI SYNDROME

This is a rare clinical syndrome caused by extensive occlusion of hepatic venous radicles by fibrosis, thrombosis, or neoplasm.

- The liver shows severe centrizonal congestion, characterized by the presence of erythrocytes both in the sinusoids and space of Disse.
- Patients present with an enlarged liver and portal hypertension.
- Ascites is often a prominent feature.

INFECTIONS OF THE LIVER

VIRAL HEPATITIS

1. ETIOLOGY

Hepatitis A (Infectious Hepatitis)

It is caused by an RNA enterovirus measuring 27 nm.

- It is usually transmitted via the fecal-oral route and has a short incubation period (2–6 weeks).
- Explosive epidemics have been recorded after fecal contamination of water, milk, and shellfish.
- It has a global incidence, highest in low socioeconomic populations.
- It is a mild acute illness with recovery occurring in a few weeks.
- It is rarely fatal, does not progress to chronic hepatitis, and there is no carrier state.
- IgM antibodies appear early in the acute phase, rise rapidly, and wane during convalescence. IgG antibodies appear later, rise rapidly, and remain elevated throughout life (Fig 42–2).

Hepatitis B (Serum Hepatitis)

It is caused by a DNA virus measuring 42 nm and is called the **Dane particle.**

- Viral replication leads to excess production of the envelope, free forms of which appear in the blood; these measure 22 nm (surface antigen).
- HBsAg itself is not infective, the core of the virus being required for infection.
- It is usually transmitted in blood or blood products from an individual with active disease or a carrier.
- Transmissions may occur:
  - By transfusion of blood or blood products from an individual with active disease or a carrier. Routine screening of blood for hepatitis B has greatly decreased the incidence of transfusion hepatitis B.
  - Among drug abusers who share needles.
  - During sexual intercourse.
  - Due to accidental spillage of specimens in the laboratory.
  - In renal dialysis units among patients and staff.

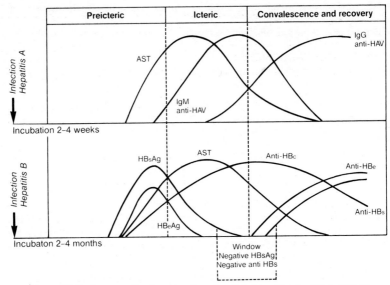

Figure 42–2. Serum antibody and antigen levels in hepatitis A and hepatitis B.

- It has a long (6 weeks to 6 months) incubation period.
- Illness is of varying severity and often subclinical. However, the risk of death, chronic disease, and a carrier state is much greater than in hepatitis A.
- HBsAg appears first in the blood late in the incubation period, and is followed by HBeAg. In patients who recover, both HBsAg and HBeAg disappear at the onset of clinical recovery.
- One sees Anti-HBc during the acute illness, followed by anti-HBe and anti-HBs (Fig 42–2).
- Testing for all antigens and antibodies permits diagnosis at all stages of the illness. If testing includes only HBsAg and anti-HBs, there is a window during the recovery phase when both of these are negative and the diagnosis may be missed.
- The presence of HBeAg and hepatitis B-DNA in the serum indicates that the patient is infective.
- The presence of anti-HBe in the blood indicates absence of the infective Dane particle; such patients are usually not infective.
- Hepatitis B-infected hepatocytes may be identified in biopsy material by:
  - Ground-glass cytoplasm of hepatocytes.
  - A positive orcein (Shikata) stain.
  - Immunoperoxidase stain using labeled antibodies against HBsAg.

Hepatitis C (Previously Hepatitis Non-A, Non-B)
It is caused by a yet unidentified virus (or viruses) and is responsible for over 90% of cases of hepatitis associated with transfusion of blood products in the United States.

- Recent development of a screening test in blood is expected to reduce transmission by transfusion of blood products.
- The disease also occurs among drug abusers, in transplant recipients, and in renal dialysis units.
- The incubation period varies between 2 weeks and 6 months.
- It has clinical features almost identical to those of hepatitis B.

Delta Hepatitis
This is caused by an RNA virus that has the envelope of hepatitis B virus but an antigenically distinct core of delta antigen. It appears to be a "defective" virus that uses hepatitis B virus as a "helper."

- It is incapable of causing infection in the absence of hepatitis B virus.
- Transmission is parenterally, by blood transfusions or intravenous drug abuse.
- Diagnosis is made by finding the delta agent in the blood or in liver cells.

2. CLINICOPATHOLOGIC SYNDROMES
The clinicopathologic features of viral hepatitis are considered here as a group (Table 42–3). Hepatitis A is a mild disease associated with few deaths and no chronic phase. The other viruses cause much more severe illness with a chronic phase and carrier state.

Acute Viral Hepatitis
This is characterized by diffuse hepatocyte swelling, focal or centrizonal necrosis, and lymphocytic and plasma cell infiltrate in the portal tracts.

- It presents with sudden onset of fever, loss of appetite, vomiting, jaundice, and tender hepatomegaly.
- Jaundice is caused by a combination of liver cell dysfunction and cholestasis. Bile is present in the urine, and urinary urobilinogen levels are increased (Table 42–2).
- Liver enzymes are elevated early in the illness.
- Acute viral hepatitis is frequently subclinical or associated with a flulike illness ("anicteric hepatitis").
- Clinical recovery usually occurs within 2–3 weeks.

Cholestatic Viral Hepatitis
This is a variant of acute viral hepatitis characterized by severe intrahepatic cholestasis, with deep jaundice, bilirubin in the urine, and absence of urobilinogen in urine and feces. Complete recovery is not threatened by this complication.

Fulminant Viral Hepatitis
This is acute liver failure associated with massive or submassive liver cell necrosis and it occurs in about 1% of cases of hepatitis B and C. The mortality rate is high. Survivors regenerate a normal liver and recover completely.

Subacute Hepatic Necrosis
This is also called **impaired regeneration syndrome,** and occurs with hepatitis B and C. It is characterized by a protracted illness lasting several months, with increasing liver dysfunction and a high mortality rate.

TABLE 42–3. HEPATITIS VIRUSES AND THE DIFFERENT CLINICOPATHOLOGIC FORMS OF LIVER DISEASE[1]

	Subclinical	Acute Hepatitis	Fulminant Hepatitis (Massive Necrosis)	Subacute Necrosis (Impaired Regeneration)	Chronic Persistent Hepatitis	Chronic Active Hepatitis	Cirrhosis	Hepatocellular Carcinoma
Hepatitis A	+	+	–	–	–	–	?	–
Hepatitis B	+	+	+	+	+	+	+	+
Non-A, non-B (NANB) hepatitis	+	+	+	+	+	+	+	?
Delta hepatitis	+	+	?	?	+	+	?	?

[1] The outcome in any given patient is dependent on age, immunologic status, "dose" of virus, and interaction of viruses such as that between hepatitis B virus and delta virus.

- Patients who survive progress to cirrhosis.
- Pathologically, there is submassive necrosis, and absence of regenerative activity.

Chronic Persistent Viral Hepatitis
This is a common clinical syndrome due to infection with hepatitis B and C.

- The patient usually has mild symptoms or slight abnormalities in liver function tests lasting for 6 months or more.
- It is a benign self-limited disease that may last for several years but does not progress to cirrhosis.
- It represents the chronic carrier state, with hepatitis B or C virus being present in the blood. The patient is infective.
- Histologically, increased numbers of lymphocytes and plasma cells are present in the portal tracts, and the limiting plate of hepatocytes is intact. There is no active necrosis of liver cells.

Chronic Active Viral Hepatitis
This is caused by hepatitis B, C, and delta agent. Clinically, it is characterized by a chronic illness associated with marked elevation of liver enzymes.

- Portal hypertension may develop.
- Chronic active hepatitis progresses to cirrhosis and chronic liver failure. It has a bad prognosis.
- Histologically, there is continuing focal necrosis of liver cells. The portal tracts show fibrosis and chronic inflammation that extends into the liver lobule, disrupting the limiting plate and causing piecemeal necrosis of hepatocytes.

BACTERIAL INFECTIONS OF THE LIVER

1. NONSUPPURATIVE INFECTIONS
These occur in many bacteremic bacterial infections.

- They are associated with miliary caseating granulomas (tuberculosis and fungal infections) or focal necrosis (typhoid fever, brucellosis, and leptospirosis).
- They produce no clinical symptoms, but may cause minor abnormalities in liver function tests.

2. PYOGENIC LIVER ABSCESS
Many different bacteria may be involved, most commonly *Escherichia coli,* other gram-negative bacilli, anaerobic bacilli, *Staphylococcus aureus,* and streptococci.

- Bacteria may reach the liver:
  - In the course of a systemic bacteremia.
  - Along the bile duct (suppurative cholangitis).
  - Along portal venous radicles (pylephlebitis suppurativa).
- Fifty percent of cases have multiple abscesses.
- Patients present with high fever, right-sided upper abdominal pain, and hepatomegaly.
- Diagnosis is by culture of the drained abscess.

PARASITIC INFECTIONS OF THE LIVER

1. HEPATIC AMOEBIASIS

This is caused by the entry of amoebic trophozoites into portal venous radicles in the colonic submucosa.

- It usually occurs in patients with subclinical or chronic intestinal amoebiasis and very rarely during an attack of acute amoebic colitis.
- About half of patients with hepatic amoebiasis give no history suggestive of preceding amoebic colitis.
- In the liver, the amoebas cause focal enzymatic necrosis leading to multiple microabscesses. These coalesce to form larger abscesses.
- Grossly, amoebic abscesses are large, lined by an irregular wall, and contain reddish brown ("anchovy paste") or yellow pus. Trophozoites of *Entamoeba histolytica* may be found.
- Patients present with high fever, right upper abdominal pain, hepatomegaly, and intercostal tenderness.
- Diagnosis is confirmed by chest X-ray, ultrasonography, CT scan, and elevated serum titers of amoebic antibodies.
- Without treatment, amoebic liver abscess has a high mortality rate. Deaths are due to:
  - Rupture into the free peritoneal cavity.
  - Rupture into the pleural cavity and lung.
  - Rupture into the pericardial sac (in left lobe abscesses), causing pericardial tamponade.
  - Systemic spread of trophozoites, resulting in amoebic abscesses in the brain and lung.
- Treatment is with metronidazole. Drainage is required for large abscesses.

2. HEPATIC SCHISTOSOMIASIS

Hepatic schistosomiasis complicates intestinal schistosomiasis. It is caused by *Schistosoma mansoni*, which causes colonic infection in the Middle East, and *Schistosoma japonicum*, which causes small intestinal infection in the Far East.

- Schistosome eggs are carried via the portal vein to the liver and are deposited in the portal areas.
- They produce portal granulomas in the acute phase followed by "pipestem fibrosis" of the portal areas.
- This causes portal hypertension and ascites.

3. HYDATID CYST

The liver is the commonest site for hydatid cysts. Infection is by *Echinococcus granulosus*.

- Hepatic hydatid cysts may reach a large size and may be multiple.
- Histologic examination shows cysts to have a thick, acellular, laminated eosinophilic wall and be filled with a fluid that contains scoleces.
- Diagnosis is made by the radiologic appearance.
- During surgical removal, care must be taken to avoid spillage of cyst contents into the peritoneal cavity, which can cause anaphylactic shock.

4. ORIENTAL CHOLANGIOHEPATITIS

This results from infection of the bile ducts with *Clonorchis sinensis*.

- It is characterized by irregular strictures, dilatation of the intrahepatic bile ducts, and fibrosis of the surrounding liver. The dilated bile ducts contain numerous black calculi, flukes, and ova.
- Patients present with episodes of fever and right upper abdominal pain.
- Diagnosis is by radiologic features.
- Surgical resection of the affected areas is curative.

Liver: II. Toxic & Metabolic Diseases; Neoplasms

43

TOXIC & METABOLIC DISEASES

ALCOHOLIC LIVER DISEASE

Incidence & Pathogenesis
Chronic alcoholism affects 10% of the population in developed countries (see Chapter 12).

- Alcoholic liver disease is most common in middle-aged men, but there is an increasing incidence among women and the young.
- Most patients with chronic alcoholic liver disease have consumed about 150 g or more of ethyl alcohol daily for over 10 years (a 750-mL bottle of 80-proof whisky contains about 300 g of alcohol).

Clinicopathologic Syndromes
A. Fatty liver:

- This is a common early manifestation of alcohol injury.
- It is caused by decreased fatty acid oxidation, increased synthesis of triglycerides, and impaired secretion of lipoproteins by the liver cell.
- Clinically, fatty liver causes diffuse liver enlargement.
- Liver function is normal even when there is severe fatty change.
- Fatty liver is reversible.

B. Acute alcoholic hepatitis:

- This is also called acute sclerosing hyaline necrosis of the liver.
- It is characterized pathologically by:
  - Focal necrosis of hepatocytes.
  - Cholestasis with jaundice.
  - Neutrophilic infiltration of the sinusoids and around necrotic liver cells.
  - Sclerosis around the central venule, initially as fine fibrils and later as course fibrosis that obliterates central veins.
  - Presence of eosinophilic waxy "alcoholic" hyalin (Mallory bodies) in the cytoplasm of liver cells.
- Clinically, patients present with acute onset of fever, jaundice, tender enlargement of the liver, and ascites, commonly after a recent bout of heavy drinking.
- Symptoms and most of the pathologic features resolve with cessation of drinking.

TABLE 43–1. CHEMICAL AND DRUG-INDUCED LIVER DISEASE

Type of Injury	Drugs or Chemicals
Dose-related ("predictable") reactions Hepatocellular necrosis	Mushroom (*Amanita phalloides*) poisoning Aflatoxin Phosphorus Carbon tetrachloride, chloroform, benzene Cytotoxic drugs (eg, methotrexate) Acetaminophen Salicylates Vitamin A (toxic levels)
Acute fatty liver	Tetracycline (intravenous)
Idiosyncratic reactions Hepatocellular necrosis (massive)	Halothane, isoniazid, methyldopa
Cholestasis	Phenothiazines, oral contraceptives, anabolic steroids, oral antidiabetic agents
Acute hepatitis-like	Isoniazid, phenytoin, salicylates
Fatty change	Methyldopa, oxyphenisatin, methotrexate
Granulomatous hepatitis	Phenylbutazone, hydralazine, allopurinol
Focal nodular hyperplasia	Oral contraceptives, anabolic steroids
Liver cell adenoma	Oral contraceptives, anabolic steroids
Angiosarcoma of the liver	Vinyl chloride, thorium dioxide (Thorotrast)
Hepatocellular carcinoma	Aflatoxin

C. Chronic alcoholic liver disease:

- This is associated with progressive fibrosis in the centrizonal region that distorts the liver architecture.
- It differs from cirrhosis in the absence of true regenerative nodules.
- Progression may slow or come to a halt if alcohol ingestion is discontinued.

D. Alcoholic cirrhosis: (See later.)

CHEMICAL- & DRUG-INDUCED LIVER DISEASE

Many drugs and other chemical substances cause many different types of liver damage (Table 43–1).

- Some agents, like acetaminophen, salicylates, methotrexate, and chloroform, cause predictable (dose-related) hepatocellular necrosis in all individuals.

■ Agents like halothane and isoniazid cause unpredictable (idiosyncratic) hepatocellular necrosis in a small percentage of susceptible individuals. This type of toxicity is not dose-related.

■ Toxic manifestations other than necrosis include cholestasis, acute hepatitis, fatty change, and granulomatous hepatitis (Table 43–1).

■ Some agents cause mass lesions, including:
● Liver cell adenoma (oral contraceptives and anabolic steroids).
● Focal nodular hyperplasia (oral contraceptives and anabolic steroids).
● Liver cell carcinoma (aflatoxin).
● Angiosarcoma (vinyl chloride and thorium dioxide).

NUTRITIONAL LIVER DISEASE

Protein-calorie malnutrition (kwashiorkor) is associated with fatty liver and nutritional cirrhosis. Obese patients treated with ileoileal bypass develop fatty change and sclerosing hyaline necrosis very similar to alcoholic liver disease.

IMMUNOLOGIC DISEASES OF THE LIVER

CHRONIC ACTIVE HEPATITIS ("Lupoid Hepatitis")

Immune-mediated and viral chronic active hepatitis have identical clinical and pathologic features.

■ Patients with immune-mediated disease are hepatitis B- and C-negative, and frequently have serum antinuclear antibodies.

■ Immune-mediated chronic active hepatitis has no relationship to systemic lupus erythematosus.

■ In contrast to its viral counterpart, immune-mediated chronic active hepatitis occurs more frequently in women.

■ The disease has a bad prognosis, progressing to cirrhosis in the majority of cases.

■ Corticosteroids are sometimes of value in treatment.

PRIMARY BILIARY CIRRHOSIS

Over 90% of cases occur in middle-aged women.

■ The exact cause is uncertain, but immunologic injury is suspected.

■ It is associated with other immunologic diseases such as progressive systemic sclerosis and Sjögren's syndrome.

■ Antimitochondrial antibody is present in the serum.

■ Histologically, the bile ductules are progressively destroyed by lymphocytes and plasma cells.

■ Epithelioid cell granulomas occur in 30% of cases.

■ In the final stage of the disease, bile ducts are absent in the portal triads.

■ Patients present with slowly progressive biliary obstruction. Pruritus and elevation of serum alkaline phosphatase occur early; jaundice occurs later, usually 6–18 months after onset.

■ Many patients have hyperlipidemia, cutaneous xanthomas, and an increased risk of atherosclerotic vascular disease.

■ Portal hypertension and liver failure may occur 5–15 years after onset.

CIRRHOSIS OF THE LIVER

Cirrhosis of the liver is a pathologic entity characterized by slow necrosis of liver cells, fibrosis, and regenerative nodules, which distort normal architecture, diffusely involving the whole liver.

Pathology

Grossly, the liver is enlarged in the early stages, but becomes progressively smaller because of cell loss and fibrous contraction.

- It is much firmer than normal and contains nodules.
- Cirrhosis is classified as macronodular, micronodular, or mixed, based on whether nodules are more or less than 3 mm.
- Histologically, there are regenerative nodules separated by broad bands of fibrous tissue; the normal lobular architecture is lost.
- Fibrous tissue obstructs portal venous radicles and cause fistulous communications between portal veins and hepatic arterioles, resulting in portal hypertension.

Clinical Features

Cirrhosis is manifested clinically by features of chronic liver failure and portal hypertension (Fig 43–1).

- Its common presenting symptoms include:
  - Hematemesis due to rupture of esophageal varices.
  - Ascites.
- Cirrhosis is an irreversible and progressive disease that ultimately causes death. The rate of progression is variable.
- Patients with cirrhosis have an increased risk of hepatocellular carcinoma.

Etiologic Types of Cirrhosis

A. Cryptogenic cirrhosis:

- Cirrhosis is defined as cryptogenic when complete evaluation of the patient has failed to identify a cause.
- It may include cirrhosis following immune-mediated chronic active hepatitis, following hepatitis due to unidentified viruses, or following injury due to drugs or chemicals.
- Its rate of progression is variable.

B. Alcoholic cirrhosis:

- It is frequently associated with evidence of fatty change or acute alcoholic hepatitis.
- Typically it is a fatty micronodular cirrhosis.
- It tends to have a slow rate of progression, particularly if the patient stops drinking.

C. Virus-induced cirrhosis:

- It follows chronic active hepatitis resulting from infection with hepatitis B and C.
- Typically, it is macronodular.
- Virus-induced cirrhosis tends to progress rapidly, with death due to chronic liver failure, portal hypertension, or hepatocellular carcinoma.

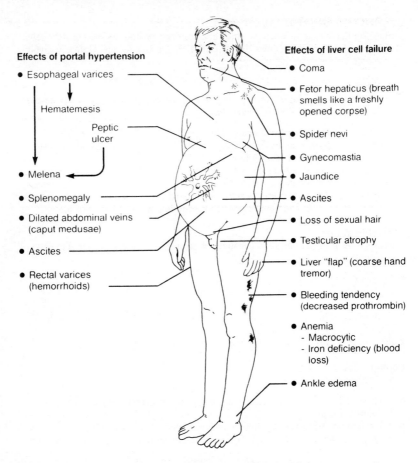

Effects of portal hypertension

- Esophageal varices

  ↓

  Hematemesis

  Peptic ulcer

- Melena

- Splenomegaly

- Dilated abdominal veins (caput medusae)

- Ascites

- Rectal varices (hemorrhoids)

Effects of liver cell failure

- Coma

- Fetor hepaticus (breath smells like a freshly opened corpse)

- Spider nevi

- Gynecomastia

- Jaundice

- Ascites

- Loss of sexual hair

- Testicular atrophy

- Liver "flap" (coarse hand tremor)

- Bleeding tendency (decreased prothrombin)

- Anemia
  - Macrocytic
  - Iron deficiency (blood loss)

- Ankle edema

Figure 43–1. Clinical effects of cirrhosis of the liver.

- Cirrhosis caused by hepatitis B virus may be identified by the presence of HBsAg in the serum and in liver cells.

D. Biliary cirrhosis:

- Primary biliary cirrhosis causes portal fibrosis, but the changes fall short of the definition of cirrhosis because regenerative nodules are absent.
- Secondary biliary cirrhosis occurs in patients with prolonged large bile duct obstruction and is characterized by a fine nodularity and slow progression.

E. Hemochromatosis:

- This results from iron overload in the body.
- Causes include:
  - Idiopathic hemochromatosis, an autosomal recessive inherited disease in which there is increased intestinal iron absorption by an uncertain mechanism.
  - Secondary hemochromatosis due to:
    - Increased dietary intake of iron, as occurs in the Bantu tribe of Africa ("Bantu siderosis").
    - Iron infusions in the form of repeated blood transfusions for chronic anemias.
    - Chronic hemolytic anemias, eg, thalassemia.
- Iron is deposited as hemosiderin in the cytoplasm of Kupffer cells and hepatocytes, and causes cell necrosis leading to cirrhosis.
- It is associated with effects of iron toxicity elsewhere:
  - Pancreas, causing diabetes mellitus.
  - Skin, causing pigmentation ("bronze diabetes").
  - Myocardium, causing heart failure.
  - Endocrine glands, causing hypofunction.

F. Wilson's disease:

- This is also called **hepatolenticular degeneration.**
- It is an autosomal recessive disorder characterized by defective excretion of copper into bile and increased total body copper.
- Copper deposition in the liver causes microvacuolar fatty change and focal liver cell necrosis, progressing to cirrhosis.
- It presents in late childhood with liver dysfunction.
- Increased copper levels in the liver can be demonstrated biochemically.
- They are associated with extrahepatic changes:
  - Extrapyramidal dysfunction due to degeneration of the basal ganglia (particularly the lenticular nucleus), thalamus, red nucleus, and dentate nucleus of the cerebellum.
  - A greenish-brown ring (Kayser-Fleischer ring) at the sclerocorneal junction due to deposition of copper in Descemet's membrane.

G. Alpha$_1$-antitrypsin deficiency:

- Severe α_1-antitrypsin deficiency occurs in homozygous PiZZ individuals (Chapter 35).
- A rare cause of cirrhosis, it usually manifests during childhood.
- The abnormal gene results in hepatic synthesis of an abnormal α_1-antitrypsin molecule that accumulates in the liver cell cytoplasm, appearing as eosinophilic globules.
- The diagnosis is made by identifying the globules by immunoperoxidase methods using antibody against α_1-antitrypsin.

H. Galactosemia:

- This is a rare inherited disease caused by deficiency of galactose-1-phosphate uridyl transferase.

- Galactose metabolites accumulate in the liver, causing fatty change and cirrhosis with rapid progression to liver failure in childhood.
- Galactosemia is also associated with cataracts and mental retardation.
- Galactosemia is routinely looked for in neonatal screening tests.
- Diagnosis in a neonate followed by a diet that contains no milk products prevents liver damage.

NEOPLASMS OF THE LIVER

BENIGN NEOPLASMS

Cavernous Hemangioma
These are common incidental findings at surgery, radiologic examination, and autopsy. Histologically, they are composed of large endothelium-lined spaces filled with blood.

Peliosis Hepatis
This is a rare degenerative condition associated with multiple blood-filled spaces in the liver, many of which lack an endothelial lining. It may be associated with use of anabolic steroids. It has an increased incidence in AIDS.

Sclerosing Bile Duct Adenoma
This is uncommon and usually presents as an incidental finding at surgery.

- It appears as a firm, gray-white subcapsular nodule, usually smaller than 1 cm.
- Histologically, it is composed of irregular glands surrounded by collagen.
- Distinction from metastatic adenocarcinoma can be difficult.

Liver Cell Adenoma
This is a rare benign neoplasm that occurs mainly in women taking oral contraceptives and athletes taking anabolic steroids.

- It is usually solitary, but may be multiple. Often it reaches a large size.
- Microscopically, it is composed of a mass of cytologically benign hepatocytes arranged in thickened cords.
- Distinction from well-differentiated hepatocellular carcinoma is based on cytologic uniformity and absence of vascular invasion.
- Patients may present with a mass, sudden pain due to infarction, or hemorrhage due to rupture through the liver capsule.

Focal Nodular Hyperplasia
Etiologically, this is related to oral contraceptives. It is not a true neoplasm and its pathogenesis is unknown.

- It presents as a solitary solid mass lesion, usually subcapsular, well-circumscribed, and only rarely larger than 5 cm.
- On cut section, it is gray-white and typically has a central scar with bands of fibrosis radiating to the periphery.
- Microscopically, nodules of liver tissue are separated by fibrous bands in which portal tracts containing bile ductules can be identified.

MALIGNANT NEOPLASMS

1. HEPATOCELLULAR CARCINOMA (Hepatoma)

Incidence
It is common in the Far East and certain parts of Africa, and uncommon in Western Europe and North America. There are about 8000 cases a year in the United States.

Etiology

- Aflatoxin, a product of the fungus *Aspergillus flavus,* which grows on improperly stored grain and nuts, is thought important in Africa and Asia.
- Hepatitis B virus infection is strongly suspected of causing hepatocellular carcinoma.
- Over 80% of patients who develop hepatocellular carcinoma have cirrhosis of the liver.
- The risk is greatest in hemochromatosis, virus-induced cirrhosis, and alcoholic cirrhosis.

Pathology
Grossly, hepatocellular carcinoma may present as a large solitary mass, as multiple nodules, or as a diffusely infiltrative lesion.

- Microscopically, the neoplasm is composed of cytologically abnormal liver cells arranged in trabeculae. Invasion of hepatic venous radicles common.
- Rarely, venous involvement is so extensive as to produce Budd-Chiari syndrome.
- Even more rarely, a tumor thrombus extends along the hepatic vein into the inferior vena cava and up into the right atrium.
- Elevated serum levels of alpha fetoprotein are present in 90% of patients.
- It metastasizes early via the bloodstream to produce lung metastases.

Clinical Features
Hepatocellular carcinoma should be suspected when a patient with known cirrhosis presents with any new symptom such as pain, loss of weight, fever, increasing liver size, or increasing ascites.

- Twenty percent of patients present with intraperitoneal hemorrhage.
- Rarely, hepatocellular carcinoma may secrete an ectopic hormone, causing:
  - Hypoglycemia (insulinlike polypeptide).
  - Polycythemia (erythropoietin).
  - Hypercalcemia (parathyroid hormone-like polypeptide).
- Progression is extremely rapid, and most patients are dead within 1 year. The median survival after diagnosis is 2 months; the 5-year survival rate is less than 1%.

2. CHOLANGIOCARCINOMA
Cholangiocarcinoma arises in the intrahepatic bile ductules. It has a high incidence in the Far East, where it follows infection with *Clonorchis sinensis.*

- It is not associated with cirrhosis.
- Grossly, it is indistinguishable from hepatocellular carcinoma.
- Histologically, it is an adenocarcinoma that shows mucin secretion. Marked sclerosis is common.

- Serum alpha-fetoprotein levels are normal.
- The clinical presentation is with a liver mass. The progress of disease is often slow.

3. MALIGNANT VASCULAR NEOPLASMS

Angiosarcoma

This is a highly malignant rare neoplasm that has been linked etiologically to vinyl chloride and to **Thorotrast,** a thorium dioxide-containing radiographic dye.

- Patients present with rapid liver enlargement.
- The tumor appears as a solid, often very large hemorrhagic mass composed of intercommunicating vascular spaces lined by malignant endothelial cells.
- It is rapidly progressive to death. There is no effective treatment.

Epithelioid Hemangioendothelioma

This is a rare malignant neoplasm of endothelial cells characterized by epithelioid-appearing endothelial cells and marked sclerosis.

- It produces a diffusely infiltrative mass in the liver.
- It progresses very slowly.
- Metastases occur late, and death occurs 10–15 years after diagnosis.

METASTATIC NEOPLASMS

Metastases account for most neoplasms involving the liver.

- Virtually any malignant neoplasm in the body can metastasize to the liver; those from the gastrointestinal tract (via the portal vein), breast, and lung and malignant melanoma are most common.
- Characteristically it produces massive liver enlargement with multiple nodules.
- It may present with a solitary lesion.
- Grossly, the nodules of metastatic carcinoma often show central necrosis and umbilication, unlike hepatocellular carcinoma.

LIVER NEOPLASMS IN INFANCY

Infantile hemangioendothelioma

This is a benign neoplasm of endothelial cells characterized by anastomosing vascular spaces. It is often large and acts as an arteriovenous fistula, leading to a hyperdynamic circulation. The usual presentation is heart failure in infancy.

Mesenchymal hamartoma

This is a benign mass composed of bile duct-like structures admixed with disorganized mesenchymal elements. It produces a large solid and cystic mass in the liver. Surgical removal is curative.

Hepatoblastoma

This is a malignant neoplasm composed of primitive cells that resemble fetal liver cells. Mesenchymal elements such as bone are present. Alpha-fetoprotein is present both in tumor cells and in the blood. It commonly presents with marked liver enlargement in infancy, and has a poor prognosis.

The Extrahepatic Biliary System

44

MANIFESTATIONS OF BILIARY TRACT DISEASE

Pain
Biliary colic is severe intermittent pain in the right upper abdomen that radiates to the back and right shoulder. It occurs when there is bile duct obstruction.

- Vague epigastric pain aggravated by ingestion of fatty foods is common in patients with gallstones and chronic cholecystitis.
- Constant right upper abdominal pain, often severe, occurs in acute cholecystitis when the inflammation extends to the parietal peritoneum.

Obstructive Jaundice
This is caused by obstruction of the common bile duct.

- In patients with a normal biliary system, there is dilatation proximal to the obstruction, and the gallbladder becomes enlarged.
- In patients who have gallstones and chronic cholecystitis with fibrosis, gallbladder enlargement does not occur (Courvoisier's law).

CONGENITAL MALFORMATIONS

ANATOMIC VARIATIONS OF THE BILIARY SYSTEM
Minor variations in the anatomy of the extrahepatic bile ducts and blood vessels are very common. Recognition of these normal variations is important at cholecystectomy in order to prevent accidental ligation of ducts and blood vessels.

- Anatomic abnormalities of the gallbladder include:
  - Congenital absence.
  - Duplication, with the presence of two gallbladders.
  - Intrahepatic location.
  - Floating gallbladder surrounded by peritoneum and connected to the inferior surface of the liver by a pedicle.
  - Focal concentric narrowing of the body of the gallbladder, producing an expanded fundus ("phrygian cap" gallbladder).

BILIARY ATRESIA
This is the most common cause of neonatal obstructive jaundice. It occurs when there is failure of development of the lumen in the epithelial cord that ultimately becomes the bile ducts; this failure may be complete or incomplete.

489

- Usually it involves the extrahepatic bile ducts only; more rarely, the intrahepatic ducts are involved.
- The liver shows the features of severe large bile duct obstruction.
- Without treatment, death occurs in infancy.
- Surgical treatment (porto-jejunostomy) has a high success rate if undertaken early and atresia is partial. In cases where atresia involves intrahepatic ducts, liver transplantation represents the only hope of survival.

CHOLEDOCHAL CYST

Though uncommon, choledochal cyst is the most frequent cause of obstructive jaundice in older children.

- Usually it is caused by focal dilatation, often massive, of the common bile duct. The wall is thick and fibrotic, and the cavity contains bile.
- Rarely, dilatation of intrahepatic bile ducts (Caroli's disease) may coexist.
- Women are more commonly affected.
- Clinical presentation is with pain, jaundice, and a cystic mass in the right upper quadrant.

CHOLELITHIASIS

Etiology & Incidence (Table 44–1)
A. Cholesterol-based gallstones:

- May be pure, mixed (cholesterol, bilirubin and calcium), or combined (cholesterol center, mixed shell).
- Formed when the concentration of cholesterol is increased or when bile salts are decreased.

TABLE 44–1. TYPES OF GALLSTONES

Type	Frequency	Chemical Composition	Gross Appearance
Mixed	80%	Cholesterol, calcium carbonate, calcium bilirubinate	Multiple, small, faceted; variable in size and shape; smooth surface, yellow; laminated on cut section.
Pure cholesterol	5%	Cholesterol	Solitary, large, oval, white; rough surface; cut section: radiating crystalline structure
Combined	10%	Pure cholesterol center, mixed shell	Solitary or 2 stones; oval or barrel-shaped, yellow; smooth surface
Pigment	Rare	Calcium bilirubinate	Multiple, very small, faceted, black
Calcium	Very rare	Calcium carbonate	Multiple, amorphous; small grains, rarely large

- It is common in:
  - Obese, middle aged, multiparous women.
  - Women using oral contraceptives.
  - Native American and South American women.
  - Patients with terminal ileal disease such as Crohn's disease, and following terminal ileal resection.
  - Patients with diabetes mellitus.

B. Pigment (bilirubin) stones:

- These are uncommon and occur in:
  - Patients suffering from chronic hemolytic anemias such as sickle cell disease and thalassemia.
  - Patients with *Clonorchis sinensis* infection.

Clinicopathologic Syndromes
A. Asymptomatic gallstones:

- Thirty percent or more of patients with gallstones have no symptoms, and gallstones are frequently found incidentally at radiologic examination.
- Only about 25% of gallstones contain sufficient calcium to be visible on plain X-rays, but ultrasonograpy and computerized tomography are highly effective at detecting gallstones.

B. Acute cholecystitis:

- Acute cholecystitis rarely occurs in the absence of gallstones.
- In 80% of cases, a stone is found obstructing the cystic duct, leading to stasis of bile in the gallbladder, followed by concentration and chemical acute inflammation.
- The damaged gallbladder is then susceptible to infection by bacteria; *Escherichia coli* and other gram-negative bacilli are cultured from the bile in 80% of cases.
- Pathologically, the gallbladder shows congestion, edema, neutrophil infiltration, and mucosal ulceration.
- Complications include:
  - Empyema of the gallbladder, where the gallbladder becomes filled with pus.
  - Gangrenous cholecystitis, with extensive necrosis, causing a greenish-black discoloration.
  - Perforation leading to local abscess formation or to generalized peritonitis.
- Clinically, acute cholecystitis produces fever and right upper quadrant pain. An enlarged, tender gallbladder is palpable in 40% of cases. Mild jaundice occurs in about 20%.
- Treatment is with antibiotics and surgical drainage or cholecystectomy.

C. Chronic cholecystitis:

- Chronic cholecystitis almost never occurs without gallstones.
- Pathologically, the gallbladder is contracted and its wall thickened by fibrosis and infiltrated by lymphocytes, plasma cells, and macrophages.
- Calcification may occur in the wall. When extensive, the gallbladder is outlined on abdominal X-ray ("porcelain gallbladder").

- The mucosa of the gallbladder may show yellow flecks due to accumulation of cholesterol-filled foamy macrophages (cholesterolosis).
- Symptoms are usually vague abdominal pain, often related to the ingestion of fatty foods. Biliary colic may occur when the cystic duct is obstructed.

D. Movement of gallstones:

- Cystic duct obstruction is characterized by distention of the gallbladder with watery bile (hydrops) or mucus (mucocele). Acute cholecystitis also complicates cystic duct obstruction.
- Common bile duct obstruction causes biliary colic, obstructive jaundice, and high fever due to cholangitis.
- Impaction of a gallstone in the ampulla of Vater may obstruct the pancreatic duct, leading to acute pancreatitis.
- Fistulous tracts develop rarely between the gallbladder and intestine. A large gallstone may pass through a cholecystoenteric fistula into the intestine, causing intestinal obstruction (gallstone ileus).

FIBROUS STRICTURES OF THE COMMON BILE DUCT

Fibrous strictures of the common bile duct are an important cause of obstructive jaundice. They occur:

- After biliary surgery, most frequently cholecystectomy.
- After external trauma (rarely).
- Following inflammation, either caused by a gallstone in the bile duct or by chronic pancreatitis.
- In infections with *Clonorchis sinensis*.
- Sclerosing cholangitis:
  - This is a rare disease that occurs mainly in patients with chronic ulcerative colitis.
  - Its cause is unknown, but immunologic injury is thought to be involved.
  - The large bile ducts both within and outside the liver undergo irregular fibrosis with narrowing, leading to obstructive jaundice.

NEOPLASMS OF THE EXTRAHEPATIC BILIARY SYSTEM

BENIGN NEOPLASMS

Benign neoplasms are rare in the biliary system.

- Papillary adenoma, which may occur at the ampulla of Vater or in the gallbladder, presenting as a polyp, is the most common type.
- The biliary tract is a site in which granular cell schwannomas occur. Though rare, they are important because they cause stenosis of the common bile duct and resemble bile duct carcinoma.

CARCINOMA OF THE GALLBLADDER

This is uncommon—less than 1% of causes of cancer in the United States. It is much more common in, and occurs with high frequency among, Native Americans and Mexicans.

- Eighty percent of patients with carcinoma have gallstones.

- Chronic cholecystitis with extensive calcification of the wall (porcelain gallbladder) is associated with a 25% incidence of carcinoma.
- Grossly, it presents as a polypoid mass that projects into the lumen, with infiltration of the wall.
- Histologically, it is an adenocarcinoma frequently associated with marked fibrosis and a tendency to perineural invasion.
- Most cases of gallbladder carcinoma are found incidentally in patients being treated for gallstones.
- In advanced disease, there is weight loss, a palpable mass, or evidence of metastases.
- The prognosis depends on the stage:
  - Tumors confined to the gallbladder have a good prognosis.
  - When there is extension through the wall of the gallbladder into the liver or peritoneum, with or without evidence of metastatic disease, the 5-year survival rate is close to zero.

CARCINOMA OF THE BILE DUCTS

Though uncommon, bile duct carcinoma represents an important cause of obstructive jaundice in adults.

- Tumors may involve the hepatic ducts at the hilum of the liver (Klatskin tumor) or common bile duct, most commonly in its terminal portion.
- Grossly, they usually cause a malignant stricture.
- Histologically, these tumors are usually well-differentiated and associated with marked sclerosis.
- Bile duct carcinoma grows slowly, with local extension along the biliary system. The ultimate prognosis is poor, though many patients have a long survival.

The Exocrine Pancreas

45

CONGENITAL DISEASES

ECTOPIC PANCREATIC TISSUE
Ectopic pancreatic tissue is present in about 2% of persons, usually discovered as an incidental finding at autopsy.

- In descending order of frequency, ectopic pancreas is found in the stomach, duodenum, jejunum, and Meckel's diverticula.
- It forms a mass composed of disorganized pancreatic acini, ducts, and muscle (sometimes called a choristoma).

MALDEVELOPMENT OF THE PANCREAS
The most common maldevelopment is annular pancreas which involves the head of the pancreas, appearing as a collar of pancreatic tissue around the second part of the duodenum. It may result in duodenal constriction and obstruction.

CYSTIC FIBROSIS (Mucoviscidosis; Fibrocystic Disease)
This is a common congenital disease that is inherited as an autosomal recessive trait and affects one in 2000 Caucasian infants. It is rare in blacks and Orientals.

- Two to five percent of the population of the United States are heterozygous carriers of the abnormal gene.
- It is characterized by abnormally viscous secretion of exocrine glands throughout the body. The basic defect has not been identified.
- Abnormal secretions contain increased sodium and chloride, increased calcium, and abnormal glycoproteins.
- The pathologic changes in cystic fibrosis are the result of obstruction of ducts of exocrine glands by the viscid mucus, and include:
  - Chronic pancreatitis with atrophy of acini, fibrosis, and dilatation of ducts in 80% of patients.
  - Pulmonary changes including collapse of the lung, recurrent pneumonia, lung abscess leading to fibrosis and bronchiectasis.
  - Intestinal obstruction in the neonatal period (meconeum ileus).
  - Bile duct obstruction, which may result in jaundice.
  - Changes in the vas deferens and seminal vesicles, which may cause infertility in the male.
- The diagnosis is established by a sweat sodium level in excess of 60 meq/L.

INFLAMMATORY LESIONS OF THE PANCREAS

ACUTE PANCREATITIS
This is a clinical syndrome resulting from the escape of activated pancreatic digestive

enzymes from the duct system into the parenchyma. It is a common medical emergency, accounting for about one in every 500 admissions to general hospital emergency rooms.

Etiology

- No etiologic factor can be identified in 25% of cases.
- Infectious agents are usually not involved, though mild nonnecrotizing acute pancreatitis occurs in mumps and cytomegalovirus infection.
- Biliary tract calculi are present in about 50% of cases.
- Acute pancreatitis complicating gallstones is chiefly a disorder of women.
- Alcoholism is a common cause of acute pancreatitis in the United States, being involved in 65% of cases. In Europe, the incidence is 5–20%.
- Other less important causes include:
  - Hypercalcemia.
  - Hyperlipidemias, particularly those types associated with increased plasma levels of chylomicrons.
  - Shock and hypothermia.
  - Drugs such as thiazide diuretics, corticosteroids, anticancer agents, and radiation.
  - Trauma, including surgical trauma.

Pathogenesis

The pathologic changes in acute pancreatitis are the result of the action of pancreatic enzymes on the pancreas and surrounding tissues. Trypsin and chymotrypsin activate phospholipase and elastase as well as kinins, complement, the coagulation cascade, and plasmin, leading to acute inflammation, thrombosis, and hemorrhage.

- Elastase contributes to vascular injury.
- Phospholipases act on cell membranes, causing cell injury.
- Pancreatic lipase acts on surrounding adipose tissue, causing enzymatic fat necrosis.
- Pancreatic enzymes flow into the bloodstream and in severe cases may cause distant effects:
  - Phospholipases contribute to the production of adult respiratory distress syndrome by interfering with the normal function of pulmonary surfactant.
  - Rarely, high serum lipase levels are associated with fat necrosis at sites distant from the pancreas.

Pathology

This is characterized by widespread necrosis and hemorrhage in pancreas and surrounding tissues.

- Fat necrosis appears as chalky white foci in and around the pancreas, omentum, and mesentery. Rarely, fat necrosis extends down the retroperitoneum and into the mediastinum.
- In severe cases, massive liquefactive necrosis of the pancreas occurs, resulting in a pancreatic abscess.
- The peritoneal cavity often contains a brownish serous fluid that contains altered blood, fat globules ("chicken broth"), and very high levels of amylase.

Clinical Features

- It usually presents as a medical emergency.
- Patients develop severe constant epigastric pain, frequently referred to the back, accompanied by vomiting and shock.
- Shock is caused by peripheral circulatory failure resulting from hemorrhage and the entry of kinins into the bloodstream.
- Mild jaundice may be present.
- In severe pancreatitis, there is discoloration due to hemorrhage in the subcutaneous tissue around the umbilicus (Cullen's sign) and in the flanks (Turner's sign).
- Activation of the plasma coagulation cascade may lead to disseminated intravascular coagulation.

Laboratory Studies

There is an immediate (within hours) elevation of the serum amylase, often to 10–20 times the normal upper level. Amylase levels return to normal in 2–3 days.

- Serum lipase is increased later, usually after 72 hours.
- Hypocalcemia is present in severe cases and is a bad prognostic sign.
- Transient glycosuria is present in the acute stage in about 10% of cases. Permanent diabetes mellitus almost never follows a single attack of acute pancreatitis.

Complications

Most patients recover from the acute attack and the pancreas returns almost to normal.

- In severe cases, death may occur as a consequence of pancreatic abscess, severe hemorrhage, shock, disseminated intravascular coagulation, or respiratory distress syndrome.
- Pancreatic pseudocyst may follow weeks to months after recovery from an acute attack.

CHRONIC PANCREATITIS

This is a chronic disease characterized by progressive destruction of the parenchyma with chronic inflammation, fibrosis, stenosis, and dilatation of the duct system.

Etiology

Chronic alcoholism is implicated in about 40% of cases in the United States. Biliary tract calculi are present in 20%. In 30–40% of cases, no etiologic factors are identified.

- Some cases follow recurrent acute episodes.
- Cystic fibrosis is a specific type of chronic pancreatitis described earlier.

Pathology

- It is characterized by fibrosis and atrophy of acini.
- The changes are usually diffuse. More rarely, a firm, localized mass forms that is difficult to distinguish grossly from carcinoma.
- The pancreatic ducts show multiple areas of stenosis with irregular dilatation distally. Ducts are filled with inspissated secretions that may undergo calcification to form calculi.

- Microscopically, there is acinar loss with marked fibrosis, duct dilatation and a variable lymphocytic infiltrate. Islets tend to be spared.

Clinical Features

Pain, either constant or intermittent, and often severe, is the dominant symptom. It may be caused by attacks of acute pancreatitis or by duct dilatation.

- Pancreatic exocrine insufficiency leads to steatorrhea, malabsorption of fat-soluble vitamins, and weight loss.
- Endocrine insufficiency (diabetes mellitus) occurs in about 30% of cases.
- Many patients have recurrent attacks of acute pancreatitis (chronic relapsing pancreatitis).
- In about 5% of patients with severe sclerosing chronic pancreatitis affecting the head of the pancreas, obstructive jaundice occurs.

Treatment & Prognosis

When pain cannot be controlled by drugs, surgery to drain the pancreatic duct by pancreaticojejunostomy often has good results. Malabsorption and diabetes mellitus can be controlled by dietary supplements and insulin if necessary.

PANCREATIC CYSTS

PANCREATIC PSEUDOCYST

This is the most common type of pancreatic cyst.

- Usually it is a solitary fluid-filled unilocular structure of variable size lined by a wall composed of collagen and inflamed granulation tissue without an epithelial lining.
- The cysts contain brownish serous fluid with a high amylase content and altered blood.
- Pseudocysts usually occur after an attack of acute necrotizing pancreatitis or during chronic relapsing pancreatitis.
- Most pseudocysts occur in and around the pancreas; rarely, pseudocysts occur at a considerable distance from the pancreas.
- Patients present with an abdominal mass, and most give a past history of abdominal pain suggestive of acute or chronic pancreatitis.
- Treatment consists of establishing surgical drainage of the cyst either into the stomach or into a loop of jejunum.
- Complications of pancreatic pseudocyst include:
  - Acute rupture of the cyst into the intestine, most commonly the stomach and transverse colon, producing intestinal hemorrhage.
  - Secondary infection, leading to an abscess.
  - Compression of the common bile duct, causing obstructive jaundice.

CONGENITAL CYSTS

Rarely, maldevelopment of the pancreatic duct system produces multiple cysts ranging in size from very small to 5 cm in diameter.

- These are true cysts, lined by epithelium and filled with serous fluid.
- Congenital pancreatic cysts are associated with

● Polycystic renal disease and congenital hepatic fibrosis.
● Von Hippel-Lindau disease (see Chapter 62).

NEOPLASTIC CYSTS

1. SEROUS CYSTADENOMA
This is a rare, benign cystic neoplasm of the pancreas. It may reach large size but rarely causes symptoms, being most commonly an incidental finding at abdominal surgery or radiography.

■ It consists of multiple small locules lined by cuboidal epithelium, the cells of which contain abundant glycogen.
■ It is also called microcystic, serous, and glycogen-rich cystadenoma.

2. MUCINOUS CYSTADENOMA & CYSTADENOCARCINOMA
This is more common than serous cystadenoma.

■ Usually it is solitary, unilocular, and very large.
■ The cysts are lined by tall, columnar epithelium and contain a glairy mucinous fluid.
■ The malignant counterpart (cystadenocarcinoma) shows cytologic atypia, stratification of cells, and invasion of the capsule.
■ Mucinous cystadenocarcinoma behaves like a low-grade malignant neoplasm. The 5-year survival rate after complete surgical removal is about 70%.

CARCINOMA OF THE PANCREAS
Carcinoma of the pancreas refers to carcinomas arising in the exocrine pancreas. Islet cell carcinomas are considered separately.

Incidence & Etiology
Approximately 20,000 patients annually in the United States die from pancreatic carcinoma, accounting for 6% of cancer deaths.

■ The incidence is slightly higher in men than in women, and is increasing.
■ Pancreatic carcinoma occurs mainly after age 50.
■ The etiology is unknown.
■ Cigarette smokers show a five-fold increase in incidence.

Pathology
Carcinomas occur throughout the pancreas: 70% in the head, 20% in the body, and 10% in the tail. Ninety-nine percent take origin from the ducts and the remainder from the acini.

■ Grossly, it presents as a hard infiltrative mass that obstructs the pancreatic duct, frequently causing chronic pancreatitis in the distal gland.
■ Carcinomas of the head tend to obstruct the common bile duct early in their course and present when the tumor is small.
■ Tumors in the body and tail tend to present late and be very large.
■ Microscopically, most cases are well-differentiated adenocarcinomas, associated with marked fibrosis.

Spread

The tumor tends to infiltrate into surrounding structures. Perineural spread is a typical feature.

- Lymphatic involvement occurs early, with metastasis to regional lymph nodes.
- Bloodstream spread also occurs early, with the liver being the commonest site of metastasis.

Clinical Features

- Carcinoma of the head of the pancreas presents with common bile duct obstruction.
- Carcinoma of the body and tail presents at a late stage with an abdominal mass, severe weight loss, and anemia.
- A high proportion of patients present with evidence of metastatic disease, most often in the liver.
- Carcinoembryonic antigen levels in the serum are elevated in some cases; this is not a specific finding.
- Percutaneous fine-needle aspiration of the mass under radiologic guidance provides tissue for cytologic examination and is an excellent method of diagnosis.
- Common paraneoplastic manifestations include:
  - Superficial thrombophlebitis in the leg veins (Trousseau's sign).
  - Disseminated intravascular coagulation.

Treatment & Prognosis

Most pancreatic carcinomas are inoperable at presentation.

- Small carcinomas confined to the head of the pancreas may be cured by total pancreaticoduodenectomy (Whipple procedure).
- Chemotherapy and radiotherapy are ineffective.
- The prognosis is dismal: Mean survival is 6 months after diagnosis, and the overall 5-year survival rate is less than 5%.

The Endocrine Pancreas (Islets of Langerhans)

DIABETES MELLITUS

Diabetes mellitus is a chronic disease characterized by relative or absolute deficiency of insulin, resulting in glucose intolerance.

- It occurs in 4–5 million persons in the United States—approximately 2% of the population.
- The incidence varies with age: 0.1% of persons under age 20 years, 2% of those between 20 and 44 years, 4% of those between 45 and 64 years, and 8–10% of those over 65 years have diabetes mellitus.

Etiology (Table 46–1)

Diabetes mellitus is caused by a relative or absolute deficiency of insulin.

- In primary diabetes (95% of cases), there is no underlying disease process to explain insulin deficiency.
- Primary diabetes is of two types, I and II (see following and Table 46–2).
- The remaining 5% of cases of secondary diabetes are due either to pancreatic destruction or to increased levels of insulin antagonists.

A. Type I diabetes mellitus:

- This is also called **insulin-dependent diabetes mellitus (IDDM)** and **juvenile onset diabetes mellitus.**
- It is caused by destruction of pancreatic beta cells.
- Plasma insulin levels are low, and there is a tendency to ketoacidosis without exogenous insulin.
- The disease affects young patients, most commonly under age 30.
- There is a significant association with HLA-B8, -B15, -DR3, and -DR4.
- There is a history of diabetes in about 20% of first-degree relatives—not as strong as in type II diabetes.
- The cause of beta cell destruction in type I diabetes is unknown:
  - A few cases have followed viral infections, most commonly with coxsackievirus B or mumps virus.
  - Autoimmunity is believed to be the major mechanism involved.
  - Islet cell autoantibodies are present in the serum of 90% of cases.

B. Type II diabetes mellitus:

- Is also called **non-insulin-dependent diabetes mellitus (NIDDM)** and **maturity or adult onset diabetes mellitus.**
- The etiology is not well understood. Two factors have been identified:

TABLE 46–1. CLASSIFICATION OF DIABETES MELLITUS

Primary diabetes mellitus (95%)
    Type I: Insulin-dependent diabetes mellitus (IDDM)
    Type II: Non-insulin-dependent diabetes mellitus (NIDDM)
    Impaired glucose tolerance: IGT ("latent diabetes")
    Gestational diabetes mellitus[1]

Secondary diabetes mellitus (5%)
    Destructive pancreatic disease
        Chronic pancreatitis (Chapter 45)
        Hemochromatosis (bronze diabetes; Chapter 43)
        Total pancreatectomy
    Endocrine diseases (high levels of insulin-antagonistic hormones)
        Acromegaly (growth hormone) (Chapter 57)
        Cushing's syndrome (cortisol) (Chapter 60)
        Hyperthyroidism (thyroxine) (Chapter 58)
        Pheochromocytoma (catecholamines) (Chapter 60)
        Glucagonoma (glucagon)
    Drug-induced diabetes (including diuretics such as thiazides, furo-
        semide; propranolol; antidepressants; phenothiazines)
    Stress diabetes[1]
    Miscellaneous genetic syndromes with an increased incidence of
        diabetes
        Down's syndrome (trisomy 21; mongolism)
        Turner's syndrome (45,XO)
        Friedreich's ataxia
        Klinefelter's syndrome (47,XXY)
        Glycogen storage disease type I
        Laurence-Moon-Biedl syndrome[2]
        Refsum's syndrome[3]

[1]Gestational and stress diabetes probably represent patients with IGT or with a genetic predisposition to diabetes who are decompensated by the physiologic changes of pregnancy or stress. The "diabetes" is often reversible, but such patients show a high incidence of diabetes in succeeding years.
[2]Retinitis pigmentosa, obesity, mental deficiency, skull defects with or without diabetes.
[3]Retinitis pigmentosa, polyneuropathy with or without diabetes.

- Impaired insulin release in response to meals.
- Insulin resistance, caused by defective insulin receptors on the target cells is believed to play a major role. Insulin resistance is associated with pregnancy and obesity.
■ Ketoacidosis is uncommon.
■ Insulin secretion can be stimulated by drugs such a sulfonylureas, and exogenous insulin is therefore not essential in treatment.
■ The genetic factor is very strong, with a history of diabetes present in about 50% of first-degree relatives.

Pathology
The changes in the pancreatic islets are variable and not specific for diabetes.

TABLE 46–2. COMPARISON OF TYPES OF PRIMARY DIABETES MELLITUS

	Type I (Juvenile Onset)	Type II (Maturity [Adult] Onset)
Incidence	15%	85%
Insulin necessary in treatment	Always	Sometimes
Age (commonly; exceptions occur)	Under 30	Over 40
Association with obesity	No	Yes
Genetic predisposition	Weak, polygenic	Strong, polygenic
Association with HLA system	Yes	No
Glucose intolerance	Severe	Mild
Ketoacidosis	Common	Rare
Beta cell numbers in the islets	Reduced	Variable
Serum insulin level	Reduced	Variable
Classic symptoms of polyuria, polydipsia, thirst, weight loss	Common	Rare
Basic cause	?Viral or immune destruction of beta cells	?Increased "resistance" to insulin

- In type I diabetes, there is frequently a lymphocytic infiltration of the islets in the early phase, followed by a decrease in the total number and size of the islets due to a progressive loss of beta cells.
- The changes in type II diabetes are often minimal in the early stages. In advanced disease, there may be fibrosis and amyloid deposition in the islets.

Clinical Features
The classic symptoms of diabetes mellitus are:

- Hyperglycemia.
- Glycosuria, which causes an osmotic diuresis, leading to increased urine production (polyuria).
- The fluid loss and hyperglycemia causes thirst.
- Stimulation of protein breakdown to provide amino acids for gluconeogenesis results in muscle wasting and weight loss.
- These classic symptoms occur only in patients with severe insulin deficiency, most commonly in type I diabetes.
- Patients with type II diabetes commonly present with one of the complications of diabetes (see following).

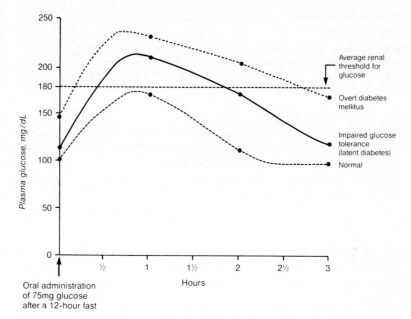

Figure 46–1. Response to an oral glucose load in normal and diabetic patients. (Normal fasting plasma glucose is 60-115 mg/dL.) Note the following points: (1) A normal glucose tolerance curve is defined as a fasting level < 115 mg/dL, 1 hour < 200 mg/dL, and 2 hours < 140 mg/dL. There is usually no glycosuria. (2) Impaired glucose tolerance is defined as a fasting level < 115 mg/dL, 1 hour > 200 mg/dL, 2 hours, > 140 mg/dL. This was formerly called "latent diabetes." Five to 10 percent of these patients develop overt diabetes mellitus within 10 years. Because the other 90% of patients do not develop overt diabetes mellitus, the term "latent diabetes" has been dropped. (3) Overt diabetes mellitus is characterized by a fasting level > 115 mg/dL, 2 hours > 200 mg/dL. Many authorities hold that a value > 200 mg/dL at 2 hours is by itself sufficient for a diagnosis of diabetes mellitus.

Diagnosis

The diagnosis of diabetes is made by detecting abnormalities ⁚ glucose metabolism. In mild cases, the patient has:

- A normal fasting plasma glucose level.
- Elevated postprandial plasma glucose concentration.
- An abnormal glucose tolerance test (Fig 46–1).
- In severe cases, there is fasting hyperglycemia and glycosuria.
- The glucose tolerance test is the most sensitive method of diagnosis.
- Estimation of glycosylated hemoglobin (HbA₁c) levels in blood is used as a guide to the serum glucose level over a long period. Normal HbA₁c is around 4% of total hemoglobin.

Acute Complications
A. Diabetic ketoacidosis:

- Is common in untreated type I diabetes but rare in type II diabetes.
- Is diagnosed by the presence of ketone bodies in blood and urine.
- Ketone bodies are moderately strong acids and cause a metabolic acidosis.
- Clinically, patients present with altered consciousness, marked fluid depletion and acidosis.

B. Hyperosmolar nonketotic coma:

Patients who develop hyperosmolar coma are usually elderly, with severe uncontrolled diabetes. This coma results from extremely high serum glucose levels that cause osmotic diuresis and marked fluid depletion, increasing plasma osmolarity.

- It is treated with aggressive fluid replacement and insulin.
- It is associated with a high mortality rate.

C. Hypoglycemic coma is a complication of therapy. It may follow overdosage of insulin or oral drugs, or when one or more meals is missed or lost by vomiting.

Chronic Complications (Table 46–3)
A. Diabetic microangiopathy (small-vessel disease):

- This is one of the most characteristic and most important pathologic changes in diabetes.
- It is characterized by diffuse thickening of the basement membranes of capillaries throughout the body.
- The kidney, retina, skin, and skeletal muscles are commonly involved.
- The thick basement membrane in diabetics contains increased amounts of collagen and laminin and decreased proteoglycans.
- Strict control of diabetes decreases the incidence and severity of microangiopathy.

B. Large-vessel disease:

- Diabetes mellitus is a major risk factor for development of atherosclerotic vascular disease.
- Myocardial infarction and cerebral arterial occlusion (stroke) represent the commonest causes of death in diabetics.
- The increased incidence of hyperlipidemia in diabetes contributes to atherosclerosis.

C. Neuropathy and cataract is believed to result from accumulation of sorbitol within nerve or lens tissue.
D. Other complications:

- General increased susceptibility to infection.
- Impaired wound healing.

Clinical Course

The average life expectancy of diabetics is reduced by 9 years for males and 7 years for females when compared with nondiabetics. The reduction is greatest when the onset of disease is at a young age.

TABLE 46–3. CHRONIC COMPLICATIONS OF DIABETES MELLITUS BY ORGAN SYSTEM

Kidney (see Chapter 48)
  Glomerular microangiopathy
    Diffuse glomerulosclerosis
    Nodular glomerulosclerosis (Kimmelstiel-Wilson disease)
  Urinary infections
    Acute pyelonephritis   Renal failure
    Necrotizing papillitis
    Emphysematous pyelonephritis
  Glycogen nephrosis (Armanni-Ebstein lesion)

Eye (see Chapter 33)
  Retinopathy
    Nonproliferative retinopathy: capillary microaneurysms,
      retinal edema, exudates, and hemorrhages
    Proliferative retinopathy: proliferation of small vessels,
      hemorrhage, fibrosis, retinal detachment   Visual failure
  Cataracts
  Transient refractive errors due to osmotic changes in lens
  Glaucoma due to proliferation of vessels in the iris
  Infections

Nervous system
  Cerebrovascular atherosclerotic disease: strokes, death
  Peripheral neuropathy: peripheral sensory and motor, cranial, autonomic

Skin
  Infections: folliculitis leading to carbuncles
  Necrobiosis lipoidica diabeticorum: due to microangiopathy
  Xanthomata: secondary to hyperlipidemia

Cardiovascular system
  Coronary atherosclerosis: myocardial infarction, death
  Peripheral atherosclerosis: limb ischemia, gangrene

Reproductive system
  Increased fetal death rate[1] (placental disease, neonatal respiratory distress syndrome, infection)

General
  Increased susceptibility to infection
  Delayed wound healing

[1]Note that elevated maternal blood glucose levels produce elevated fetal blood glucose levels; the fetal pancreas often shows islet hyperplasia due to increased beta cells responding to the demand for more insulin.

■ Quality of life is seriously affected because of disabling complications, strict diet, and drug treatment.
■ Causes of death in diabetes (in order of frequency) are myocardial infarction, renal failure, cerebrovascular accidents, infections, ketoacidosis, hyperosmolar coma, and hypoglycemia.

HYPERFUNCTION OF THE PANCREATIC ISLETS

ISLET CELL NEOPLASMS

Adenomas derived from the islet cells are relatively common. In 10–15% of cases, multiple adenomas are present.

- Islet cell carcinomas occur, but less frequently.
- Grossly, islet cell neoplasms are firm nodules that vary in size from microscopic (microadenomas) to large masses that may weigh several kilograms.
- Microscopically, islet cell neoplasms are composed of uniform small cells arranged in nests and trabeculae separated by endothelium-lined vascular spaces.
- The islet cell origin of a pancreatic neoplasm can be established by:
  - The presence of membrane-bound, electron-dense neurosecretory granules in the cytoplasm on electron microscopy.
  - Positive staining for neuron-specific enolase, chromogranin, or specific hormones by immunoperoxidase techniques.
- Differentiation of adenomas from carcinomas of islet cells is difficult by light microscopic examination.
- Features that favor a diagnosis of carcinoma are extensive invasion, venous involvement, and perineural invasion. The only definite evidence of malignancy is the presence of metastatic lesions.
- Islet cell adenomas are cured by surgical excision; carcinomas tend to grow slowly, but are difficult to control if surgery fails.
- Most islet cell neoplasms are composed of one cell type. Less commonly, multiple cell types are involved.
- The diagnosis of the cell type requires:
  - Electron microscopy, which demonstrates the characteristic granules of the different cells.
  - Serum assay for the different pancreatic hormones.
  - Demonstration of hormone in the tumor cells by immunoperoxidase techniques.

ISLET CELL HYPERPLASIA

Diffuse hyperplasia of the islets is a rare cause of hypersecretion of pancreatic hormones.

- It is characterized by the presence of islets in the size range 300–700 μm.
- Microscopically, hyperplastic islets resemble normal islets. Immunohistochemical studies sometimes show a dominance of one cell type.
- Marked islet cell hyperplasia (of insulin-producing beta cells) is also seen in fetuses born of diabetic mothers.

CLINICAL FEATURES OF PANCREATIC HORMONE EXCESS

Hyperinsulinism

This is the commonest clinical syndrome associated with hyperfunctioning islets.

- Seventy percent of cases are caused by solitary beta cell adenomas (insulinomas), 10% by multiple adenomas, 10% by carcinomas, and 10% by islet cell hyperplasia.
- It is characterized by Whipple's triad of symptoms:

- Hypoglycemia, precipitated by fasting or exercise.
- Prompt relief of symptoms by glucose administration.
- A plasma glucose level under 40 mg/dL during an attack.
■ Diagnosis is established by the finding of an inappropriately high serum insulin level during a period of hypoglycemia.

B. Glucagon excess:

■ Hyperfunction of alpha cells is rare and caused by an islet cell neoplasm (glucagonoma), 70% of which are carcinomas and 30% adenomas.
■ Two-thirds of patients with carcinomas present with evidence of metastases, commonly in the liver.
■ Patients have mild diabetes mellitus and a typical erythematous necrotizing migratory skin eruption.
■ Alopecia, increased skin pigmentation, and glossitis are less common manifestations.
■ Diagnosis is made by finding an elevated serum glucagon level.

C. Gastrin excess (Zollinger-Ellison syndrome):
This is second in frequency to hyperinsulinism among this group of diseases.

■ It is usually caused by an islet cell neoplasm composed of G cells (gastrinoma), 70% of which are malignant.
■ Secretion of large amounts of gastrin leads to:
  - Continuous hypersecretion of gastric acid. The resting acid secretion is greater than 60% of the maximum acid secretion in response to an injection of histamine or pentagastrin.
  - Unrelenting, recurrent peptic ulcers occur in the stomach, duodenum, esophagus, and jejunum in 90% of patients.
  - Severe diarrhea and hypokalemia are present in 30% of patients.
  - Diarrhea may be associated with steatorrhea due to inactivation of lipase by the low pH in the duodenum.
■ Diagnosis of Zollinger-Ellison syndrome is made by:
  - High serum gastrin levels.
  - A paradoxic increase in gastrin levels in response to intravenous secretin and calcium injections.

D. Somatostatin excess:

■ D cell neoplasms of the pancreas (somatostatinomas) are very rare. Eighty percent are malignant.
■ Clinically, mild diabetes mellitus is the most constant feature. Diarrhea and gallstones also occur.
■ Diagnosis by demonstration of an elevated serum level is difficult because of the short half-life of somatostatin.

E. Vasoactive intestinal polypeptide excess:

■ This is rare and usually caused by a D_1 cell neoplasm of the islets (VIPoma).
■ Clinically, patients develop watery diarrhea with hypokalemia and alkalosis (WDHA syndrome; Verner-Morrison syndrome).

■ Diagnosis is established by demonstrating elevated VIP levels in the serum and in an extract of the tumor.

F. Pancreatic polypeptide excess: Pancreatic polypeptide (PP)-producing neoplasms are extremely rare. Some patients have watery diarrhea and hypokalemia; others have peptic ulcer disease.

Section XI. The Urinary Tract & Male Reproductive System

The Kidney: I. Congenital Diseases; Tubulointerstitial Diseases

47

CLINICAL MANIFESTATIONS OF RENAL DISEASE

Pain

Stretching of the renal fascia causes poorly localized pain in the flank. Severe muscular contraction of the ureters associated with ureteral obstruction produces ureteral colic.

Hematuria

When bleeding is severe, hematuria causes red discoloration of urine. Hematuria is diagnosed by the presence of erythrocytes in a sample of urinary sediment. Hematuria has many causes (Table 47–1).

Proteinuria

Proteinuria is a common finding in many renal diseases, and testing for it is a useful screening test for renal disease. Urinary casts are formed when protein and other organic matter in the renal tubules solidifies.

Nephrotic Syndrome

Nephrotic syndrome is characterized by massive proteinuria (over 5 g/24 h), hypoproteinemia, and edema. Hypercholesterolemia is frequently also present. Nephrotic syndrome may result from any condition that causes increased glomerular capillary permeability to proteins (Table 47–2).

Acute Nephritic Syndrome

Acute nephritic syndrome is characterized by decreased urinary volume (oliguria), hematuria, mild proteinuria, and elevation of serum urea and creatinine. Acute glomerular disease associated with a decreased glomerular filtration is the major cause.

Acute Renal Failure

Acute renal failure is defined as marked diminution of urine output to less than 400

TABLE 47–1. CAUSES OF HEMATURIA

	Additional Urinary Findings[1]
Renal diseases	
Acute and chronic glomerulonephritis	Red cell casts, granular casts,[2]
Primary types, including Goodpasture's syndrome	leukocytes, protein
Secondary to systemic lupus erythematosus, polyarteritis nodosa, Henoch-Schönlein purpura	
Acute and chronic pyelonephritis	Proteins, leukocytes, white cell and epithelial cell casts, organisms
Tumor	Protein, sometimes malignant cells
Calculi	Leukocytes
Trauma	None
Drug/chemical toxicity	Protein, casts
Papillary necrosis	Necrotic papillae occasionally
Polycystic disease	None
Diseases of bladder, ureters, urethra	
Cystitis	Leukocytes, organisms
Urethritis	Leukocytes, organisms
Tumor	Sometimes malignant cells
Calculi	Leukocytes
Trauma	None
Systemic disease causing bleeding from genitourinary tract	
Malignant hypertension	Protein
Systemic emboli as in bacterial endocarditis	Protein
Bleeding diathesis or anticoagulant therapy	None
Osler-Weber-Rendu disease	None
Hemoglobinopathies, hemolysis	Hemoglobinuria[3]
Exercise hematuria (after violent exercise)	None

[1]All hematurias by definition contain red cells, ranging from few (microscopic hematuria, detectable only by microscopic examination of urine) to many (grossly visible blood in urine).

[2]Hyaline casts indicate increased protein loss; white cell, epithelial cell, and granular casts indicate tubular or glomerular disease; they are formed in the damaged tubules.

[3]Red cells may be present in some hemoglobinopathies (eg, sickle cell disease). However, free hemoglobin will also cause red coloration of urine and give a positive result with the usual colorimetric and "dipstick" tests for hematuria. Microscopic examination for red cells is essential to differentiate hematuria from hemoglobinuria.

TABLE 47–2. CAUSES OF NEPHROTIC SYNDROME

Primary renal disease
Minimal change glomerulonephritis (lipoid nephrosis)
Other forms of glomerulonephritis
Renal vein thrombosis
Nephrotoxins such as gold, bismuth, mercury

Systemic disorders with renal damage
Diabetes
Amyloidosis
Systemic lupus erythematosus
Allergic responses, poison ivy, insect stings, tumors
Infections, malaria, syphilis
Myeloma kidney
Goodpasture's syndrome, Henoch-Schönlein purpura,
    and other forms of secondary glomerulonephritis

mL/d. It leads to elevation of serum creatinine and urea plus hypertension due to retention of sodium and water. It has many causes (Table 47–3).

Chronic Renal Failure

Chronic renal failure is characterized by a variety of abnormalities (Fig 47–1) resulting from a decrease in the total number of nephrons. There are many causes (Table 47–4).

- It is most accurately assessed by the creatinine clearance test.
- Serum urea and creatinine become elevated only when creatinine clearance decreases to 30–40% of normal.

Hypertension

Hypertension occurs in both acute and chronic renal failure and may be the presenting feature of renal disease. The principal mechanism is retention of sodium and water by the nephron.

METHODS OF EVALUATING RENAL STRUCTURE & FUNCTION

Physical Examination

When the kidney is enlarged (eg, in cystic disease, neoplasms), it can be palpated by bimanual examination.

Radiologic Examination

- Plain abdominal X-ray provides an estimate of renal size and shape.
- Intravenous and retrograde pyelography outlines the pelvicaliceal system.
- Ultrasonography and computerized tomography are sensitive methods of detecting cysts and neoplasms within the kidney.
- Renal arteriography provides information regarding the vasculature of the kidney.

Examination of Urine

Routine urine examination should be part of every complete physical examination. Most of the chemical tests and microscopic examination of the sediment can be easily performed by the physician in an office or ward laboratory.

TABLE 47–3. CAUSES OF OLIGURIA OR ANURIA

Prerenal
  Shock due to any cause: hypovolemia, renal vasoconstriction, and decreased renal blood flow
  Postoperative oliguria (antidiuresis)
  Dehydration (antidiuresis)

Renal
  Acute glomerulonephritis
  Acute tubular necrosis
    Nephrotoxic
      Drugs: aminoglycosides,[1] sulfonamides
      X-ray contrast media[1]
      Gold, mercury, arsenic
      Industrial: carbon tetrachloride, ethylene glycol
    Ischemic
      Prolonged hypotension in shock
      Includes trauma (crush syndrome),[2] incompatible transfusion,[2] burns,[2] eclampsia, hepatorenal syndrome
    Transplant rejection
  Acute cortical necrosis
    Severe ischemia: Extreme shock, especially with infections, burns, and hemorrhage in pregnancy
    Disseminated intravascular coagulation: Again, shock is usually present
    Snakebite
  Acute pyelonephritis when associated with papillary necrosis (rare)

Postrenal obstruction
  To cause anuria, obstruction must involve both ureters, the bladder neck, or the urethra. Common causes include tumor, prostatic hyperplasia, calculus, and trauma (including abdominal surgery).

[1]Aminoglycosides (kanamycin, neomycin, etc) and x-ray contrast media are 2 of the most common causes in modern hospital practice.
[2]It has been argued that precipitation of hemoglobin, myoglobin, or fragmented red cell membranes in the tubules in these conditions may aggravate the effects of hypotension.

Renal Biopsy

Percutaneous renal biopsy is a safe procedure that provides a cylindric core of renal tissue for histologic examination. Samples are also processed for electron microscopy and immunofluorescence.

CONGENITAL RENAL MALFORMATIONS

RENAL AGENESIS

Renal agenesis is the failure of development of the renal anlage, resulting in complete absence of the kidney.

- Bilateral renal agenesis:
  - Is a rare anomaly resulting in death, either in utero or soon after delivery.
  - Infants have renal failure associated with characteristic facial features (wide-set eyes, prominent inner canthi, a broad, flattened nose, large and low-set ears, and a receding chin (Potter facies).

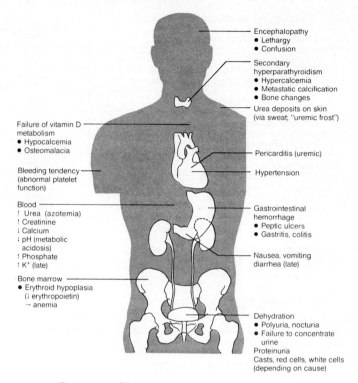

Figure 47–1. Clinical sequelae of chronic renal failure.

■ Unilateral renal agenesis is more common, occurring in 0.1% of the population. It is asymptomatic.

RENAL HYPOPLASIA
Renal hypoplasia is defined as a small kidney (<50 g in an adult) with five or fewer calices (normal is 7–13) but otherwise normal in structure. The anomaly is rare and usually unilateral.

ECTOPIC KIDNEY
Ectopic position of one or both kidneys is common. The most common location is at the pelvic brim or in the pelvis. Renal ectopia is usually asymptomatic but may cause obstruction and infection if there is kinking of the ureter.

HORSESHOE KIDNEY
Horseshoe kidney consists of an abnormal fusion of the lower poles across the midline by a broad band of renal tissue. It occurs in 0.4% of individuals. The ureters pass anterior to the isthmus of the horseshoe kidney and may be narrowed. Most patients are asymptomatic, but there is an increased incidence of urinary infection.

TABLE 47-4. CAUSES OF CHRONIC RENAL FAILURE[1]

Chronic glomerulonephritis: many causes	30%
Chronic pyelonephritis	15%
Obstructive nephropathy, hydronephrosis	10%
Hypertensive renal disease	10%
Polycystic disease	10%
Diabetic nephropathy	10%
Amyloidosis	5%
Multiple myeloma	rare
Nephrolithiasis, hypercalcemia	rare
Analgesic nephropathy, drugs, and chemicals	rare

[1]Note that many of these conditions occur together, eg, obstructive nephropathy, nephrolithiasis (stones), and pyelonephritis.

RENAL DYSGENESIS (Renal Dysplasia)

Renal dysgenesis is a maldevelopment of the renal anlage. It may be total or segmental and many involve one or both kidneys. Cysts are commonly present. Renal failure may develop in severe cases.

CYSTIC DISEASES OF THE KIDNEY

ADULT POLYCYSTIC DISEASE

This is a relatively common inherited disorder affecting one of every 500 individuals. It accounts for 5-10% of chronic dialysis patients and 5-10% of transplantation procedures for chronic renal failure. The pathogenesis is unknown.

■ Grossly, both kidneys are replaced by a mass of cysts involving both cortex and medulla.
■ Microscopically, the cysts are lined by renal tubular epithelium.
■ Residual nephrons are progressively destroyed.
■ Patients with adult polycystic disease have increased frequency of cysts in the liver, pancreas, and spleen and, congenital (berry) aneurysms of cerebral arteries.
■ Clinically, patients present in adult life with hypertension, chronic renal failure, or hematuria.

INFANTILE POLYCYSTIC DISEASE

This is a rare autosomal recessive disorder causing severe renal failure in infancy. The cut surface of the kidney shows innumerable radially oriented fusiform cysts lined by cuboidal epithelium. It is believed to result from failure of communication between the nephron and the pelvicaliceal system during development. Many patients have associated bile duct microhamartomas and congenital hepatic fibrosis.

MEDULLARY CYSTIC DISEASE
Medullary cystic disease affects the medulla selectively.

- Medullary sponge kidney is relatively common:
  - It occurs in one or both kidneys of older patients (ages 40–60).
  - Small cysts are present in the renal papillae.
  - Pathogenesis is unknown, and there are usually no symptoms. Some patients have defective sodium reabsorption.
- Uremic medullary cystic disease:
  - This is a rare disease of children and young adults.
  - It is characterized by the presence of multiple cysts in the medulla, cortical tubular atrophy, and interstitial fibrosis.
  - Pathogenesis is unknown.
  - Chronic renal failure progresses to death in 5–10 years.

GLOMERULOCYSTIC DISEASE
This is a rare lesion of infants and young children. The entire cortex of both kidneys is replaced by small cysts (< 1 cm) composed microscopically of dilated Bowman spaces in glomeruli. It is associated with progressive renal failure.

SIMPLE RENAL CYSTS
Simple cortical cysts are present in over 50% of patients after age 50. They may be multiple and large. They are of no clinical significance. Large cortical cysts may be difficult to differentiate clinically and radiologically from cystic renal adenocarcinoma.

DIALYSIS CYSTIC DISEASE
Multiple renal cysts occur in as many as 60% of patients receiving long-term hemodialysis for chronic renal failure. The cause is unknown. There is an increased incidence of renal adenocarcinoma.

TUBULOINTERSTITIAL DISEASES
Tubulointerstitial diseases are a group of renal disorders characterized by primary abnormalities in the renal tubules or interstitium. There are four principal causes: infectious, toxic, metabolic, and immunologic.

- The morphologic changes in tubulointerstitial disease include:
  - Acute tubular necrosis.
  - Atrophy of tubules, with interstitial fibrosis.
  - Interstitial inflammation, either acute or chronic.
  - Tubular basement membrane thickening.
  - Deposition of abnormal substances such as calcium, amyloid, urate, myeloma proteins, and oxalate in the tubules and interstitium.

Infectious Diseases

ACUTE PYELONEPHRITIS

Incidence
This is extremely common—more so in females than in males (10 : 1). It occurs at all ages, with highest frequency during early sexual activity and during pregnancy.

Etiology

- Usually it appears after an ascending bacterial infection. Hematogenous infection is uncommon.
- Factors important in etiology:
  - A short urethra, as in females.
  - Stasis of urine from any cause.
  - Structural abnormalities in the urinary tract.
  - Vesicoureteral reflux of urine.
  - Catheterization of the bladder.
  - Diabetes mellitus.
- Seventy-five percent of cases of acute pyelonephritis are caused by *Escherichia coli.*
- Other organisms include *Klebsiella, Proteus, Streptococcus faecalis,* and *Pseudomonas aeruginosa.*

Pathology

- Grossly, acute pyelonephritis may be unilateral or bilateral.
- The kidney is enlarged and shows areas of suppuration (abscesses) in the cortex with radial yellow streaks traversing the medulla.
- The renal pelvis is erythematous and frequently covered with exudate.
- Extension to the perinephric space to form a perinephric abscess is not uncommon.
- Microscopically, there is an acute suppurative inflammation involving the renal tubules.

Clinical Features

- Onset is with high fever, chills, rigors, and flank pain. Dysuria and increased frequency are present in most cases.
- The urine shows mild proteinuria, with neutrophils, white cell casts, and bacteria in the sediment.
- Diagnosis is made by quantitative urine culture. A positive culture with over 100,000 organisms/mL is diagnostic.

Complications

- Gram-negative sepsis with shock.
- Renal papillary necrosis, particularly in diabetics.
- Emphysematous pyelonephritis, characterized by anaerobic bacterial fermentation with gas formation in the renal parenchyma, occurs rarely in diabetic patients.

CHRONIC PYELONEPHRITIS

Incidence & Etiology

- Infectious pyelonephritis accounts for 15–20% of cases of chronic renal failure.
- Etiologic factors include:
  - Chronic obstruction of the urinary tract by calculi, prostatic hyperplasia, tumors, congenital anomalies, retroperitoneal fibrosis, and in neurogenic bladder.
  - Vesico-ureteral reflux in children, leading to chronic pyelonephritis in half the cases.

Pathology

- Kidneys show asymmetric involvement, with irregular scarring and contraction.
- Deformity of the pelvicaliceal system and hydronephrosis may be present.
- Microscopically, there is marked patchy chronic inflammation and fibrosis of the interstitium.
- Periglomerular fibrosis is followed by global sclerosis.
- Immunofluorescence and electron microscopy do not show immune complex deposition in the glomeruli.
- Xanthogranulomatous pyelonephritis:
  - Is a variant of chronic pyelonephritis characterized by sheets of lipid-laden foamy histiocytes.
  - Is associated with caliceal staghorn calculi.
  - The inflammatory process frequently extends into the perinephric tissues and may involve adjacent organs.

Clinical Features

Chronic pyelonephritis usually manifests as hypertension or chronic renal failure. Pyuria (neutrophils in urine), mild proteinuria, and bacteriuria are present.

RENAL TUBERCULOSIS

This is uncommon in the United States and Western Europe, but still occurs frequently in parts of the world where tuberculosis is endemic. It results from reactivation of dormant bacilli.

- It is most common in patients aged 20–50.
- Approximately half of patients with renal tuberculosis have a normal chest X-ray.
- The kidney is grossly enlarged, and shows several caseating granulomas in the corticomedullary region. Cavitation and fibrosis are common.
- Acid-fast bacilli can be demonstrated in most cases.
- Clinically, patients present with low-grade fever, weight loss, hematuria, frequency, and lumbar pain.
- The urine shows numerous neutrophils and routine urine culture is negative ("sterile pyuria"); culture for mycobacteria is positive and diagnostic.

LEPTOSPIROSIS (Weil's Disease)

This is an uncommon infection caused by a spirochete of the genus *Leptospira,* most commonly *L icterohaemorrhagiae.*

- Humans are infected by contact with infected rat urine, usually in occupations that necessitate working in open trenches, fields, or sewers.
- Pathologically, there is focal renal tubular necrosis with interstitial inflammation.
- Clinical onset is abrupt, with high fever, oliguria, proteinuria, and hematuria. Jaundice may occur as a result of liver involvement.
- Diagnosis is made by blood culture and demonstration of rising titers of specific agglutinating antibody.

MALARIA

Plasmodium falciparum malaria may cause acute glomerulonephritis of immune complex type, or blackwater fever resulting from hemoglobinuria. *Plasmodium malariae* malaria causes nephrotic syndrome and chronic renal failure.

Toxic Tubulointerstitial Disease

RADIATION NEPHRITIS

This occurs when the kidneys are in the field of radiation during treatment of malignant neoplasms. The dose required to produce radiation nephritis is about 23 Gy in adults. Pathologically, the small arteries show fibrinoid necrosis. Tubular atrophy and interstitial fibrosis follow.

ANALGESIC NEPHROPATHY

Excessive use of analgesics is a relatively common cause of chronic renal disease in Australia and Europe but is rare in the United States.

- Phenacetin is believed to be the main offender.
- Pathologically, there is renal papillary necrosis, with interstitial medullary fibrosis and calcification.
- Clinically, there is hematuria, ureteral colic, hypertension, and progressive renal failure.
- In some cases, the shed necrotic renal papilla may be identified in a sample of urine.

DRUG-INDUCED NEPHROTOXICITY

Acute Interstitial Nephritis

This is caused by methicillin, other penicillin derivatives, sulfonamides, and various diuretics.

- Pathologically, there is tubular degeneration and necrosis and marked interstitial inflammation.
- Clinically, patients develop fever, hematuria, and proteinuria about two weeks after exposure to the drug.
- Acute renal failure develops in 50%.
- Recovery usually occurs when the drug is withdrawn.

Acute Renal Tubular Necrosis

Drug-induced acute renal tubular necrosis has been reported with aminoglycosides (gentamicin, kanamycin), amphotericin B, an antifungal agent, cephaloridine, and methoxyflurane, an anesthetic agent.

Nephrotic Syndrome

Nephrotic syndrome may be caused by mercurial compounds used as skin ointments and diuretics, trimethadione (an antiepileptic drug), and gold, used in the treatment of rheumatoid arthritis.

METAL TOXICITY

Mercurial compounds cause proximal convoluted tubule damage. **Lead poisoning** damages the entire tubule. The presence of intranuclear eosinophilic inclusions in the cells is characteristic.

"Metabolic" Tubulointerstitial Diseases

GOUT (Urate Nephropathy)
Acute urate nephropathy occurs with very high serum uric acid levels; urate crystals deposited in the tubules cause obstruction. Chronic urate nephropathy occurs with protracted hyperuricemia, resulting in tubulointerstitial inflammation and fibrosis.

HYPOKALEMIA
Hypokalemia causes tubular dysfunction with inability to concentrate urine, polyuria, loss of sodium in urine, and failure to excrete acid (renal tubular acidosis).

HYPERCALCEMIA
Acute hypercalcemia damages the distal convoluted tubular epithelium, resulting in failure to concentrate urine.

- With prolonged hypercalcemia, metastatic calcification occurs in the renal interstitium (nephrocalcinosis) and may lead to chronic renal failure.
- Increased calcium excretion in the urine increases the risk of urinary calculi.

MYELOMATOSIS ("Myeloma Kidney")
This is characterized by an interstitial granulomatous reaction to immunoglobulin light chains (Bence Jones proteins) in the renal tubules. Amyloidosis may also complicate myelomatosis.

IMMUNOLOGIC TUBULOINTERSTITIAL DISEASE
Immunologic mechanisms involving the renal tubules include:

- Transplant rejection (see Chapter 8).
- Some cases of drug-induced acute interstitial nephritis (see preceding page).

The Kidney: II. Glomerular Disease

48

INTRODUCTION

Glomerular diseases are characterized by primary abnormalities of the glomerulus. Their classification uses a combination of clinical (congenital or acquired; acute or chronic), morphologic (proliferative, membranous, minimal change), and immunologic criteria (Table 48–1 and 48–2).

Pathologic Changes

Glomerular diseases may be focal, showing abnormality in some but not all of the glomeruli, or diffuse, where all glomeruli are affected. They can be further divided into segmental, when only a portion of each individual glomerulus is affected, and global, where entire glomeruli are involved.

- Diagnosis of specific diseases frequently depends on the identification of morphologic changes in the glomerulus in renal biopsy specimens (Fig 48–1):
  - Proliferation of epithelial, mesangial, or endothelial cells (proliferative glomerulonephritis).
  - Crescent formation, which occurs when epithelial cell proliferation is extensive. (A crescent is a mass of cellular or collagenized tissue that obliterates Bowman's space.)
  - Infiltration of the glomerulus by inflammatory cells. Acute inflammation is accompanied by fluid exudation and swelling of the glomerulus.
  - Capillary basement membrane thickening. This may be detected by light microscopy when severe, but requires electron microscopy in early stages.
  - Increased mesangial matrix material.
  - Epithelial foot process fusion, which can be seen only by electron microscopy.
  - Fibrosis (equals sclerosis).
  - Deposition of amyloid.

Pathogenesis of Glomerular Disease (Fig 48–2)
A. Immune complex disease:

- This is the most common cause of glomerular injury.
- Immune complexes may be deposited on the glomerular filtration membrane or in the mesangium.
- Immune complex deposition may produce any or all of the pathologic features described above, one or the other predominating in different diseases.
- Immunoglobulin and complement are demonstrable by immunofluorescence. The staining pattern on immunofluorescence is "lumpy-bumpy" (irregular).

TABLE 48-1. CLASSIFICATION OF GLOMERULAR DISEASES

Congenital glomerulonephritis
Hereditary nephritis (includes Alport's syndrome)
Congenital nephrotic syndrome

Primary acquired glomerulonephritis (primary indicates that the renal involvement is the main manifestation of the disease)
Diffuse glomerulonephritis
  Minimal change glomerulonephritis (glomerular epithelial cell disease)
  Proliferative glomerulonephritis
    Postinfectious (poststreptococcal) glomerulonephritis
    Crescentic glomerulonephritis
    Antiglomerular basement membrane disease (Goodpasture's syndrome)
  Mesangial proliferative glomerulonephritis
Membranous glomerulonephritis
Membranoproliferative (mesangiocapillary) glomerulonephritis
Focal glomerulonephritis

Secondary acquired glomerulonephritis (secondary indicates that the renal involvement is part of a systemic disease such as systemic lupus erythematosus or progressive systemic sclerosis).

Chronic glomerulonephritis

Other glomerular diseases
Diabetic nephropathy
Amyloidosis

■ Immune complexes are visible with the electron microscope as electron-dense deposits.

B. Anti-glomerular basement membrane antibody:

■ Deposition of anti-glomerular basement membrane antibodies on the basement membrane leads to lesions that by light microscopy are identical to those seen in some immune complex diseases.
■ Immunofluorescence shows linear deposition of immunoglobulin and complement in the basement membrane (Fig 48-2).

MINIMAL CHANGE GLOMERULAR DISEASE (Epithelial Cell Disease)
Minimal change glomerular disease occurs most often in young children and is relatively rare in adults. The cause and pathogenesis are unknown. A significant association with allergic diseases is present.

Pathology (Fig 48-3 and Table 48-2)

■ Light microscopy shows no abnormality.
■ Immunofluorescence shows absence of immunoglobulin or complement deposition.

TABLE 48–2. DIFFERENTIAL FEATURES OF GLOMERULAR DISEASE

Disease	Usual Clinical Findings	Proliferative	Membranous	Immunofluorescence				Electron Microscope	Diffuse/ Focal	Mechanism
				Pattern	Ig	Complement	Fibrin			
Minimal change glomerular disease (lipoid nephrosis)	Nephrotic syndrome	-	-	-	-	-	-	Foot process fusion	Diffuse	Unknown
Proliferative glomerulonephritis Poststreptococcal glomerulonephritis	Acute nephritic syndrome, nephrotic syndrome	+ Crescents (occasionally)	-	Granular	IgG	+	-	Subepithelial humps	Diffuse	Immune complex
Crescentic glomerulonephritis	Acute nephritic syndrome, rapidly progressive	+ Crescents	-	Granular or linear	IgG/ IgA	+	+	Variable deposits	Diffuse	Immune complex or basement membrane antibody
Anti-basement membrane disease (Goodpasture's syndrome)	Acute nephritic syndrome	+ Crescents	±	Linear	IgG	+	+	Thick basement membrane	Focal → diffuse	Basement membrane antibody (also lung)
Mesangioproliferative glomerulonephritis IgG	Proteinuria, hematuria				IgG	+	-			
IgA (Buerger's disease)	Nephrotic syndrome, proteinuria, hematuria, acute nephritic syndrome	+ Mesangial	-	Mesangial	IgA	+	-	Mesangial deposits	Diffuse	Immune complex
IgA (Henoch-Schölein purpura)	Nephrotic syndrome, proteinuria, hematuria, acute nephritic syndrome				IgA	+	+			

Disease	Clinical			Immunofluorescence	Ig			Morphology	Distribution	Pathogenesis
Membranous glomerulonephritis	Proteinuria, nephrotic syndrome, chronic renal failure	–	+	Granular	IgG	±	–	Subepithelial deposits, spikes, split basement membrane	Diffuse	Immune complex; probably formed in situ
Membranoproliferative glomerulonephritis (mesangiocapillary) I	Acute nephritic syndrome, nephrotic syndrome	+ Endothelial, mesangial	+	Granular	IgG	+	–	Subendothelial deposits, split basement membrane	Diffuse	Immune complex
II	Nephrotic syndrome, chronic renal failure			Granular	–	+	–	Thick basement membrane, dense deposits	Diffuse	Immune complex; probably alternative pathway
Focal glomerulonephritis	Proteinuria, nephrotic syndrome	Focal +	±	Granular	IgM, IgA	+	+	Foot process fusion	Focal plus segmental	?Immune complex
Secondary glomerulonephritis, systemic lupus erythematosus, polyarteritis nodosa, etc	Variable	Variable +	Variable + (wireloops + in systemic lupus erythematosus)	Granular	IgG	+	+	Variable	Diffuse/focal	Immune complex
Chronic glomerulonephritis	Chronic renal failure	Any of above		Granular, linear: variable				Variable	Diffuse	Immune complex/antibasement membrane antibody
Diabetic nephropathy	Nephrotic syndrome, chronic renal failure	–	Focal sclerosis	None	–	–	–	Sclerosis	Diffuse/focal	Unknown
Amyloidosis	Nephrotic syndrome, chronic renal failure	–	+	None	–	–	–	Fibrillar amyloid	Diffuse	Deposition of amyloid protein

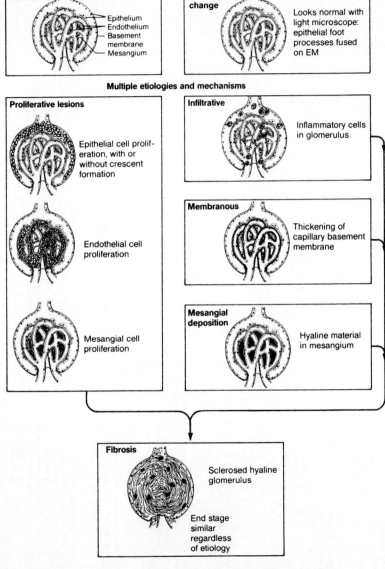

Figure 48–1. Basic pathologic changes that occur in glomerular diseases.

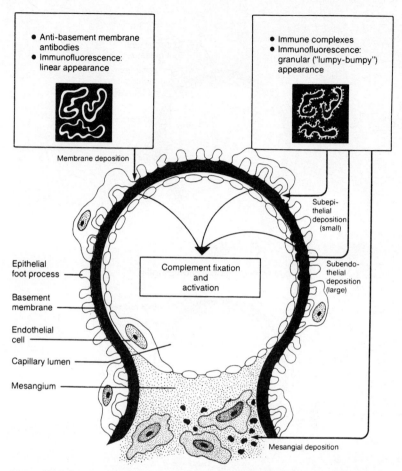

- Anti-basement membrane antibodies
- Immunofluorescence: linear appearance

- Immune complexes
- Immunofluorescence: granular ("lumpy-bumpy") appearance

Membrane deposition

Subepithelial deposition (small)

Epithelial foot process

Complement fixation and activation

Subendothelial deposition (large)

Basement membrane

Endothelial cell

Capillary lumen

Mesangium

Mesangial deposition

Figure 48–2. Basic types of glomerular injury resulting from (at left) the action of anti-glomerular basement membrane antibody, and (at right) immune complex deposition. In both instances, complement activation results in damage. These 2 types of injury can be distinguished by their different staining patterns on immunofluorescence.

■ Electron microscopy shows fusion of the foot processes of the epithelial cells. This change is not specific for the disease.

Clinical Features

This is one of the most common causes of nephrotic syndrome, particularly in the young.

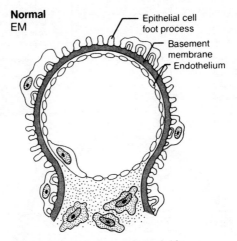

Normal
EM

Epithelial cell
foot process

Basement
membrane

Endothelium

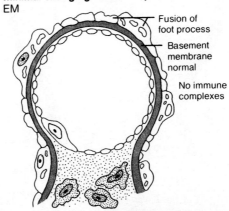

Minimal change glomerulonephritis
EM

Fusion of
foot process

Basement
membrane
normal

No immune
complexes

Immunofluorescence
● No immunoglobin or
   complement detectable
● Light microscopy looks
   normal

Figure 48–3. Minimal change glomerular disease. The only abnormality is fusion of epithelial foot processes, which is visible only by electron microscopy. Note that fusion of foot
processes is not a specific abnormality.

- The proteinuria is almost always highly selective, with loss of only low-molecular-weight proteins (high transferrin:IgG ratio in urine).
- Hematuria, hypertension, and azotemia are absent.

Treatment & Prognosis

- High-dosage corticosteroid therapy causes a dramatic decrease in proteinuria, with patients showing complete remission within 8 weeks.
- After withdrawal of steroids, about 50% of patients relapse intermittently for up to 10 years. Relapses respond well to steroid therapy.
- Resistance to steroids or development of renal failure is rare and should prompt a search for some other diagnosis, usually focal glomerulosclerosis or membranoproliferative glomerulonephritis.
- Prognosis for life and renal function is almost the same as that of the general population.

POSTINFECTIOUS (STREPTOCOCCAL) GLOMERULONEPHRITIS (Acute Diffuse Proliferative Glomerulonephritis)

This is one of the most common renal diseases in childhood. It is less common in adults. Occurrence is worldwide, at times in epidemics.

- An infection precedes the glomerulonephritis by 1–3 weeks.
- In most cases, the infection is a group A β-hemolytic streptococcal infection of the throat or skin.
- Other organisms are very rarely involved and include *Staphylococcus aureus,* pneumococcus, meningococcus, and some viruses.
- Deposition of immune complexes formed between bacterial antigens and host antibody in the glomerulus causes the disease.

Pathology (Fig 48–4 and Table 48–2)

- Grossly, the kidneys are slightly enlarged, with a smooth surface which may show petechial hemorrhages.
- Light microscopic examination shows diffuse glomerulonephritis. The glomeruli are enlarged, edematous, and hypercellular (due to proliferation of endothelial and mesangial cells), and infiltrated with neutrophils.
- A few crescents may be present. Rarely, crescent formation is extensive.
- The immune complexes appear as large, dome-shaped electron-dense deposits on the epithelial side of the basement membrane ("subepithelial humps").
- Immunofluorescence shows a granular ("lumpy-bumpy") deposition of IgG and C3 along the glomerular basement membrane and in the mesangium.

Clinical Features

Most patients present with an abrupt onset of the acute nephritic syndrome, characterized by mild periorbital edema, hypertension, proteinuria, and elevated serum urea and creatinine.

- A few patients present with nephrotic syndrome.

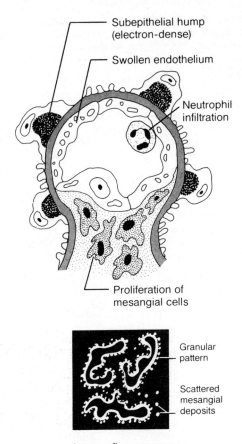

Figure 48–4. Poststreptococcal glomerulonephritis, characterized by the deposition of electron-dense immune complexes in the subepithelial and mesangial regions. Complement activation leads to proliferation of cells and inflammation.

- Throat and skin cultures are usually negative because the streptococcal infection has usually resolved.
- Serum levels of antistreptococcal antibodies such as antistreptolysin O and antihyaluronidase are often elevated.

Treatment & Prognosis

Treatment is supportive. The short-term prognosis is excellent, most patients resuming normal renal function and blood pressure within a year.

- A small number of patients progress rapidly to renal failure within 1–2 years. These cases are associated with the presence of numerous epithelial crescents.
- The long-term prognosis is controversial. A few studies report an increased incidence of chronic renal failure after initial resolution.

CRESCENTIC GLOMERULONEPHRITIS (Rapidly Progressive Glomerulonephritis)

This is a rare disease defined by the presence of epithelial crescents in more than 80% of the glomeruli. In most cases of crescentic glomerulonephritis there is no known cause.

- A few cases occur secondary to other diseases such as postinfectious glomerulonephritis and Goodpasture's syndrome.
- In a few cases, anti-glomerular basement membrane antibodies are found in the serum.

Pathology (Table 48–2)

Eighty percent of glomeruli must show crescent formation for this diagnosis to be made. Immunofluorescence studies show variable findings. IgA and C3 may be present in some cases. Electron microscopy shows varying destructive changes in the glomeruli.

Treatment & Prognosis

Treatment is unsatisfactory, and the prognosis is very poor. A few cases of recurrence of the disease in transplanted kidneys have been reported.

ANTI-GLOMERULAR BASEMENT MEMBRANE DISEASE (Goodpasture's Syndrome)

Goodpasture's syndrome is rare. It occurs in young adults, with males affected more frequently than females.

- The serum contains anti-glomerular basement membrane antibodies of IgG type.
- These antibodies bind to both kidney and pulmonary alveolar basement membrane. Antibody binding in the lungs causes pulmonary hemorrhage (see Chapter 35).

Pathology (Table 48–2)

Light microscopy initially shows a focal proliferative glomerulonephritis. In the later stages, diffuse glomerular involvement occurs.

- Proliferative changes are frequently associated with necrosis and epithelial crescent formation.
- Sclerosis becomes prominent in the late stages.
- Immunofluorescence shows IgG and C3 deposition in a characteristic diffuse linear pattern along the basement membrane.
- Electron microscopy shows diffuse and irregular thickening of the glomerular basement membrane. The electron microscopic findings are nonspecific.

Clinical Features

It commonly presents with proteinuria and hematuria followed by progressive renal failure. Patients with pulmonary involvement have recurrent hemoptysis, with dyspnea, cough, and bilateral pulmonary infiltrates on X-ray. Chronic loss of blood in the urine and lungs may cause severe iron deficiency anemia.

Treatment & Prognosis

Treatment of Goodpasture's syndrome is unsatisfactory, and the prognosis is poor. Most cases progress to renal failure within 1 year after diagnosis.

MESANGIAL PROLIFERATIVE GLOMERULONEPHRITIS

Proliferation of mesangial cells as the only abnormality in a renal biopsy specimen is a nonspecific finding. It is classified according to the type of immunoglobulin present in the glomerulus.

A. With IgG in mesangium:

- Mesangial IgG deposition is common and may occur as an isolated finding or in the healing phase of postinfectious glomerulonephritis.
- The pathogenesis is unknown in most cases.
- Light microscopy shows increased numbers of mesangial cells in the glomeruli (more than the normal three nuclei per lobule).
- The mesangial matrix material is increased.
- Immunofluorescence shows the presence of IgG and C3 in the mesangium.
- Electron microscopy shows the presence of mesangial electron-dense deposits in some cases.

B. With IgA in mesangium (Table 48–2).

1. IgA nephropathy (Berger's disease) accounts for 2–5% of all cases of primary glomerulonephritis in the United States and England. The incidence is much higher (up to 20%) in France and Australia.

- It is most common in the age group from 10 to 30 years and has a marked male predominance.
- On light microscopy, there is mesangial hypercellularity and increased matrix material.
- Immunofluorescence shows IgA deposits in the mesangium as confluent masses or discrete granules. C3 is frequently present.
- Electron microscopy shows mesangial hypercellularity, sclerosis, and electron-dense mesangial deposits.
- Clinically, patients present with recurrent episodes of hematuria.
- Though progression of the disease is very slow, the ultimate prognosis is not good. Most patients progress to chronic renal failure after a mean interval of 6 years.

2. Henoch-Schönlein purpura:

- This is a rare disease, mainly affecting children.
- It is characterized clinically by a systemic vasculitis affecting skin, joints, intestine, and kidneys.
- Renal involvement is common and may cause hematuria, proteinuria, acute renal failure, or nephrotic syndrome.
- Light microscopy shows mesangial hypercellularity and epithelial crescents.
- Immunofluorescence shows the presence of IgA deposition in the mesangium.
- Electron microscopy shows mesangial deposits and hypercellularity.
- Henoch-Schönlein purpura is a progressive disorder. About 20% of patients develop chronic renal disease.

MEMBRANOUS NEPHROPATHY (Membranous Glomerulonephritis)

Membranous nephropathy is an important and common cause of nephrotic syndrome in adults (mean age 35). It is rare in children.

- It is believed to result from accumulation of circulating immune complexes in the glomerular capillary.
- The nature of the antigen involved is unknown.
- A few cases are associated with:
  - Systemic infections, including hepatitis B, malaria, schistosomiasis, syphilis, and leprosy.
  - Drugs such as penicillamine and heroin.
  - Toxic metals such as gold and mercury.
  - Neoplasms, including carcinomas, malignant lymphomas, and Hodgkin's lymphoma.
  - Collagen diseases such as systemic lupus erythematosus, progressive systemic sclerosis, and mixed connective tissue disease.
  - Miscellaneous conditions including renal vein thrombosis and sickle cell disease.

Pathology (Fig 48–5 and Table 48–2)

Light and electron microscopy permit recognition of three stages of the disease:

- Stage I is characterized by the deposition of dome-shaped subepithelial electron-dense deposits. At this stage, the basement membrane is near normal.
- Stage II is characterized by spikes of basement membrane material protruding outward toward the epithelial side between the deposits.
- Stage III: The spikes fuse on the epithelial side around the deposits, giving the basement membrane a bilayered appearance on silver stain.
- There is no hypercellularity of the glomerulus.
- With progression, increasing thickness of the basement membrane converts the glomerulus into a hyaline mass.
- The changes of idiopathic membranous nephropathy are identical to those of secondary disease.
- Immunofluorescence shows granular deposits of IgG and C3 corresponding to the subepithelial deposits.

Clinical Features

Patients present with either the nephrotic syndrome or asymptomatic proteinuria. The proteinuria is nonselective. Most patients have a slow progression to chronic renal failure; 70% of patients are alive at 10 years. The prognosis is better in females and in children.

MEMBRANOPROLIFERATIVE GLOMERULONEPHRITIS (Mesangiocapillary Glomerulonephritis)

This is characterized by the presence of a combination of thickening of the capillary wall and proliferation of mesangial cells. Two distinct patterns are recognized (Fig 48–6 and Table 48–2).

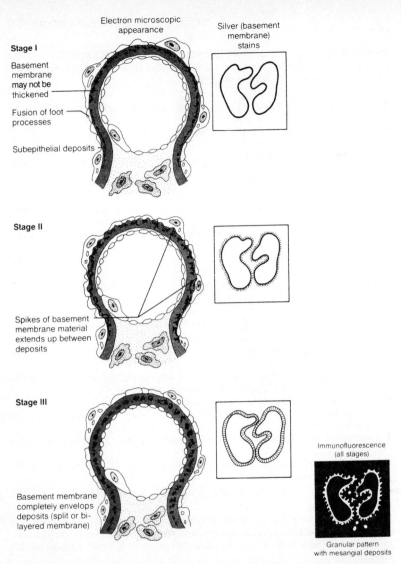

Electron microscopic appearance

Silver (basement membrane) stains

Stage I

Basement membrane may not be thickened

Fusion of foot processes

Subepithelial deposits

Stage II

Spikes of basement membrane material extends up between deposits

Stage III

Basement membrane completely envelops deposits (split or bi-layered membrane)

Immunofluorescence (all stages)

Granular pattern with mesangial deposits

Figure 48–5. Membranous nephropathy. In stage I disease, light microscopy resembles minimal change disease but can be differentiated on electron microscopy and immunofluorescence because of the presence in membranous nephropathy of immune complexes. In later stages of the disease, protrusion of basement membrane material around the immune complexes produces spikes (stage II) and a bilayered appearance (stage III) when the basement membrane is stained with silver stains. Light microscopy shows thickened basement membrane in these later stages.

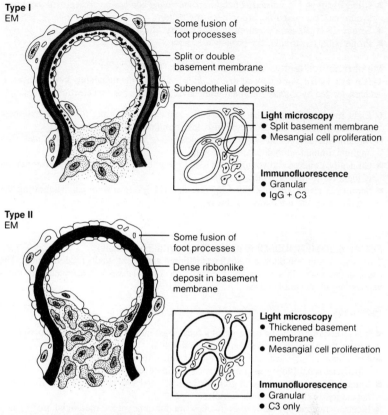

Type I
EM

- Some fusion of foot processes
- Split or double basement membrane
- Subendothelial deposits

Light microscopy
- Split basement membrane
- Mesangial cell proliferation

Immunofluorescence
- Granular
- IgG + C3

Type II
EM

- Some fusion of foot processes
- Dense ribbonlike deposit in basement membrane

Light microscopy
- Thickened basement membrane
- Mesangial cell proliferation

Immunofluorescence
- Granular
- C3 only

Figure 48–6. Membranoproliferative glomerulonephritis. Type I disease is characterized by subendothelial immune complexes, a split ("tram track") basement membrane, and deposition of IgG and C3. Type II is characterized by a densely thickened, ribbonlike basement membrane and the presence of C3 only on immunofluorescence.

Membranoproliferative Glomerulonephritis, Type I

Type I accounts for 65% of cases. It is characterized by deposition of subendothelial immune complexes in the glomerular capillary.

- Most cases have no known cause.
- Light microscopy shows mesangial cell proliferation and diffuse thickening of the basement membrane, which appears to be split (double-contour or tram-track appearance).
- Immunofluorescence shows granular deposition of IgG and C3 in the capillary wall.
- Electron microscopy shows the diagnostic subendothelial deposits.

- Clinically, type I is a disease of children and young adults who present with nephrotic syndrome or a mixed nephrotic-nephritic pattern.
- Serum C3 levels are decreased in the majority of cases.
- Progression is variable; the prognosis is poor.

Membranoproliferative Glomerulonephritis, Type II

This is also called dense deposit disease. It accounts for the remaining 35% of cases. It is characterized by a dense intramembranous ribbonlike deposit on electron microscopy.

- Light microscopy shows an eosinophilic, refractile, uniformly thickened basement membrane. Mesangial proliferation is less prominent than in type I.
- Immunofluorescence shows granular deposition of C3 in the capillary wall and mesangium. Immunoglobulins are not found.
- Clinically, children and young adults tend to be affected most frequently. Presentation is identical to that of type I.
- Serum C3 levels are low, but Clq, C2, and C4 levels are normal, suggesting C3 activation by the alternative pathway.
- The prognosis is poor.

FOCAL GLOMERULOSCLEROSIS (Segmental Hyalinosis)

This is an uncommon disease that affects children and young adults predominantly. The cause is unknown. In some patients, focal glomerulosclerosis is associated with intravenous heroin abuse or AIDS.

Pathology

- It is characterized by the presence of a focal segmental sclerotic area in the peripheral part of the glomerulus, frequently near the hilum.
- The glomeruli affected first are in the juxtamedullary (deep cortical) region, and a superficial renal biopsy may easily miss the involved glomeruli.
- Immunofluorescence shows a granular IgM, C3 and sometimes IgA, and fibrinogen deposition in the affected glomeruli.
- Electron microscopy shows an increase in the amount of mesangial matrix and collapse of the glomerular capillaries in areas of glomerulosclerosis.

Clinical Features

Patients present with nephrotic syndrome or asymptomatic proteinuria. The proteinuria is nonselective.

- Prognosis is poor, with slow progression to chronic renal failure.
- There is no response to corticosteroid therapy.
- A few patients have disease recurring in the allografts after renal transplantation.

SECONDARY ACQUIRED GLOMERULONEPHRITIS

1. SYSTEMIC LUPUS ERYTHEMATOSUS (SLE)

Renal involvement is the most common cause of death in SLE, and the presenting feature in 5% of patients with SLE.

TABLE 48-3. WORLD HEALTH ORGANIZATION CATEGORIES OF GLOMERULAR DISEASE IN SYSTEMIC LUPUS ERYTHEMATOSUS

Class	Pathologic Change	% With Glomerulonephritis	Clinical Features
I	No change		Mild disease with microscopic hematuria or proteinuria; slow progression
II	Mesangial glomerulonephritis	10%	
III	Focal proliferative glomerulonephritis	30%	
IV	Diffuse proliferative glomerulonephritis	50%	Severe disease with rapid progression to renal failure
V	Diffuse membranous glomerulonephritis	10%	Nephrotic syndrome; slow progression to renal failure

- Clinical manifestations include proteinuria, microscopic hematuria, nephrotic syndrome, acute nephritic syndrome, and renal failure.
- Light microscopy shows:
  - Focal and diffuse proliferation of capillary endothelial cells, which is the most serious microscopic abnormality.
  - Mesangial hypercellularity, which is commoner but less ominous.
  - Diffuse or segmental basement membrane thickening due to subepithelial immune complex deposition.
  - Large subendothelial immune complexes that produce wire loop lesions.
  - Glomerular sclerosis.
- Immunofluorescence shows lumpy IgG and C3 in the glomerular basement membrane and mesangium.
- Electron microscopy shows large immune complexes in the subendothelial, mesangial, and subepithelial regions.
- The clinical features and prognosis depend on the histologic class of disease (Table 48-3).

2. PROGRESSIVE SYSTEMIC SCLEROSIS (Scleroderma)
The kidneys are frequently involved in progressive systemic sclerosis, causing proteinuria and nephrotic syndrome, with progression to renal failure.

- Light microscopy shows:
  - Fibrinoid necrosis of the afferent arteriole and intimal fibrosis ("onionskin" change) of the interlobular arteries.
  - Segmental basement membrane thickening and wire loop lesions in the glomeruli.
  - Glomerular sclerosis.
- Immunofluorescence shows granular deposits of IgM and C3 in the glomerular capillaries.
- Electron microscopy shows nonspecific changes.

3. MIXED CONNECTIVE TISSUE DISEASE (MCTD)

Renal involvement occurs in about 20–30% of cases of MCTD. Changes are mainly in glomeruli, which show a combination of proliferative and membranous glomerulonephritis.

4. POLYARTERITIS NODOSA

Renal involvement is present in 80% of cases of polyarteritis nodosa. Thirty percent of patients with polyarteritis nodosa die of renal failure.

- A minority of patients are positive for hepatitis B surface antigen in serum.
- Grossly, the kidneys are reduced in size and show evidence of infarction and multiple hemorrhages.
- Light microscopy shows fibrinoid necrosis, inflammation, thrombosis, aneurysm formation, and rupture of the segmental and arcuate arteries.
- Glomeruli show fibrinoid necrosis and proliferative changes with crescents.
- Immunofluorescence shows immunoglobulin (mainly IgG) and fibrin in areas of fibrinoid necrosis.
- Clinically, patients present with hematuria, proteinuria, hypertension, and rapidly progressive renal failure.

5. WEGENER'S GRANULOMATOSIS

Renal involvement is one part of the classic triad of features of Wegener's granulomatosis—the others being upper respiratory tract and lung involvement.

- Renal disease occurs in 90% of cases and is characterized by proteinuria, hematuria, and rapidly progressive renal failure.
- Light microscopy shows a necrotizing granulomatous arteritis involving small and medium-sized arteries.
- The glomeruli show a focal segmental proliferative glomerulonephritis.
- Fibrinoid necrosis, capillary thrombosis, and epithelial crescent formation are common.
- Immunofluorescence shows granular deposits of IgA, C3, and fibrinogen in the glomerular capillary wall.

CHRONIC GLOMERULONEPHRITIS

Chronic glomerulonephritis is a common pathologic lesion in the kidney that probably represents the end stage of many diseases affecting glomeruli. Some patients give a history suggestive of glomerular disease.

- Grossly, the kidneys are greatly reduced in size, and the cortex shows a finely irregular surface ("granular contracted kidney").
- The cortex is narrowed, corticomedullary demarcation is obscured, and the arteries have thickened walls.
- Microscopically, the narrowed cortex shows a great decrease in number of nephrons.
- Glomeruli show diffuse sclerosis, many being converted to hyaline balls.
- There is atrophy of intervening tubules, and residual tubules often show dilatation and are filled with pink proteinaceous material ("thyroidization").
- Interstitial fibrosis is present and may be severe.

- Immunofluorescence and electron microscopy may show evidence of electron-dense deposits containing IgG, IgA, and C3 in affected glomeruli.
- Clinically, patients show chronic renal failure and hypertension and frequently have microscopic hematuria, proteinuria, and sometimes nephrotic syndrome.

DIABETIC NEPHROPATHY

Ten percent of patients with type II (adult-onset) diabetes mellitus die of chronic renal failure. The incidence of renal disease is still higher in type I (juvenile onset) diabetes. Diabetic nephropathy is the result of diabetic microangiopathy (see Chapter 46), and is almost invariably associated with diabetic retinopathy.

Pathology

- Grossly, the kidney shows little abnormality in all but the most severe cases, when the organ may be contracted and show fine scarring.
- Light microscopy shows focal and diffuse glomerulosclerosis and hyalinization of the afferent and efferent arterioles.
- Electron microscopy of the focal nodular lesions shows them to be composed of increased mesangial matrix material. There are no electron-dense deposits.
- Immunofluorescence is negative.

Clinical Features

Diabetic nephropathy presents with proteinuria, which may be sufficient to lead to nephrotic syndrome. Hypertension is commonly present. The renal lesion is progressive and causes progressive chronic renal failure.

RENAL AMYLOIDOSIS (See Chapter 2)

The kidneys are almost always affected in secondary amyloidosis, and in about 30% of cases of primary amyloidosis.

- Amyloid deposition occurs mainly in the glomerular capillaries, where it appears as a homogeneous thickening of the basement membrane.
- Amyloidosis can be diagnosed by the presence of apple-green birefringence when Congo-red–stained sections are examined under polarized light.
- Electron microscopy shows the diagnostic amyloid fibrillary material.
- Clinically, patients present with proteinuria and the nephrotic syndrome.
- Amyloidosis is a progressive disease that usually results in chronic renal failure, a common cause of death in amyloidosis.

The Kidney: III. Vascular Diseases; Neoplasms

49

RENAL VASCULAR DISEASES

Hypertensive Renal Disease (Nephrosclerosis)

BENIGN NEPHROSCLEROSIS
This disease occurs in most patients with essential hypertension.

- There is bilateral symmetric reduction in the size of the kidneys. The renal surface has a fine, even granularity, and there is uniform thinning of the renal cortex.
- Microscopically, there is hyaline thickening of the walls of small arteries and arterioles, global sclerosis of glomeruli, and atrophy of nephrons with interstitial fibrosis.
- Immunofluorescence and electron microscopy show no evidence of immune deposits.
- The changes of benign nephrosclerosis are usually mild. Chronic renal failure occurs in less than 5% of cases.

MALIGNANT NEPHROSCLEROSIS
This occurs with malignant hypertension (see Chapter 20), which is a complication that occurs in about 5% of patients with hypertension.

- The kidneys are normal in size or slightly enlarged and have a smooth surface with numerous small petechial hemorrhages ("fleabitten kidneys").
- Microscopically, there is fibrinoid necrosis of arterioles and glomeruli. Interlobar arteries show intimal cellular proliferation and laminated (onionskin) fibrosis.
- Clinically, malignant nephrosclerosis is manifested by proteinuria and hematuria, rapidly followed by acute renal failure.
- Without treatment, 90% of patients die within 1 year.
- With modern antihypertensive therapy, over 60% of patients are alive 5 years after diagnosis.

Renal Artery Stenosis

Etiology
Atherosclerosis is the most common cause, particularly in older patients.

- Fibromuscular dysplasia of the renal artery is a rare condition of unknown cause, occurring in younger patients (aged 20–40), particularly in women.
- Posttransplantation stenosis occurs in 10–20% of patients after renal transplantation, most commonly as a manifestation of rejection.

Pathology & Clinical Features

When a significant degree (> 75%) of narrowing of the renal artery is present, diffuse ischemia of the kidney occurs. This causes increased renin secretion leading to hypertension.

- Intravenous pyelography shows a delay in excretion of dye on the affected side, but later films show an increased dye concentration.
- The diagnosis is made by renal arteriography.

Treatment & Prognosis

Transluminal balloon dilatation and surgical excision of the stenotic segment produces cure rates of 80–90%. In long-standing stenoses, significant hypertensive changes in the opposite kidney prevent complete reversal of hypertension after treatment.

Renal Changes in Shock

Prerenal Uremia

Renal vasoconstriction in early shock leads to decreased glomerular filtration and oliguria, which may be severe (< 400 mL/d).

- The urine is highly concentrated, with high levels of urea and creatinine, reflecting normal tubular function.
- Serum urea levels rise.
- No morphologic changes are seen in the kidney.
- Reversal of shock leads to return of normal renal function.

Acute Renal Tubular Necrosis (ATN)

Severe shock with prolonged renal vasoconstriction is the commonest cause of acute tubular necrosis. The tubules show patchy necrosis affecting both proximal and distal convoluted tubules.

- Disappearance of the brush border of proximal convoluted tubular epithelial cells is an early microscopic feature.
- If the patient survives, tubular epithelial regeneration is seen in the second week.
- Clinically, acute tubular necrosis is characterized by:
  - Acute renal failure, with oliguria and azotemia.
  - Decreasing osmolality of urine, approaching that of glomerular ultrafiltrate (specific gravity 1.010, ie, isosthenuria).
  - Red cells and tubular epithelial casts in urine.
- The oliguric phase of tubular necrosis usually lasts 10–14 days.
- In patients who recover, this is followed by the diuretic phase, in which:
  - Urine output increases without tubular regulation.
  - There is a risk of fluid and electrolyte imbalance.
- Normal tubular function is restored only 2–3 weeks after the occurrence of tubular necrosis.

Renal Cortical Necrosis

This is a rare complication of shock, caused by severe, prolonged shock (hypotension). It is characterized by necrosis of the entire renal cortex, including the glomeruli.

- It is irreversible.
- Clinically, there is acute renal failure. The oliguric phase is profound and prolonged and the diuretic phase does not appear.
- It has a very high mortality rate unless hemodialysis or transplantation is undertaken.

Renal Infarction

Etiology
Arterial occlusion by emboli, usually originating in the heart (in infective endocarditis, myocardial infarction, mitral stenosis, or atrial fibrillation), is the commonest cause.

- Less common is arterial occlusion by thrombosis, usually secondary to atherosclerosis, and more rarely in polyarteritis nodosa.
- Renal vein occlusion by thrombosis or neoplasms may rarely cause ischemia to the degree that hemorrhagic infarction occurs.

Pathologic & Clinical Features

- Grossly, arterial infarcts are pale and wedge-shaped, with the occluded vessels at the apex of the wedge. Venous infarcts are hemorrhagic and often involve large areas, frequently the entire kidney.
- Microscopically, the infarcted area shows coagulative necrosis.
- The infarct heals by progressive enzymatic liquefaction, macrophage phagocytosis of debris, and scar formation.
- Clinically, infarction produces sudden-onset flank pain followed by hematuria.

NEOPLASMS OF THE KIDNEYS (Table 49-1)

Benign Neoplasms

RENAL CORTICAL ADENOMA
This is a common incidental finding at autopsy. It is a well-circumscribed, round, yellowish nodule in the cortex, less than 3 cm, composed of cytologically benign cells arranged in a papillary or solid pattern. When found during life, differentiation from early carcinoma is impossible.

RENAL ONCOCYTOMA
This is a special kind of cortical adenoma believed to be derived from proximal tubular cells.

- It may reach a large size but remain benign.
- Oncocytomas have a uniform mahogany brown color without necrosis or hemorrhage, though frequently there is a central scarred area.
- Microscopically, they are composed of a uniform population of large cells having small round nuclei and abundant pink, granular cytoplasm.

ANGIOMYOLIPOMA
This is an uncommon neoplasm. It may be solitary or multiple and bilateral. If bilateral, it is often part of the syndrome of tuberous sclerosis (Chapter 62).

TABLE 49–1. RENAL NEOPLASMS

	Frequency	Gross Features	Microscopic Features	Clinical Features	Comments
Benign					
Renal cortical adenoma	Common	< 3 cm; firm circumscribed yellowish nodule in cortex	Cytologically benign cells; papillary or solid pattern	Asymptomatic; usually an incidental autopsy finding	When found during life, difficult to differentiate from a small renal adenocarcinoma
Renal oncocytoma	Rare	May be large; circumscribed, mahogany brown, uniform; central scar	Uniform large cells with small, regular nuclei and abundant granular cytoplasm	Mass, slowly growing; hematuria	Difficult to differentiate from oncocytic renal carcinoma
Angiomyolipoma	Uncommon	May be large; solitary or multiple; circumscribed yellow mass; may be bilateral	3 components; mature fat cells, abnormal blood vessels, and smooth muscle cell proliferation	Mass, hematuria; CT scan shows fat density	Associated with tuberous sclerosis
Juxtaglomerular apparatus tumor	Very rare	Small, solid cortical mass	Small, round, uniform cells arranged in nests and sheets	Hypertension due to increased renin secretion by tumor	Rare cause of secondary hypertension in a young patient
Congenital mesoblastic nephroma	Rare	May be large; circumscribed, firm, pale mass; whorled surface	Benign fibroblastic spindle cell proliferation	Mass during neonatal period	Occurs in first 3 months of life
Medullary fibroma	Common	< 1 cm/ firm, circumscribed mass in medulla	Benign fibroblastic spindle cell proliferation	Asymptomatic; incidental finding at autopsy	Of little clinical significance

(continued)

TABLE 49–1. (Continued)

	Frequency	Gross Features	Microscopic Features	Clinical Features	Comments
Malignant					
Renal adenocarcinoma	Common	Usually large; variegated appearance; pseudoencapsulated, may invade renal vein	Clear cells of varying cytologic malignancy; solid, papillary, cystic, oncocytic variants	Mass; hematuria, metastatic disease	1–2% of all cancers in adults
Nephroblastoma (Wilms's tumor)	Common in children	Large; firm, solid mass; frequently replaces kidney	Primitive small spindle cells; tubular differentiation; mesenchymal elements	Mass in childhood; abdominal enlargement	25–30% of cancers in children under age 10 years
Transitional cell neoplasms of renal pelvis	Common	Papillary mass in renal pelvis; may invade kidney	Papillary urothelial neoplasms of varying grades	Hematuria; mass; malignant cells in urine	Multiple tumors may be present
Primary sarcomas	Very rare	Large masses; usually in capsule and perinephric fat	Depends on type of sarcoma; liposarcoma, leiomyosarcoma, and fibrosarcoma most common	Mass	
Primary renal malignant lymphoma	Very rare	Large mass; solid and fleshy	Commonly aggressive large cell and immunoblastic lymphomas	Mass; hilar nodes commonly involved	Renal involvement in systemic lymphoma is more common

- It may produce a large mass that clinically resembles carcinoma.
- Its content of fat gives it a characteristic appearance on computerized tomography.
- Microscopically, it is composed of a variable admixture of mature adipose tissue, proliferating smooth muscle cells, and abnormal blood vessels.
- Renal angiomyolipoma is a benign lesion.

Malignant Neoplasms

RENAL ADENOCARCINOMA (Hypernephroma; Grawitz's Tumor)

Incidence and Etiology
The most common malignant neoplasm of the kidney, this accounts for 1–2% of all cancers in adults. It occurs most frequently in the sixth decade but is not rare in younger patients. No strong etiologic factors have been identified. Associated diseases include von Hippel-Lindau syndrome and dialysis cystic disease.

Pathology
Grossly, renal adenocarcinoma varies in size from small to massive, and may be solid or cystic. The cut surface is yellow-orange mottled with hemorrhagic and fibrous areas.

- It may infiltrate locally through the capsule of the kidney and, rarely, through Gerota's fascia into surrounding organs.
- Invasion into the renal vein is common; occasionally, tumor extends along the lumen of the inferior vena cava to the right atrium.
- Microscopically, it is composed of a mixture of clear cells and pink granular cells.
- It is highly vascular.
- Tumors are classified into four histologic grades, based on the degree of nuclear pleomorphism.

Clinical Features
The usual presentation is with hematuria. A renal mass may be palpable when it becomes large.

- Metastases occur early and may be the reason for clinical presentation. Common metastatic sites are lungs, bone, liver, brain, and skin.
- Extension of the neoplasm into the renal vein may cause:
  - Obstruction of the testicular vein on the left side, causing a scrotal varicocele.
  - Venous infarction of the kidney.
- Extension into the inferior vena cava may occlude it, leading to edema in the lower extremities.
- A few renal adenocarcinomas secrete hormones:
  - Parathyroid hormone-like substances that cause hypercalcemia, low serum phosphate, and a clinical syndrome resembling primary hyperparathyroidism.
  - Erythropoietin, causing polycythemia.
  - Prolactin causing galactorrhea.
  - Renin causing hypertension.
- The diagnosis is made by intravenous pyelography, CT scan, or angiography, which show the presence of a renal mass.
- Treatment is surgical removal.

TABLE 49–2. RENAL ADENOCARCINOMA: STAGING

Stage	Criteria	5-Year Survival Rate[1]
I	Confined to kidney; no capsular invasion	70%
II	Invades perinephric fat	30%
III	Involvement of renal vein[2] or regional nodes	< 10%
IV	Extension beyond perinephric fat (Gerota's fascia) or distant metastases	< 5%

[1]Five-year survival rate following aggressive surgery, radio- and chemo-therapy where appropriate.
[2]Recent evidence suggests that survival rates in patients with renal vein involvement, including cases where the tumor thrombus extends into the inferior vena cava, are much higher than 10% if patients are treated with radical surgery. Reevaluation of renal vein involvement as a criterion for stage III disease is necessary.

■ Prognosis correlates well with clinical stage (Table 49–2). Histologic grade is a relatively minor prognostic indicator.

NEPHROBLASTOMA (Wilms's tumor)
Nephroblastoma constitutes about 25–30% of cancers in childhood, being second in frequency to leukemia and lymphoma as a cause of cancer in childhood. Most cases occur between ages 1 and 7.

Genetic Features
All bilateral and approximately one-third of unilateral nephroblastomas are hereditary. Molecular studies suggest that homozygous recessive genes are responsible, both of which must have undergone mutation for the neoplasm to develop.

■ In the hereditary form of the disease, one recessive gene is inherited in the mutant form (creating a predisposition to the disease); the second gene undergoes an acquired mutation (leading to neoplasia).
■ Some patients with nephroblastoma show deletion of part of the short arm of chromosome 11. This may be accompanied by aniridia.

Pathology
Grossly, nephroblastoma is commonly a large, firm tumor. Bilateral tumors occur in about 8% of cases.

■ Microscopically, it is composed of small, spindle-shaped cells with hyperchromatic nuclei and scant cytoplasm that resemble renal blastema.
■ Undifferentiated neoplasms that display anaplasia, necrosis, and a high mitotic rate have a bad prognosis.
■ Differentiation into epithelial tubular structures, primitive glomeruli, and mesenchymal tissues indicate a good prognosis.
■ Rarely, tumors of childhood resembling Wilms's tumor are composed of cells resembling primitive skeletal muscle (rhabdoid sarcoma) or clear cells (clear cell sarcoma).

These histologic subtypes have a more aggressive behavior than the usual Wilms tumor.

Clinical Features & Treatment

Most patients present with a large abdominal mass that is usually felt by a parent.

- Clinical staging according to the size of tumor, the presence of tumor on either side of the midline, and distant spread, determine treatment and prognosis.
- Treatment combines surgery, radiation, and chemotherapy.
- Prognosis has improved dramatically with increasingly effective chemotherapeutic agents.
- Currently, the 5-year survival rate exceeds 50%, even when metastases are present. For tumors confined to the kidney and resected surgically, the 5-year survival rate exceeds 80%.

The Ureters, Urinary Bladder, & Urethra

50

THE RENAL PELVIS & URETERS

Congenital Anomalies

ANATOMIC ANOMALIES
Anatomic anomalies of the urinary tract occur in about 2% of autopsies as incidental findings. They include abnormalities in position and number of ureters (eg, double and bifid ureter).

URETEROCELE
A ureterocele is a thin-walled cystic swelling of the lowermost part of the ureter in its course through the bladder muscle. The cyst usually protrudes into the bladder lumen.

- It is believed to be the result of congenital stenosis of the ureteral orifice in the bladder wall.
- It is common in children and young adults and is bilateral in 10% of cases.
- Frequently it is asymptomatic, but it may be associated with ureteral obstruction, hydroureter, and hydronephrosis.

MEGAURETER
This is a rare anomaly characterized by marked dilatation of the ureter associated with increased thickness of the muscle wall. The ureteral lumen is patent. It is believed to be caused by an abnormal arrangement of the muscle in the lower ureter, which results in abnormal peristalsis and functional obstruction.

IDIOPATHIC HYDRONEPHROSIS
This is characterized by functional obstruction at the ureteropelvic junction, leading to massive hydronephrosis. The lumen is patent.

- In a few cases, an abnormal renal artery draped around the ureteropelvic junction has been incriminated in causing obstruction.
- In most other cases, it has been suggested that congenital abnormalities in innervation or arrangement of muscle fibers result in failure of peristalsis at the ureteropelvic junction.
- Surgical removal of the junction zone is curative.

Urinary Tract Calculi (Urolithiasis)
Urolithiasis is a common clinical problem, occurring in about 0.5–2% of the general

population. It accounts for 1 of every 1000 hospital admissions in the United States. The vast majority of urinary calculi form in the renal pelvis (renal calculi) or bladder.

Etiology & Classification (Table 50–1)

A. Calcium oxalate calculi account for 70% of urinary calculi.

- In most of these patients, there is no biochemical abnormality to account for the calculi.
- Hypercalciuria or hyperoxaluria is present in a minority of patients.
- Calcium oxalate calculi are small, hard calculi with jagged edges.

B. Phosphate calculi account for 15% of urinary calculi.

- They tend to be associated with urinary infections caused by urea-splitting organisms such as *Proteus* that produce ammonia and make the urine alkaline.
- Phosphate calculi tend to be solitary, large, and soft and may fill the pelvicaliceal system (staghorn calculus).

C. Uric acid calculi account for 10% of urinary calculi. They are radiolucent and therefore not seen on plain abdominal X-rays.

Clinical Features & Diagnosis

- They present with acute ureteral obstruction, ureteral colic, and hematuria due to mucosal trauma.
- Small stones are successfully pushed down the ureter by peristalsis into the bladder and then passed out with urine.
- Urinary tract obstruction occurs when a stone becomes impacted in the ureter. Hydronephrosis, urinary stasis, and acute pyelonephritis commonly follow.
- Diagnosis of ureteral calculi is made by plain X-ray (radiopaque calculi—90%) or intravenous retrograde pyelography (radiolucent stones).
- Serum and urinary studies are necessary to identify a predisposing cause (hypercalcemia, hyperoxaluria, cystinuria, gout, urinary infection).
- The presence of crystals in the urine does not correlate with the presence of urinary calculi.

Treatment

It consists of observation of the stone as it passes down the ureter, combined with alleviation of pain. With large and impacted calculi, surgery or lithotripsy is necessary to remove the calculi.

Fibrous Stricture of the Ureters

A variety of nonneoplastic conditions cause fibrosis and narrowing of the ureters.

- Chronic nonspecific ureteritis with fibrosis of the wall, associated with cystic dilatation of epithelial nests in the submucosa (ureteritis cystica) is a rare cause of stricture.
- Tuberculosis of the ureter, usually secondary to renal tuberculosis, is another.
- Injury to the ureter occurs relatively frequently in extensive pelvic operations for gynecologic cancer and may be followed by fibrous strictures.

TABLE 50–1. URINARY TRACT CALCULI

Type	Frequency	Predisposing Factors	Urine pH	Morphology
Calcium oxalate	70%	Hypercalcemia: Primary hyperparathyroidism Metastatic neoplasms in bone Idiopathic hypercalciuria Hyperoxaluria: Inherited Intestinal diseases (Crohn's ileitis, ileoileal bypass) High dietary intake of green vegetables, decaffeinated coffee High vitamin C intake Ethylene glycol poisoning	Any pH	Hard, small ($<$ 5 mm), multiple stones; may be smooth, round, or jagged; radiopaque
Phosphate calculi (mixture of calcium phosphate and magnesium ammonium phosphate)	15%	Urinary infections by urea-splitting bacteria, commonly *Proteus* spp.	Alkaline	Soft, gray-white; often large and solitary, filling the pelvicaliceal system ("staghorn calculus"); radiopaque
Uric acid (urates)	10%	Most cases occur in patients with normal serum uric acid levels Gout; frequency has decreased after allopurinol therapy	Acidic	Yellow-brown; small, hard, smooth; often multiple; radiolucent—not visible on plain x-ray
Cystine and xanthine stones	Rare	Cystinuria, xanthinuria	Any pH	Yellowish; soft, waxy, small; smooth, round, multiple; cystine stones are slightly radiopaque; xanthine stones are radiolucent

- Radiation of the retroperitoneum can cause stricture.
- Retroperitoneal fibrosis is a form of idiopathic fibromatosis that involves the retroperitoneum, producing strictures and medial displacement of both ureters.
- Endometriosis of the ureteral wall associated with cyclic hemorrhage and fibrosis is a rare cause of ureteral stricture in women.
- It presents with ureteral obstruction, hydronephrosis, and acute pyelonephritis.

Urothelial Neoplasms
Primary urothelial neoplasms occur fairly frequently in the renal pelvis but are rare in the ureters. They have features identical with those of urothelial neoplasms of the bladder (see following). Involvement of the ureters by retroperitoneal neoplasms, both primary and metastatic, is more common.

THE URINARY BLADDER

Congenital Anomalies

ANATOMIC ABNORMALITIES
Anatomic abnormalities, such as duplication and congenital fistulas caused by abnormal development of the cloaca and urogenital sinus, are rare.

URACHAL ABNORMALITIES

- Persistence of the entire urachus causes a vesicoumbilical fistula.
- Persistence of parts of the urachus predisposes to infection, sinuses, and fistula formation.
- Urachal cysts and neoplasms occur rarely.

EXSTROPHY OF THE BLADDER
This is a rare congenital anomaly associated with failure of development of the anterior wall of the bladder and the overlying abdominal wall, including the pubic symphysis.

- The bladder is open to the skin surface as a large defect (complete exstrophy). Lesser defects also occur.
- The exposed bladder is red and granular at birth and is covered by transitional epithelium.
- Repeated infections cause epithelial metaplasia of the squamous or intestinal type.
- Isolated defects can be corrected surgically.
- A higher incidence of cancer (usually adenocarcinoma) is reported in exstrophic bladders.

Inflammatory Lesions

ACUTE CYSTITIS

Etiology
A. Acute bacterial cystitis:

- This is a common ascending infection caused by coliform bacteria, often *Escherichia coli*, *Proteus* species, or *Streptococcus faecalis*.

- It occurs more commonly in females and is etiologically related to sexual intercourse, pregnancy, and instrumentation.
- In older men, chronic retention of urine in patients with prostatic hyperplasia is the major predisposing factor.
- The etiologic agent can be cultured from urine, which also contains protein, red cells, and neutrophils.
- Many cases are associated with acute pyelonephritis.

B. Acute radiation cystitis: This occurs in cases where the bladder is included in the field of pelvic irradiation for malignant neoplasms.

C. Drug effects: Drugs used in the treatment of cancer (eg, cyclophosphamide) cause acute hemorrhagic cystitis.

Pathology
It is characterized by hyperemia of the mucosa with neutrophilic infiltration of the lamina propria.

- Encrusted cystitis denotes an acute cystitis in which alkalinity of the urine causes precipitation of crystalline phosphates on the bladder mucosa.
- Bullous cystitis is a variant of acute cystitis in which large fluid-filled spaces form in the submucosa.

Clinical Features
It is characterized by fever, low abdominal pain, frequency of micturition, and dysuria. The diagnosis is established by quantitative culture (colony count) of a midstream urine specimen. Specific antibiotic treatment depends on the results of culture and sensitivity tests. The prognosis is excellent.

TUBERCULOSIS
Vesical tuberculosis occurs in 70% of patients with renal tuberculosis.

- The trigone is affected first, the early lesions appearing as small submucosal granulomas. Extensive caseous granulomas may cause nodules and ulceration.
- The associated fibrosis may cause:
  - Retraction of the ureteral orifice into the wall of the bladder ("golf-hole ureter").
  - Marked fibrous contraction of the bladder ("thimble bladder").
- Clinically, there is frequency, pain, dysuria, and pyuria. Low-grade fever and weight loss may be present.
- Cultures for mycobacteria are positive.

SCHISTOSOMIASIS
The perivesical venous plexus is the favored habitat of *Schistosoma haematobium,* a species that is common in Egypt and the Middle East.

- The ova pass through the bladder wall to enter the lumen and are excreted in urine. Finding typical ova in the urine is diagnostic.
- In their passage through the wall, the ova cause marked inflammation, with abscesses and granulomas in which there are large numbers of eosinophils.
- Clinically, there is fever, frequency, dysuria, and hematuria.

- Cystoscopic examination shows scarring and small nodules in the bladder mucosa. Marked fibrosis occurs in the chronic stage.
- The bladder epithelium frequently shows squamous metaplasia. There is a greatly increased risk of squamous carcinoma.

CHRONIC NONSPECIFIC CYSTITIS
It is characterized by infiltration of the bladder mucosa with lymphocytes and plasma cells. Glandular metaplasia (cystitis glandularis) and cystic dilatation of glands (cystitis cystica) are common.

- In patients with neurogenic bladders, the epithelium may undergo a peculiar metaplastic change with a papillary clear cell appearance (nephrogenic "adenoma").
- A form of chronic nonspecific cystitis characterized by ulceration of the mucosa with submucosal fibrosis, vasculitis, and infiltration by eosinophils is called Hunner's interstitial cystitis.

MALAKOPLAKIA
Malakoplakia is a peculiar chronic inflammation characterized by yellowish plaques, nodules, or polyps in the bladder mucosa.

- Microscopically, there are dense collections of macrophages with abundant granular cytoplasm. Within the cytoplasm are round, laminated concretions called **Michaelis-Gutman bodies.**
- Malakoplakia is most commonly found in the bladder; other sites include the renal pelvis, ureter, prostate, epididymis, colon, and lungs.

BLADDER CALCULI
Calculi may form in the bladder (primary) or descend from the kidney (secondary). They have the same composition and causes as renal calculi.

AMYLOIDOSIS OF THE BLADDER
Amyloidosis rarely presents as a localized mucosal plaque or nodule in the bladder.

- Hemorrhage caused by rupture of amyloid-affected vessels is common.
- Clinically, patients present with hematuria.
- Diagnosis is made by identifying amyloid in Congo-red–stained sections of a biopsy sample.

Neoplasms of the Bladder

UROTHELIAL NEOPLASMS
Bladder cancer is responsible for about 2% of cancer deaths in the United States and Europe. In Japan, the incidence is extremely low, while in Egypt it accounts for 40% of cancers (because of the high incidence of schistosomiasis).

Etiology

- Several chemical carcinogens have been identified:
  - Aniline dyes containing benzidine and 2α-naphthylamine, in workers in the dye, rubber, and insulating cable industries.

- Cigarette smoking is the most important factor.
- In Egypt, schistosomiasis is important, producing squamous metaplasia, dysplasia, and squamous carcinoma.

Pathology
Urothelial neoplasms may occur anywhere in the bladder mucosa. The most common locations are near the trigone or in a diverticulum.

- The better-differentiated urothelial neoplasms commonly project into the lumen and have a delicate papillary appearance.
- Poorly differentiated neoplasms are solid ulcerative lesions that show evidence of infiltration.
- Microscopically, most are transitional cell carcinomas. Squamous or glandular differentiation commonly occurs.
- Four histologic grades are recognized, based on the degree of cytologic abnormality present in the neoplasm:
  - Transitional cell papilloma.
  - Grades I, II and III transitional cell carcinoma.
- Infiltration of lamina propria, smooth muscle, or blood vessels has adverse prognostic significance.
- Dysplasia and carcinoma in situ commonly co-exists with high-grade carcinomas, and represents a precursor lesion.

Clinical Features
Dysplasia and carcinoma in situ are asymptomatic and can be diagnosed by cytologic examination of urine and random mucosal biopsies.

- Painless hematuria is the commonest presenting symptom of bladder carcinoma.
- Involvement of the trigone may cause frequency and dysuria.
- Involvement of the ureteral orifice may lead to hydronephrosis and infection.
- Rarely, invasion of adjacent organs (most commonly the colon) leads to fistulous tracts.
- Diagnosis is made by cystoscopy and biopsy.
- Clinical staging depends on the degree of invasion by the neoplasm and the presence of lymph node and distant metastases (Table 50-2).

Treatment & Prognosis
Radical cystectomy is indicated for poorly differentiated carcinomas and well-differentiated carcinomas in which there is muscle invasion.

- Local resection or partial cystectomy suffices for better-differentiated noninvasive neoplasms.
- The prognosis depends on both clinical stage and histologic grade.
- With appropriate surgical resection, 50-80% of patients with stage B neoplasms survive 5 years. With local extension outside the bladder, the 5-year survival rate drops to 20-30%.

TABLE 50–2. STAGING OF TRANSITIONAL CELL CARCINOMA OF THE BLADDER[1]

Stage 0	PIS	Carcinoma in situ
	Pa	Papillary neoplasm without invasion
Stage A	P1	Invasion of lamina propria
Stage B1	P2	Invasion of superficial half of the muscle wall
Stage B2	P3a	Invasion of deep half of the muscle wall
Stage C	P3b	Invasion through bladder wall into perivesical fat
Stage D1	P4a	Invasion of prostate, vagina, or uterus
	P4b	Tumor fixed to pelvic or abdominal wall
	N1-3	Pelvic nodes involved
Stage D2	M1	Distant metastases
	N4	Involvement of lymph nodes above the aortic bifurcation

[1]These designations are based on the TNM staging system which is being used more frequently. In this system, P = characteristics of the primary tumor based on pathologic examination; N = node status; M = metastatic status.

OTHER EPITHELIAL NEOPLASMS

Pure Squamous Carcinoma
This is rare except where schistosomiasis is endemic; then it represents the commonest type.

- Well-differentiated keratinizing squamous carcinoma tends to form large, bulky exophytic masses that protrude into the lumen.
- They tend to remain confined to the bladder until a late stage and have a better prognosis than transitional carcinomas of similar size.

Pure Adenocarcinoma
Adenocarcinoma is rare but may arise:

- In urachal epithelial remnants in the dome of the bladder.
- In bladder mucosa that has undergone glandular metaplasia.
- In cystitis glandularis.

NONEPITHELIAL NEOPLASMS

Paraganglioma (Pheochromocytoma)
These originate in paraganglionic structures in the bladder wall. They resemble pheochromocytomas of the adrenal gland. Most are nonfunctioning. Functioning paragangliomas secrete bursts of catecholamines during urination, causing palpitations and hypertension.

Mesenchymal Neoplasms
Mesenchymal neoplasms are rare. Smooth muscle tumors (leiomyoma and leiomyosarcoma) are the most common of these in adults. Embryonal rhabdomyosarcoma occurs in young children.

THE URETHRA

Congenital Anomalies

POSTERIOR URETHRAL VALVE
Posterior urethral valve occurs mainly in males. It is characterized by the presence of folds of mucous membrane in the posterior urethra that causes partial valvular obstruction. It leads to infection and hydronephrosis in childhood.

ECTOPIC URETERS
Ectopic ureters opening into the urethra are rare. Continuous dribbling of urine results.

Urethral Infections (Urethritis)
Most infections of the urethra are sexually transmitted (see Chapter 54). Gonorrhea and nonspecific urethritis, which is probably caused by chlamydiae, are the most common. Urethral strictures may follow chronic infections.

Urethral Neoplasms

URETHRAL CARUNCLE
This is a common lesion of the urethra, occurring mainly in older women. It usually presents as a small, red, friable mass situated at the external urethral orifice. Frequently it becomes ulcerated and bleeds.

- Microscopically, it is composed of inflamed, highly vascular granulation tissue.
- The cause is uncertain, but it is more apt to be a reactive change than a neoplasm.
- Surgical excision is curative.

CARCINOMA OF THE URETHRA

- This is extremely rare. The most common form is transitional cell carcinoma of the prostatic urethra in males. Lower urethral squamous and adenocarcinomas are highly malignant, with a 5-year survival rate close to zero.

The Testis, Prostate, & Penis

51

THE TESTIS & EPIDIDYMIS

Manifestations of Testicular Disease

Infertility
Male infertility is usually recognized by absence of spermatozoa (azoospermia) or decreased numbers of spermatozoa in semen (oligozoospermia). It may result from:

- Pretesticular causes, most commonly hypopituitarism.
- Posttesticular causes, leading to bilateral obstruction to the overflow of spermatozoa. Obstructive infertility is responsible for 50% of cases of male fertility.
- Testicular atrophy and failure of spermatogenesis.

Testicular Masses or Enlargement
Acute inflammatory lesions cause painful enlargement. Chronic inflammatory lesions and neoplasms are usually painless. Any testicular mass should be considered to be a neoplasm until proved otherwise.

Abnormal Production of Hormones
Hormones from functioning testicular stromal tumors may produce precocious puberty (androgens) or gynecomastia (estrogens).

Congenital Testicular Anomalies
Absence of one or both testes and fusion of testes are very rare anomalies. **Klinefelter's syndrome** (testicular dysgenesis) results in failure of normal testicular development at puberty (Chapter 15).

Abnormalities of Testicular Descent
A. Undescended testis:

- This is a testis that remains arrested at an extrascrotal location along the normal path of migration.
- It presents in 3% of full-term male infants; in most of these cases, complete descent occurs in the first year of life.
- Surgical correction before age 6 assures normal development and function.
- After puberty, testicular atrophy occurs.

- There is a greatly increased risk of malignant germ cell neoplasms in an undescended testis.
- Trauma and torsion occur more commonly in undescended testes.

B. Ectopic testis:

- This is a testis that is located outside its normal descent route, eg, at the root of the penis or the medial thigh.
- Trauma, torsion and neoplasia are common.

Inflammatory Lesions of the Testis & Epididymis

ACUTE EPIDIDYMO-ORCHITIS

This is a common infection caused by bacteria that reach the epididymis from the urethra.

- *Escherichia coli* and the gonococcus are the most common.
- Pathologically, there is an acute pyogenic inflammation of the epididymis that commonly extends into the testis.
- Clinically, patients present with acute onset of fever, pain, tenderness, and redness of the scrotum extending along the spermatic cord.
- Resolution occurs rapidly with specific antibiotic therapy.
- Complications include:
  - Fibrosis leading to obstruction of the epididymis.
  - Sterility only in those cases where both sides are affected.
  - Vascular compromise leading, rarely, to infarction of the testis.
  - Abscess formation in the scrotum.

TUBERCULOUS EPIDIDYMO-ORCHITIS

Tuberculosis of the epididymis is common wherever there is a high incidence of tuberculosis.

- Eighty percent have urinary tract tuberculosis. Tubercle bacilli gain access to the epididymis from the urethra.
- Pathologically, there is a chronic caseating granulomatous inflammation with fibrosis, involving the epididymis and testis.
- Clinically, patients present with enlargement of the scrotum. Pain is usually not a major complaint.
- The caseous granulomas may ulcerate and drain through the skin of the scrotum, usually the posterior aspect.
- Diagnosis is made by culture or by demonstration of acid-fast bacilli in caseous granulomas on tissue sections.

MUMPS ORCHITIS

Orchitis occurs in 10–20% of cases of mumps in postpubertal males. It usually causes mild acute inflammation with pain and mild swelling that resolves rapidly. In a small number of cases, severe inflammation results in testicular atrophy and sterility.

SYPHILIS

Syphilis affects the testis in the tertiary (late) stage and is characterized by formation of a gumma. It is rare today because of better treatment of early syphilis.

IDIOPATHIC GRANULOMATOUS ORCHITIS

This uncommon inflammatory lesion of the testis is of unknown cause. Autoimmunity has been suggested.

- Grossly, the testis is enlarged, with a smooth capsule. The cut surface is firm, grayish-white and multinodular.
- Microscopically, there is destruction of seminiferous tubules and the presence of multiple epithelioid granulomas with giant cells. Caseation does not occur.
- Patients are usually postpubertal and present with enlargement of the testis.
- Clinically, differentiation from a neoplasm is difficult without biopsy.

SPERM GRANULOMA

This is a fairly common lesion that occurs in the testis and epididymis when there is leakage of spermatozoa into the interstitium. It is characterized by a granulomatous response around sperms with progressive fibrosis. Diagnosis is made by identification of spermatozoa within the inflammatory lesion.

FOURNIER'S SCROTAL GANGRENE

This is a rare disease of adults characterized by necrotizing cellulitis and fasciitis of the scrotum. It is usually caused by anaerobic bacteria.

- Acute inflammation with marked edema progresses rapidly to vascular thrombosis and gangrene of the scrotal skin, which then ulcerates and sloughs, leaving the testes exposed.
- The mortality rate is high unless treatment is started expeditiously.

HYDROCELE

This is a collection of fluid within the space between the two layers of the tunica vaginalis.

- The usual causes are trauma, infection, or tumor of the underlying testis.
- Hydrocele fluid is usually clear and straw-colored; if it contains much blood, it is called a hematocele.

Testicular Torsion

This is a common condition caused by twisting of the spermatic cord, leading to vascular obstruction.

- Abnormalities of the testis (eg, undescended testis) or its ligaments are predisposing factors.
- Pathologically, there is edema and hemorrhage, followed by venous infarction of the testis.
- Clinically, there is sudden onset of severe pain with marked swelling of the scrotum. The testis is intensely tender.
- Orchiectomy is required in cases that have progressed to necrosis of testicular tissue.

Testicular Neoplasms (Table 51–1)

GERM CELL NEOPLASMS

These account for over 95% of testicular tumors. They occur with an incidence of 2 per 100,000 males. In the age group from 15 to 34 years, they cause 10–12% of cancer deaths.

Etiology

- The etiology of testicular germ cell neoplasms is unknown. Known etiologic factors include:
  - Extrascrotal position of the testes; 5% of testes in the abdominal cavity and 1% of testes in the inguinal canal develop cancer.
  - An undescended testis detected early in life and surgically placed in the scrotum slightly increases the risk of germ cell neoplasia.
  - Diethylstilbestrol (DES) ingestion by the mother during pregnancy (rare).

Classification (Table 51–1)

Germ cell tumors are presumed to arise in a primitive germ cell in the seminiferous tubules.

- They are classified as:
  - Seminoma.
  - Non-seminomatous germ cell tumors, which are classified according to their differentiation into embryonal carcinoma, teratoma, choriocarcinoma, and yolk sac carcinoma.
- Forty percent of germ cell tumors have more than one component.

Pathology

A. Gross appearance:

- They appear as masses causing destruction of testicular substance.
- Seminomas are firm, solid, and yellowish, circumscribed lesions.
- Teratomas are cystic with cartilaginous foci.
- Embryonal carcinoma and yolk sac carcinoma are fleshy tumors with areas of necrosis.
- Choriocarcinoma is markedly hemorrhagic.

B. Microscopic appearance:

- Seminoma is characterized by nests of uniform large round cells separated by fibrous trabeculae infiltrated by numerous lymphocytes.
- Embryonal carcinoma is characterized by sheets of undifferentiated cells showing frequent mitoses and necrosis.
- Teratomas contain tissues derived from all three germ layers. The tissues may be mature or immature.
- Yolk sac carcinoma is characterized by a delicate reticular or papillary pattern in which structures that resemble glomeruli (glomeruloid or Schiller-Duval bodies) are present.

TABLE 51–1. CLASSIFICATION OF TESTICULAR NEOPLASMS

Tumor Type	Frequency	Age	Gross
Germ cell tumors Seminoma	30%	30–50	Solid, yellowish-white, firm.
Embryonal carcinoma[1]	20%	15–30	Solid, fleshy, soft, friable, hemorrhagic.
Teratoma[1]	10%	10–30	Cystic, solid area, cartilage.
Yolk sac (entodermal sinus) carcinoma	Rare	10–30	Solid, fleshy, soft, friable.
Choriocarcinoma[1]	Rare	10–30	Solid, hemorrhagic.
Mixed germ cell neoplasms[1]	35%	10–50	Variable, usually have a cystic teratomatous component.
Gonadal stromal tumors Undifferentiated	1%	Any age	Usually small round circumscribed nodule
Leydig cell	1%	Any age	Usually small round circumscribed nodule
Sertoli (granulosa-theca) cell	1%	Any age	Usually small round circumscribed nodule
Mixed stromal	Rare	Any age	Usually small round circumscribed nodule
Mixed germ cell and stromal	Rare	10–50	Variable
Lymphoma	2%	60–80	Solid nodules
Metastasis and other	Rare	Any age, usually elderly	Solid nodules

[1]Note that the British Testicular Tumor Panel classifies these neoplasms as varieties of teratoma: embryonal carcinoma = malignant teratoma undifferentiated; teratoma = teratoma differentiated (mature); mixed germ cell neoplasms = malignant teratoma intermediate; choriocarcinoma = malignant teratoma trophoblastic.

■ Choriocarcinoma shows cytotrophoblastic cells and syncytiotrophoblastic giant cells. There is almost always extensive hemorrhage.

Tumor Markers

■ High levels of βHCG are present in the serum in patients with choriocarcinoma.
■ Mildly elevated serum βHCG levels occur in patients with other germ cell neoplasms containing syncytiotrophoblastic giant cells.
■ Alpha-fetoprotein levels in serum are markedly elevated in patients with yolk sac carcinoma and embryonal carcinoma.

- These two tumor markers are very useful in monitoring the treatment of patients with germ cell neoplasms.

Biologic Behavior

- All germ cell neoplasms of the testis should be considered malignant. The only exception is teratoma in children, which behaves as a benign neoplasm.
- The metastatic potential is very high for these neoplasms.
- They spread by lymphatics to the retroperitoneal and para-aortic lymph nodes and via the bloodstream to the lungs and liver.

Clinical Presentation

They usually present as a painless mass in the testis, often associated with a hydrocele. Not uncommonly, the first manifestation of the neoplasm is at a metastatic site (retroperitoneum, lung).

Treatment

- Seminomas are extremely radiosensitive.
- All germ cell neoplasms are highly sensitive to modern chemotherapy.
- Orchiectomy and surgical removal of metastases from the lungs and retroperitoneum combined with aggressive chemotherapy has greatly improved the prognosis.
- The 5 year survival rate is close to 90%.

GONADAL STROMAL NEOPLASMS

Interstitial (Leydig) cell tumors constitute about 2% of testicular neoplasms. They occur mainly in children and young adults.

- They often produce androgens, causing precocious puberty in children.
- They vary from 0.5 cm to over 10 cm in diameter and are usually well-circumscribed and yellowish-brown.
- Microscopically, there are sheets of large cells resembling interstitial cells. Immunoperoxidase stains for steroid hormones are positive in the tumor cells.
- The biologic behavior of these tumors is usually benign, but about 10% are malignant.

MALIGNANT LYMPHOMA

Primary malignant lymphoma of the testis occurs most often in patients over age 60. It accounts for 2% of all testicular neoplasms. B-immunoblastic sarcoma is the most common type.

ADENOMATOID TUMOR

This is a benign neoplasm that usually arises in the epididymis, probably from mesothelial cells in the tunica vaginalis. A similar tumor occurs also in the pelvic cavity in females, commonly on the external surface of the uterus and uterine tubes.

- They appear as small circumscribed, firm nodules with a homogeneous grayish-white cut surface.

■ Microscopically, they are composed of slitlike spaces lined by mesothelial cells in a fibroblastic stroma.

THE PROSTATE

Inflammation of the Prostate

ACUTE PROSTATITIS
This is a common disease caused by gram-negative coliform bacteria, most commonly *Escherichia coli*, and the gonococcus.

■ Acute inflammation—sometimes with suppuration—involves the gland focally or diffusely.
■ Clinically, it presents with pain associated with urination or ejaculation. Marked tenderness is present over the enlarged prostate on rectal examination.

CHRONIC PROSTATITIS
In many cases the cause is uncertain ("abacterial prostatitis"). The gland is irregularly enlarged, firm, and infiltrated by numerous lymphocytes, plasma cells, and macrophages.

■ In some cases, a granulomatous reaction dominates (granulomatous prostatitis).
■ The symptoms are vague. On examination, the gland feels irregular and firm, arousing a suspicion of cancer.
■ Diagnosis is by biopsy.

Nodular Hyperplasia of the Prostate (Benign Prostatic Hyperplasia; BPH)
BPH is present in 50% of men between ages 40 and 60 and 95% of men over 70. In most of these individuals, the condition is symptomless. Clinically significant BPH is present in about 5–10% of men over age 60.

Etiology
The cause of prostatic hyperplasia is unknown. Declining levels of androgens relative to estrogen levels are believed to stimulate glandular and stromal hyperplasia.

Pathology
The periurethral part of the gland is most commonly involved. The gland is enlarged, often reaching massive size, and has a firm, rubbery nodular consistency.

■ Microscopically, the nodules are composed of a variable mixture of hyperplastic glandular and stromal elements.
■ Infarction of a nodule is common and may cause-
  ● Acute swelling that may precipitate acute pain and urinary retention.
  ● Hematuria.

Clinical Features
Obstruction to urinary outflow causes difficulty initiating urination and decreased urinary stream. Incomplete emptying of the bladder leads to chronic retention of urine and frequency.

- Complications include:
  - Chronic retention of urine, hypertrophy of bladder musculature, and the development of bladder diverticula.
  - Acute retention of urine, often due to swelling of the prostate caused by infarction.
  - Hematuria, also the result of infarction.
  - Urinary infection, because of urinary stasis.
  - Hydronephrosis and chronic renal failure.
- Treatment of prostatic hyperplasia is surgical removal of the obstructing part of the glands, either by transurethral resection or open prostatectomy.

Neoplasms of the Prostate

CARCINOMA OF THE PROSTATE

This is a common incidental finding at autopsy, being present in 15–20% of men over age 50 and over 70% of men at age 90.

- Tumors not manifested clinically during life are called latent or occult cancers.
- The incidence of clinically evident carcinoma is about 30 per 100,000 in the United States (about 75,000 cases per year).
- Prostatic cancer is most common in American blacks, fairly common in whites, and uncommon in Orientals.

Etiology

The etiology of prostatic carcinoma is unknown. The low incidence in Japanese men increases to approach that of American whites when they emigrate to the United States, suggesting an important role for environmental factors.

- The fall in androgen levels in later life leads to involutionary changes in the outer part of the gland, and it is in this region that cancer arises.
- The growth of prostatic carcinoma is androgen-dependent.

Pathology

Prostatic cancer appears grossly as a hard, irregular, ill-defined gray or grayish-yellow mass. Nearly all cancers occur in the peripheral part of the gland—about 75% in the posterior part.

- The size of the neoplasm varies from microscopic to massive.
- Histologically, prostatic carcinomas are adenocarcinomas that may be graded into five histologic grades based on the architectural and cytologic pattern.
- Perineural invasion is a common feature.

Spread

Local extension through the prostatic capsule into pelvic fat occurs early.

- Local structures such as the seminal vesicles, the base of the bladder, and the ureters are commonly involved.
- Lymphatic spread to the regional lymph nodes (iliac, periaortic, inguinal) is common.

- Hematogenous spread to the lumbosacral spine occurs early, via communications that exist between the prostatic and vertebral venous plexuses.
- Systemic hematogenous spread occurs late in the course of prostatic cancer, mainly in high-grade lesions.
- The clinicopathologic stage, which depends on the size of the tumor and the extent of spread (Table 51–2), is the most reliable prognostic indicator.

Clinical Features

Urinary symptoms such as altered flow, hematuria, and frequency occur late because of the usual peripheral posterior location of the tumor.

- Diagnosis can often be made by rectal examination, where the cancerous area can be felt as a hard, irregular nodule.
- Back pain due to vertebral metastases is a common presenting feature, and is associated with sclerotic lesions on X-rays.
- Serum prostatic acid phosphatase becomes elevated when the tumor infiltrates outside the capsule.
- Serum prostate-specific antigen level is increased even in early prostate cancer.
- Diagnosis is made by needle biopsy (guided manually or by transrectal ultrasound examination) or fine-needle aspiration cytology.

Prognosis

Prognosis depends on the clinicopathologic stage and to a lesser extent on histologic grade.

- With early disease (stage B), 80% of patients survive 5 years and 60% survive 10 years.
- With advanced disease (stage D), the prognosis is poor, only 20% surviving 5 years.

OTHER PROSTATIC NEOPLASMS

Neoplasms other than prostatic adenocarcinoma are rare. Embryonal rhabdomyosarcoma is the most common prostatic neoplasm in childhood. It is highly malignant.

TABLE 51–2. STAGING OF PROSTATE CARCINOMA

Stage A: Occult or latent carcinoma
Found by the pathologist in a prostatectomy specimen from a patient in whom carcinoma was not suspected prior to surgery. Latent carcinoma is subdivided into stages A1 and A2 depending on extent.

Stage B: Clinically suspected carcinoma
Confined within the prostatic capsule: stage B1, a tumor less than 1.5 cm in diameter, involving only one lobe; stage B2, a larger tumor or involvement of more than one lobe.

Stage C: Extracapsular extension

Stage D: Distant metastases

THE PENIS

CONGENITAL PENILE ANOMALIES

Hypospadias
Hypospadias is the opening of the urethra on the ventral aspect of the penis. It is common, and usually minor in degree.

- The most extreme form of hypospadias, where the urethra opens at the root of the penis, resembles the female genitalia (ambiguous genitalia).
- Epispadias (uncommon) is the opening of the urethra on the dorsal aspect of the penis.

Phimosis
Phimosis is a common condition that may be congenital or acquired by trauma or recurrent infection. It is characterized by an excessively small preputial orifice that prevents retraction over the glans and in extreme cases obstructs urinary outflow.

Penile Neoplasms

CONDYLOMA ACUMINATUM
This is a common benign neoplasm caused by human papilloma virus, which is transmitted sexually.

- They occur commonly on the coronal sulcus of the glans or the inner surface of the prepuce.
- They vary in size from 1 mm to several centimeters and appear grossly as wartlike masses; they are frequently multiple.
- Microscopically, they appear as benign squamous papillomas showing vacuolization of the cytoplasm of the virus-infected cells ("koilocytosis").

PENILE CARCINOMA IN SITU (Bowen's Disease; Erythroplasia of Queyrat)
This appears clinically as a red plaque on the glans or prepuce. There is a high risk of subsequent invasive carcinoma.

CARCINOMA OF THE PENIS
This is uncommon in the United States, representing less than 1% of cancers in males.

- The incidence is low in the circumcised male. Penile carcinoma is almost nonexistent in Jews, in whom circumcision is performed at birth, and is seen very infrequently in Moslems, in whom circumcision is performed in the early teens.
- Penile carcinoma is common in Oriental races, accounting for as much as 10% of male cancers in some Asian countries.
- It occurs in the age group from 40 to 70 years.

Pathology & Clinical Features
The common sites for carcinoma of the penis are the glans and inner surface of the prepuce.

- The early lesion is a white plaque followed by formation of an elevated white papule. Ulceration follows, producing the characteristic indurated, painless ulcer with raised, everted edges.
- Less commonly, carcinoma appears as a papillomatous or warty growth.
- Microscopically, penile carcinoma is a squamous carcinoma of variable differentiation.

Behavior & Treatment

Penile carcinoma usually shows slow infiltrative growth locally, with invasion of the corpora cavernosa occurring early. At the time of presentation, about 25–30% of patients have regional (inguinal) lymph node involvement.

- Distant metastases occur only at a late stage.
- With penectomy and excision of regional inguinal lymph nodes, the overall 5-year survival approaches 50%.
- Radiation therapy is useful in controlling recurrent disease.

THE SCROTUM

Scrotal disease is commonly secondary to underlying disorders of the testis or epididymis (eg, tuberculous epididymo-orchitis). The scrotum may be involved by skin diseases, most commonly epidermal cysts, which frequently calcify. Necrotizing fasciitis of the scrotum (Fournier's gangrene) has been described earlier in this chapter. The scrotum may rarely be the site of squamous carcinoma.

Section XII. The Female Reproductive System

The Ovary & Uterine Tubes

52

THE OVARIES

MANIFESTATIONS OF OVARIAN DISEASE

- Infertility may result from failure of ovulation.
- Menstrual irregularities may result from abnormal patterns of secretion of ovarian hormones.
- Mass lesions also occur, but are usually asymptomatic until they become very large.

NONNEOPLASTIC OVARIAN CYSTS & TUMORS

1. FOLLICULAR CYST
These are extremely common variations of developing or atretic graafian follicles. They contain serum fluid, rarely exceed 1–5 cm in diameter, and are lined by flattened layers of granulosa cells. They are of no clinical significance, disappearing spontaneously in 1–2 months.

2. POLYCYSTIC OVARY SYNDROME
This syndrome is characterized by:

- Bilaterally enlarged ovaries containing multiple follicular cysts in the outer, subcapsular region.
- Absence of corpora lutea resulting from failure of ovulation.
- Hyperplastic ovarian stroma with thickening of the capsule.
- It is associated clinically with amenorrhea, infertility, and virilism (Stein-Leventhal syndrome).
- There is excess androgen secretion, with normal or elevated estrogen levels.
- It is associated with endometrial hyperplasia, causing abnormal uterine bleeding and an increased incidence of endometrial carcinoma.
- The cause is probably abnormal secretion of pituitary gonadotropins; the normal luteinizing hormone (LH) surge that causes ovulation is lacking.
- Treatment with clomiphene, which stimulates ovulation, is effective.

3. LUTEINIZED FOLLICULAR CYSTS (Theca Lutein Cysts)

Multiple luteinized follicular cysts occur in patients with abnormally elevated secretion of chorionic gonadotropins, as occurs in:

- Hydatidiform mole.
- Choriocarcinoma.
- hCG stimulates luteinization of granulosa and theca interna cells in normal and atretic follicles.

4. VARIATIONS RELATING TO THE CORPUS LUTEUM

Rarely, a corpus luteum may be large enough to be palpable—particularly when it becomes hemorrhagic (corpus luteum hematoma) or cystic (luteal cyst).

- Luteoma of pregnancy:
  - Is an extreme form of luteal hyperplasia that produces a nodular mass in the ovary in the last trimester.
  - May reach a large size and may be bilateral.
  - Is commonly encountered during cesarean sections and should not be mistaken for neoplasms.
  - Rarely, luteomas produce androgens and cause virilization.
  - They involute spontaneously within a few weeks after delivery.

5. ENDOMETRIOTIC CYSTS

The ovary is the commonest site for extrauterine endometriosis (see Chapter 53). Ovarian endometriosis manifests as multiple hemorrhagic cysts ("chocolate cysts") characterized microscopically by a lining of endometrial epithelium and stroma.

NEOPLASMS OF THE OVARIES

Incidence

- They are relatively common; 75–80% are benign.
- Malignant ovarian neoplasms account for about 5% of all cancers in women (the fifth most common cancer in American women).
- Benign neoplasms occur in a younger age group (20–40 years) than malignant ones (40–60 years), but there is considerable overlap.

Classification (Table 52–1)

Primary ovarian neoplasms are classified according to their histogenesis into:

- Neoplasms of celomic epithelium.
- Germ cell neoplasms.
- Stromal neoplasms.
- Mixed germ cell and stromal neoplasms.
- Metastatic carcinoma, mainly from the gastrointestinal tract, is common.

Clinical Features

They are often found incidentally during pelvic examination, radiography, or abdominal surgery.

TABLE 52–1. CLASSIFICATION OF OVARIAN NEOPLASMS

Tumor Type	Frequency[1] (%)	Age[2] (Years)	Gross
Tumors of coelomic (germinal) epithelium	75		
Serous tumors	40	15–50	Solid or cystic, may be large; often bilateral
Benign serous cystadenoma			
Borderline serous tumor			
Serous cystadenocarcinoma			
Mucinous tumors	20	15–50	Large solid or cystic
Benign mucinous cystadenoma			
Borderline mucinous tumor			
Mucinous cystadenocarcinoma			
Endometrioid tumors	5	30–70	Large solid or cystic
Borderline type (rare)			
Carcinoma			
Clear cell carcinoma	2	50–70	Usually unilateral, solid or cystic
Brenner tumors	2	30–70	Usually small and solid; small cystic areas
Benign			
Borderline (rare)			
Malignant (very rare)			
Undifferentiated carcinoma	5–10	30–70	Bilateral, necrotic, hemorrhagic
Germ cell tumors	20		
Teratoma	15	1–80	Frequently cystic; may be large, occasionally bilateral
Benign ("dermoid cyst")		> 20	
Immature (rare)		< 20	
Dysgerminoma	5	1–80	Solid, occasionally bilateral
Yolk sac carcinoma	Rare	1–30	Solid with necrosis
Embryonal carcinoma	Very rare	—	Solid with necrosis; associated with teratoma
Choriocarcinoma[3]	Very rare	—	Associated with teratoma
Gonadal stromal tumors	5	1–80	
Granulosa-theca cell	2	Especially 50+	Solid, often hemorrhagic; hormonal effects
Undifferentiated	Rare	Especially 50+	Aggressive, often bilateral
Fibrothecoma	3	Especially 50+	Solid with or without ascites

(*continued*)

TABLE 52–1. (Continued)

Tumor Type	Frequency[1] (%)	Age[2] (Years)	Gross
Sertoli-Leydig cell	Rare	10–30	Solid, with necrosis
Mixed germ cell and stromal (gonadoblastoma)	Rare		Occurs in dysgenetic ovaries in patients with chromosomal abnormalities
Metastatic neoplasms	Common	Usually 40+	Often bilateral

[1]Frequencies are approximate percentages of all primary ovarian tumors; the text also gives figures as a percentage of malignant tumors only.
[2]Represents the usual age range; occasional tumors will occur outside the range given.
[3]Choriocarcinoma also occurs in the ovary secondary to gestational choriocarcinoma.

- Large neoplasms may produce a sensation of "heaviness" or discomfort in the lower abdomen.
- Pressure on the bladder may cause frequency of micturition.
- Malignant neoplasms often remain silent until they have metastasized.
- Hormone-secreting ovarian neoplasms present with manifestations of hormone excess:
  - Estrogen-secreting granulosa-theca cell tumors cause endometrial hyperplasia and adenocarcinoma, leading to abnormal uterine bleeding.
  - Androgen-secreting tumors cause virilization.

Spread
Malignant ovarian neoplasms tend to spread locally in the peritoneal cavity, leading to ascites.

- Cytologic examination of aspirated peritoneal fluid may offer a diagnosis in such cases.
- Lymphatic spread, to iliac and para-aortic lymph nodes, and bloodstream spread, most commonly to the lungs, occurs in the high-grade malignant neoplasms.

Treatment
Surgical removal represents the primary mode of therapy for treatment of ovarian neoplasms.

- With benign and most borderline neoplasms, surgery is curative.
- For malignant neoplasms, radiation therapy and chemotherapy are used in conjunction with surgery.

1. COELOMIC (GERMINAL) EPITHELIAL NEOPLASMS
These neoplasms are classified according to their differentiation (Table 52–2). Within these groups, three biologic types of tumor may be recognized based on histologic criteria (Table 52–2 and Fig 52–1).

TABLE 52–2. NOMENCLATURE OF OVARIAN NEOPLASMS OF COELOMIC EPITHELIAL ORIGIN

Cell Differentiation	Benign	Borderline[2]	Malignant
Tubal (serous tumors)	Serous cystadenoma (100%)	Borderline tumor (95%)	Cystadenocarcinoma (20%)
Endocervical (mucinous tumors)	Mucinous cystadenoma (100%)	Borderline tumor (95%)	Cystadenocarcinoma (45%)
Endometrial	?Endometriosis[3]	Very rare	Endometrioid carcinoma (50%)
Uncertain			Clear cell carcinoma (40%)
Urothelial	Brenner tumor	Proliferating Brenner tumor (rare)	Malignant Brenner tumor (very rare)
Undifferentiated	...	...	Undifferentiated carcinoma (10%)

[1] Figures in parentheses are 5-year survival rates. Note that 10-year survival rates are generally lower, because late recurrence of tumor is not uncommon in ovarian neoplasms. Survival figures are not available for the very rare tumor types.

[2] Borderline tumors are also called tumors of low malignant potential.

[3] The origin of endometrial tissue in endometriosis is uncertain, whether by displacement from the uterus or by differentiation of the ovarian coelomic epithelium.

Serous Tumors

Serous tumors are the commonest ovarian neoplasms, accounting for approximately 40% of primary ovarian neoplasms and 20% of primary cancers.

- They occur in the age group from 15 to 50 years.
- Twenty-five percent of benign, 50% of borderline, and 70% of malignant serous tumors are bilateral.
- Based on the microscopic appearance, three different biologic types are recognized (Fig 52–1).

A. Benign serous cystadenoma:

- Vary in size from small cysts in the ovary to large multilocular cystic neoplasms reaching a size of over 40 cm.
- Have a smooth external surface and a smooth or papillary internal lining of cuboidal or flattened epithelium.
- Do not infiltrate the capsule or metastasize.
- Surgical removal is curative.

B. Borderline serous tumor:

- Are also called serous tumors of low malignant potential.

Benign serous cystadenoma
- Single layer of epithelial cells
- No atypia

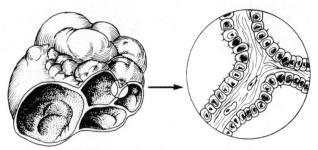

Borderline serous tumor
- Mild atypia
- Stratification of cells less than 3 layers deep

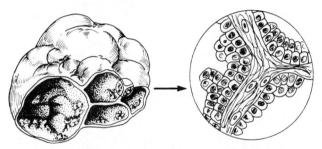

Malignant serous cystadenocarcinoma
- Stratified epithelium with marked cytologic atypia
- Invasion of stroma

Hemorrhage and necrosis

Cystic areas

Solid areas

Tumor on surface

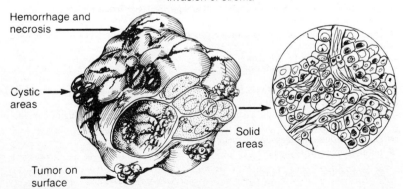

Figure 52–1. Serous tumors of the ovary, showing criteria used for differentiating benign, borderline, and malignant counterparts of these tumors.

- Are distinguished from benign serous cystadenomas in having a more complex histologic pattern, and stratification and cytologic atypia of lining cells.
- Are distinguished from serous cystadenocarcinoma by the lack of infiltration of the stroma.
- Behave in a low-grade malignant manner, metastasizing to the peritoneal cavity and rarely to the lungs.
- Have a good prognosis (5-year survival rate of 95%) even in the presence of peritoneal metastases.

C. Serous cystadenocarcinoma:

- Shows irregular solid and cystic areas and may show gross infiltration.
- Is a highly malignant neoplasm, infiltrating and metastasizing early in its course.
- Spread locally to the peritoneum and omentum occurs early.
- Commonly has calcification in the form of round, laminated psammoma bodies.
- Microscopically, the cyst epithelial lining is highly complex, with marked cell stratification (more than three cell layers), marked cytologic atypia, and stromal or capsular invasion.
- Lymph node involvement also occurs early, with metastases in pelvic and para-aortic lymph nodes.
- Distant metastases occur late, with lung and liver being the main sites.
- The 5-year survival rate is about 20%.

Mucinous Tumors

- Account for 20% of ovarian neoplasms.
- Occur most often in the age group from 15 to 50 years.
- Most are benign.
- Mucinous cystadenocarcinoma accounts for less than 5% of ovarian cancers.
- Mucinous tumors are less frequently bilateral than serous tumors (20% bilaterality for borderline and malignant mucinous tumors).
- Based on their histologic features in a manner similar to serous tumors, mucinous tumors are classified into cystadenoma, borderline, and cystadenocarcinoma.
- Microscopically, the lining epithelium is composed of tall columnar cells with flattened basal nuclei, and the apical part of the cell is distended with mucin.
- The behavior, treatment, and prognosis are analogous to the corresponding serous tumors.
- Extensive peritoneal involvement in borderline mucinous tumors has a typical myxomatous appearance ("pseudomyxoma peritonii").

Endometrioid Carcinoma

- Accounts for 15% of malignant ovarian neoplasms.
- Resembles endometrial carcinoma microscopically.
- Associated endometriosis is found in about 25% of cases.
- In most cases, the tumor represents endometrioid differentiation of a celomic epithelial neoplasm. In a few cases, an origin from endometriosis can be shown.
- Grossly, appear as solid and cystic masses that frequently show areas of hemorrhage and necrosis.

- Borderline endometrioid tumors are very rare.
- Endometrioid carcinoma has the best prognosis among ovarian carcinomas, with a 5-year survival rate of 50%.

Clear Cell Carcinoma
Clear cell carcinoma is derived from the coelomic epithelium.

- It accounts for 5% of malignant primary ovarian neoplasms.
- It is characterized histologically by large cells with clear cytoplasm arranged in solid, glandular, tubular, or papillary patterns.
- It has a prognosis similar to that of endometrioid carcinoma.

Brenner Tumor
This is uncommon, accounting for 2% of ovarian neoplasms.

- It occurs at all ages, but is most frequently encountered as an incidental finding in older patients.
- Grossly, it is a solid, firm white neoplasm that varies from 1 to 30 cm in size.
- Small cysts containing mucinous material are common.
- Microscopically, it is characterized by a cellular fibroblastic stroma in which there are epithelial islands composed of uniform, cytologically benign cells that resemble transitional epithelium.
- It is usually benign. Rare Brenner tumors show epithelial proliferation and are analogous to borderline tumors.
- Malignant Brenner tumors are very rare and resemble transitional cell carcinoma.

Undifferentiated Carcinoma
This is an epithelial neoplasm of the ovary that does not show any kind of differentiation. It is composed of solid masses of cells with necrosis, hemorrhage, and a high mitotic rate. It has the poorest prognosis, with a 5-year survival rate of less than 10%.

2. GERM CELL NEOPLASMS

Benign Cystic Teratoma (Dermoid Cyst)
Dermoid cyst is common, accounting for 15% of ovarian neoplasms. It is bilateral in 10% of cases and occurs in all age groups, most commonly over 20 years.

- Benign teratoma appears grossly as a cyst containing thick sebaceous material and hair. Cartilage, bone, and well-formed teeth may be present.
- Microscopically, skin elements dominate, but structures of entodermal (respiratory and gastrointestinal epithelia) and mesodermal (muscle, fat, cartilage) origin are present.
- Rare ovarian teratomas are composed almost entirely of thyroid tissue ("struma ovarii") or tissue resembling carcinoid tumor.
- Cystic teratomas of the ovary are benign.
- Very rarely, malignant transformation occurs in one of the elements of a benign teratoma, most commonly the squamous epithelium, giving rise to squamous carcinoma.

Immature Teratoma (Malignant Teratoma)

This is a rare malignant variant of teratoma that occurs mainly in patients under age 25.

- Grossly, immature teratomas are usually solid neoplasms with minimal cystic change.
- Microscopically, they are composed of immature elements derived from all three germ layers. Primitive neuroectodermal (neuroblastic) elements are especially common.
- Tumors with large areas of primitive neuroectodermal tissue have the worst prognosis.

Dysgerminoma

This is the ovarian counterpart of seminoma of the testis. It accounts for about 2% of ovarian cancers, and commonly occurs in the age group from 10 to 30 years.

- Grossly, masses are usually solid, rarely (5–10%) bilateral, and range in size from very small to huge.
- Microscopically, nests of round germ cells are separated by fibrous trabeculae infiltrated by lymphocytes.
- The overall prognosis is good, with a 5-year survival rate of 80%.

Yolk Sac Tumor (Entodermal Sinus Tumor)

Yolk sac tumors are rare, accounting for 1% of ovarian cancers. They occur mainly in females under age 20.

- Grossly, they are solid neoplasms with areas of necrosis and hemorrhage.
- Histologically, yolk sac tumors are composed of a reticular arrangement of primitive cells containing structures resembling immature glomeruli (Schiller-Duval bodies).
- They are highly malignant neoplasms with a bad prognosis.
- Serum alpha-fetoprotein is elevated and provides a mechanism for following therapy.

3. GONADAL STROMAL NEOPLASMS

These neoplasms account for 5% of ovarian neoplasms. They are composed of variable mixtures of granulosa cells, theca cells, stromal fibroblasts, and cells resembling testicular Sertoli cells and Leydig cells.

Granulosa-Theca Cell Tumors

These tumors occur at any age, but are most frequently seen in postmenopausal women. About 5% are bilateral.

- Grossly, they are solid, yellowish fleshy masses that frequently show hemorrhage and cystic change.
- Microscopically, they are composed of small, uniform cells arranged in solid masses; the formation of spaces filled with eosinophilic fluid (Call-Exner bodies), is characteristic.
- Typically they secrete estrogens, which produce hyperplasia of the endometrium and predispose to endometrial adenocarcinoma.
- Abnormal uterine bleeding is the most common mode of presentation.

- Twenty-five percent behave in a locally aggressive manner. Distant metastases occur in about 10–15% of cases.
- The 5-year survival rate is 85%.

Fibroma (Fibrothecoma)

Benign neoplasms that arise in the ovarian mesenchymal stroma. They account for 3% of ovarian neoplasms and occasionally (5%) are bilateral. They are most often seen in postmenopausal women.

- Grossly, they form encapsulated white to yellow masses, usually less than 20 cm in diameter.
- Microscopically, they are composed of fibroblasts and interspersed theca cells.
- Approximately 20% are associated with marked ascites, and a small proportion also show pleural effusions (Meig's syndrome).

Sertoli-Leydig Cell Tumor (Androblastoma; Arrhenoblastoma)

These are neoplasms occurring most commonly in the 10- to 30-year age group. Less than 5% are bilateral.

- Grossly, they are solid grayish-white neoplasms with areas of hemorrhage, necrosis, and cystic degeneration.
- Histologically, they are composed of large cells with abundant eosinophilic cytoplasm arranged in nests or tubules.
- Commonly, they produce androgens and cause virilization.
- Most have a benign biologic behavior; the 5-year survival rate is 90%.

4. GONADOBLASTOMA

This is a rare ovarian neoplasm composed of a mixture of stromal cells (usually Sertoli-Leydig cells) and germ cells (usually dysgerminoma).

- It occurs almost exclusively in dysgenetic ovaries in patients with sex chromosome abnormalities (usually in streak ovaries of phenotypic females who have a Y chromosome in their karyotype, eg, XX,XY mosaics).
- The biologic behavior of gonadoblastoma depends on the amount of germ cell neoplasm.

5. METASTATIC NEOPLASMS

The ovary is a common site for metastases, particularly in carcinoma of the endometrium, breast, stomach, and colon.

- Metastatic carcinoma causes solid enlargement of one or both ovaries, which may reach a large size.
- Differentiation from primary ovarian carcinoma can be difficult, particularly in undifferentiated carcinoma and metastatic colon and endometrial carcinoma, which resemble endometrioid carcinoma of the ovary.
- Krukenberg's tumor is a bilateral involvement of the ovaries by a desmoplastic signet ring cell carcinoma of gastric origin.

THE UTERINE (FALLOPIAN) TUBES

Inflammatory Lesions

ACUTE SALPINGITIS
Acute salpingitis is also called **acute pelvic inflammatory disease (PID).** It is most commonly the result of gonococcal infection.

- In the past, acute streptococcal salpingitis was a frequent complication of abortion or childbirth.
- It is characterized by hyperemia and edema of the tube. The external surface is covered by a fibrinopurulent exudate, and the lumen contains pus.
- Suppuration occurs frequently, producing an abscess that involves the tube and ovary (tubo-ovarian abscess).
- Patients present with fever and lower abdominal pain.
- Treatment with appropriate antibiotics is effective.

CHRONIC SALPINGITIS
Chronic salpingitis follows recurrent attacks of acute inflammation.

- It is characterized by luminal adhesions and progressive fibrosis.
- Complete luminal obliteration may also occur, resulting in dilatation of the distal ampullary part of the tube, which is filled with serous fluid (hydrosalpinx).
- Clinically, it is characterized by recurrent lower abdominal pain.
- Luminal narrowing may cause infertility and predisposes to tubal ectopic pregnancy (see Chapter 55).

TUBERCULOUS SALPINGITIS
The uterine tube is a relatively common site for tuberculosis. Gross appearance differs little from that of nonspecific chronic salpingitis. Diagnosis is made by microscopic examination, which shows caseating granulomas with acid-fast bacilli.

Neoplasms of the Uterine Tubes
Neoplasms of the uterine tube are rare. The commonest benign neoplasm is adenomatoid tumor, which arises in the mesothelial covering of the tube. Carcinoma of the uterine tube is very rare. It resembles papillary serous cystadenocarcinoma of the ovary.

The Uterus, Vagina, & Vulva   53

THE UTERUS (BODY & ENDOMETRIUM)

MANIFESTATIONS OF UTERINE DISEASE

Abnormal Uterine Bleeding
Abnormal uterine bleeding may be an increased amount of regular bleeding (**menor-rhagia**) or irregular noncyclic bleeding (**epimenorrhea**).

- In some instances, an organic cause can be identified.
- In others, bleeding is the result of abnormal hormonal stimulation (dysfunctional uterine bleeding).

Pain Associated with Menstruation
Menstruation is commonly associated with a dull ache or with cramping pain.

- Severe pain during menstruation is called **dysmenorrhea.**
  - Primary dysmenorrhea appears with the onset of menstruation at menarche, and there is usually no organic basis.
  - Secondary dysmenorrhea begins later in life and is often associated with underlying organic disease (eg, endometriosis).

Infertility & Spontaneous Abortion
Infertility may be caused by congenital anatomic uterine anomalies, uterine neoplasms, or endometrial disease that interfere with implantation and development of the embryo.

Uterine Masses
Neoplasms of the uterus often cause uterine enlargement; they must become large before they produce clinical symptoms.

METHODS OF EVALUATING THE UTERUS

Physical Examination
Vaginal examination permits direct palpation of the cervix and assessment of the uterine body for changes in position and in size, and for the presence of masses.

Cervical (Pap) Smears (Table 53–1)
Pap smears taken with a spatula from the surface epithelium of the cervix provide material for cytologic evaluation of:

TABLE 53–1. PAPANICOLAOU ("PAP") SMEAR OF CERVIX

Involves cytologic evaluation of exfoliated cells stained by the Papanicolaou method.

A cervical smear is taken by lightly sweeping the surface of the cervix with a spatula (Ayre's spatula) through a vaginal speculum or at colposcopy. The spatula covers the ectocervix, squamocolumnar junction, and lower endocervix. An endocervical smear is usually obtained additionally with a cotton swab.

A Pap smear report may include the following:

Degree of estrogen effect (stage of cycle, or post-menopausal). The evaluation of hormonal status by Pap smear is not accurate.

Presence of any infectious agent (eg, *Trichomonas, Chlamydia, Candida,* evidence of papillomavirus cytomegalovirus, or herpevirus).

A description of the cervical epithelial cells:

This may use the following grading system:

Class I	Normal
Class II	Slightly abnormal or inflammatory change
Class III	Marked abnormality, uncertain significance
Class IV	Dysplasia (mild, moderate, severe, carcinoma in situ)
Class V	Squamous carcinoma or adenocarcinoma

A class II result requires a repeat smear. A class III, IV, or V report requires formal cervical biopsy to confirm diagnosis histologically.

More commonly, the Pap smear report describes the cytologic changes observed without a numerical grade (eg, inflammatory atypia, repair, dysplasia, squamous carcinoma), using the Berthesda system.

- The phase of the cycle.
- The presence of certain infections.
- Epithelial dysplasia or neoplasia.

Colposcopy & Biopsy of Cervix & Endometrium

The cervix can be directly visualized and biopsied by colposcopy. Biopsy of the endometrium can be performed through the endocervical canal.

- Endometrial biopsies provide information on:
  - The phase of the cycle, which can be correlated with the menstrual history (Table 53–2).
  - The presence of endometrial disease.

TABLE 53–2. FEATURES OBSERVED IN NORMAL ENDOMETRIUM AT DIFFERENT STAGES OF THE ENDOMETRIAL CYCLE THAT ARE USEFUL IN ASCRIBING A "DATE" TO THE ENDOMETRIUM

Date[1]	Changes[2]
Proliferative phase 1st–4th day	Menstruation; neutrophils, necrosis, and a mixture of late secretory and early proliferative glands
4th–7th day (early proliferative)	Thin regenerating surface epithelium; straight, short glands; compact stroma; few mitotic figures in epithelium and stroma
8th–10th day (mid proliferative)	Columnar surface epithelium; long glands; numerous mitotic figures in epithelium and stroma; moderately dense stroma
11th–14th day (late proliferative)	Long glands showing stratification of nuclei with numerous mitoses; dense stroma with numerous mitotic figures
Secretory phase 14th–15th day	No microscopic changes from late proliferative endometrium
16th–17th day	Subnuclear vacuoles appear in the epithelium, which loses its nuclear stratification; mitotic activity in epithelium and stroma disappears
18th–20th day	Subnuclear vacuoles shrink, and the nuclei of the orderly row of epithelial cells in the glands move toward the base; intraluminal eosinophilic secretions appear; glands tortuous
21st–22nd day	Stromal edema appears; gland tortuosity increased with serrated lumens
23rd day	Spiral arterioles become prominent
24th–25th day	Stromal cells show predecidual changes with an increase in cytoplasm
26th–28th day (premenstrual)	Neutrophils appear; increasing necrosis and hemorrhage of the endometrium

[1]The date is given with day 1 being the onset of menstruation. Note that the date of ovulation is assumed to be day 14 of the cycle. Because the date of ovulation varies considerably, it is probably more accurate to date the secretory phase changes as days after ovulation rather than day of the cycle; eg, the 18th to 20th days in this table will become the 4th to 6th days after ovulation.

[2]Note that the changes in the proliferative phase do not permit accurate dating; however, in the secretory phase it is possible to date a given endometrium within 2 days of its actual date.

ABNORMAL ENDOMETRIAL CYCLES

Exogenous Progestational Hormone Effect

This effect is due to exogenous administration either of progesterone or of a combined progesterone-estrogen oral contraceptive. The stroma becomes abundant and shows predecidual change and edema, but the endometrial glands remain small and show minimal secretory activity due to lack of priming by estrogen.

Unopposed Estrogen Effect

Prolonged estrogen stimulation of the endometrium, unopposed by progesterone, occurs:

- Due to exogenous estrogen administration.
- With estrogen-secreting neoplasms, most commonly granulosa cell tumor of the ovary and, more rarely, adrenal cortical neoplasms.
- In anovulatory cycles, which tend to occur at the extremes of reproductive life (postmenarcheal and premenopausal).
- In polycystic ovary (Stein-Leventhal) syndrome.
- Unopposed estrogen effect causes prolongation of the proliferative phase of the endometrial cycle, followed by irregular breakdown to produce excessive uterine bleeding. In these cases, endometrial biopsy during the bleeding phase shows proliferative phase endometrium.
- With more intense estrogen stimulation, various degrees of **endometrial hyperplasia** occur:
  - Mild endometrial hyperplasia, with increased numbers of glands showing stratitifed epithelium and cystic dilatation (simple hyperplasia).
  - Moderate endometrial hyperplasia, which shows a greater increase in the number and complexity of glands and marked stratification of cells. There is no cytologic atypia (complex hyperplasia without atypia).
  - Severe endometrial hyperplasia, where the complex glandular hyperplasia is accompanied by cytologic atypia (complex hyperplasia with atypia).

- Unopposed estrogen stimulation predisposes to endometrial adenocarcinoma. The risk of carcinoma varies from less than 1% for mild hyperplasia to 15% for severe atypical hyperplasia.
- Clinically, prolonged estrogenic excess produces prolonged periods of amenorrhea followed by excessive irregular bleeding.
- Treatment consists of administering progestogens.

Inadequate Luteal Phase

Inadequate function of the corpus luteum leads to low progesterone output and a poorly developed secretory endometrium.

- The abnormal endometrium breaks down irregularly, resulting in abnormal uterine bleeding late in the cycle.
- Endometrial biopsy shows poorly formed secretory endometrium, which lags 4 or more days behind that predicted by the menstrual history.
- Serum progesterone, FSH, and LH levels are low.

Persistent Luteal Phase; Irregular Shedding of Menstrual Endometrium

Rarely, the corpus luteum maintains low levels of progesterone secretion after onset of menstruation, causing protracted and irregular shedding of the menstrual endometrium.

- Clinically, the patient has regular periods, but menstrual bleeding is excessive and prolonged, frequently lasting 10–14 days.
- Diagnosis is made by the finding of persistent secretory endometrium after the fifth day of menstruation.

ENDOMETRIOSIS

This is defined as the occurrence of endometrial tissue at a site other than the lining of the uterine cavity. The ectopic endometrial tissue is composed of both glands and stroma and responds to ovarian hormones.

Pathology
A. Adenomyosis (endometriosis interna):

- Is the presence of endometrial glands and stroma situated deep in the myometrium (more than 3 mm from the base of the endometrium).
- Is common in older women (over age 40) and is seen in about 40% of uteri at autopsy.
- The diffuse form of adenomyosis involves much or all of the uterus, causing uterine enlargement.
- Focal adenomyosis (adenomyoma) forms a nodular mass that resembles a leiomyoma grossly.

B. Extrauterine endometriosis (endometriosis externa): Endometriosis occurring outside the uterus is pathogenetically unrelated to adenomyosis.

- In order of decreasing frequency, endometriosis externa is found in:
  - An ovary.
  - The wall of a uterine tube.
  - Parametrial soft tissue.
  - The serosa of the intestine, most commonly the sigmoid colon and appendix.
  - The umbilicus.
  - The urinary tract.
  - The skin at the site of laparotomy scars, usually after surgery on the uterus and most commonly after cesarian section.
  - Extra-abdominal sites such as the lungs, pleura, and bones.
- Pathologically, foci of endometriosis appear as cysts that contain areas of new and old hemorrhage ("chocolate cysts").
- Microscopically, characterized by the presence of endometrial glands surrounded by stroma.

Pathogenesis

Adenomyosis is believed to be the result of abnormal downgrowth of the endometrium into the myometrium, with entrapment of endometrium deep in the uterine muscle.

- Endometriosis externa results from one of two mechanisms:
  - Metaplasia of the coelomic epithelium into endometrial tissue.
  - Transport of fragments of normal menstrual endometrium from the uterus, through the uterine tubes into the peritoneal cavity.

Clinical Features

Patients with endometriosis are in the reproductive phase of life; endometriotic foci regress after menopause when the hormone levels decrease.

- Endometriosis may be asymptomatic.
- The commonest symptoms of adenomyosis are dysmenorrhea, menorrhagia, and infertility.
- Repeated episodes of bleeding result in fibrosis, which may cause peritoneal adhesions and intestinal obstruction.
- Endometriosis of the uterine tubes results in infertility and an increased risk of tubal pregnancy.

INFLAMMATORY LESIONS OF THE ENDOMETRIUM

1. ACUTE ENDOMETRITIS

Acute endometritis occurs at a postpartum or postabortion infection, where the usual organisms are streptococci, or as an ascending gonococcal infection. The diagnosis of postpartum or postabortal endometritis is suggested by fever 2–4 days after delivery, with offensive lochia (uterine discharge).

2. CHRONIC NONSPECIFIC ENDOMETRITIS

This is common in patients harboring foreign material in the uterine cavity, such as an intra-uterine contraceptive device, and retained products of conception.

- Culture for bacteria is rarely positive.
- Chronic endometritis interferes with the cyclic development of the endometrium.
- The endometrial glands remain small throughout the cycle, while the stromal reaction is often heightened.
- The endometrium is unstable and irregular uterine bleeding results.
- Diagnosis depends on the finding of plasma cells in the endometrium.

3. TUBERCULOUS ENDOMETRITIS

This is rare, even in regions where tuberculosis is endemic. It is usually associated with tuberculous salpingitis.

- It may cause irregular uterine bleeding and infertility.
- Diagnosis is usually made by finding caseating epithelioid cell granulomas in an endometrial biopsy.
- Mycobacteria can be demonstrated in tissue sections or by culture.

NEOPLASMS OF THE ENDOMETRIUM

1. ENDOMETRIAL POLYPS

Endometrial polyps are common, particularly around menopause. They vary in size from 0.5 to 3 cm and are covered by endometrial epithelium.

- Microscopically, they are composed of endometrial glands—which may or may not show cyclic changes—and a fibrovascular stroma.

■ Clinically, they may be asymptomatic or may cause excessive uterine bleeding.
■ Very rarely, they undergo carcinomatous transformation.

2. ENDOMETRIAL CARCINOMA

Endometrial carcinoma is common, accounting for about 10% of cancers in women, and the incidence is increasing in many countries. Ninety percent of cases occur in postmenopausal women, the most common ages being 55–65 years. The epidemiology of carcinoma of the endometrium is very different from that of carcinoma of the cervix (Table 53–3).

Etiology

Prolonged unopposed estrogen stimulation of the endometrium is believed to be the major etiologic factor.

■ Endometrial hyperplasia precedes cancer in most cases.
■ It is associated with obesity, diabetes mellitus, and hypertension (corpus cancer syndrome).
■ There is a decreased incidence in multiparous, as compared with nulliparous, women.

Pathology

Most endometrial carcinomas present as polypoid fungating masses in the endometrial cavity.

■ The uterus is often asymmetrically enlarged.
■ Invasion into the myometrium occurs early.
■ Microscopically, endometrial carcinoma is an adenocarcinoma. Most are well-differentiated, with irregular glands lined by malignant columnar epithelial cells.

TABLE 53–3. CARCINOMA OF THE UTERUS AND CERVIX

	Carcinoma of Body (Corpus)	Carcinoma of Cervix
Incidence in USA	39,000/year	16,000/year
Deaths	4000/year	8000/year
Site	Body of uterus	Cervix
Age	50 plus	40 plus
Etiologic factors	Nulliparity, obesity, hypertension, diabetes	Multiparity, human papilloma virus, herpes simplex virus; multiple sexual partners
5-year survival rate (overall)	80%	60%
Histology	Adenocarcinoma (occasionally with squamous metaplasia)	Squamous carcinoma (except endocervical carcinoma which is adenocarcinoma)

- They are graded according to their degree of histologic differentiation into grades 1 (well-differentiated) to 3 (poorly differentiated).
- Areas of squamous differentiation are common.
- The pathologic stage of the neoplasm, determined by the degree of spread is the most important prognostic factor.

Clinical Features
Abnormal uterine bleeding is the earliest symptom. This may be postmenopausal bleeding or irregular menstrual bleeding.

- Physical examination may be normal or may disclose enlargement of the uterus.
- Examination of a cervical (Pap) smear may be diagnostic but is not reliable unless special techniques are used to obtain material from the endometrium.
- Endometrial biopsy or curettage is usually diagnostic.

Prognosis
Prognosis depends mainly on the stage of disease.

- With treatment, 90% of patients with stage I (carcinoma restricted to uterine body), 40% with stage II (limited extension into pelvic fat or cervix), and 10–20% with more advanced disease, survive 5 years.
- The histologic grade of the neoplasm is of secondary importance; the overall 5-year survival rate is 70% in grade 1 and 20% in grade 3 carcinomas.

3. MIXED MESODERMAL TUMOR (Malignant Mixed Müllerian Tumor)
This is a rare neoplasm that usually occurs in women over age 55.

- Grossly, these tumors appear as bulky, fleshy masses that fill the uterine cavity. They often show extensive necrosis and hemorrhage.
- Microscopically, they are composed of a malignant epithelial component (usually an adenocarcinoma) and a malignant mesenchymal component (usually leiomyosarcoma; occasionally rhabdomyosarcoma, chondrosarcoma, or osteosarcoma).
- Clinically, they present with uterine bleeding, which is usually postmenopausal.
- They are highly malignant neoplasms that tend to metastasize early. The overall 5 year-survival rate is about 20%.

4. ENDOMETRIAL STROMAL NEOPLASMS

Benign Stromal Nodule
This is a small nodular collection of stromal cells. The nodule is well circumscribed. Microscopically, nodules are composed of well differentiated stromal cells with a very low mitotic rate.

Endolymphatic Stromal Myosis
This is a low grade stromal sarcoma. It is characterized by collections of well-differentiated stromal cells lying between myometrial bundles or penetrating lymphatic spaces.

- It has a low mitotic rate.
- It tends to spread outside the uterus, but to a very limited extent.
- It almost never metastasizes, but local recurrence is common after hysterectomy.

Stromal Sarcoma

This is a high grade malignant neoplasm. It is characterized by stromal cells which show marked cytologic atypia and a high mitotic rate (over 10 mitoses per 10 high-power fields).

- Grossly, it appears as a bulky, infiltrating, friable mass.
- Hematogenous metastases occur early.
- Clinically, presents with postmenopausal bleeding.
- The prognosis is poor.

NEOPLASMS OF THE MYOMETRIUM

1. LEIOMYOMA

Leiomyoma is a benign neoplasm of uterine smooth muscle. It is one of the most common neoplasms in females, being found in 1 of every 4 women in the reproductive years.

- Leiomyomas are responsible for 30% of gynecologic admissions to hospitals.
- They are most common between ages 20 and 40, and tend to stop growing actively or to regress after menopause.
- Growth appears to be dependent on estrogens and may be rapid during pregnancy.
- Leiomyomas may be solitary or multiple and may be located anywhere in the uterine smooth muscle.
- Grossly, leiomyomas are circumscribed, firm, grayish-white masses with a characteristic whorled appearance. They may reach a large size.
- Histologically, they are composed of a uniform proliferation of spindle-shaped smooth muscle cells.
- Degenerative changes occur frequently:
  - Red degeneration (necrobiosis) is typically seen during pregnancy, when the neoplasm undergoes necrosis and develops a beefy-red color.
  - Cystic degeneration.
  - Hyalinization, with broad bands of collagen appearing in the tumor, may be associated with marked cytologic atypia ("bizarre leiomyoma").
  - Calcification, sometimes extensive.
- Malignant change is very rare.
- Leiomyomas are a common cause of excessive uterine bleeding (menorrhagia) and an important cause of infertility. However, most patients are asymptomatic.

2. LEIOMYOSARCOMA

This is a rare uterine neoplasm, accounting for 3% of uterine malignant neoplasms. It is nonetheless the most common uterine sarcoma.

- Grossly, they appear as bulky, fleshy masses that show hemorrhage and necrosis.
- Microscopically, they are composed of a highly cellular mass of smooth muscle cells with marked cytologic atypia and a high mitotic rate (over 10 mitoses per 10 high-power fields).
- They are most common in older women, presenting as postmenopausal bleeding or a uterine mass.
- Local recurrence after hysterectomy and hematogenous metastases are frequent. The 5-year survival rate is about 40%.

THE UTERINE CERVIX

INFLAMMATORY CERVICAL LESIONS

1. ACUTE CERVICITIS
This is a common condition characterized by erythema, swelling, neutrophilic infiltration, and focal epithelial ulceration, commonly of the endocervix.

- Usually it is a sexually transmitted infection, commonly with gonococci, *Trichomonas vaginalis*, and herpes simplex (see Chapter 54).
- Non-sexually-transmitted agents such as *Escherichia coli* and staphylococci may also be isolated from acutely inflamed cervices, but their role is not clear.
- Clinically, there is a purulent vaginal discharge and pain. The severity of symptoms does not correlate well with the degree of inflammation.

2. CHRONIC CERVICITIS
Moderate numbers of lymphocytes, plasma cells, and histiocytes are present in the cervix in all females. Chronic cervicitis is therefore difficult to define pathologically. Clinically, chronic cervicitis is often an incidental finding. It may rarely produce a vaginal discharge, and in a few cases associated fibrosis of the endocervical canal may cause stenosis, leading to infertility.

NONNEOPLASTIC CERVICAL PROLIFERATIONS

1. SQUAMOUS METAPLASIA
Squamous metaplasia of the endocervical epithelium is common, probably representing a response to irritation.

2. MICROGLANDULAR HYPERPLASIA
Microglandular hyperplasia is an unusual proliferation of endocervical glands associated with the use of oral contraceptive agents.

- It presents grossly as a polypoid lesion that protrudes into the endocervical canal.
- Microscopically, it is characterized by an abnormal mass of endocervical glands lined by a flattened cuboidal epithelium.
- It has no clinical significance.

3. ENDOCERVICAL POLYP
Polyps are common lesions of the endocervical canal. When large, a polyp may protrude out of the external os. Microscopically, endocervical polyps contain hyperplastic endocervical glands and a highly vascular stroma and may show marked chronic inflammation. Endocervical polyps are benign, with no increased incidence of neoplasia.

NEOPLASMS OF THE CERVIX

1. CONDYLOMA ACUMINATUM
This is a common lesion of the cervix caused by the human papilloma virus, which is transmitted by sexual contact.

- It occurs in two forms:

- As a wartlike, papillomatous lesion that resembles condylomata in other sites.
- As elevated flat areas in the epithelium.

■ Flat condylomas, which are commonly caused by types 16 and 18 human papilloma virus, are frequently associated with epithelial dysplasia, and are believed to be precursor lesions for cervical carcinoma.

■ They are characterized by hyperplasia of the squamous epithelium with marked cytoplasmic vacuolation and nuclear chromatin condensation (koilocytosis).

■ Immunoperoxidase studies using antibodies against human papilloma virus are positive.

2. SQUAMOUS CARCINOMA

Cervical squamous carcinoma is common, causing 8000 deaths annually in the United States. It ranks sixth as a cause of cancer death in women.

Etiology

Evidence suggests that carcinoma of the cervix is caused by a sexually transmitted carcinogenic agent, probably viral (Table 53–3).

■ The risk of developing carcinoma increases with early onset of sexual activity, frequency of coitus, and greater number of sexual partners. (It is common in multiparous women who have married early and in prostitutes, but vanishingly rare in nuns).

■ Cervical carcinoma tends to affect the lower socioeconomic stratum of society.

■ Two viruses have been suspected of having an etiologic role in cancer of the cervix:
  - Herpes simplex virus type 2 (HSV-2), which is not believed to be a major etiologic factor.
  - Human papilloma virus, particularly serologic types 16 and 18, is presently considered to be an important etiologic agent.

Dysplasia of the Cervix (Fig 53–1)

Dysplasia and cervical intraepithelial neoplasia (CIN) are synonymous terms.

■ Most cervical carcinomas are preceded by squamous epithelial dysplasia.

■ Dysplasia commonly involves the region of the squamocolumnar junction and the endocervical canal that has undergone squamous metaplasia.

■ Dysplasia is recognized by:
  - The presence of cytologic abnormalities in a cervical (Pap) smear.
  - Histologic features in a cervical biopsy.

■ Dysplasia is graded (in order of increasing severity) as mild, moderate, or severe dysplasia and carcinoma in situ (Fig 53–1):
  - CIN I = mild dysplasia; CIN II = moderate dysplasia; and CIN III = all dysplasias more severe than moderate.

■ Dysplasias are reversible lesions, but the more severe the degree of dysplasia, the less the tendency to reverse.

■ Twenty-five percent of patients with carcinoma in situ develop invasive carcinoma within 5 years if left untreated.

■ The median time for carcinoma to develop is 7 years for mild dysplasia and 1 year for severe dysplasia.

■ Dysplasia and carcinoma in situ produce no symptoms.

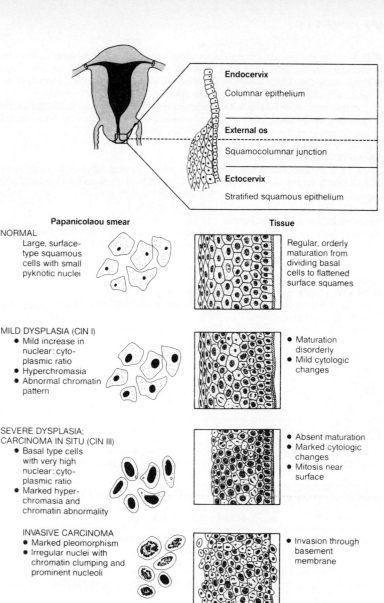

Endocervix
Columnar epithelium

External os
Squamocolumnar junction

Ectocervix
Stratified squamous epithelium

Papanicolaou smear		Tissue	

NORMAL
Large, surface-type squamous cells with small pyknotic nuclei

Regular, orderly maturation from dividing basal cells to flattened surface squames

MILD DYSPLASIA (CIN I)
- Mild increase in nuclear:cytoplasmic ratio
- Hyperchromasia
- Abnormal chromatin pattern

- Maturation disorderly
- Mild cytologic changes

SEVERE DYSPLASIA; CARCINOMA IN SITU (CIN III)
- Basal type cells with very high nuclear:cytoplasmic ratio
- Marked hyperchromasia and chromatin abnormality

- Absent maturation
- Marked cytologic changes
- Mitosis near surface

INVASIVE CARCINOMA
- Marked pleomorphism
- Irregular nuclei with chromatin clumping and prominent nucleoli

- Invasion through basement membrane

Figure 53–1. Squamous epithelial dysplasia and carcinoma of the cervix, showing criteria used to grade dysplasia. Dysplasia commonly occurs at the squamocolumnar junction.

- Changes in the mucosa on inspection are minimal, but changes such as abnormal vascular pattern, thickening, and white coloration, may be visible at colposcopy.
- Colposcopy and biopsy should be performed in all patients in whom dysplasia of any grade is found on routine cytologic examination.
- The treatment of dysplasia is local and conservative. Cryosurgery, electrocoagulation, laser coagulation, and conization—removal of a cone of cervical tissue, including the entire squamocolumnar junction—are all effective.

Microinvasive Carcinoma (Stage IA)

Stage 1A is defined as cervical carcinoma in which the total depth of invasion is less than 3 mm from the basement membrane (Table 53–4). It is rarely associated with metastases, and local surgical excision is curative.

Invasive Squamous Carcinoma

This is defined as carcinoma infiltrating a depth of greater than 3 mm from the basement membrane. It occurs most frequently in the age group from 30 to 50 years.

- Grossly, it may present as an exophytic, fungating, necrotic mass, as a malignant ulcer, or as a diffusely infiltrative lesion with minimal surface ulceration.
- Microscopically, there are three different types:
  - Large cell, nonkeratinizing squamous carcinoma—the most common type, with the best prognosis.
  - Keratinizing squamous carcinoma—next most common, with an intermediate prognosis.

TABLE 53–4. CLINICAL STAGING OF CERVICAL CARCINOMA[1,2]

Stage 0:	Carcinoma in situ (100%)
Stage 1A:	Microinvasive carcinoma; invasion to a depth less than 3 mm from the basement membrane (> 95%)
Stage 1B:	Invasive carcinoma, infiltrating to a depth greater than 3 mm but confined to the cervix (90%)
Stage II:	Extension of tumor beyond the cervix to involve the endometrium, vagina (but not the lower third), or paracervical soft tissue (but has not extended to the pelvic side wall) (75%)
Stage III:	Extension to the pelvic side wall or involvement of the lower third of the vagina or the presence of hydronephrosis from ureteral involvement (35%)
Stage IV:	Extension beyond the pelvis or clinical involvement of bladder or rectal mucosa (10%)

[1] Adapted from American Joint Committee for Cancer Staging and End-Results Reporting; Task Force on Gynecologic Sites: Staging System for Cancer at Gynecologic Sites, 1979.
[2] Figures in parentheses represent 5-year survival rates for the stage.

- Small cell undifferentiated (neuroendocrine) carcinoma-rare, with a poor prognosis.
- Clinically, it is manifested as abnormal uterine bleeding or vaginal discharge.
- Obstruction of the cervical canal may cause blood to accumulate in the uterine cavity and result in infection (pyometron).
- Diagnosis is by direct visualization and biopsy.
- Cervical carcinoma is staged according to the degree of spread (Table 53–4).
- Treatment is a combination of surgery and radiation therapy, depending on the extent of disease.
- Prognosis depends primarily on the clinical stage of the disease (Table 53–4).

3. ENDOCERVICAL ADENOCARCINOMA
Endocervical adenocarcinoma accounts for 10–15% of cervical cancers. It arises in the endocervical glands, presenting as a mass in the endocervical canal.

- It frequently obstructs the endocervical canal, predisposing to pyometron.
- Microscopically, it is usually a well-differentiated adenocarcinoma, often with a papillary appearance.
- Prognosis is less favorable than that of squamous carcinoma.

THE VAGINA

INFLAMMATORY VAGINAL LESIONS

1. ACUTE VAGINITIS (Non-Sexually-Transmitted)
Acute vaginitis is rare during the reproductive years. It may be caused by *Gardnerella (Haemophilus) vaginalis*, *Trichomonas vaginalis*, and *Candida albicans*.

- Atrophic vaginitis is a specific form of acute inflammation that occurs in postmenopausal women due to estrogen withdrawal.
- It presents clinically with vaginal discomfort and discharge.
- Diagnosis may be established by examination of a smear and culture.

TUMORS (MASS LESIONS) OF THE VAGINA

1. GARTNER'S DUCT CYST
These cysts are derived from vestigial remnants of the mesonephric ducts. They occur in the anterolateral wall of the vagina and are lined by cuboidal or columnar epithelium.

2. VAGINAL ADENOSIS
Vaginal adenosis is the occurrence of endocervical type glands in the vaginal wall in women. It occurs mainly in women whose mothers received diethylstilbestrol (DES) during pregnancy. In most cases, there is no visible lesion, and the condition is of little significance clinically except for its yet uncertain relationship to clear cell adenocarcinoma of the vagina.

3. SQUAMOUS CARCINOMA

Squamous carcinoma is the most common vaginal neoplasm. It is rare, and accounts for only 1–2% of cancers in the female genital tract.

- Grossly, it presents as a polypoid, fungating, exophytic mass or as an ulcerative, infiltrative tumor.
- Microscopically, it is usually a well-differentiated squamous carcinoma with keratinization.
- Local extension beyond the vagina occurs early.
- Lymphatic spread occurs early. Tumors in the lower third tend to involve inguinal nodes.
- Vaginal carcinoma is staged according to its degree of spread (Table 53–5).
- Treatment is by a combination of surgery and radiation therapy.
- The overall prognosis is poor, with a 5-year survival rate of 30–40%.

4. CLEAR CELL ADENOCARCINOMA

Clear cell adenocarcinoma of the vagina is rare, accounting for about 0.1–0.2% of cancers in the female genital tract. It occurs in young females, usually between ages 10 and 35. It is associated with exposure of the mother to diethylstilbestrol (DES) during pregnancy.

- Grossly, appears as a polypoid mass.
- Microscopically, it is composed of clear cells arranged in a tubuloglandular pattern. The neoplastic cells have a "hobnail" appearance.
- Treatment is with surgery and radiation.

5. EMBRYONAL RHABDOMYOSARCOMA (Sarcoma Botryoides)

Embryonal rhabdomyosarcoma is the commonest sarcoma of the vagina. It occurs in the first 5 years of life.

- Grossly appears as a large, lobulated tumor mass that frequently protrudes at the vaginal orifice.
- Microscopically, it is an anaplastic embryonal rhabdomyosarcoma.
- It is a highly malignant neoplasm with early hematogenous dissemination.
- Prognosis is poor, though recent chemotherapy regimens have improved the outlook.

TABLE 53–5. CLINICAL STAGING OF VAGINAL CARCINOMA

Stage 0:	Carcinoma in situ (intraepithelial neoplasia)
Stage I:	Carcinoma limited to vaginal wall
Stage II:	Involvement of subvaginal tissues without extension to the pelvic side walls
Stage III:	Extension to one or both pelvic side walls
Stage IV:	Involvement of mucosa of bladder or rectum (stage IVA) or extension beyond the true pelvis (stage IVB)

THE VULVA

INFLAMMATORY VULVAL LESIONS
Inflammatory lesions of the vulva are similar to those occurring in the skin.

- The sexually transmitted diseases may produce lesions in the vulva (Chapter 54).
- Acute bartholinitis:
  - Is a common lesion, frequently complicated by abscess formation.
  - *Staphylococcus aureus, Streptococcus pyogenes, Neisseria gonorrhoeae,* and *Escherichia coli* are the common organisms.
  - Presents as a painful, tender, erythematous swelling in the inferior part of the labium majus.
  - Treatment with surgical drainage and appropriate antibiotics is effective.

VULVAL DYSTROPHIES

1. LICHEN SCLEROSUS (Kraurosis Vulvae)
Lichen sclerosus is a chronic, progressive disease of unknown cause usually occurring in postmenopausal women.

- It is characterized by scaly and pruritic white plaques.
- Sclerosis and shrinkage of the dermis causes the vulva to be smooth, glazed, and parchmentlike.
- Microscopically, it is characterized by thinning of the epidermis, with hyperkeratosis and basal layer degeneration. A band of dense hyaline collagen is present in the upper dermis.
- It is not premalignant.

2. HYPERPLASTIC DYSTROPHY
Hyperplastic dystrophy is a common lesion occurring mainly in postmenopausal women.

- Clinically, it appears as leukoplakia.
- Microscopically, there is hyperplasia of the epidermis, with hyperkeratosis and chronic dermal inflammation.
- In some cases, dysplasia is present.
- Hyperplastic dystrophy is a premalignant lesion, the risk being proportionate to the degree of dysplasia.

NEOPLASMS OF THE VULVA

- Condyloma acuminatum is a common benign, verrucous lesion caused by the sexually transmitted papilloma virus.
- Adnexal skin tumors occur commonly in the vulva. The most common of these is hidradenoma papilliferum.
- Melanocytic lesions of all types occur in the vulva. Most frequently, these are benign compound nevi. Vulval malignant melanoma is rare.

1. SQUAMOUS CARCINOMA IN SITU (Bowen's Disease)

Squamous carcinoma in situ of the vulva (vulvar intraepithelial neoplasia, grade III) occurs both in hyperplastic dystrophy and de novo.

- It presents clinically as leukoplakia, indistinguishable from hyperplastic dystrophy.
- In cases without preceding vulval dystrophy, it appears as a slightly elevated, red-brown plaque.
- It may be associated with carcinoma in situ in the cervix and vagina, suggesting a common etiologic agent.
- Microscopically, it is characterized by absence of normal maturation and cytologic features of dysplasia. Invasion of the basement membrane is absent.
- Carcinoma in situ of the vulva carries a high risk of squamous carcinoma, but the latent period may vary from 1 to 10 years.
- Treatment of carcinoma in situ of the vulva is complete surgical excision of the involved area.

2. INVASIVE SQUAMOUS CARCINOMA

This is the commonest malignant neoplasm of the vulva. It accounts for only 4% of female genital tract cancers, usually occurring in women over age 60.

- The cause is unknown; human papilloma virus infection may be involved.
- Grossly, the early lesion is an indurated plaque, progressing to a firm nodule that ulcerates.
- Microscopically, squamous carcinoma of the vulva is usually well differentiated.
- Lymphatic spread to inguinal and pelvic nodes occurs early, with bilateral involvement being common. About 60% of patients have involved nodes at the time of diagnosis.

TABLE 53–6. CLINICAL STAGING OF VULVAR CARCINOMA[1]

Stage 0:	Carcinoma in situ (100%)
Stage I:	Lesion less than 2 cm in diameter and confined to vulva, with no suspicious groin nodes (80%)
Stage II:	Lesion greater than 2 cm in diameter and confined to vulva, with no suspicious groin nodes (70%)
Stage III:	Lesion of any size with extension beyond vulva to involve urethra, vagina, perineum, and anus without suspicious groin nodes, or lesion confined to vulva with suspicious or positive groin nodes (40%)
Stage IV:	Extension beyond vulva with positive groin nodes, or involvement of mucosa of rectum, bladder, or upper urethra, or distant metastases (20%)

[1] Figures in parentheses represent 5-year survival rates for the stage.

- Hematogenous dissemination occurs in advanced disease.
- The clinical stage of the disease (Table 53–6) correlates well with prognosis.

3. VERRUCOUS CARCINOMA

Verrucous carcinoma is a variant of well-differentiated squamous carcinoma, characterized by a polypoid growth pattern with little infiltrative tendency. They tend to remain localized and are cured by wide excision. They are resistant to radiation therapy, which may induce aggressive behavior.

4. EXTRAMAMMARY PAGET'S DISEASE

The vulva is the most common site for extramammary Paget's disease.

- Clinically, it presents as an eczemalike red, crusted lesion in the labia majora, usually in elderly women.
- Microscopically, large anaplastic tumor cells are present singly or in small groups in the epidermis.
- Thirty percent of cases have an associated underlying carcinoma in vulval glands.
- Prognosis is poor if it is associated with an underlying invasive cancer.

Sexually Transmitted Infections

54

GONORRHEA

Gonorrhea is one of the most common sexually transmitted diseases, with a reported incidence of over 300 per 100,000 population in the United States. Approximately 1% of the US population (ie, 2–3 million persons) have had gonorrhea.

Pathology

It is caused by the gram-negative diplococcus, *Neisseria gonorrhoeae.*

- In the male, the organism infects chiefly the urethra, producing acute urethritis.
- In the female, the cervix is the main site of infection.
- Infection occurs also at other sites in the genital tract:
  - In men, the prostate, seminal vesicles, and epididymides are commonly involved.
  - In women, the urethra, Bartholin's and Skene's glands, and the uterine tubes are commonly involved.
- With varied sexual practices, gonococcal pharyngitis and anal gonorrhea may occur. Gonococcal proctitis is common in male homosexuals.
- Entry of gonococci into the pelvic peritoneum in the female via the uterine tubes may cause peritonitis.
- Entry of gonococci into the bloodstream may cause:
  - Gonococcal bacteremia, with fever and a skin rash.
  - Gonococcal endocarditis, which tends to affect both the right- and left-sided valves of the heart.
  - Gonococcal arthritis, frequently monarticular, affecting large joints, most commonly the knee joint.
- Gonococcal infection of the fetus by an infected birth canal during delivery produces neonatal ophthalmitis, which may cause blindness.

Clinical Features & Diagnosis

- In men, the common presentation is with dysuria and purulent urethral discharge.
- In women, cervicitis may produce a vaginal discharge.
- Systemic symptoms are usually absent.
- In both sexes, gonorrhea may be asymptomatic, constituting a source of apparently healthy carriers.
- The risk of infection during a single act of intercourse with an infected partner is estimated to be 10–20%.

TABLE 54–1. MAJOR SEXUALLY TRANSMITTED DISEASES

Disease	Clinical Features	Organism
Gonorrhea	Urethritis, cervicitis, pelvic inflammatory disease, prostatitis, epididymitis, arthritis	*Neisseria gonorrhoeae*
Syphilis Primary syphilis	Chancre	*Treponema pallidum*
Secondary syphilis	Fever, lymph node enlargement, skin rashes, mucosal patches and ulcers, condyloma latum	
Tertiary syphilis	Gumma, tabes dorsalis, general paresis (dementia paralytica), aortitis	
Congenital syphilis	See text	
Herpes genitalis	Penile, vulvular, or cervical ulcers	Herpes simplex type 2
Chancroid	Soft chancres, lymphadenopathy	*Haemophilus ducreyi*
Chlamydial urethritis/cervicitis	Conjunctivitis, Reiter's syndrome, pelvic inflammatory disease	*Chlamydia trachomatis* (D–K)
Lymphogranuloma venereum	Ulcers, lymphadenopathy, rectal strictures	*C trachomatis* (L1–L3)
Granuloma inguinale	Ulcerating nodules, lymphadenopathy	*Calymmatobacterium donovani*
Trichomonas vaginitis	Vaginitis	*Trichomonas vaginalis*
Acquired immune deficiency syndrome (AIDS)	Opportunistic infections, Kaposi's sarcoma, lymphoma	Human immunodeficiency virus (see Chapter 7)
Condyloma acuminatum	Cervical cancer	Human papilloma virus
Viral B hepatitis	(See Chapter 42)	Hepatitis B virus

- Diagnosis is made by direct smear of the urethral or vaginal discharge. Gram staining reveals gram-negative diplococci.
- The diagnosis should be confirmed by culture, because *Neisseria* species other than gonococci may be present as commensals in the vagina.
- The gonococcus is sensitive to penicillin in most cases.
- Spectinomycin and trimethoprim-sulfamethoxazole are used against penicillin-resistant strains.

SYPHILIS

Syphilis is caused by *Treponema pallidum*, a spirochete. While the incidence of syphilis has increased, the incidence of late syphilis has declined because of effective antibiotic treatment of early disease.

- It is probable that there are about 1 million active cases of syphilis in the United States.
- The common age for contracting syphilis is shifting from the mid 20s to the teen years.
- There has been a recent increase in the incidence of syphilis among individuals that are at high risk for developing AIDS (male homosexuals, intravenous drug users).
- Routine testing of transfused blood and pregnant women for syphilis has resulted in a decline of transfusion syphilis and congenital syphilis, respectively.

1. PRIMARY SYPHILIS

The incubation period after infection is 9–90 days.

- The first visible lesion is termed the **primary chancre,** which appears at the site of initial invasion—usually the penis (glans or shaft) in the male and the vulva in the female.
- Other sites for primary chancre include the cervix, scrotum, anus, rectum, and oral cavity.
- The primary chancre is a painless, punched-out ulcer with an indurated base consisting of chronic inflammatory tissue.
- Its surface exudes a serous fluid containing large numbers of treponemes.
- Painless enlargement of the inguinal lymph nodes may be present, but there are no systemic symptoms and the patient feels well.
- The diagnosis is best made at this stage by identifying spirochetes in the serous exudate from the chancre by dark-field microscopy.
- Serologic tests for syphilis may be negative in the early primary stage (Table 54–2), and the organism cannot be cultured.
- The primary chancre heals spontaneously in 3–6 weeks.

2. SECONDARY SYPHILIS

Secondary syphilis usually follows the primary stage after 2–20 weeks, but may begin before the primary chancre heals.

TABLE 54–2. SYPHILIS SEROLOGY[1]

Test	Percent Serum Positivity by Stage of Disease			Neurosyphilis	
	Primary	Secondary	Late Tertiary	Serum	CSF
VDRL (reagin)	70%	99%	<5%	50%	60%
FTA-ABS	85%	100%	98%	95%	80%[2]

[1]Congenital syphilis is difficult to diagnose because maternal IgG antibodies cross the placenta; the fetus will give positive serology whether infected or not. An IgM FTA-ABS test, measuring only fetal IgM, has been developed; however, its use is not fully accepted.

[2]FTA-ABS test should not be used alone because it yields up to 5% of technical false-positives in cerebrospinal fluid.

- It is characterized by:
  - Fever.
  - Generalized lymph node enlargement.
  - A red, maculopapular skin rash.
  - Orogenital mucosal lesions such as mucous membrane patches, irregular ("snail track") ulcers in the mouth, and plaquelike lesions in the perineum (condylomata lata).
  - Hepatitis, meningitis, nephritis (immune complex type), and osteochondritis may also occur.
- Microscopically, these lesions are characterized by a nonspecific inflammatory response with numerous plasma cells.
- Spirochetes are present in large numbers and can be demonstrated in tissue sections with silver stains.
- Diagnosis is by demonstration of the organism in smears made from lesions and examined by dark-field microscopy.
- Serologic tests are positive (Table 54–2).

3. TERTIARY OR LATE SYPHILIS

Manifestations of late syphilis appear any time after 4 years following primary infection. Even without treatment, only 30% of cases of early syphilis ever develop tertiary syphilis. Tertiary syphilis takes one of three forms: gumma, aortitis, or neurosyphilis.

- **Gumma:**
  - Is a localized destructive granuloma.
  - Is most common in the liver, bones, oral cavity, and testes.
  - Grossly, produces a large mass that may be mistaken for a neoplasm.
  - Microscopically, a gumma is an epithelioid granuloma with central gummatous necrosis. Spirochetes cannot usually be demonstrated.
- **Syphilitic aortitis** (see Chapter 20) leads to the development of aneurysms in the ascending thoracic aorta, aortic valve incompetence, and myocardial ischemia.
- **Neurosyphilis** (see Chapter 63) is manifested as chronic meningovascular inflammation, tabes dorsalis, or general paresis. Organisms are not demonstrable except in general paresis.

CONGENITAL SYPHILIS

Transplacental infection of the fetus occurs if the mother has untreated early (first 4 years) syphilis.

- Routine serologic testing and treatment of women in early pregnancy prevents congenital syphilis, which now occurs only when prenatal care is deficient.
- Intrauterine infection causes disease of varying degree:
  - Abortion and intrauterine death of the fetus.
  - Neonatal or infantile congenital syphilis, characterized by skin rashes, ulcerating patches on mucous membranes, osteochondritis and perichondritis (causing nasal bridge collapse (saddle nose), and tibial deformity (sabre shins).
  - Late childhood congenital syphilis, characterized by interstitial keratitis (causing blindness), nerve deafness, and abnormalities in permanent teeth (Hutchinson's teeth, Moon's molars).
- Diagnosis of congenital syphilis is based on clinical manifestations, dark-field microscopy, and serologic tests (Table 54–2).

HERPES GENITALIS

Infection with herpes simplex virus type 2 is currently at epidemic level (500,000 cases per year in the USA for a total of more than 5 million infected).

- Herpes simplex virus causes painful shallow ulcers on the penis, vulva, and cervix.
- The ulcers heal spontaneously, but the virus remains latent in lumbar and sacral ganglia and may cause lifelong recurrent infections.
- Active herpes genitalis in a pregnant woman is an absolute indication for cesarian section because of the risk of fetal infection during vaginal delivery.

CHANCROID

Chancroid is an uncommon sexually transmitted disease caused by *Haemophilus ducreyi*, a gram-negative bacillus.

- Clinically, it is characterized by the development of one or more painful, shallow, necrotic ulcers (soft chancres) at the site of inoculation on the external genitalia.
- Regional lymph nodes are enlarged and tender and show suppurative acute inflammation.
- Systemic symptoms are mild.
- Diagnosis is established by culture from either an ulcer or a lymph node aspirate.
- Treatment with antibiotics (tetracycline, trimethoprim-sulfamethoxazole) is effective.

CHLAMYDIAL URETHRITIS & CERVICITIS

Chlamydia trachomatis serotypes D–K are increasingly being recognized as a cause of sexually transmitted disease. In some studies, chlamydial infection ranks as the commonest sexually transmitted disease in the United States.

- It causes urethritis and cervicitis that clinically resembles gonorrhea. In male homosexuals, chlamydial proctitis is common.
- Because bacterial cultures are negative, this infection was called **nonspecific or nongonococcal urethritis.**
- Reiter's syndrome—conjunctivitis, arthritis, skin lesions, and urethritis—may complicate chlamydial infection in men.
- Diagnosis may be made by culturing the organism in living cell culture media or by demonstration of intracytoplasmic inclusions in smears from lesions.
- Chlamydial infections respond to treatment with tetracyclines.

LYMPHOGRANULOMA VENEREUM

Lymphogranuloma venereum (LGV) is an uncommon sexually transmitted disease caused by *Chlamydia trachomatis* L1–L3 (LGV serotype).

- The acute phase is characterized by an ulcerative lesion at the site of entry.
- Enlarged, tender, fluctuant regional lymph nodes develop 1–2 weeks later.
- Microscopically, the nodes show distinctive stellate granulomas containing central suppuration.
- Chronic LGV is characterized by extensive fibrosis, which extends into pelvic soft tissues causing:
  - Rectal strictures.

- Extensive lymphatic obstruction, leading to chronic lymphedema ("elephantiasis") of the vulva and penis.
- Diagnosis is made by a combination of clinical, histologic, and serologic findings.

GRANULOMA INGUINALE

Granuloma inguinale is a rare sexually transmitted disease caused by *Calymmatobacterium donovani*, a small gram-negative coccobacillus.

- The lesion at the site of inoculation begins as a papule that slowly enlarges, ulcerates, and spreads, resulting in a nodular mass with extensive scarring and regional lymph node involvement.
- Intracellular organisms may be identified with some difficulty in the involved lymph nodes using Giemsa's stain or silver stains.
- Diagnosis is based on the clinical presentation and may be confirmed by demonstrating Donovan bodies in smears or biopsies of the lesions.
- Culture is possible but difficult.
- Treatment with antibiotics (eg, tetracycline, erythromycin) is effective.

Diseases of Pregnancy; Trophoblastic Neoplasms

55

ECTOPIC PREGNANCY

TUBAL PREGNANCY
Tubal pregnancy is common, representing about 0.3–0.5% of all pregnancies.

- Common etiologic factors are:
  - Pelvic inflammatory disease
  - Endometriosis involving the uterine tube.
- In many cases of tubal pregnancy, however, no etiologic factor is identified.

Pathology
In spite of the abnormal implantation site, the ovum develops normally in the first few weeks, forming a placenta, an embryo, and an amniotic sac.

- Rupture of the tube containing the pregnancy frequently occurs 2–6 weeks after fertilization, causing massive, potentially fatal intraperitoneal hemorrhage.
- In most cases, the released embryo dies soon after tubal rupture.
- When rupture of a tubal pregnancy releases a live embryo into the peritoneal cavity, it can move to a secondary implantation site on the peritoneal surface (secondary abdominal pregnancy).
- If the tubal pregnancy does not rupture, death of the embryo occurs at about 10 weeks, with one of several consequences:
  - Absorption of the products of conception.
  - Calcification of the fetus to form a lithopedion.
  - Extrusion of the dead fetus into the peritoneum through the fimbrial end of the tube—again associated with severe intraperitoneal hemorrhage.

Clinical Features
Patients with tubal pregnancy present with evidence of early pregnancy (missed menstrual period, vomiting, or a positive pregnancy test). On examination, there is absence of appropriate uterine enlargement and the presence of a tender mass in the adnexa.

- Rupture of a tubal pregnancy produces severe abdominal pain and intraperitoneal bleeding, often rapid and severe.
- Many patients are in a state of hypovolemic shock at the time of presentation.
- Death of the fetus in a tubal pregnancy results in rapid decline in the serum level of chorionic gonadotropin, leading to a negative pregnancy test.
- Decline in hCG levels causes the corpus luteum to degenerate. This leads to de-

creased estrogen and progesterone levels, which causes the endometrium to break down. Uterine bleeding results.
■ Diagnosis of tubal pregnancy is established by clinical examination.

Treatment
The diagnosis and treatment of tubal pregnancy is urgent.

■ Treatment is surgical and may consist of:
  ● Removal of the tube (salpingectomy).
  ● Salpingostomy and removal of the products of conception from the tube. This preserves fertility, particularly if bilateral tubal disease is present.

SPONTANEOUS ABORTION
Delivery of the embryo or fetus before 20 weeks is termed *abortion*.

■ Spontaneous abortion is common, and the causes are many (Table 55–1).
■ It has been estimated that 25% of fertilized ova abort, many so early that the pregnancy is never recognized.
■ It is characterized clinically by:
  ● Vaginal bleeding, which may be rapid and severe, leading to hypovolemia and shock.
  ● Lower abdominal pain due to uterine contraction.
  ● The pregnancy test becomes negative.

TABLE 55–1. CAUSES OF SPONTANEOUS ABORTION

Ovular/fetal
  Failure to implant
  Lethal chromosomal defects
  Hydatidiform mole

Maternal/uterine
  Uterine abnormalities, eg, leiomyoma, septate uterus
  Ectopic pregnancy
  Incompetent cervix
  Endocrine abnormalities: failure of the corpus luteum, daibetes, hypertension, hyperthyroidism, hypothryoidism
  Various systemic diseases, including renal failure, hypertension, malnutrition, severe anemia
  Infections: toxoplasmosis, rubella, *Chlamydia*, cytomegalovirus, herpes simplex virus, syphilis, brucellosis
  Drugs and chemicals: lead poisoning, thalidomide, anticoagulants
  Chemotherapy for cancer in the mother

Physical agents
  Severe maternal trauma and shock
  Irradiation
  Electric shock: lightning

- It is not uncommon for products of conception to be retained in the uterus (incomplete abortion). This may cause continued irregular bleeding.
- Most patients with spontaneous abortion require surgical evacuation of the uterus (dilatation and curettage).

PLACENTAL ABNORMALITIES

PLACENTA PREVIA
The fertilized ovum normally implants in the fundus, and the placenta forms in that location. Placenta previa is an abnormally low implantation of the placenta such that part of it is over the internal os.

- Placenta previa causes severe antepartum hemorrhage at the onset of labor when there is effacement of the cervix, leading to premature separation of the placenta.
- Diagnosis is by placental localization by ultrasonography.
- Treatment is elective cesarian section before the onset of labor.

ABRUPTIO PLACENTAE
Abruptio placentae is premature separation of a normally situated placenta after 20 weeks of gestation, leading to antepartum hemorrhage.

- In 20% of cases, blood is retained in the placental bed as concealed hemorrhage.
- In the remainder, severe bleeding occurs vaginally due to opening of the retroplacental hematoma into the cervical os (revealed hemorrhage).
- In both instances, there may be:
  - Extensive blood loss resulting in shock.
  - Disseminated intravascular coagulation.
  - Fetal death and premature labor.

PLACENTA ACCRETA
The normal placental villi are separated from the myometrium by a decidual plate, which is the plane of separation of the placenta in the third stage of labor. Placenta accreta is absence of a plane of separation between the placental villi and myometrium.

- The placenta fails to separate in labor, leading to severe postpartum hemorrhage.
- Placenta increta and percreta are increasingly more severe degrees of this abnormality in which the villi actually penetrate the myometrium.
- In this group of placental abnormalities, hysterectomy is frequently necessary to arrest postpartum bleeding.

PLACENTAL INFECTION
Infection of the fetal membranes (chorioamnionitis) represents ascending infection from the vagina and cervix. *Escherichia coli,* β-hemolytic streptococci, and anaerobes are the usual organisms.

- Rupture of the membranes not followed by delivery of the fetus within 24–48 hours almost always leads to chorioamnionitis.
- Maternal hematogenous infections involving the placenta include syphilis, tuber-

culosis, cytomegalovirus infection, toxoplasmosis, listeriosis, rubella, and herpes simplex.
- These organisms cause focal abscesses, granulomas, and necrosis of the placenta.

AMNIOTIC FLUID EMBOLISM

Amniotic fluid and debris may gain entry to uterine veins at the time of placental separation in labor. Though amniotic fluid embolism is rare, it accounts for a significant percentage of maternal deaths in developed countries, where maternal mortality rates are very low.

- Predisposing factors include premature placental separation and a dead fetus.
- Amniotic debris, which consists mainly of fetal squames, may be found in the lungs.
- Diagnosis is by the identification of squamous epithelial cells in pulmonary capillaries at autopsy.
- The amniotic fluid contains thromboplastic substances that cause disseminated intravascular coagulation, which is responsible for the main clinical features.

RUPTURE OF THE UTERUS

A normal uterus in normal labor "never" ruptures.

- Factors that predispose to rupture during labor are:
  - Uterine leiomyomas.
  - Placenta increta or percreta.
  - The presence of a fibrous scar from a previous cesarian section.
  - Prolonged labor due to malposition (eg, breech presentation).
  - Instrumentation (eg, forceps delivery).
  - Extensive uterine stimulants (oxytocin, prostaglandins, ergot infusions).
- Uterine rupture not associated with labor may be associated with choriocarcinoma, invasive hydatidiform mole, or endometrial carcinoma.

PREECLAMPSIA-ECLAMPSIA

Preeclampsia is a syndrome consisting of:

- Hypertension.
- Proteinuria (albuminuria).
- Generalized edema.
- The term *gestational edema with proteinuria and hypertension* (GEPH) is used synonymously with preeclampsia.

Incidence

Preeclampsia complicates about 5% of pregnancies in the United States.

- Ten percent of patients with preeclampsia develop seizure symptoms (eclampsia).
- Presentation is usually in the third trimester.
- Predisposing factors include:
  - Primigravida status. Two-thirds of cases of preeclampsia occur in first pregnancies.
  - Multiple pregnancies.

- Hydramnios (excess amniotic fluid).
- Preexisting diabetes or hypertension.
- Hydatidiform mole.
- Malnutrition and familial factors.

Etiology

The cause of preeclampsia-eclampsia is unknown.

■ Theories as to etiology include:
  - Placental ischemia.
  - Immunologic reaction against placental vessels.
  - Deficient production of prostaglandin E by the placenta, resulting in increased sensitivity to the hypertensive effects of renin and angiotensin.

Pathology

■ The placenta shows degeneration, hyaline deposition, calcification, and congestion (premature aging).
■ Placental infarcts may occur.
■ In eclampsia:
  - The maternal kidneys show features of cortical ischemia. Renal cortical necrosis may rarely occur.
  - The liver shows periportal necrosis and congestion.
  - Hemorrhages and edema may also occur in the brain, heart, lungs, and pituitary.

Clinical Findings

Edema is common in pregnancy and does not of itself warrant a diagnosis of preeclampsia.

■ Hypertension is the most critical feature.
■ Proteinuria is usually last to appear.
■ Fetal growth may be less than expected because of placental insufficiency (small-for-gestational age fetus).
■ Eclampsia is preceded by increasing hypertension. Individual twitchings of muscles are followed by generalized clonic contractions.

Treatment

Treatment is aimed at reducing the blood pressure and preventing eclampsia. Induction of labor or cesarian section when the fetus is judged sufficiently mature is dramatically effective.

TROPHOBLASTIC NEOPLASMS

HYDATIDIFORM MOLE

The incidence of hydatidiform mole varies greatly in different parts of the world. It occurs in 1 in every 2000 pregnancies in the United States, but has a much higher frequency (1:150) in India and the Far Eastern countries.

Etiology
It represents a benign neoplasm of trophoblastic tissue.

- Edematous (hydropic) villi are commonly associated with blighted or degenerated ova, but probably as an entity distinct from hydatidiform mole.
- Cytogenetic studies show that most have an XX karyotype, with both X chromosomes being derived from the male, suggesting an abnormal zygote.

Pathology

- The uterus is usually enlarged.
- The uterine cavity is filled with a mass of grapelike structures—thin-walled, translucent, cystic, and grayish-white.
- The weight of this evacuated mass is usually in excess of 200 g.
- In most cases, no normal fetal parts are identified.
- Microscopically, the cysts are composed of dilated chorionic villi with an avascular stroma and trophoblastic proliferation.
- Hydatidiform mole is associated with:
  - Greatly elevated levels of chorionic gonadotropin.
  - Multiple bilateral theca lutein cysts in the ovary, in about 30% of cases.

Clinical Features
The initial features are those of early pregnancy, including amenorrhea, vomiting of pregnancy—often severe—and a positive pregnancy test.

- Uterine enlargement is usually greater than in the case of normal pregnancy.
- Vaginal bleeding usually begins in the third to fourth month.
- Ultrasound examination is usually diagnostic, showing the enlarged, multicystic placenta and the absence of a fetus.
- Treated by evacuation of the mole from the uterine cavity by curettage.
- After evacuation, the serum βHCG level falls rapidly to normal; failure to do so indicates residual mole.

Complications
About 2.5% of molar pregnancies lead to subsequent choriocarcinoma. The most precise method of detecting cancer after molar pregnancy is by follow-up determination of serum βHCG.

CHORIOADENOMA DESTRUENS (Invasive Mole)
Chorioadenoma destruens is a hydatidiform mole that shows extensive penetration of the villi and trophoblast into the myometrium.

- Extension often reaches the serosal surface.
- Spontaneous uterine rupture may occur.
- Villi may embolize to distant sites—commonly the lungs—but regress spontaneously.
- Invasive mole is associated with persistent elevation of βHCG levels after evacuation of the uterine cavity.

- Without treatment, the mortality rate from hemorrhage or uterine rupture is about 10%.
- Treatment with chemotherapy is effective.

GESTATIONAL CHORIOCARCINOMA

Gestational choriocarcinoma of the uterus is rare, complicating about one in 40,000 pregnancies. About half follow a hydatidiform mole; others occur after abortion (25%), normal pregnancy (23%), or ectopic pregnancy (2%). It has a relatively high incidence in some parts of Asia and Africa.

Pathology

- Grossly, it appears as a friable hemorrhagic mass in the uterine cavity.
- It infiltrates the myometrium extensively, and vascular invasion occurs early, with widespread metastases in lungs, brain, liver, and bone marrow.
- Microscopically, it is composed of cytologically malignant sheets of cytotrophoblastic and syncytiotrophoblastic cells associated with necrosis and hemorrhage.
- Formed chorionic villi are absent.
- βHCG can often be demonstrated in the tumor cells.

Clinical Features & Treatment

- They present with abnormal uterine bleeding, commonly occurring within a few months after normal pregnancy, abortion, or hydatidiform mole.
- Many patients have metastatic lesions at the time of diagnosis.
- Serum βHCG is markedly elevated.
- Diagnosis is made by histologic examination of a biopsy specimen, which shows malignant trophoblastic cells.
- Prognosis has markedly improved with aggressive combined chemotherapy. The 5-year survival rate has improved to over 50%, even in patients with widespread metastases at presentation.
- Serum βHCG levels are extremely useful in monitoring treatment.

PLACENTAL SITE TROPHOBLASTIC TUMOR (PSTT)

This is a rare lesion characterized by the diffuse proliferation in the uterus of sheets of intermediate trophoblastic cells. It occurs most commonly after abortion or normal pregnancy.

- The neoplastic cells contain human placental lactogen, demonstrable by immunoperoxidase techniques.
- Unlike choriocarcinoma, PSTT shows only a slight elevation of βHCG and no syncytiotrophoblastic cells.
- The biologic behavior of PSTT is usually benign. Most cases are cured by curettage.
- A few cases have demonstrated a more aggressive biologic behavior, and rare cases with metastases have been reported.

The Breast

56

MANIFESTATIONS OF BREAST DISEASE

Breast Mass
A mass in the breast is the earliest manifestation of breast carcinoma and therefore the most important symptom of breast disease.

Nipple Discharge
This is a common symptom of a variety of breast diseases.

- Discharge of milk occurs in pregnancy and lactation and rarely at other times (galactorrhea).
- Nonhemorrhagic nipple discharge is a common symptom in breasts showing fibrocystic change.
- Bloody discharge occurs in fibrocystic change and intraductal neoplasms, most commonly intraductal papilloma and carcinoma.

Skin Changes
Skin changes over an advanced cancer include:

- Tethering and dimpling of the skin over the mass.
- Ulceration.
- Lymphedema with thickening and peau d'orange.
- Acute inflammation with erythema and pain (inflammatory carcinoma).
- Acute inflammatory signs may also be present overlying a breast abscess.
- Paget's disease of the nipple is an eczemalike appearance of the nipple and surrounding skin caused by intraepidermal spread of cancer cells.

Pain
Diffuse mild pain in the breast occurs commonly during the premenstrual phase in many women. Pain is rare in early breast carcinoma, but its presence in relation to a breast mass should not prevent the mass from being evaluated for carcinoma.

METHODS OF EVALUATING BREAST DISEASE

Physical Examination
Physical examination of a breast mass is useful in differentiating carcinoma from other causes only in advanced disease. Fixation of the mass to skin or to the chest wall, ulceration of the skin, nipple retraction, and lymphedema are late signs of breast carcinoma.

Mammography
Mammography is of value in identifying the presence of breast carcinoma before it is

palpable. It is extremely useful as a screening procedure for patients at high risk for breast carcinoma.

Biopsy
Microscopic examination of a sample of tissue is the definitive means of diagnosis of a breast mass. Tissue may be obtained by:

- Fine needle aspiration.
- Core needle biopsy.
- Incisional or excisional open biopsy.

CONGENITAL BREAST ANOMALIES
The commonest anomaly is the presence of a supernumerary breast or nipple along the milk line from the axilla to the groin. Absence of the breast is extremely rare. In ovarian dysgenesis (Turner's syndrome), the breasts remain rudimentary.

INFLAMMATORY BREAST LESIONS

ACUTE MASTITIS & BREAST ABSCESS
Acute inflammation of the breast, often with abscess formation, occurs commonly at the onset of lactation (puerperal mastitis).

- Cracks in the nipple and stasis of milk predispose to infection.
- *Staphylococcus aureus* is the most common infecting agent.
- Acute mastitis causes redness, swelling, pain, and tenderness in the affected area of the breast.
- Abscess formation is common and requires drainage of puss.

CHRONIC MASTITIS
This is uncommon. It usually occurs in perimenopausal women as a result of obstruction of the lactiferous ducts by inspissated luminal secretions.

- Obstruction leads to dilatation of the ducts (**mammary duct ectasia**) and periductal chronic inflammation.
- In most cases, the inflammatory cells are predominantly plasma cells (**plasma cell mastitis**).
- Rarely the inflammatory response includes numerous foamy histiocytes and fibrosis (**granulomatous mastitis**).
- Grossly, both plasma cell mastitis and granulomatous mastitis produce irregular masses with induration that closely mimics breast carcinoma.

FAT NECROSIS
This is an uncommon disease of unknown cause. Ischemia resulting from stretching and narrowing of arteries in pendulous breasts may be a factor.

- It is characterized by collection of neutrophils and histiocytes around the necrotic fat cells. Later, fibrosis and calcification occur.
- Grossly, fat necrosis appears as an ill-defined grayish-white nodular lesion that resembles carcinoma.

FIBROCYSTIC CHANGES

Incidence
This is a very common change of the female breast, affecting about 10% of women. Many of the same changes have been found at autopsy in up to 50% of women who had no symptoms of breast disease during life, suggesting that they may be physiologic variations rather than disease.

- The changes occur after puberty, reach a maximum during the late reproductive period, and persist into the postmenopausal period.
- Some of the histologic features observed in fibrocystic change indicate an increased risk of future breast carcinoma (Table 56–1).

Etiology
Fibrocystic changes are believed to result from response of the breast to cyclic changes in levels of female sex hormones, mainly estrogens. No constant endocrine abnormality has been identified. Oral contraceptives do not increase the incidence of fibrocystic changes.

Pathology (Table 56–1)
Changes not associated with an increased risk of breast carcinoma include:

- Fibrosis.
- Cyst formation.
- Inflammation, either acute or chronic.
- Mild ductal or lobular hyperplasia.

TABLE 56–1. RELATIVE RISK FOR INVASIVE BREAST CARCINOMA BASED ON PATHOLOGIC EXAMINATION OF BREAST TISSUE WITH FIBROCYSTIC CHANGES[1]

No increased risk
Adenosis, sclerosing or florid
Apocrine metaplasia
Cysts, macro- or micro- (or both)
Duct ectasia
Fibrosis
Hyperplasia, mild
Mastitis (inflammation)

Slightly increased risk (1½–2 times[2])
Hyperplasia, moderate or florid, solid or papillary

Moderately increased risk (4–5 times[2])
Atypical hyperplasia (borderline lesion)
    Ductal
    Lobular

[1] Modified from Consensus Meeting: Is "fibrocystic disease" of the breast precancerous? October 3–5, 1985, New York. *Arch Pathol Lab Med* 1986;110:171.
[2] Risk is expressed as the risk compared with the general female population.

- Sclerosing adenosis and microglandular adenosis.
- Apocrine metaplasia of the ductal epithelium.
- Changes associated with a slightly increased (2 times the general population) risk of carcinoma include ductal hyperplasia of the usual type, moderate to severe degree.
- Changes associated with a moderately increased (4–5 times the general population) risk of carcinoma are:
  - Atypical lobular hyperplasia.
  - Atypical ductal hyperplasia.

Clinical Features

Patients with fibrocystic changes may present with pain, nipple discharge, and an irregular "lumpy" consistency of the breast. Bilateral involvement is common. The occurrence of a breast mass that is suspicious for carcinoma needs aspiration or biopsy.

NEOPLASMS OF THE BREAST

Benign Neoplasms

FIBROADENOMA OF THE BREAST

This is a common benign neoplasm that occurs at all ages, with the highest incidence in young women. It presents as a discrete, firm, freely movable nodule in the breast.

- Multiple fibroadenomas occur in 10% of cases.
- Grossly, they are encapsulated, firm, and uniformly grayish-white.
- They are usually 1–5 cm in diameter but may be larger ("giant fibroadenoma").
- Histologic examination reveals proliferation of both gandular and stromal elements.
- Simple removal is curative.

LACTATING ADENOMA

Lactating adenoma is probably a fibroadenoma in which lactational changes have supervened. It may be associated with rapid increase in size during pregnancy, raising a suspicion of carcinoma.

INTRADUCTAL PAPILLOMA

Ductal papillomas are benign neoplasms, commonly originating in a major lactiferous duct near the nipple. They commonly present with a bloody nipple discharge.

- Most ductal papillomas are small—about 1 cm in diameter. The large tumors are palpable as a subareolar mass.
- Grossly, the tumor appears as a papillary mass projecting into the lumen of a large duct.
- Histologically, there are numerous delicate papillae composed of a fibrovascular core, covered by a layer of epithelial and myoepithelial cells.
- In complex papillomas, distinction from papillary carcinoma may be difficult.

GRANULAR CELL TUMOR

This is a rare, benign neoplasm of the breast, probably derived from neural Schwann cells. It presents clinically and on gross pathologic examination as a hard infiltrative mass that resembles breast cancer. Microscopic examination shows large cells with small nuclei and abundant granular cytoplasm.

Malignant Neoplasms

CARCINOMA OF THE BREAST

Incidence
There are more than 100,000 new cases of breast cancer every year in the United States, and 35,000 deaths. It has been estimated that 1 of every 10 women in the United States will develop breast carcinoma during her lifetime.

- It is second to lung cancer as a cause of cancer mortality in women.
- It is very common in North America and Western Europe but rare in Japan, where the incidence is about 20% that in the United States.
- It is rare before age 25 and uncommon before age 30. The incidence increases sharply after 30 years, with a mean and median age of 60 years.

Risk Factors
Statistically, the risk of breast cancer is increased in:

- Nulliparous women (nuns have a high incidence).
- Women who have early menarche and late menopause.
- Women who have their first pregnancy after age 30.
- Breastfeeding appears to have a protective effect.
- A few studies suggest a very slightly increased incidence in women who use oral contraceptives.
- The presence of moderate or severe ductal epithelial hyperplasia in a biopsy slightly increases the risk.
- The presence of atypical lobular and ductal hyperplasia in a breast biopsy increases the risk four- to five-fold.
- A positive family history of breast carcinoma (in a first-degree relative) increases the risk five-fold. The risk is greatest for relatives of premenopausal women with bilateral breast cancer.
- The increased risks resulting from atypical hyperplasia and family history are additive (ie, the presence of both increases the risk eight- to ten-fold).
- The occurrence of carcinoma in one breast increases the risk of carcinoma in the other breast about six-fold.

Etiology
The cause of breast carcinoma is unknown but is probably multifactorial.

- Genetic factors are suggested by:
  - The strong familial tendency.
  - A marker chromosome (1q+) has been reported.
  - Increased expression of the oncogene (*HER2/NEU*) has been detected in some cases.
- Hormones are widely believed to play a role in the etiology of breast cancer.
  - Estrogen has been the most studied, because of the epidemiologic evidence that

prolonged estrogen exposure (early menarche, late menopause, nulliparity, and delayed pregnancy) increases the risk of breast cancer.
- ● Prolactin may also be involved.
- ■ Viruses are also suspected of causing breast carcinoma. While this has been demonstrated to be important in animals, there is little evidence in humans.

Pathology

Based upon histologic criteria, several different types of breast carcinoma are recognized (Table 56–2).

  A. In situ (noninvasive) carcinoma.
    1. Lobular carcinoma in situ (LCIS):

TABLE 56–2. PATHOLOGIC TYPES OF BREAST CARCINOMA

Lobular carcinoma (10%)
  Lobular carcinoma in situ (LCIS)
    Does not produce a mass; often discovered incidentally in breast biopsies
    Multifocal, bilateral in 70%
    Long in situ phase
    High risk (10–12 fold) of breast carcinoma (either infiltrating ductal or lobular) in both ipsilateral and contralateral breast

  Invasive lobular carcinoma
    Approximately 10% of infiltrating breast carcinoma
    Differentiated from infiltrating ductal carcinoma by histologic features only
    More frequently bilateral than infiltrating ductal carcinoma
    More frequently estrogen receptor-positive than ductal carcinoma
    Prognosis similar to that of infiltrating ductal carcinoma

Ductal carcinoma (85%)
  Ductal carcinoma in situ (DCIS)
    Produces a breast mass or is detected by mammography
    Short in situ phase
    Multifocal, bilateral in 20%
    Type of carcinoma most often associated with Paget's disease of the nipple

Infiltrating ductal carcinoma (lacking other specific features)
    Diagnosis made by histologic features; invasion present

Histologic variants of breast carcinoma
  With a better prognosis than regular infiltrating ductal carcinoma
    Medullary carcinoma
    Tubular carcinoma
    Mucinous (colloid) carcinoma
    Papillary carcinoma
With a worse prognosis than regular infiltrating ductal carcinoma
    Inflammatory carcinoma (dermal lymphatic carcinomatosis)

Others (5%)
  Paget's disease of the nipple
  Unclassifiable and anaplastic types
  Mixed lobular and ductal carcinoma

- Is a neoplastic proliferation of lobular epithelial cells that fills and distends at least one complete lobular unit, obliterating their lumens.
- Tends to be multifocal and bilateral.
- Does not produce a palpable lesion and is not apparent on mammography.
- Is usually an incidental pathologic finding in a patient who has had breast tissue removed for some other reason.
- The presence of LCIS increases the risk of future development of invasive breast carcinoma 10- to 12-fold. Both breasts are at risk. Invasive carcinoma associated with LCIS may be either ductal or lobular.
- The management of a patient with LCIS is highly controversial. Recommended treatment ranges from careful follow-up to bilateral simple mastectomy.

2. Intraductal carcinoma (ductal carcinoma in situ; DCIS)

- Is a neoplastic proliferation of ductal epithelial cells confined within the basement membrane.
- Is frequently multifocal, and is bilateral in 15–20% of cases.
- Is detectable by mammography.
- Grossly, DCIS may produce a hard mass composed of thickened, cordlike structures. Calcification is a common feature.
- Histologically, the involved ducts are distended by malignant cells that may be arranged in cribriform, papillary, or solid patterns. Central necrosis is a common feature ("comedo" carcinoma).
- When large, DCIS is treated similarly to infiltrating carcinoma.

B. Invasive (infiltrating) carcinoma.
1. Invasive ductal carcinoma:

- This is the most common type of breast cancer, comprising more than 80% of all cases.
- Grossly, it forms a gritty, rock-hard, grayish-white infiltrative mass. Yellowish-white chalk streaks are characteristic.
- Microscopically, highly pleomorphic ductal epithelial cells infiltrate the fibrous stroma. Lymphatic invasion is common.

2. Infiltrating lobular carcinomas:

- Constitute 5–10% of all breast carcinomas.
- Are similar to infiltrating ductal carcinomas except for:
  - A different histologic pattern.
  - A higher incidence of bilaterality.
  - A greater frequency of estrogen receptor positivity.

3. Morphologic variants of breast carcinoma:

- Variant histologic forms of breast carcinoma are recognized (Table 56–2).
- Medullary carcinoma, mucinous (colloid) carcinoma, and tubular carcinoma have a better prognosis than the usual infiltrating ductal carcinoma.

Clinical Features
Most patients present with a painless mass, which enlarges, sometimes rapidly. Fixity to the chest wall and skin, retraction of skin and nipple, and ulceration are late features.

- A few patients present with a bloody nipple discharge.
- Early detection of breast carcinoma is very important, because the smaller the lesion is, the greater the likelihood of cure.
- Methods for early detection are:
  - Self-examination of the breast.
  - Mammography is currently recommended for women over age 40, women with a family history or a previous breast biopsy showing atypical hyperplasia, or women with a previous history of breast carcinoma.
- A small number of breast carcinomas have a distinctive clinical presentation:
  - Paget's disease of the nipple, which presents as an eczematous change in the nipple and surrounding skin, and is characterized microscopically by the presence of carcinoma cells in the epidermis.
  - Inflammatory breast carcinoma, which is characterized by swelling, redness, pain, and tenderness of the skin over a breast that shows diffuse induration. Microscopically, there is extensive dermal lymphatic carcinomatosis.

Mode of Spread

- **Direct spread** occurs
  - Along the ductal system and into lobules. Intraductal extension to the nipple results in Paget's disease.
  - Into the connective tissue of the breast.
  - Into overlying skin.
  - Into underlying pectoralis major.
- **Lymphatic spread** is commonly to axillary lymph nodes.
  - Nodes along the internal mammary artery may be involved in carcinomas located in the medial half of the breast.
  - Spread beyond the axillary node into supraclavicular and cervical nodes is evidence of advanced disease.
- **Bloodstream spread** with metastatic deposits in bone, liver, and lungs occurs in the later stages.
- **Spread via the pleural or peritoneal cavity** occurs when the pleura or peritoneum is secondarily involved by the breast cancer.

Diagnosis

Cytologic examination of an aspiration specimen is an accurate method of diagnosing carcinoma. Histologic examination of a biopsy of the mass is the definitive diagnostic method.

- A complete pathologic diagnosis of breast carcinoma provides the following information:
  - The histologic type and grade of carcinoma.
  - The size of the tumor.
  - The stage of disease (Table 56–3).
  - The estrogen and progesterone receptor status.
- Hormone receptor status is currently established by bioassay, for which a sample of tumor must be frozen immediately after excision.

TABLE 56–3. CLINICOPATHOLOGIC STAGING OF BREAST CANCER[1]

Stage	Tumor Size and Metastasis	5-Year Survival Rate
I	Tumor < 5 cm diameter; no involved nodes, no distant metastases	85%
II	Tumor < 5 cm diameter; involved axillary nodes, no distant metastases	66%
III	Tumor > 5 cm diameter, or any size with attachment to skin or chest wall; no distant metastases	41%
IV	Distant metastases (includes lymph nodes outside axilla)	10%

[1]Several slightly different staging systems exist; all are based on similar principles.

Treatment

Surgery is the mainstay of treatment of breast cancer.

- Modified radical mastectomy is necessary for tumors over 4 cm in size.
- For smaller tumors, equivalent results are obtained with either modified radical mastectomy or complete lump excision followed by radiotherapy.
- Radiotherapy is very useful as an adjunct to surgery, particularly when it is necessary to control locally recurrent disease in the chest wall.
- Chemotherapy has improved the prognosis in breast carcinoma and is used after surgical treatment (adjuvant chemotherapy) in several groups of patients.
- Hormonal therapy, usually antiestrogen therapy (tamoxifen) is most effective in patients with estrogen receptor-positive carcinomas.

Prognosis

- Infiltrating carcinoma of the breast has a 5-year survival rate of about 70%.
- About 20% of patients who survive 5 years will develop late recurrences.
- Factors influencing prognosis include:
  - The clinicopathologic stage (Table 56–3).
  - The histologic type (Table 56–2) and grade.
  - The presence of *NEU* oncogene, especially when large numbers (more than 20 copies per cell) are present, indicates a poor prognosis.
  - Absence of steroid hormone receptors indicates a poor prognosis.

CYSTOSARCOMA PHYLLODES (Phyllodes Tumor)

Cytosarcoma phillodes is (in 80–90% of cases) a low-grade malignant neopolasm that is locally infiltrative, with a tendency to recur locally after simple excision.

- In 10–20% of cases, the tumor behaves like a high-grade neoplasm, metastasizing to distant sites, mainly the lungs.

- Typically it forms a large mass, commonly over 5 cm in diameter.
- Grossly, it is a fleshy tumor with poorly circumscribed margins and areas of cystic degeneration.
- Histologically, it is composed of epithelial and stromal components. The stroma is highly cellular.
- Features that indicate likelihood of metastasis are:
  - High mitotic rate in the stroma (>3 mitotic figures per 10 high-power fields).
  - Stromal overgrowth at the expense of the epithelial component.
- Cystosarcoma phyllodes must be removed with a margin of breast tissue. With large tumors, simple mastectomy may be necessary.
- Tumors that metastasize usually cause death, since chemotherapy and radiotherapy are not very effective.

OTHER MALIGNANT NEOPLASMS

Primary malignant neoplasms other than carcinomas and cystosarcoma phyllodes occur very rarely in the breast.

- Rare primary tumors include:
  - Angiosarcoma.
  - Acute myeloblastic leukemia (granulocytic sarcoma).
  - Malignant lymphomas.
  - Sarcomas derived from stromal cells.
- Metastases to the breast from cancers in other organs are rare.

DISEASES OF THE MALE BREAST

GYNECOMASTIA

Enlargement of the male breast may be unilateral or bilateral. It is uncommon.

- It usually presents as a nodule or plaque of firm tissue under the nipple, and may be painful.
- Most cases have no identifiable cause.
- In a few cases, a cause can be identified:
  - Testicular atrophy or destruction, as in Klinefelter's syndrome, cirrhosis of the liver, and lepromatous leprosy.
  - Estrogen-secreting tumor of the testis or adrenal. Increased gonadotropin levels, as in choriocarcinoma of the testis.
  - Increased prolactin levels, as in diseases of the hypothalamopituitary axis, where breast enlargement may be accompanied by galactorrhea.
  - Drugs, most commonly digoxin.
- Histologically, gynecomastia is characterized by proliferation of the ducts of the breast, which become surrounded by proliferating edematous stroma.
- Gynecomastia is a benign condition and carries no increased risk of malignancy.

CARCINOMA OF THE MALE BREAST

Carcinoma of the male breast is extremely rare.

- It presents with a painless breast mass.

- Histologic features are identical to those of infiltrating ductal carcinomas in the female.
- Diagnosis of male breast carcinoma is usually delayed. Fifty percent of patients have axillary lymph node metastases at the time of diagnosis.
- Male breast cancer has a worse overall prognosis than female breast cancer.

Section XIII. The Endocrine System

The Pituitary Gland 57

HYPERSECRETION OF ANTERIOR PITUITARY HORMONES

PITUITARY ADENOMA
Nearly all cases of anterior pituitary hypersecretion are due to a benign neoplasm (pituitary adenoma).

- Pituitary adenomas are uncommon, constituting about 10% of primary intracranial neoplasms.
- They occur at all ages but are most common in the age group from 20 to 50 years.
- They occur in men slightly more frequently than in women.
- About 30% are nonfunctional, causing destruction of the normal gland and presenting with hypopituitarism.
- About 30% secrete prolactin, 25% growth hormone, and 10% ACTH. The remainder secrete thyrotropin or gonadotropins.
- Occasionally, pituitary adenoma occurs as part of the multiple endocrine adenoma syndrome (MEA, Werner's syndrome; see Chapter 60).

Pathology
Grossly, pituitary adenomas vary greatly in size from microscopic to very large.

- Microadenomas (diameter <1 cm) are commonly found in autopsy glands, but their significance is unclear.
- ACTH- and prolactin-secreting adenomas tend to be small at the time of presentation. Nonfunctioning and growth hormone-secreting adenomas tend to be large.
- Larger tumors expand the sella turcica and compress surrounding structures, especially the optic chiasm (Table 57–1).
- Pituitary adenomas are circumscribed and often have a thin fibrous capsule.
- In a few cases—particularly when the adenoma recurs after surgical removal—the neoplasm is locally infiltrative (invasive adenomas).
- Diagnosis of carcinoma is made only when distant metastases are documented, which is extremely rare.
- Grossly, pituitary adenomas are fleshy, gray to red masses with frequent cystic degeneration and hemorrhage.
- Microscopically, the cells are small, round and uniform, and arranged in nests and trabeculae separated by sinusoidal blood vessels.
- The characterization of cell type requires either immunohistochemical or electron microscopic study.

TABLE 57–1. PITUITARY ADENOMA: CLINICAL EFFECTS

Mass Effects	Excessive Hormone Secretion (Only Manifestation in Small Adenomas)
Large adenomas Usually nonfunctioning or growth-hormone producing ↓ Destruction of normal pituitary cells → hypopituitarism, diabetes insipidus Expansion of sella turcica → visible on x-ray Suprasellar extension through diaphragma sella ↓	Absent in 30% of cases 30% Prolactin → galactorrhea 25% Growth hormone → gigantism (child) → acromegaly (adult)
Compression of optic chiasm or nerves → visual field defects Compression of hypothalamus → diabetes insipidus Interference with outflow of CSF from 3rd ventricle → raised intracranial pressure → hyrdocephalus Compression of vessels → headache Cranial nerve compression (rare) May invade brain ("invasive adenoma"), paranasal sinuses, cavernous sinus	10% Corticotropin → Cushing's syndrome 5% Thyrotropin, gonadotropins

Clinical Features (Table 57–1)
A. Local effects:

- Depend on the size of the tumor.
- In large tumors, enlargement of the sella turcica can be detected by plain X-ray.
- As the neoplasm expands into the suprasellar cistern, it:
  - Impinges on the large blood vessels causing dull headache.
  - Compresses the central inferior part of the optic chiasm leading to visual field defects, typically superior quadrantic bitemporal hemianopia.
  - Compresses the hypothalamus, with variable changes.
  - Compresses the third ventricle, resulting in hydrocephalus.
- Infiltrative neoplasms may extend into:
  - The paranasal sinuses with a high risk of meningitis.
  - The cavernous sinus, producing thrombosis with orbital edema and congestion.

B. Systemic effects due to hormone excess
1. Hyperprolactinemia:

- Prolactin secreting lactotroph adenoma is the commonest type of pituitary adenoma (30% of cases).
- In women, prolactin causes amenorrhea, infertility, and galactorrhea (milk secretion in the absence of pregnancy).
- In men, it causes decreased libido, impotence, and galactorrhea.

2. Growth hormone (somatotropin) excess:

- Growth hormone producing somatotroph adenomas account for 25% of pituitary adenomas.
- Increased growth hormone levels cause increased growth of nearly every tissue in the body.
- In children, there is excessive uniform bone growth at the epiphyses, resulting in a massive but proportionate increase in height (gigantism).
- In adults, there is generalized enlargement of:
  - Bones, causing spadelike hands, protruding jaw, enlarging skull.
  - Cartilages, causing enlargement of nose and ears.
  - Nearly all organs, eg, cardiomegaly, hepatomegaly.
  - Soft tissues, causing coarsening of facial features.
- Joint abnormalities occur, particularly in the vertebral column, causing osteoarthritis.
- Decreased secretion of other pituitary hormones, because of compression of normal pituitary cells, causes impotence (in men), amenorrhea (in women), and infertility (both sexes).
- Growth hormone antagonizes insulin and causes secondary diabetes mellitus. Ten percent of patients with acromegaly have overt diabetes; over 40% have abnormalities in the glucose tolerance test.
- Diagnosis is established by a finding of elevated serum levels of growth hormone that cannot be suppressed by glucose administration.

3. Corticotropin (ACTH) excess:

- Ten percent of pituitary adenomas are corticotroph adenomas.
- Increased corticotropin (ACTH) stimulates bilateral hyperplasia of the adrenal cortex, causing excessive secretion of cortisol (Cushing's syndrome).
- The high serum cortisol levels fail to depress ACTH secretion by the partially autonomous adenoma.
- Increased skin pigmentation is variously attributed to increased production of MSH or to the melanogenic effect of high ACTH levels.
- High serum levels of both cortisol and ACTH strongly suggest a diagnosis of corticotroph adenoma.
- Diagnosis is made by demonstrating the pituitary adenoma by radiographic studies.
- Most ACTH-secreting adenomas are very small.

4. Thyrotropin (TSH) and gonadotropin excess: These disorders are very rare.

Treatment & Prognosis
The treatment of pituitary adenoma is surgical removal. The adenoma recurs in a small percentage of cases and may show locally aggressive behavior. Metastasis (ie, carcinoma) is very rare.

HYPOSECRETION OF PITUITARY HORMONES

Incidence & Etiology (Table 57–2)
Hypopituitarism in adults (Simmonds' disease) is rare.

- The commonest cause in the past was ischemic necrosis of a gland that had undergone hyperplasia during pregnancy (Sheehan's syndrome). This is now very uncommon in developed countries.

■ Nonfunctioning neoplasms involving the sella represent the commonest cause of hypopituitarism in developed countries (Table 57–2).

Pathology

Over 90% of the gland must be destroyed before clinical evidence of hypopituitarism is manifested. The pathologic changes in the gland depend on the cause.

Clinical Features

A. Hypopituitarism in children: Results in a proportionate failure of growth due to absence of growth hormone (pituitary dwarfism). These children have normal intelligence and remain childlike, failing to develop sexually (Lorain type of dwarfism).

B. Hypopituitarism in adults:

■ Is characterized mainly by the effects of gonadotropin deficiency.

■ In the female, there is amenorrhea and infertility.

■ In the male, there is infertility and impotence.

■ Decrease in growth hormone, thyrotropin, and corticotropin rarely produces clinical abnormality in the adult.

TABLE 57–2. CAUSES OF HYPOPITUITARISM

Ischemic necrosis of the pituitary
    Postpartum necrosis (Sheehan's syndrome)
    Head injury
    Vascular disease, commonly associated with diabetes mellitus

Neoplasms involving the sella turcica
    Nonfunctioning adenoma
    Craniopharyngioma
    Suprasellar chordoma
    Histiocytosis X (eosinophilic granuloma; Hand-Schüller-Christian disease)

Intrasellar cysts

Chronic inflammatory lesions
    Tuberculosis, syphilis, sarcoidosis

Infiltrative diseases
    Amyloidosis
    Hemochromatosis
    Mucopolysaccharidoses

Congenital pituitary dwarfism
    Lorain type: normal proportions and intelligence but delayed sexual development
    Fröhlich type: obese with stunted growth, mental retardation, and abnormal sexual development

Treatment

Treatment of hypopituitarism is by replacement of all the deficient hormones. When a neoplasm is responsible, surgical removal of the mass is necessary.

DISEASES OF THE POSTERIOR PITUITARY

DIABETES INSIPIDUS

Diabetes insipidus is caused by failure of the hypothalamus and posterior pituitary to secrete antidiuretic hormone (ADH).

- Deficient water reabsorption in the kidney causes polyuria of very low specific gravity, increased serum osmolality, thirst, and polydipsia (excessive water intake).
- May be caused by any condition that interferes with the hypothalamopituitary axis:
  - Hypothalamic or pituitary neoplasms.
  - Traumatic disruption of the pituitary stalk.
  - Meningeal disease (metastatic carcinoma, sarcoidosis, tuberculous meningitis).
  - Bone disease affecting the sellar region (eg, Hand-Schüller-Christian disease).
- Diagnosis is based on the clinical features with confirmation by the water deprivation test.

EXCESSIVE SECRETION OF ANTIDIURETIC HORMONE

Inappropriate excessive secretion of ADH (SIADH; Schwartz-Bartter syndrome) by the posterior pituitary is a common phenomenon seen in:

- Pulmonary disorders, eg, tuberculosis and pneumonia.
- Cerebral neoplasms and trauma.
- Drugs, eg, vincristine and chlorpropamide.
- Cirrhosis of the liver.
- Adrenal and thyroid insufficiency.
- ADH may also be produced by several different malignant neoplasms, most commonly small-cell undifferentiated (oat cell) carcinoma of the lung and pancreatic carcinoma (ectopic ADH syndrome).
- High levels of ADH cause water to be retained, with excretion of a highly concentrated urine, leading to decreased serum osmolality (<275 mosm/kg) and hyponatremia.
- The clinical manifestations are those of hyponatremia and include weakness, lethargy, confusion, convulsions, and coma.

The Thyroid Gland

DISORDERS OF THYROID SECRETION

EXCESSIVE SECRETION OF THYROID HORMONE (Hyperthyroidism; Thyrotoxicosis)

Etiology
Over 95% of cases of hyperthyroidism are caused by Graves' disease, an autoimmune thyroid disease in which autoantibodies stimulate the cells.

■ Rare causes of hyperthyroidism other than Graves' disease are:
- Toxicity in a multinodular goiter.
- Functioning follicular adenoma or, rarely, carcinoma.
- Thyrotropin-secreting pituitary adenoma.
- Choriocarcinoma, which may rarely produce a TSH-like substance.
- Teratoma, usually ovarian, that contain functioning thyroid tissue.
- Thyroiditis, both subacute and Hashimoto type, which may be associated with transient hyperthyroidism in the early phase.
- Hypothalamic disease with production of excess TRH (thyrotropin-releasing hormone).

Pathology
Pathologic changes in the thyroid depend on the cause (see individual diseases, following).

Clinical Features (Table 58–1)
Hyperthyroidism results in a general increase in cellular metabolism of target cells, which causes:

■ Nervousness, anxiety, insomnia, and fine tremors.
■ Weight loss, despite a good appetite, because of increased basal metabolic rate.
■ Heat intolerance and increased sweating.
■ Palpitations, tachycardia, atrial fibrillation, and cardiac failure, as a result of the effect of thyroxine on myocardial cells.
■ Amenorrhea and infertility.
■ Muscle weakness, particularly involving the limb girdles (proximal myopathy).
■ Osteoporosis with bone pain.

Laboratory Diagnosis (Tables 58–1 and 58–2)

■ Elevated total serum T_4 and T_3 are not reliable indices of thyroid hyperfunction because of variations in levels of binding proteins.

TABLE 58–1. CONTRASTING FEATURES IN DISORDERS OF THYROID FUNCTION

	Hyperthyroid	Hypothyroid
Laboratory Free thyroxine index	↑	↓
T_4 and T_3 levels	↑[1]	↓
TSH[2] levels	↓[3]	↑[3]
Physiologic mechanisms Cellular metabolism and protein synthesis	↑	↓
Potentiation of β-adrenergic effects	↑	↓
Insulin antagonism	↑	↓
Clinical effects Basal metabolic rate	↑	↓
Goiter	Usually present	May be present
Body weight	↓	N or ↑
Activity	Hyperactive, insomniac	Lethargic, somnolent
Reflexes	Brisk	Slow
Cardiovascular	Tachycardia, arrhythmias	Bradycardia
Gastrointestinal	Mild diarrhea	Constipation
Hair	Fine	Coarse, brittle; hair loss
Myxedema[4]	Circumscribed patches, mainly pretibial	Generalized, especially extremities and face
Temperature tolerance	Heat-intolerant	Cold-intolerant
Other	Exophthalmos (in Graves' disease)	Mental and growth retardation (in childhood cretinism); anemia, hypercholesterolemia

[1]Occasionally only T_3 is elevated.
[2]TSH = thyroid-stimulating hormone.
[3]Reflects changes in biofeedback in primary thyroid disease; in hyperthyroidism caused by pituitary disease, the TSH level will be increased; if hypothyroidism is due to pituitary failure, TSH will be decreased.
[4]The term myxedema refers to accumulation of mucopolysaccharides in the dermis. Although myxedema occurs in both hyper- and hypothyroidism, the distribution and pathogenesis are different.

TABLE 58–2. DIFFERENTIAL FEATURES IN THYROID DISEASE

	Thyroid Gland	Thyroid Hormones	Thyroid-Stimulating Hormone	Autoantibodies
Hyperthyroidism **Primary** Graves' disease	Diffuse enlargement	Elevated	Decreased	Thyroid-stimulating Ig; exophthalmos-producing factor
Toxic nodular goiter	Multinodular goiter	Elevated	Decreased	None
Toxic adenoma	Solitary nodule	Elevated	Decreased	None
Subacute thyroiditis	Tender enlargement	Elevated	Normal	None
Secondary Pituitary thyrotropic adenoma	Diffuse enlargement	Elevated	Elevated	None
Hypothyroidism **Primary** Thyroid agenesis	Absent	Absent	Elevated	None
Enzyme deficiency	Diffuse enlargement	Decreased	Elevated	None
Iodine deficiency	Diffuse/nodular goiter	Decreased	Elevated	None
Hashimoto's thyroiditis	Diffuse enlargement	Decreased	Elevated	Antithyroglobulin, anti-microsomal, anticolloid
Secondary Pituitary failure	Atrophy	Decreased	Decreased	None

[1]Thyroid hormone levels may be assessed by total T_4, total T_3, and free T_4 index. In most thyroid diseases, all 3 are elevated; free T_4 index is more reliable than total T_4 and total T_3 levels. In a few cases of hyperthyroidism, T_4 levels are normal and only T_3 is elevated ("T_3 toxicosis").

■ Free thyroxine index is elevated in hyperthyroidism and is currently the best diagnostic test.
■ In about 10% of cases, T_4 secretion is within normal limits, the hyperthyroidism being the result of elevated T_3 levels (T_3 toxicosis).

- Graves' disease is distinguished from other causes of hyperthyroidism by the presence of eye changes and serum thyroid-stimulating autoantibodies (see following).
- Serum TSH levels are decreased in all cases of hyperthyroidism, except in those rare cases where the hyperthyroidism is secondary to a thyrotroph adenoma of the pituitary.

DECREASED SECRETION OF THYROID HORMONE (Hypothyroidism)

Decreased secretion of thyroid hormones results in cretinism if deficiency is present from birth, and myxedema if it develops in an adult.

- Hypothyroidism may be broadly classified as:
  - Primary, due to decrease in thyroid hormone resulting from a disease process in the thyroid gland (common).
  - Secondary, resulting from failure of pituitary TSH secretion (rare).
- Diagnosis of hypothyroidism may be confirmed in the laboratory (Tables 58–1 and 58–2) by:
  - Decreased levels of T_4 (not very reliable) and a decreased free thyroxine index (reliable).
  - The T_3 level is of little value, since it only falls in extreme hypothyroidism.
  - Elevation of serum thyrotropin (TSH) concentration, which is a sensitive test for primary hypothyroidism.

CRETINISM

Etiology

Cretinism is an uncommon disease of childhood. Diagnosis is important because thyroxine administration soon after birth can in many cases prevent severe consequences.

- The causes of cretinism are:
  - Failure of development of the thyroid (thyroid agenesis).
  - Failure of hormone synthesis due to severe iodine deficiency in the diet of both the mother during pregnancy and the baby after birth. This is rare in countries in which table salt is iodized, but still occurs in some mountainous Third World countries (endemic cretinism).
  - Failure of hormone synthesis due to the presence of dietary substances (goitrogens) that block hormone synthesis, eg, thiocyanate in the cassava plant eaten in Central Africa.
  - Failure of hormone synthesis due to autosomal recessive deficiency (sporadic cretinism). Many enzyme deficiencies are reported. They are all rare.

Pathology

The appearance of the thyroid depends on the cause.

- In cretinism due to thyroid agenesis, the gland is absent.
- In cretinism caused by failure of thyroid hormone synthesis, the gland undergoes enlargement owing to increased secretion of pituitary thyrotropin resulting from decreased feedback inhibition (goitrous cretinism).

Clinical Features

Babies with cretinism show lethargy, somnolence, hypothermia, feeding problems, and persistent neonatal jaundice. A hoarse cry, hypotonia of muscles, large protruding tongue, and umbilical hernia are common.

- If the diagnosis is not made at birth, there is growth retardation (failure to thrive, delayed bone growth) and irreversible mental retardation.
- Replacement of thyroid in the perinatal period prevents mental retardation to a large extent.

MYXEDEMA

Etiology

Causes of hypothyroidism in the adult include:

- Hashimoto's autoimmune thyroiditis, which is responsible for most cases and is discussed later.
- Pituitary failure is an uncommon cause, but may be recognized by the markedly decreased thyrotropin level in the blood.
- Iatrogenic hypothyroidism may result from administration of antithyroid drugs or ablation of the gland by surgery (total thyroidectomy) or radiation.
- Failure of thyroid hormone synthesis due to extreme dietary iodine deficiency very rarely results in hypothyroidism.
- Dietary goitrogens also rarely cause hypothyroidism.

Pathology

The changes in the thyroid depend on the cause of hypothyroidism (see Hashimoto's thyroiditis, later).

Clinical Features (Table 58–1)

Decreased thyroid hormones cause a decreased rate of metabolism in all target cells. Typical clinical features include:

- Lethargy, cold intolerance, weight gain, and constipation.
- Loss of hair all over the body, but typically in the scalp and eyebrows.
- Neurologic manifestations, including psychomotor retardation and overt psychosis (myxedema madness).
- Anemia, usually normochromic normocytic, due to decreased erythropoiesis.
- Pleural and pericardial effusions.
- Increased serum cholesterol and atherosclerosis.
- The term *myxedema* is used because of the deposition of increased amounts of mucopolysaccharides in:
  - The skin, where it causes a diffuse, nonpitting doughy swelling.
  - The larynx, causing hoarseness.
  - The interstitium between myocardial fibers causing cardiac enlargement and heart failure.

DISEASES OF THE THYROID

IMMUNOLOGIC DISEASES OF THE THYROID

GRAVES' DISEASE
Graves' disease is responsible for the great majority of cases of hyperthyroidism.

- It is a relatively common disease affecting females 4–5 times more commonly than males.
- It has its highest incidence in the 15- to 40-year age group.
- There is a familial tendency and an association with the histocompatibility antigen HLA-DR3.
- Patients with Graves' disease frequently suffer from other autoimmune diseases such as pernicious anemia.

Etiology
Graves' disease is characterized by the presence in serum of thyroid-stimulating immunoglobulins (TSI), which are autoantibodies of the IgG class, and include:

- Long-acting thyroid stimulator (LATS).
- Human thyroid stimulator (HTS).
- LATS protector (LATS-P).
- The TSIs combine with cell membrane receptors. This stimulates thyroid hormone production.
- The precipitating cause is unknown.
- Serum levels of antibodies do not correlate precisely with severity of disease.
- The IgG antibodies cross the placenta in pregnancy and cause neonatal hyperthyroidism. This condition spontaneously reverses after delivery.

Pathology
The thyroid gland is diffusely and symmetrically enlarged and extremely vascular.

- Microscopically, thyroid follicular epithelial cells show marked hyperplasia with decreased colloid.
- Lymphocytic infiltration of the interstitium is common, and lymphoid follicles with germinal centers may be present.

Clinical Features & Diagnosis (Tables 58–1 and 58–2)

- The thyroid gland is diffusely enlarged. A bruit resulting from the greatly increased blood flow is often present over the gland.
- Eye changes are present in most patients, and include:
  - Exophthalmos (see following).
  - A staring gaze due to decreased blinking.
  - Impaired eye muscle function.
- Laboratory evidence of hyperthyroidism is present. Ten percent of patients show normal T_4 but elevated levels of free T_3 (T_3 toxicosis).

- Thyroid scan shows increased uptake of radioiodine but is rarely needed for diagnosis.
- Most patients have TSI in their blood.

Associated Lesions
A. Exophthalmos is a forward protrusion of the eyeballs.

- It occurs in 70% of patients with Graves' disease.
- Its presence is unrelated to the severity of Graves' disease, and it may rarely occur in the absence of hyperthyroidism.
- It is related to the presence in serum of an autoantibody known as exophthalmos-producing factor (EPF) that is independent of TSI.
- It is caused by infiltration of the orbital soft tissue by edema, mucopolysaccharides, and lymphocytes.
- When it is severe, there is risk of ocular infections and blindness.

B. Pretibial myxedema occurs in 5% of patients with Graves' disease.

- It is due to localized accumulation of mucopolysaccharide, forming circumscribed patches, in the pretibial skin.
- It causes no symptoms other than itching.

Treatment
Graves' disease may be treated with:

- Antithyroid drugs such as propylthiouracil, which blocks the synthesis of thyroid hormones, or propranolol, which blocks the peripheral effects of thyroxine.
- Surgical removal (subtotal thyroidectomy).
- Radioactive ablation with therapeutic doses of radioactive iodine.
- Radioiodine therapy has an increased risk of hypothyroidism and future thyroid carcinoma.
- Treatment of Graves' disease has no effect on the exophthalmos. The eye changes usually remit spontaneously, but may require corticosteroids and surgical decompression of the orbit in severe cases.

HASHIMOTO'S AUTOIMMUNE THYROIDITIS
Hashimoto's thyroiditis is responsible for most cases of primary hypothyroidism. It is common in middle-aged individuals. Females are affected 10 times more frequently than males.

Etiology
It is caused by an autoimmune response against the thyroid.

- Most patients with Hashimoto's disease have in their serum several IgG autoantibodies:
  - Antithyroglobulin antibody.
  - Antimicrosomal antibody.
  - An antibody directed against a component of colloid other than thyroglobulin.
- Serum levels of these antibodies do not correlate with severity of disease.

Pathology

In the early stages, the thyroid is enlarged diffusely, firm and rubbery, with a coarsely nodular ("bosselated") appearance. As the disease progresses, the gland becomes smaller. The end result is a markedly atrophic fibrosed thyroid.

- Microscopically, there is destruction of thyroid follicles associated with severe lymphocytic infiltration of the gland.
- Large lymphoid follicles with germinal centers are commonly present. Hürthle cell metaplasia and fibrosis are present.

Clinical Features

Most patients present with gradual enlargement of the thyroid that may raise a suspicion of neoplasm.

- Thyroid function is variable; patients are commonly either euthyroid or mildly hypothyroid. Rarely, there is mild hyperthyroidism in the early phase.
- In most cases, the disease progresses with increasing degrees of hypothyroidism.
- Thyroid autoantibodies can be detected in the serum of almost all patients. High titers of these antibodies are diagnostic of Hashimoto's disease.

Treatment and Prognosis

Thyroid hormone replacement is necessary in the later stages. Five percent of patients with long-standing Hashimoto's disease develop malignant neoplasms of the thyroid, either papillary carcinoma or malignant B cell lymphoma.

INFLAMMATORY THYROID DISEASES

1. SUBACUTE THYROIDITIS

Subacute thyroiditis—also called granulomatous thyroiditis and DeQuervain's thyroiditis—is an uncommon disease.

- It affects both sexes and all ages.
- A viral origin is considered most likely.
- Thyroid inflammation frequently follows upper respiratory infection.
- Coxsackieviruses are the most commonly implicated.
- Neither culture nor electron microscopy has demonstrated the virus in affected thyroid.
- Subacute thyroiditis has no relationship to either Graves' disease or Hashimoto's thyroiditis.

Pathology

The thyroid is diffusely enlarged, firm, and often adherent to surrounding structures. Microscopically, there is extensive destruction and fibrosis of thyroid follicles with aggregates of macrophages and giant cells around free colloid.

Clinical Features

There is acute onset of painful enlargement of the thyroid, often associated with fever, malaise, and muscle aches.

■ Most patients are euthyroid but in a few cases there is a transient hyperthyroidism.
■ The disease is self-limited and does not lead to hypothyroidism.

2. RIEDEL'S THYROIDITIS
Riedel's thyroiditis is a rare chronic disorder occurring in older patients.

■ Women are affected more frequently than men.
■ Thyroid autoantibodies are usually not present.
■ It is sometimes associated with similar fibrosing lesions in the retroperitoneum and mediastinum, suggesting that it may be a systemic disorder involving fibroblasts.

Pathology
The gland is usually mildly enlarged and replaced wholly or in part by stony hard, grayish-white fibrous tissue ("woody" or "ligneous" thyroiditis) that extends beyond the capsule. Microscopically, there is atrophy of thyroid follicles, which are replaced by dense scarlike collagen. Scattered lymphocytes and plasma cells are present.

Clinical Features
Clinically and at surgery, Riedel's thyroiditis resembles anaplastic carcinoma of the thyroid. It presents with painless rock-hard enlargement of the thyroid.

■ The fibrosis may constrict:
  ● The trachea, producing dyspnea and stridor.
  ● The esophagus, causing dysphagia.
  ● The recurrent laryngeal nerve, causing hoarseness.
■ Patients are usually euthyroid.
■ Treatment is difficult. In most cases the disorder causes slowly increasing fibrosis of the neck structures.

DIFFUSE NONTOXIC & MULTINODULAR GOITER
Goiters represent the culmination of mild deficiency of thyroid hormone production, which causes feedback increase of TSH secretion by the pituitary, resulting in thyroid hyperplasia. Hyperplasia of the gland corrects the hormone deficiency and maintains the euthyroid state at the expense of thyroid enlargement.

Etiology
A. Endemic goiter:

■ Is the result of chronic dietary deficiency of iodine.
■ Occurs mainly in inland mountainous regions of the world such as the Alps, Andes, and Himalayas and inland regions of Asia and Africa, away from coastal waters.
■ In these populations, up to 5% of individuals may have thyroid enlargement, sometimes massive.
■ Endemic goiter is not common in coastal communities because of the high iodine content of seawater and seafood.
■ Endemic goiter is more common in women, because of increased iodine requirements in pregnancy and lactation.

- The incidence of endemic goiter has decreased greatly in countries where table salt is iodized.
- Much less commonly, goitrogens are responsible for endemic goiter.

B. Sporadic goiter:

- May occur anywhere, and is usually due to increased physiologic demand for thyroxine at puberty or during pregnancy.
- Less commonly, sporadic goiter may result from mild deficiency of enzymes involved in thyroid hormone synthesis.
- In some patients, no cause can be identified.

Pathology
Changes in the thyroid gland progress through diffuse enlargement (diffuse nontoxic goiter) to multinodular goiter. The gland may reach a massive size.

- Microscopically, there is a combination of TSH-induced hyperplasia (small follicles lined by tall columnar cells) and involution (macrofollicles distended with colloid and lined by flattened cells), and fibrosis.
- Degenerative changes like hemorrhage, cystic degeneration, and calcification are common.

Clinical Features
Patients present with painless diffuse enlargement of the thyroid. As the disease progresses, the thyroid becomes larger and more nodular.

- Patients are euthyroid.
- In a few patients, the presence of a dominant nodule may mimic a neoplastic process.
- Rarely, hyperthyroidism occurs in multinodular goiter due to the development of autonomous hyperplastic nodules (toxic nodular goiter).
- The risk of developing carcinoma in a multinodular goiter is small.

Treatment
In the earliest stage, providing iodine or thyroxine will remove the TSH stimulus and result in cessation of the hyperplastic process. In the later stages, where gland enlargement has resulted in a large neck mass, surgery (subtotal thyroidectomy) may be indicated.

Thyroid Neoplasms (Fig 58–1)

FOLLICULAR ADENOMA
The commonest neoplasm of the thyroid, accounting for about 30% of all cases of solitary thyroid nodules. It may occur at any age; females are affected 4 times as frequently as males.

Pathology

- Grossly, thyroid adenomas present as a solitary, firm gray or red nodule up to 5 cm in

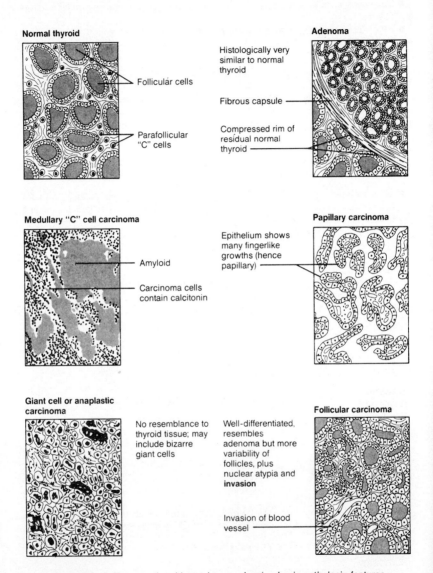

Figure 58–1. Common thyroid neoplasms, showing basic pathologic features.

diameter. Hemorrhage, fibrosis, calcification, and cystic degeneration may be present.

- Microscopically, follicular adenomas are usually composed of follicles of varying size or solid nests of thyroid epithelial cells.
- Follicular adenomas are surrounded by a complete fibrous capsule of varying thickness, and the normal thyroid parenchyma around the adenoma is compressed.
- Absence of capsule and vascular invasion are the criteria used to differentiate follicular adenoma from follicular carcinoma.

Clinical Features, Diagnosis, & Treatment

- Patients usually present with a solitary thyroid nodule.
- Patients are usually euthyroid. Rare "toxic" adenomas cause hyperthyroidism.
- Thyroid scan shows the presence of a circumscribed cold nodule.
- Fine-needle aspiration usually shows a cellular smear with many microfollicles. Adenoma cannot be differentiated from carcinoma on fine needle aspiration.
- Treatment is surgical excision (thyroid lobectomy).

CARCINOMA OF THE THYROID

Thyroid carcinoma is uncommon, with an incidence in the United States of about 25–30 cases per million population. It is responsible for about 2000 deaths per year, or 0.5% of all cancer deaths in the United States.

- Thyroid cancer affects females about 3 times as frequently as males.
- The incidence has increased greatly in the last 50 years, probably as a result of increased exposure to radiation.
- Three types of radiation are known to cause thyroid cancer:
  - External neck radiation when used during childhood.
  - Radioiodine therapy for treatment of Graves' disease.
  - Nuclear mishaps that release radioactive isotopes of iodine, as occurred at Hiroshima and Nagasaki; among the Marshall Islanders exposed to nuclear tests in the South Pacific; and more recently, the nuclear accident at Chernobyl in the Soviet Union.

Pathology (Fig 58–1 and Table 58–3)

Papillary, follicular, and anaplastic carcinomas are derived from thyroid follicular epithelium. Medullary carcinoma arises in the parafollicular calcitonin-secreting cells.

A. Papillary carcinoma: Papillary carcinoma is the most common type (Table 58–3).

- It affects females 3 times more commonly than males.
- Individuals in the age range 15–35 years are predominantly affected.
- Grossly, papillary carcinomas range from microscopic lesions to large masses over 10 cm in diameter. They are usually infiltrative, but may appear as circumscribed nodules.
- Microscopically, they are characterized by:
  - A papillary arrangement of cells.
  - Clear nuclei (Orphan Annie nuclei).

TABLE 58–3. DIFFERENTIAL FEATURES OF THYROID CARCINOMAS

Neoplasm	Cell of Origin	Frequency[1]	Age/Sex Incidence	Local Features	Lymphatic Metastasis	Blood-Borne Metastasis	5-Year Survival Rate	Tumor Markers
Papillary carcinoma	Follicular epithelial cell	70%	F > M = 3:1 15–35 yrs	Infiltrative masses; multifocal and bilateral; lymph nodes often +	+ + +	Late/ uncommon	90%	Thyroglobulin
Follicular carcinoma	Follicular epithelial cell	20%	F > M all ages; > 30 yrs	May be grossly infiltrative or "encapsulated" angioinvasive	+	+ + +	65%	Thyroglobulin
Anaplastic carcinoma	Follicular epithelial cell	5%	F > M; > 50 yrs	Massively infiltrating locally	+ + +	+ + +	0%	None
Medullary carcinoma	Parafollicular or "C" cell	5%	F = M; 30–60 yrs	Slowly growing mass; infiltrative	+	+	50%	Calcitonin

[1]Percentages relate to frequency among thyroid carcinomas.

- Intranuclear inclusions caused by cytoplasmic invaginations into the nucleus.
- Psammoma bodies, which are round, laminated, calcified bodies, are present in about 40% of papillary carcinomas.
- Thyroglobulin can be demonstrated in the neoplastic cells by immunoperoxidase.
- Papillary carcinomas grow very slowly.
- They commonly spread by local invasion, and most have invaded the thyroid capsule at the time of presentation.
- Lymphatic spread causes:
  - Multiple intraglandular metastatic nodules. In 60% of cases, tumor is present in the opposite lobe.
  - Cervical lymph node metastases, which are present in 40% of cases at the time of presentation.
- Bloodstream dissemination is rare in papillary carcinoma.

B. Follicular carcinomas comprise 20% of thyroid carcinomas.

- Females are affected more commonly than males.
- All ages are vulnerable, but the disease is more common after age 40.
- Grossly, follicular carcinoma may be:
  - Apparently encapsulated and indistinguishable from an adenoma.
  - A large infiltrative mass.
- Microscopically, follicular carcinomas are composed of follicles of varying size lined by thyroid epithelial cells of varying differentiation.
- The diagnosis of follicular carcinoma depends on the presence of invasion of the capsule or vascular structures.
- Thyroglobulin can be demonstrated in the neoplastic cells by immunoperoxidase technique.
- Follicular carcinoma is a slowly growing neoplasm.
- Bloodstream spread tends to occur at an early stage, producing metastases in bone and lungs.
- Lymphatic metastasis to cervical nodes also occurs but to a lesser extent than in papillary carcinoma.

C. Anaplastic carcinoma:

- Is rare, comprising 5% of thyroid carcinomas.
- Occurs most commonly over age 50.
- Grossly, appears as a massive infiltrative lesion. It is hard, gritty, and grayish-white and frequently shows areas of necrosis and hemorrhage.
- Microscopically, it is composed of highly malignant-appearing spindle or giant cells, showing extreme pleomorphism and frequent mitotic figures.
- Anaplastic carcinomas are highly malignant, rapidly growing neoplasms that disseminate extensively.
- Death usually occurs within a year after diagnosis and is mainly due to local invasion of neck structures.

D. Medullary carcinoma is uncommon, accounting for about 5% of thyroid carcinomas.

- They are derived from the calcitonin-secreting C cells of the thyroid.

- Ninety percent of medullary carcinomas occur as sporadic lesions.
- Ten percent are familial and may form part of the multiple endocrine adenomatosis (MEA type II) syndrome (see Chapter 60).
- Grossly, medullary carcinoma forms a hard, grayish-white infiltrative mass.
- Microscopically, composed of small spindle-shaped and polygonal cells arranged in nests, cords, and sheets. The stroma contains amyloid.
- Electron microscopy shows membrane-bound dense-core neurosecretory granules in the neoplastic cells and fibrillar amyloid material in the stroma.
- Calcitonin can be demonstrated in the neoplastic cells by the immunoperoxidase technique.
- Medullary carcinomas have a slow but progressive growth pattern.
- Local invasion of neck structures is common.
- Both lymphatic and bloodstream metastasis occurs.

Clinical Features

Thyroid carcinomas commonly present with a painless solitary nodule in the thyroid.

- Thyroid scan commonly shows a lack of uptake (cold nodule).
- Fine-needle aspiration may be diagnostic of papillary carcinoma, medullary carcinoma, and anaplastic carcinoma, but the distinction of follicular carcinoma from follicular adenoma is not possible.
- Patients with thyroid carcinoma are euthyroid as a rule. Very rarely, hyperthyroidism occurs.
- Local invasion of neck structures may cause:
  - Stridor and respiratory obstruction due to invasion of the trachea.
  - Hoarseness due to recurrent laryngeal nerve involvement.
  - Dysphagia due to invasion of the esophagus.
- Patients may also present with distant metastases. In papillary carcinoma, cervical lymph node enlargement is common.
- In follicular carcinoma, patients may present with a metastasis in bone or lung.

Tumor Markers

Medullary carcinoma is associated with elevated serum levels of calcitonin. Serum calcitonin assay is useful in diagnosis and following response to treatment.

- Well-differentiated thyroid carcinomas (papillary and follicular types) are associated with increased serum levels of thyroglobulin, which are useful in diagnosis and monitoring treatment.
- Anaplastic carcinomas commonly do not have tumor markers in the blood.

Treatment & Prognosis

Surgery (total thyroidectomy or lobectomy) is the primary mode of treatment for well-differentiated thyroid carcinoma and medullary carcinoma.

- Papillary and follicular carcinomas are TSH-dependent. Suppression of TSH secretion by thyroxine slows neoplastic growth.
- Papillary and follicular carcinomas can also be treated with radioactive iodine.
- External radiation is useful for temporary control only, but it is the only feasible therapy for most anaplastic carcinomas.

- The prognosis of papillary carcinoma is good, with a 5-year survival rate of 90% and a 20-year survival rate of 85%.
- Follicular carcinoma has a 5-year survival rate of about 65% and a 20-year survival rate of 30%.
- Medullary carcinoma has a 5-year survival rate of 50%.
- Anaplastic carcinoma is a highly malignant neoplasm, and most patients die within a year after diagnosis; the 5-year survival rate is almost zero.

MALIGNANT LYMPHOMA

Primary malignant lymphoma of the thyroid is extremely rare. It occurs mainly in elderly persons, particularly as a complication of Hashimoto's thyroiditis. The commonest type of malignant lymphoma is B-cell immunoblastic sarcoma.

The Parathyroid Glands   59

EXCESS PTH SECRETION (Hyperparathyroidism)

Hyperparathyroidism is defined as elevated serum PTH due to increased secretion.

- **Primary hyperparathyroidism** is most commonly due to a solitary adenoma involving one gland. Less often, multiple adenomas or diffuse hyperplasia of all four glands occurs (Table 59–1).
  - In about 10% of cases, the gross findings at surgery are atypical, with 2 or 3 slightly enlarged glands being found (Fig 59–1).
  - Serum calcium level is elevated.
- **Secondary hyperparathyroidism** is excessive secretion of PTH by a normal parathyroid gland in response to a lowered serum ionized calcium level.
  - It is characterized by hyperplasia of all four glands.
  - In most cases, serum calcium levels are corrected toward normal but are not elevated.
  - Rarely, overcorrection occurs, and serum calcium level is elevated.
- **Ectopic PTH:** PTH- or PTH-like polypeptides may be secreted by a variety of malignant neoplasms, producing a syndrome that is very similar to primary hyperparathyroidism. Squamous carcinomas of the lung, adenocarcinomas of the kidney and endometrium, and bladder carcinoma are the common sources of ectopic PTH.

Pathology (Fig 59–1)
A. Parathyroid adenoma:

- Is a benign solitary neoplasm that involves one gland only; very rarely, multiple adenomas are present.
- Grossly, they are usually small (commonly 1–2 cm in diameter and weighing 1–3 g) and well-encapsulated masses.
- Microscopically, they are composed of a mixed population of chief, water-clear, and oxyphil cells, arranged in sheets, trabeculae, or glandular structures. Mitotic activity is absent.
- Parathyroid adenoma is differentiated from a normal gland by:
  - The increased size (the maximum weight of a normal parathyroid gland is 40 mg).
  - The absence of fat.
  - The presence of a compressed rim of normal parathyroid tissue around the mass.
- In patients with a solitary adenoma, the other three parathyroid glands are normal in size and microscopic appearance (Fig 59–1).

B. Parathyroid hyperplasia:

- The pathologic changes in parathyroid hyperplasia in primary and secondary hyperparathyroidism are identical.

TABLE 59-1. CAUSES OF HYPERPARATHYROIDISM

Primary hyperparathyroidism	
Single adenoma	80–90%
Multiple adenomas	1–4%
Diffuse hyperplasia	3–15%
Carcinoma	1–4%
Secondary hyperparathyroidism	
Chronic renal failure	
Malabsorption syndrome	
Vitamin D deficiency	
Medullary carcinoma of the thyroid	
Ectopic parathyroid hormone (PTH) syndromes[1]	
Squamous carcinoma of lung	
Renal adenocarcinoma	
Others	

[1]Most malignant neoplasms secrete a hormone that activates PTH receptors on target cells but does not cross-react with immunologic testing reagents used in PTH assays. These patients have high urinary cAMP levels (indicating activation of cells) and low (suppressed) plasma PTH levels associated with marked hypercalcemia.

- Hyperplasia usually affects all glands equally with uniform enlargement of all four glands. Rarely, one or two glands are disproportionately enlarged. (Fig 59–1).
- Microscopically, parathyroid hyperplasia is characterized by proliferation of all three cell types at the expense of the intraglandular fat.
- Microscopic examination of a single enlarged gland does not permit differentiation of parathyroid adenoma from hyperplasia except in cases where a rim of compressed normal gland is present in an adenoma.
- Differentiation of hyperplasia from adenoma requires biopsy of a second parathyroid gland. In hyperplasia, the second gland is microscopically abnormal, whereas in adenoma the second gland is normal.
- Normality of the second gland is established by:
  - Weight, when the entire gland is available.
  - The presence of cytoplasmic lipid.
- Lipid is absent in hyperplastic and neoplastic parathyroid cells.

C. Parathyroid carcinoma is very rare.

- Patients with parathyroid carcinoma tend to have higher serum calcium and PTH levels.
- Carcinoma differs pathologically from adenoma in the following respects:
  - It tends to infiltrate outside the capsule, so that it is difficult to remove at surgery.
  - Mitotic figures are present.
  - Broad bands of collagen, which are frequently present in the substance of a carcinoma.
- Parathyroid carcinoma tends to recur locally after excision and metastasize to regional lymph nodes and distant sites.

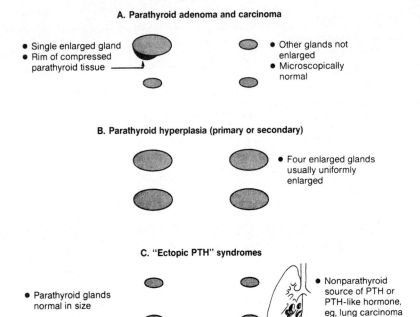

A. Parathyroid adenoma and carcinoma

- Single enlarged gland
- Rim of compressed parathyroid tissue ⟶

- Other glands not enlarged
- Microscopically normal

B. Parathyroid hyperplasia (primary or secondary)

- Four enlarged glands usually uniformly enlarged

C. "Ectopic PTH" syndromes

- Parathyroid glands normal in size

- Nonparathyroid source of PTH or PTH-like hormone, eg, lung carcinoma

D. Cases causing diagnostic difficulty at surgery (10%)

- Two or 3 glands enlarged
- One or 2 normal in size

- ? Multiple adenomas
- ? Irregular hyperplasia

Figure 59–1. Operative findings in hyperparathyroidism. In cases that are atypical, where 2 or 3 glands are enlarged (D), the diagnosis is facilitated by biopsy of a normal-appearing gland. In adenoma, this will be a histologically normal gland; in hyperplasia, it will be histologically abnormal.

Clinical Features & Diagnosis (Table 59–2)

A. Primary hyperparathyroidism is characterized by elevated serum PTH, elevated serum calcium, and decreased serum phosphate (Table 59–2).

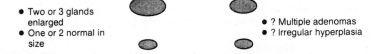 The degree of elevation of serum calcium is usually not great, being in the 11–12 mg/dL range (normal = 9–11 mg/dL).

- When serum calcium and PTH levels are considered together, the PTH level is seen to be inappropriately increased.
- In rare patients with parathyroid carcinoma, serum calcium levels may be very high (15–20 mg/dL).
- Determination of the active N-terminal PTH is more accurate than total serum PTH level.
- Urinary calculi of calcium phosphate type occur in 25% of patients with primary hyperparathyroidism.
- Metastatic calcification occurs as a result of elevated serum levels of ionized calcium in:
  - The renal interstitium (nephrocalcinosis), causing renal failure.
  - The walls of small blood vessels throughout the body, causing ischemic changes.
- Increased calcium levels also interfere with cellular function:
  - In the distal convoluted tubule, resulting in inability to concentrate urine and causing polyuria, nocturia, and thirst.
  - In the nervous system, causing disturbances in level of consciousness, convulsions, and coma.
  - In the heart, producing arrhythmias and electrocardiographic abnormalities.
- Bone changes are characteristic and may be the presenting feature. They include:
  - Osteoporosis, fibrosis of the intertrabecular zone, and cyst formation (osteitis fibrosa cystica).
  - Compensatory osteoblastic proliferation causes elevation of serum alkaline phosphatase.
  - Brown tumors, which are solid masses of osteoclastic giant cells, fibroblasts, and collagen.

B. Secondary hyperparathyroidism is characterized by normal or slightly decreased serum calcium with high PTH (Table 59–2) and low serum phosphate levels.

- Bone changes caused by high PTH concentrations are similar to those in primary hyperparathyroidism.
- A few patients have high serum calcium levels and are liable to develop all the renal, vascular, and neurologic complications that are caused by hypercalcemia.

Treatment

Treatment of severe hypercalcemia is a medical emergency because death may occur from neurologic or cardiac dysfunction.

- Control of hypercalcemia is by:
  - Hydration with saline solution, which is usually adequate.
  - Diuretics, which may increase calcium excretion.
  - Mithramycin, which inhibits bone resorption—but this toxic drug should only be used in the short term.
- The definitive treatment of symptomatic hyperparathyroidism is surgery:
  - If one gland is found to be enlarged and the others normal, the diagnosis of parathyroid adenoma may be made and the involved gland excised.
  - If more than one gland is enlarged, a diagnosis of parathyroid hyperplasia is made, and three and a half glands are removed.

TABLE 59–2. PATHOLOGIC ABNORMALITIES IN DISEASES ASSOCIATED WITH ABNORMAL CALCIUM AND PHOSPHORUS METABOLISM

	Size of Parathyroid Glands	Serum Ca	Serum Phosphate	Serum PTH	Alkaline Phosphatase	Urine Ca	Urine cAMP[1]	Comments
Primary Hyperparathyroidism Adenoma	Only 1 enlarged	↑	↓	↑	↑	↑	↑	Bone lesions and urinary calculi, peptic ulcer, metastatic calcification
Hyperplasia	All 4 large	↑	↓	↑	↑	↑	↑	Bone lesions and urinary calculi, peptic ulcer, metastatic calcification
Ectopic parathyroid hormone (PTH)	All 4 normal	↑↑	↓	↑[2]	N(↑)	↑	↑	Bone lesions, calculi rare; underlying malignant neoplasm
Secondary Hyperparathyroidism	All 4 large	N, ↑ or ↓	N(↓ ↑)	↑	N(↑)	N ↑ →	↑	Features of underlying disease[3]
Other causes of hypercalcemia Lytic metastases to bone, including myeloma	All 4 normal	↑	↑	↓	↑	↑	↓	Caused by (a) bone lysis, (b) production of vitamin D-like molecule by tumor, (c) production of osteoclast-activating factor (myeloma)

Sarcoidosis	All 4 normal	←	←	→	N(↑)	←	→	Systemic granulomas: hypersensitivity to vitamin D with high 1,25-(OH)$_2$D$_3$ levels[4]
Vitamin D intoxication	All 4 normal	←	←	→	N	←	→	Elevated 25(OH)D levels
Milk-alkali syndrome	All 4 normal	←	←	→	N	←	→	Associated with alkalosis
Familial hypercalcemia with hypocalciuria	All 4 slightly enlarged	←	→	←	N	→	←	Autosomal dominant
Hypoparathyroidism Idiopathic	All 4 normal	→	←	→	N	N→	→	Metastatic calcification
Pseudo-	All 4 normal	→	←	N↑	N	N→	→	Albright's dystrophy

[1] Urine cAMP is increased when there is excessive renal cell stimulation by PTH or PTH-like hormones that combine with cell membrane PTH receptors.

[2] In most cases PTH-like hormone is not detected by PTH assays; PTH levels may then be decreased.

[3] Findings vary with underlying causal disease (see Table 59–1).

[4] Vitamin D is converted in the liver to 25(OH)D(hydroxycholecalciferol), which is further changed to biologically active 1,25-(OH)$_2$D$_3$(dihydroxycholecalciferol) in the kidney; this latter step appears to be accelerated in sarcoidosis.

- Parathyroid tissue may be cryopreserved for later reimplantation in case hypoparathyroidism develops after surgery.
- If a diagnosis of adenoma or hyperplasia cannot be made after neck exploration, a search must be made for ectopic parathyroid tissue:
  - In the mediastinum.
  - Within the substance of the thyroid gland.

DECREASED PTH SECRETION (Hypoparathyroidism)

Etiology & Pathology
A. Hypoparathyroidism complicating neck surgery:

- Neck surgery (usually total thyroidectomy) is the commonest cause of hypoparathyroidism.
- Two to 10 percent of patients undergoing total thyroidectomy develop permanent hypoparathyroidism after surgery.
- Postoperative hypoparathyroidism results from:
  - Accidental removal of multiple glands.
  - Infarction of the glands, caused by interference with their arterial supply during surgery.

B. Idiopathic hypoparathyroidism is a rare disease with slight female predominance.

- It is believed to be the result of autoimmune destruction of the parathyroid cells.
- Parathyroid-specific autoantibodies are demonstrable in about 40% of patients.
- There is an association with other autoimmune diseases, such as pernicious anemia, Addison's disease, and Hashimoto's thyroiditis.
- Microscopically, there is atrophy of parathyroid cells, lymphocytic infiltration, and fibrosis.

C. Congenital absence of parathyroids is a result of generalized failure of development of the third and fourth branchial arches.

- It is associated with thymic agenesis and marked deficiency of cellular immunity (DiGeorge's syndrome; see Chapter 7).
- Patients with congenital absence of parathyroids present with hypocalcemia and convulsions soon after birth.

D. Pseudohypoparathyroidism is a group of rare inherited disorders characterized by lack of end-organ response to PTH due to abnormal PTH receptors.

- There is clinical hypoparathyroidism, but serum PTH levels are normal.
- Both autosomal and X-linked inheritance have been reported.
- Pseudohypoparathyroidism is commonly associated with Albright's osteodystrophy, which is characterized by short stature, short neck, abnormally developed metacarpal and metatarsal bones, and subcutaneous ossification.
- Rarely, these skeletal abnormalities are present in a patient who has no evidence of clinical hypoparathyroidism (psuedopseudohypoparathyroidism).

Clinical Features & Diagnosis (Table 59–2)

Hypoparathyroidism is characterized by decreased serum levels of ionized calcium, which cause:

- Increased irritability of nerves, leading to numbness and tingling of the hands, feet, and lips.
- Tetany, which is manifested as carpopedal spasms.
- Laryngeal spasm may cause respiratory obstruction.
- Trousseau's sign and Chvostek's sign are positive.
- Generalized convulsions, particularly in children.
- Serum phosphate is increased because of defective renal excretion of phosphate when PTH is deficient. High phosphate levels are associated with:
  - Increased bone density.
  - Calcification of the basal ganglia.
  - Mineral deposition in the lens to form cataracts.

Treatment

Treatment consists of correction of hypocalcemia by the administration of vitamin D analogues and by ensuring adequate intake of calcium in the diet.

The Adrenal Cortex & Medulla

60

CONGENITAL ADRENAL HYPERPLASIA

This is a group of uncommon diseases that result from inherited deficiency of one of the several enzymes in the cortisol synthetic pathway.

- Decreased secretion of cortisol stimulates pituitary ACTH secretion, leading to hyperplasia of the zona fasciculata and reticularis.
- There is excessive secretion of precursor hormones.
- Clinical effects depend on the enzyme that is deficient and upon the products that accumulate prior to the block induced by the deficiency.

Complete 21-hydroxylase deficiency

This accounts for 30% of cases of congenital adrenal hyperplasia. It is a severe disease manifested in early childhood by failure of cortisol and aldosterone secretion (Fig 60–1). There is marked sodium loss in urine, leading to severe hypotension. Increased androgen synthesis from the 17-hydroxyprogesterone that accumulates results in virilism in females.

Partial 21-hydroxylase deficiency

This accounts for 60% of cases. It is the commonest type of congenital adrenal hyperplasia.

- 21-Hydroxylase levels are adequate to maintain normal aldosterone secretion under the renin-angiotensin stimulus, so that there is no sodium loss.
- Cortisol levels are also normal, the tendency to hypocortisolism having been compensated by adrenal hyperplasia via increased pituitary ACTH levels.
- The main effects of partial 21-hydroxylase deficiency are:
  - Bilateral adrenal hyperplasia.
  - High serum ACTH levels.
  - Increased secretion of androgens by the overstimulated zona reticularis, producing virilism in the female and precocious puberty in the male.
- Diagnosis is by detecting elevated serum levels of 17-hydroxyprogesterone and androgens.

11-Hydroxylase deficiency

This is rare, accounting for 5% of cases. The enzyme deficiency leads to accumulation of 11-deoxycortisol and deoxycorticosterone, both of which are strong mineralocorticoids.

- It is characterized by sodium retention and hypertension.

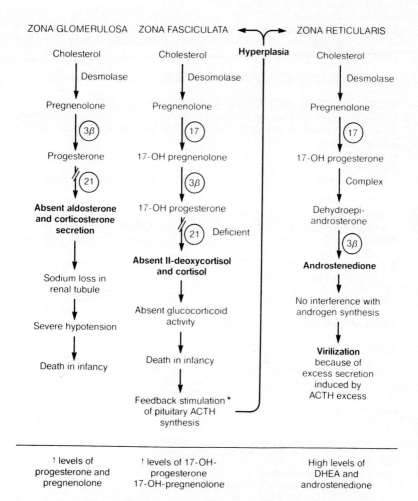

Figure 60–1. Pattern of abnormal steroid synthesis in a patient with complete 21-hydroxylase deficiency. Patients with complete 21-hydroxylase deficiency die in early life as a result of failure of synthesis of both mineralocorticoids and glucocorticoids. Note that partial 21-hydroxylase deficiency which is compatible with longer survival is more common.

- Virilization due to androgen excess is also present as a result of increased ACTH stimulation of the zone reticularis.

Other enzyme deficiencies

These are extremely rare. They include deficiency of desmolase, 17-hydroxylase, and 3β-dehydrogenase.

EXCESS SECRETION OF ADRENOCORTICAL HORMONES

EXCESS CORTISOL SECRETION (CUSHING'S SYNDROME)

Cushing's syndrome is a relatively common clinical abnormality, usually affecting middle-aged individuals, women more often than men. It is caused by several different diseases (Table 60–1).

Pathology

    A. Adrenocortical adenoma accounts for 25% of cases of Cushing's syndrome.

- Grossly, adrenocortical adenomas appear as well-circumscribed nodular masses that are usually small (<5 cm in greatest diameter and 5–50 g in weight). They are bright yellow and may show areas of cystic degeneration, fibrosis, and hemorrhage.
- Microscopically, adenomas are composed of uniform large clear cells with small nuclei arranged in nests and trabeculae.
- Pathologic examination does not permit differentiation of nonfunctioning adenomas and those that secrete different hormones.

    B. Adrenocortical carcinoma is a rare cause of Cushing's syndrome. They are large (>6 cm and >50 g), poorly circumscribed masses that commonly show infiltration of the kidney, perinephric fat, and adrenal vein.

- Microscopically, adrenal carcinomas are composed of large, pleomorphic cells arranged in diffuse sheets. Mitotic figures are frequent and abnormal. Areas of necrosis, capsular invasion, and vascular invasion are common.

TABLE 60–1. ETIOLOGY OF EXCESS CORTISOL SECRETION

Iatrogenic
Glucocorticoid administered in high doses in the treatment of nonendocrine diseases
Noniatrogenic
Functioning adrenocortical neoplasms (25%)
Adenoma (20%)
Carcinoma (5%)
Bilateral adrenal hyperplasia (75%)
ACTH-secreting pituitary adenoma (60%)
ACTH-secreting nonpituitary neoplasms (ectopic ACTH syndrome; 15%)

ACTH = adrenocorticotropic hormone.

- The pathologic features of nonfunctioning carcinomas are similar to those that secrete hormones.
- Adrenal carcinoma behaves as a highly malignant neoplasm, metastasizing both to lymph nodes and via the bloodstream.

C. Bilateral adrenal hyperplasia is the commonest cause of Cushing's syndrome.
- It is almost always secondary to increased ACTH production, either from:
  - A corticotroph adenoma of the pituitary (common).
  - A malignant nonpituitary neoplasm (usually small-cell undifferentiated carcinoma of lung).
- Both adrenal glands are enlarged to greater than their aggregate upper weight limit of 8 gm. The enlarged glands may be nodular or diffuse.
- Microscopically, the zona fasciculata and reticularis are greatly widened.

D. Iatrogenic hypercortisolism: In cases where hypercortisolism is the result of exogenous glucocorticoid administration, both adrenal cortices show diffuse atrophy due to inhibition of pituitary ACTH secretion.

Clinical Features
Cortisol excess causes an extensive array of metabolic abnormalities:

- Redistribution of body fat from the extremities to the trunk results in moon facies, truncal obesity and thin extremities.
- Hypercholesterolemia and aggravated atherosclerosis. The insulin antagonistic effect of cortisol produces diabetes mellitus.
- Protein catabolism is increased, leading to muscle wasting. Growth retardation occurs in children.
- Thinning of the skin with development of striae, easy bruising, and delayed wound healing.
- Osteoporosis.
- Retention of sodium in the distal renal tubule at the expense of potassium and hydrogen causes hypertension and hypokalemic alkalosis.
- Inhibitory effect on lymphocyte, macrophage, and neutrophil function, results in increased susceptibility to infections.
- Psychiatric symptoms such as euphoria, mania, and psychosis (steroid encephalopathy).
- Androgen excess often coexists with cortisol excess in many patients, leading to hirsutism, acne, infertility, and menstrual disturbances in females.

Diagnosis (Table 60–2)
The first step in the diagnosis is to establish the presence of excess cortisol secretion.

- Plasma levels of cortisol and its metabolites, the 17-hydroxycorticosteroids, are high.
- The 24-hour urinary free cortisol level is elevated.
- The diurnal rhythm of cortisol secretion is lost. A high cortisol level in a midnight sample is typical.
- Once it has been established that a given patient has hypercortisolism, it is necessary to determine the cause.

TABLE 60–2. LABORATORY DIAGNOSIS OF CUSHING'S SYNDROME

Step A: Establishment of presence of hypercortisolism
Plasma cortisol: elevated
Loss of normal diurnal variation: high level in a midnight sample when cortisol
levels are normally very low

Urinary 24-hour free cortisol level is elevated: a very good screening test

Low-dose 2-day dexamethasone suppression:
Suppresses plasma cortisol in all but patients with Cushing's syndrome[1]

Step B: Differential diagnosis of Cushing's syndrome

	Plasma ACTH[2]	Suppression With High-Dose Dexamethasone[1]	CT Scan Findings
Pituitary-induced adrenal hyperplasia	Elevated	Yes	Pituitary adenoma (may be small); bilateral adrenal hyperplasia
Adrenal adenoma	Low	No	Adrenal neoplasm: small
Adrenal carcinoma	Low	No	Adrenal neoplasm: large
Ectopic ACTH[2] production	Very high	No	Bilateral adrenal hyperplasia; normal pituitary; some other malignant neoplasm

[1]Dexamethasone is a synthetic glucocorticoid that suppresses ACTH secretion. At low doses suppression is not adequate to decrease excess cortisol secretion in any patient with Cushing's syndrome. At high doses it suppresses excessive ACTH secretion by pituitary adenomas.
[2]ACTH = adrenocorticotropic hormone.

- Plasma ACTH is elevated in patients with pituitary adenoma and ectopic ACTH syndrome.
- High-dose dexamethazone suppression test permits distinction between adrenocortical neoplasms and pituitary induced adrenal hyperplasia.
- Radiologic studies of the pituitary and adrenal are sensitive in detecting neoplasms.

Treatment
Functioning adrenal neoplasms and pituitary neoplasms that produce ACTH are surgically removed. In the ectopic ACTH syndrome, therapy is aimed at the tumor responsible, eg, chemotherapy for small-cell carcinoma of the lung.

EXCESS ALDOSTERONE SECRETION

Incidence & Etiology
A. Primary hyperaldosteronism (Conn's syndrome) is a rare disease.

- Most commonly, it is the result of an aldosterone-secreting adrenocortical adenoma.

- Less commonly, it may result from bilateral hyperplasia of the zona glomerulosa.
- Adrenal carcinomas only very rarely secrete aldosterone.
- In a few cases of hyperaldosteronism, no definite abnormality is detected in the gland.

B. Secondary hyperaldosteronism is very common.

- It is caused by a high renin output from the juxtaglomerular cells of the kidney in response to:
  - Renal ischemia, such as occurs in renal artery stenosis and malignant hypertension.
  - Reduced effective plasma volume, as occurs in cardiac failure and hypoproteinemic states.
  - Juxtaglomerular cell hyperplasia (Bartter's syndrome) or neoplasia.

Pathology

- Aldosterone-producing adenomas are indistinguishable from adenomas that produce cortisol except that they tend to be smaller (usually <2 cm in diameter).
- The adrenals appear grossly normal in patients with secondary hyperaldosteronism. Microscopic demonstration of hyperplasia of the zona glomerulosa is difficult.

Clinical Features

Aldosterone causes sodium retention in the distal renal tubule in exchange for potassium and hydrogen ions, resulting in hypertension and hypokalemic alkalosis. Less than 1% of patients with hypertension have primary hyperaldosteronism.

- Hypokalemia may cause muscle weakness, fatigue, paralyses, and paresthesias.
- Alkalosis may cause a decrease in serum ionized calcium, leading to tetany.
- Secondary hyperaldosteronism causes sodium retention, contributing to edema in many cases. Hypokalemic alkalosis may also be present.
- Edema is uncommon in primary hyperaldosteronism.

Diagnosis

The diagnosis of primary hyperaldosteronism may be suspected in any hypertensive patient who has hypokalemia without an apparent cause. The combination of elevated serum aldosterone and low serum renin is characteristic of primary aldosteronism.

- Salt-loading tests and furosemide stimulation tests are being less widely used.
- Preoperative localization of the adrenal adenoma responsible for primary hyperaldosteronism is by:
  - Computerized tomography, which is successful in demonstrating the adrenal adenoma in about 95% of cases.
  - Measurement of adrenal vein aldosterone, which is elevated on the side of the adenoma.
  - Iodocholesterol scan. Iodocholesterol (tagged with radioiodine) is taken up by the zona glomerulosa and delineates an adenoma (unilateral) and hyperplasia (bilateral).

Treatment

Primary hyperaldosteronism is best treated by surgical removal of the adrenal gland that contains the adenoma. Aldosterone antagonist drugs (eg, spironolactone) are useful in the management of patients with secondary hyperaldosteronism.

EXCESS SEX HORMONE SECRETION

Excessive secretion of sex hormones by the adrenals is very rare.

- Excess androgen secretion may be due to:
  - Adrenocortical neoplasms (particularly carcinomas).
  - Congenital adrenal hyperplasia.
  - Cushing's syndrome, where androgen excess is associated with cortisol excess.
- Excessive estrogen secretion occurs very rarely with adrenocortical carcinomas.

DECREASED SECRETION OF ADRENOCORTICAL HORMONES (Addison's Disease)

Etiology

A. Acute insufficiency (Addisonian crisis) may follow destruction of the adrenal glands in severe bacteremias, most commonly meningococcal bacteremia (Waterhouse-Friderichsen syndrome).

- Most commonly seen today in patients on high-dose glucocorticoids which suppress ACTH and result in atrophy of the adrenal cortex. Crises occur:
  - If there is a sudden increased demand for cortisol (as during stress or an infection).
  - If the exogenous steroids are withdrawn rapidly.

B. Chronic insufficiency (Addison's disease): Autoimmune destruction of the adrenal gland is the commonest cause of Addison's disease in developed countries. Fifty percent of these patients have antiadrenal antibodies in their serum.

- Other causes:
  - Infections, such as tuberculosis and histoplasmosis.
  - Metastatic carcinoma, particularly lung carcinoma.
  - Metabolic diseases such as hemochromatosis and amyloidosis.
  - Congenital adrenal hyperplasia, particularly that due to complete 21-hydroxylase deficiency.
  - Deficient ACTH secretion in hypopituitarism.

Pathology

When the adrenals are the site of a disease (tuberculosis, fungal infection, metastatic carcinoma, hemochromatosis, amyloidosis, etc), the gland shows the specific morphologic features associated with those disorders. In autoimmune Addison's disease, the adrenals are markedly atrophic, with fibrosis and lymphocytic infiltration.

Clinical Features

The dominant clinical features of Addison's disease are caused by decreased mineralocorticoid activity.

- Sodium loss in the kidney results in hyponatremia, contraction of plasma volume, and hypotension.

- Serum chloride is decreased.
- There is hyperkalemic acidosis.
- Hyperkalemia may cause muscular weakness and electrocardiographic abnormalities.
- A decreased cortisol level in plasma does not cause immediate symptoms. Addisonian crisis may be precipitated by stresses such as infections, surgery, and trauma.
- Plasma ACTH levels are increased by feedback. This causes increased skin pigmentation.

THE ADRENAL MEDULLA

Neoplasms represent the only significant diseases of the adrenal medulla (Table 60-3).

PHEOCHROMOCYTOMA (Paraganglioma)

Pheochromocytoma is a catecholamine-producing neoplasm of the adrenal medulla or extra-adrenal paraganglia. It is an uncommon neoplasm.

- It usually occurs sporadically, but occasional patients give a positive family history for:
  - Familial pheochromocytoma, with an autosomal dominant pattern of inheritance, is very rare.
  - Generalized neurofibromatosis (von Recklinghausen's disease).
  - Multiple endocrine neoplasia types IIa and IIb (see following).

TABLE 60-3. PRIMARY NEOPLASMS OF THE ADRENAL MEDULLA

	Pheochromocytoma	Ganglioneuroma	Neuroblastoma[1]
Age	Adults	Adults/children	Children
Biologic behavior	90% benign; 10% malignant	Benign	Highly malignant
Secretion	High levels of catecholamines	Slight increase in catecholamines	Slight increase in catecholamines
Clinical presentation	Hypertension, sweating, palpitations	Abdominal mass	Abdominal mass, metastases
Macroscopic features	Mass, often hemorrhagic	Solid, firm mass	Mass, often necrotic
Microscopic features	Nests of large cells, vascular	Ganglion cells and neural tissue	Primitive small neuroblasts
Immunohistochemical markers	Chromogranin, NSE[2]	S100 protein	NSE[2]

[1]Neuroblastomas may spontaneously show evidence of maturation characterized by the appearance of multinucleated ganglion cells. The end result of maturation resembles a benign ganglioneuroma and has a benign biologic behavior.
[2]NSE = neuron-specific enolase.

Pathology

Pheochromocytoma occurs most commonly in the adrenal medulla. Ten percent of pheochromocytomas occur in extra-adrenal paraganglia—most often intra-abdominal, occasionally in the mediastinum, neck, or wall of the urinary bladder.

- Ten percent of patients with pheochromocytoma have multiple tumors, most commonly involving both adrenal glands but also the extra-adrenal paraganglia.
- Most pheochromocytomas behave as benign neoplasms, but 10% are malignant, with metastasis.
- Pheochromocytomas vary in size from very small (1 cm) to massive tumors, are well circumscribed, and frequently show areas of hemorrhage and necrosis.
- Microscopically, the tumor consists of large, often pleomorphic cells arranged in sheets and nests separated by a rich vascular stroma.
- Invasion of capsule and vessels is common even in those neoplasms that behave in a benign fashion.
- Electron microscopy shows membrane-bound, dense-core neurosecretory granules in the cytoplasm.
- Immunologic studies show markers for neuroendocrine cells such as neuron-specific enolase and chromogranin.
- The biologic behavior of a pheochromocytoma cannot be predicted by pathologic examination.
- Diagnosis of malignant pheochromocytoma is made only when metastasis is demonstrated.

Clinical Features

The clinical manifestations are due to increased catecholamine secretion.

- Hypertension is the commonest presenting feature. Hypertension is commonly persistent but may be paroxysmal, with return of the blood pressure to normal between paroxysms.
- Paroxysms of hypertension are caused by sudden release of hormone from the neoplasm and may be precipitated by:
  - Postural changes such as bending.
  - Increased abdominal pressure (as during physical examination).
  - Meals.
  - Angiographic studies.
  - Micturition in those rare cases in the bladder wall.
- During a hypertensive crisis, the systolic pressure can rise to 300 mm Hg.
- Hypertension is accompanied by other manifestations of catecholamine excess such as:
  - Palpitations and tachycardia. Feelings of anxiety and panic.
  - Excessive sweating.
- Impaired glucose tolerance (diabetes mellitus) is common, as a result of the insulin-antagonistic action of catecholamines.
- Untreated, patients with pheochromocytomas die of cardiac failure or cerebral hemorrhage during a hypertensive crisis.

Diagnosis

Patients with hypertension—particularly if they are under age 40—must be evaluated for the possibility of pheochromocytoma.

- The best screening tests are urinary metanephrine and vanillylmandelic acid, one or both of which is elevated in almost all cases.
- The diagnosis may be confirmed by urinary and serum catecholamine assays.
- Localization of the neoplasm or neoplasms by radiologic studies is very accurate.

Treatment

It is treated by surgical removal of the tumor. Surgical removal is a complex procedure that requires sympathetic blockade, expert anesthesiologic support, and meticulous fluid balance. Removal of the neoplasm may cause a sudden drop in blood pressure. If some fall in blood pressure does not occur at surgery, the possibility of a second pheochromocytoma must be suspected.

NEUROBLASTOMA

This is a malignant neoplasm composed of primitive neural crest cells. It occurs chiefly in very young children. The median age is 2 years, and 80% of cases occur under the age of 5 years. Neuroblastoma is rare past puberty.

- The adrenal medulla is by far the most common site, followed by neural crest derivatives in the retroperitoneum.
- Neuroblastoma is the third most common malignant neoplasm in childhood, following leukemia-lymphoma and nephroblastoma.
- Most cases are sporadic. Very rarely, neuroblastoma occurs in families.

Genetic Abnormalities

Most cases of neuroblastoma show a near-terminal deletion of part of the short arm of chromosome 1 (partial monosomy 1).

- Chromosome 2 frequently shows a dense homogeneously stained region (HSR).
- Multiple double-minute (DM) chromatin bodies may be observed apart from the chromosomes (Fig 60–2).
- Both HSR and DM chromatin bodies are believed to represent amplification sites of an oncogene (N-*MYC*).

Pathology

- Grossly, neuroblastomas tend to be very large infiltrative tumors. They are soft and friable and often show extensive hemorrhage and necrosis.
- Microscopically, the primitive neuroblastic cells are arranged in diffuse sheets with very little intervening stroma. The formation of rosettes is characteristic.
- Electron microscopy shows neurosecretory granules in the cytoplasm.
- Immunohistochemical studies show positivity for neuron-specific enolase.
- Maturation is signified by the presence of large multinucleated ganglion cells (ganglioneuroblastoma).

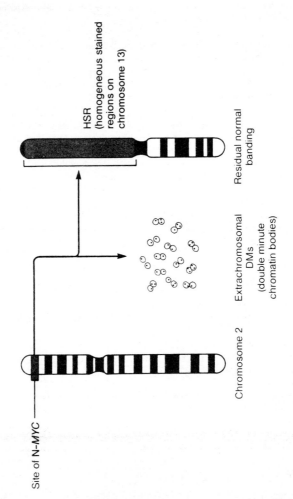

Figure 60–2. Effects of N-*MYC* oncogene amplification in human neuroblastoma. N-*MYC*, which is normally present on the short arm of chromosome 2, becomes amplified either as extrachromosomal double minute (DM) chromatin bodies or as a chromosomally integrated homogeneously stained region (HSR). In this figure, the HSR is shown on chromosome 13.

Clinical Features

Most patients with neuroblastoma present with an enlarging mass in the abdomen.

- Seventy-five percent of patients have slightly increased catecholamine secretion. Clinical evidence of catecholamine excess is rare.
- Hematogenous dissemination occurs very early. Bone, liver and bone marrow are favored sites of metastasis.

Treatment & Prognosis

Treatment is with combined surgery, chemotherapy, and radiation.

- Surgery is necessary to provide tissue for diagnosis and reduce tumor bulk.
- The increased effectiveness of chemotherapy has greatly improved the survival statistics.
- The prognosis of a patient with neuroblastoma depends on:
  - The age at presentation. The younger the patient, the better the prognosis. Patients under 2 years have a high survival rate.
  - The clinical stage of the disease (see following).
- Histologic evidence of ganglionic differentiation is a good prognostic sign.
- Amplification of N-*MYC* oncogene in the cancer cells is a bad prognostic sign.
- Neuroblastomas are staged as follows (according to the degree of spread of tumor):
  - Stage I: Tumor confined to the organ of origin.
  - Stage II: Local spread, confined to one side.
  - Stage III: Local spread across the midline, with involved regional lymph nodes.
  - Stage IV: Distant metastasis.

MULTIPLE ENDOCRINE NEOPLASIA SYNDROMES

The multiple endocrine neoplasia (MEN) or multiple endocrine adenomatosis (MEA) syndromes are characterized by the familial occurrence of multiple endocrine neoplasms. They are rare and are inherited as an autosomal dominant trait with variable penetrance.

1. MEN (MEA) TYPE I

Type I consists of pituitary adenoma, parathyroid hyperplasia or adenoma, and pancreatic islet cell neoplasms, including gastrinoma. Peptic ulcers also occur in these patients, probably related to gastrin production (Zollinger-Ellison syndrome).

2. MEN TYPE IIa (Sipple syndrome)

Type IIa consists of medullary carcinoma and parafollicular cell hyperplasia of the thyroid and adrenal medullary hyperplasia or pheochromocytoma. Parathyroid hyperplasia or adenoma may also be present.

3. MEN TYPE IIb

Type IIb is a subgroup of MEN type II that is associated with mucocutaneous (tongue, eyelids, bronchus, intestine) neuromas in addition to the thyroid and adrenal neoplasms. This is sometimes also called MEN type III.

TABLE 60–4. "APUDOMAS" (NEUROENDOCRINE TUMORS)

Site	Tumor	Secretory Products[1]
Anterior pituitary	Pituitary adenoma	GH, ACTH, prolactin, FSH, LH, TSH
Bronchus	Carcinoid, small cell undifferentiated carcinoma	5HT, ACTH, ADH, parathormone
Gastrointestinal tract	Carcinoid	5HT, VIP, gastrin
Pancreas	Islet cell adenoma and carcinoma	Insulin, glucagon, VIP, PP, somatostatin, 5HT, ACTH, bombesin
Thyroid	Medullary carcinoma	Calcitonin
Parathyroid	Adenoma, carcinoma	Parathormone
Adrenal medulla and autonomic ganglia	Pheochromocytoma, neuroblastoma	Catecholamines
Paraganglia, glomus jugulare, carotid body	Paraganglioma, glomus tumor, chemodectoma	Catecholamines
Skin	Merkel cell tumor	Calcitonin, parathormone

[1]GH = growth hormone; ACTH = adrenocorticotropic hormone; FSH = follicle-stimulating hormone; LH = luteinizing hormone; TSH = thyroid-stimulating hormone; 5HT = 5-hydroxytryptamine; ADH = antidiuretic hormone; VIP = vasoactive intestinal polypeptide; PP = pancreatic polypeptide.

THE APUD (NEUROENDOCRINE CELL) SYSTEM

The occurrence of multiple neoplasms involving several endocrine glands as a consequence of the inheritance of a single abnormal gene suggests that these cells are related in some way.

- The terms *APUD* or *neuroendocrine cell system* have been applied to these interrelated cells.
- These cells are distributed throughout the body in virtually all organs.
- They have certain characteristics in common:
  - They are believed to be derived embryologically from neuroectodermal cells of the neural crest.
  - They have the ability to take up amine precursors and possess a decarboxylase that converts these into amines. Hence the acronym **APUD** for **amine precursor uptake and decarboxylation.**
  - They secrete physiologically active amines (serotonin, catecholamines) or polypeptide hormones.

- They contain membrane-bound dense-core neurosecretory granules in their cytoplasm, by electron microscopy.
- By immunoperoxidase techniques, they stain positively for neuroendocrine markers such as neuron-specific enolase and chromogranin.

APUDomas (neuroendocrine tumors)

These are neoplasms derived from neuroendocrine (APUD) cells and retain the features that characterize these cells. They are classified by the cell of origin or the principal cell product (Table 60–4).

Section XIV. The Skin

Diseases of the Skin   **61**

MANIFESTATIONS OF SKIN DISEASE

General Responses

Acute inflammation may involve the epidermis and the dermis.

- Accumulation of fluid in the epidermis between the keratinocytes is called spongiosis. Extreme spongiosis leads to a vesicle (a localized fluid collection).
- Dermal swelling causes elevation of the epidermis (wheal formation).
- Epidermal necrosis leads to ulceration.
- Dermal necrosis produces a variety of clinical appearances depending on the structures involved and the extent of necrosis.
- The changes of chronic inflammation in the skin are less obvious, but include thickening of the epidermis (acanthosis), thickening of the stratum corneum (hyperkeratosis), and dermal fibrosis.

Specific Responses

The skin may show a variety of specific changes (Table 61–1). These responses in varying combinations produce the histologic changes seen in the various skin diseases.

INFECTIONS OF THE SKIN

BACTERIAL INFECTIONS

Impetigo

This is a superficial epidermal infection caused by *Staphylococcus aureus*. Streptococci may also be present, probably as secondary invaders.

- Most commonly, it occurs in children—particularly on the face, whence it may spread by scratching.
- Transmission is by direct contact. Impetigo is highly contagious.
- Grossly, it begins as a pustule (a blister filled with pus) that ruptures to form the typical thick, yellow, translucent crust.
- Microscopically, the pustule is in the superficial part of the epidermis.
- Antibiotic therapy leads to rapid healing without scarring.
- Neonatal impetigo:
  - Is an extremely serious specific variant in infants caused by strains of staphylococci that produce an epidermolytic toxin.

TABLE 61–1. SKIN RESPONSES TO INJURY

Response	Terminology	Clinical Appearance
Hyperplasia of keratinocytes → thickening of the epidermis	Acanthosis	Diffuse thickening or localized elevated plaque (papule)
Increased rate of maturation of keratinocyte → thickening of stratum corneum	Hyperkeratosis	Silvery surface scales
Increased rate of maturation of keratinocytes with premature shedding → nucleated cells in stratum corneum	Parakeratosis	None
Abnormal keratinization	Dyskeratosis	None
Epidermal atrophy → thin epidermis	Atrophy	Thinning of skin
Degeneration of basal layer	. . .	Subepidermal vesicle[1]
Separation of epidermal cells	Acantholysis	Intraepidermal vesicle[1]
Epidermal edema	Spongiosis	Intraepidermal vesicle[1]
Dysplasia of keratinocytes	Dysplasia	Papule[2]
Inflammatory cells in epidermis	Exocytosis	None
Epidermal abscess formation	Pustule	Pus-filled vesicle[1]
Dermal inflammation, edema	. . .	Macule;[2] wheal
Dermal hemorrhage	. . .	Petechiae, purpura

[1]Vesicles appear clinically as blisters, or bullae (see Table 61–3).
[2]Macule = a change in the skin that is flat and level with the skin surface; papule = an elevated, flat lesion.

- Bullae extend and enlarge, resulting in denudation of large areas of the superficial epidermis ("scalded skin syndrome").

Hair Follicle Infections
Folliculitis is extremely common, occurring in any part of the body where there is hair, often the face and upper trunk.

- *Staphylococcus aureus* is the usual pathogen.
- Acute inflammation with pain, swelling, and erythema is followed by abscess formation (furuncle).
- A carbuncle:
  - Is a much more serious infection that begins as a folliculitis, but spreads deep and laterally to form a large inflammatory mass with multiple areas of suppuration.
  - Commonly occurs in diabetics.

Acne Vulgaris

While not primarily an infection, the lesions of acne vulgaris frequently become infected by low-grade pathogens such as *Propionibacterium acnes*.

- The lesion of acne vulgaris is the comedo, which consists of a pilosebaceous structure plugged with keratin and lipids.
- Secondary infection is common and may cause an abscess very similar to a furuncle.
- Acne affects most adolescents at about the age of puberty.
- Its cause is uncertain. Elevated sex hormone levels at puberty may be involved.

Hidradenitis Suppurativa

This is a staphylococcal infection of apocrine glands associated with acute suppurative inflammation with abscess formation. The axillas and anogenital regions are the usual sites. Recurrent infection leads to chronic disease with increasing fibrous scarring and recurrent abscesses.

Erysipelas

This is an acute, spreading inflammation of the skin, commonly of the face or scalp.

- It is usually caused by streptococci.
- The involved skin is red, hot, swollen, and thickened.
- The dermis shows hyperemia and neutrophil infiltration. Abscess formation does not occur.
- Patients have systemic signs of acute inflammation, with high fever.

Cellulitis

Cellulitis is a rapidly spreading acute inflammation of subcutaneous tissue, commonly occurring as a complication of wound infection.

- The usual infecting organism is *Streptococcus pyogenes*.
- The inflamed area is red, hot, and swollen.
- Bacteremia is frequent, and the patient is febrile.
- Two severe forms of necrotizing cellulitis caused by anaerobic bacteria are:
  - Ludwig's angina, affecting the floor of the mouth and neck.
  - Fournier's gangrene of the scrotum.

Necrotizing Fasciitis

This is an uncommon spreading infection of the deep subcutaneous tissue, deep fascia, and underlying skeletal muscle, most commonly affecting the extremities and abdominal wall.

- It is usually caused by anaerobic bacteria.
- It is characterized by extensive necrosis of muscle, fascia, and overlying skin. The skin shows necrosis and large bullous lesions filled with blood-stained fluid.
- The lesion spreads rapidly and requires emergent and aggressive surgical debridement.
- A specific type of necrotizing fasciitis is caused by *Vibrio vulnificans*, which is a frequent contaminant of fish in coastal waters. This is characterized by:

- A history of ingestion of raw oysters is present in 90% of the cases.
- Occurs mainly in patients with chronic liver disease.

Anthrax
This is a rare infection caused by *Bacillus anthracis,* a spore-bearing gram-positive bacillus found mainly in and around farm animals.

- It has a strong occupational relationship to industries dealing with animal products and hides (farming, textile and leather industries).
- Ninety-five percent of cases are cutaneous as a result of skin inoculation. Five percent are pulmonary due to inhalation of spores.
- It causes a severe necrotizing hemorrhagic acute inflammation of the skin.
- Clinically, it is characterized by a large hemorrhagic blister that ruptures, leaving an ulcer with a black crust.
- The course varies from mild localized infection to severe bacteremia ending in death.

Leprosy (Hansen's Disease)
This is a common disease in tropical countries. In the United States, leprosy is seen in Southern California, Hawaii, and the southern states. It is caused by *Mycobacterium leprae.*

A. Tuberculoid leprosy (Table 61–2) occurs in patients who develop T cell immunity and hypersensitivity to the bacillus.

- The lepromin test is positive.
- Clinically, patients develop a hypopigmented hypoesthetic macule.
- Involvement of large peripheral nerves (ulnar, common peroneal, greater auricular) produces palpable thickening and nerve palsies (wristdrop and footdrop are common presenting features).
- Histologically, the skin lesion is characterized by epithelioid cell granulomas, numerous lymphocytes, and small numbers of leprosy bacilli.
- Tuberculoid leprosy has a slowly progressive course.
- It can often be successfully treated.

B. Lepromatous leprosy (Table 61–2) occurs in patients who have a low level of cellular immunity. The lepromin test is negative.

- The bacillus multiples unchecked in skin macrophages, forming large foamy "lepra cells" in which are found many acid-fast bacilli.
- Aggregation of macrophages causes thickening and nodularity of the skin.
- The bacillus also spreads via the bloodstream, causing widespread lesions in the skin, eye, upper respiratory tract, and testis.
- Internal viscera are rarely involved.
- Lepromatous leprosy is a serious disease that causes extensive destruction of tissue and disfigurement.
- Treatment is unsatisfactory.

C. Borderline leprosy has features intermediate between lepromatous and tuberculous leprosy (Table 61–2).

TABLE 61–2. CLINICOPATHOLOGIC TYPES OF LEPROSY[1]

	Lepromatous	Borderline	Tuberculoid
Cell-mediated immunity	Deficient	Intermediate	Present
Lepromin test[2]	Negative	Positive or negative	Positive
Number of lesions	Numerous	Many	Few
Visceral lesions	Common	Uncommon	Absent
Skin lesion appearance	Nodular	Variable	Macular
Hypoesthesia of lesions	Rare	Rare	Common
Number of lymphocytes	Few	Intermediate	Numerous
Number of organisms	Numerous	Many	Few
Lepra cell	Numerous	Present	Absent
Distribution of macrophages	Diffuse	Aggregates	Granulomas
Erythema nodosum leprosum	Common	May occur	Rare

[1]Leprosy is characterized by a clinicopathologic spectrum whose extremes are called lepromatous and tuberculoid leprosy. Borderline leprosy is an intermediate form. Other intermediate forms, borderline-tuberculoid and borderline-lepromatous, are also recognized.
[2]The lepromin test consists of an intradermal injection of *Mycobacterium leprae* antigens. A positive response (induration) indicates the presence of type IV hypersensitivity against leprosy antigens.

D. Reactional forms of leprosy occur in patients with lepromatous leprosy. They include:

- Erythema nodosum leprosum, which is characterized by tender erythematous skin nodules due to a panniculitis (inflammation of the subcutaneous fat).
- Lucio's phenomenon, which is a vasculitis that affects small to medium-sized arteries.

Other Mycobacterial Infections

- Rarely, tuberculosis infects the skin, causing:
  - Lupus vulgaris, in which reddish patches occur on the face.
  - Scrofuloderma, which represents skin involvement over a tuberculous lymph node, usually in the neck.
- *Mycobacterium marinum* causes a chronic granulomatous nodular or ulcerative skin lesion in skin exposed to sea water, swimming pools, and aquaria.
- *Mycobacterium ulcerans* causes **Buruli ulcer,** which is common in parts of Africa.

Spirochetal Infections
Syphilis (see Chapter 54) causes skin lesions in both early and late stages.

- Yaws:
  - Is caused by *Treponema pertenue,* is endemic in humid, tropical countries around the world.
  - Is transmitted by direct contact, and is most common in children.
  - The early stage of the disease is characterized by multiple raspberrylike papillomas of the skin that tend to heal with scarring.
  - The late stage of yaws, which occurs many years after onset, is characterized by ulcerative nodular masses resembling syphilitic gummas.
- Pinta, similar to yaws, is caused by *Treponema carateum.*

VIRAL INFECTIONS

1. EPIDERMOTROPIC VIRUSES

Viral infection of the epidermal cells leads to cellular degeneration and necrosis, resulting in formation of an intraepidermal vesicle (Fig 61-1).

- It is caused by:
  - Smallpox (variola), which has been eradicated from the world.
  - Chicken pox, caused by Herpes varicella.
  - Herpes zoster.
  - Herpes simplex, types I and II.
- The differential diagnosis between these agents is by:
  - Clinical examination, including contact and travel history, incubation period, and distribution of lesions.
  - Skin biopsy, looking for specific histologic changes such as inclusions and giant cells (Fig 61-1).
  - Demonstration of antigens by immunohistochemical techniques.
  - Demonstration of virus by electron microscopy.
  - Viral culture.
  - Serologic testing to detect the specific antibody response.

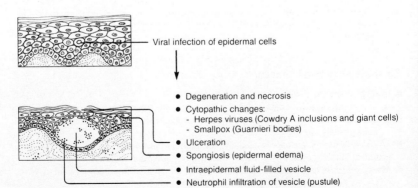

Viral infection of epidermal cells

- Degeneration and necrosis
- Cytopathic changes:
  - Herpes viruses (Cowdry A inclusions and giant cells)
  - Smallpox (Guarnieri bodies)
- Ulceration
- Spongiosis (epidermal edema)
- Intraepidermal fluid-filled vesicle
- Neutrophil infiltration of vesicle (pustule)

Figure 61-1. Epidermal viral infection leading to formation of an intraepidermal vesicle (as occurs in herpes simplex, chickenpox, zoster, and smallpox infections).

2. DERMOTROPIC VIRUSES

Measles and rubella produce lesions in the skin, but in the dermis rather than the epidermis. They do not produce vesicles. Involvement and inflammation around dermal small blood vessels produces an erythematous maculopapular rash.

FUNGAL INFECTIONS

Dermatophyte Infections (Tinea, "Ringworm")

Dermatophytes are a group of mycelial fungi that infect keratin of the stratum corneum, hair, and nails.

- They do not penetrate deeper parts of the skin.
- The three main species involved are *Trichophyton, Epidermophyton,* and *Microsporum.*
- Clinically, they cause circular, elevated, red, scaly lesions that may exude fluid. Severe itching is present.
- Sites affected are the scalp (tinea capitis), the glabrous skin of the body (tinea corporis), the groin (tinea cruris), the feet (tinea pedis, or "athlete's foot"), the nails (tinea unguium), and the beard (tinea barbae).
- Diagnosis is made by identifying the fungus in a KOH preparation of a scraping from a lesion.

Deep Fungal Infections

Deep cutaneous infections may result from:

- Local inoculation (puncture wounds, etc). This is the common route of infection in chromoblastomycosis and sporotrichosis.
- Superinfection of burnt or ulcerated skin. *Candida* and *Aspergillus,* are the most common.
- Skin involvement secondary to bloodstream spread, usually from a primary focus in the lung. Coccidioidomycosis, histoplasmosis, blastomycosis, and cryptococcosis all cause skin lesions of this group.
- Clinically, the skin lesions may be papular, pustular, or verrucous (wartlike). Lymphangitic spread is characteristic.
- Histologic sections show a mixed granulomatous and suppurative inflammation. In most cases, the fungus can be identified in tissue sections.
- Culture is diagnostic.

Mycetoma

This is a specific form of chronic suppurative inflammation with extensive local tissue destruction and fibrosis.

- The organisms rarely disseminate in the body.
- It is caused by:
  - *Actinomyces* and *Nocardia* species (filamentous gram-positive bacteria).
  - Mycelial fungi, most commonly *Allescheria boydii.*
- Clinically, mycetoma presents as an indurated abscess with multiple sinuses draining sulfur granules.
- Diagnosis is made by culture of the granules.

PARASITIC INFECTIONS

Leishmaniasis
Leishmania trophozoites multiply in macrophages and result in diffuse accumulation of macrophages causing enlargement of affected tissues.

- Diagnosis is made by finding the organisms (after Giemsa staining) in a biopsy specimen or smear.
- Three forms of leishmaniasis are recognized:
  - Cutaneous leishmaniasis, caused by *Leishmania tropica*, is localized to the skin.
  - Mucocutaneous leishmaniasis, caused by *Leishmania braziliensis*, affects the face, nose, and oral cavity.
  - Visceral leishmaniasis (kala-azar) is caused by *Leishmania donovani* and is characterized by involvement of the liver and spleen.

Filariasis
Onchocerciasis (due to *Onchocerca volvulus* infection) is a common cause of skin and eye disease in Africa and a frequent cause of blindness. Lymphatic filariasis (due to infection with *Wuchereria bancrofti* and *Brugia malayi*) is common in South and Southeast Asia. It causes lymphatic obstruction leading to elephantiasis.

Larva Migrans
This is caused by larval forms of animal nematode parasites, most commonly hookworms and roundworms of dogs and cats. Migration of the larvae in the skin (cutaneous larva migrans) or viscera (visceral larva migrans) evokes a granulomatous reaction with numerous eosinophils.

Scabies
This is a common infection caused by the itch mite *Sarcoptes scabiei*. The mite burrows in the stratum corneum, where it lays eggs, which causes pruritus, scratching, excoriation, and secondary bacterial infection.

IMMUNOLOGIC DISEASES OF THE SKIN

Allergic Dermatitis (Eczema; Contact Dermatitis)
A large number of allergens produce dermatitis, acting either directly on the skin or via the bloodstream (after ingestion). In many cases, multiple allergens are involved, and in others the allergen is obscure.

- Type I and type III hypersensitivity mechanisms are involved.
- In type I reactions, patients have a high incidence of associated atopic disorders such as asthma and hay fever.
- Acute dermatitis, characterized by erythema and edema, is followed by chronic dermatitis with thickening of the skin (Fig 61–2).

Pemphigus Vulgaris
This is a chronic, severe, potentially fatal disease of middle age (40–60 years). It is characterized by formation of bullae (large blisters) in the skin and oral mucosa (Table 61–3).

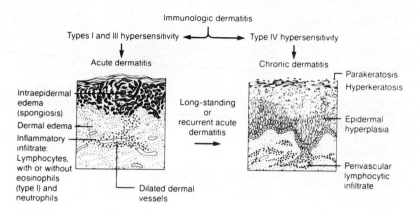

Figure 61-2. Immunologically mediated (allergic) dermatitis. In acute dermatitis, spongiosis, frequently accompanied by the formation of intraepidermal vesicles (not shown in this diagram), is the dominant feature. In chronic dermatitis, epidermal hyperplasia predominates. These histologic appearances are not specific.

- It is associated with IgG autoantibodies in the serum, which react against intercellular attachment sites of keratinocytes (Fig 61-3A).
- Separation of keratinocytes (acantholysis) and intraepidermal (suprabasal) vesicles are typical.
- Clinically, the bullae of pemphigus vulgaris are large and flaccid and appear to arise on otherwise normal skin. They easily rupture, leaving tender, raw areas.

TABLE 61-3. COMMON CAUSES OF BLISTERS (BULLAE) IN THE SKIN[1]

Site of Blister	Disease	Pathogenesis
Upper epidermal (subcorneal)	Impetigo (pustules)	Infection
	Burns, friction blisters	Physical injury
Intraepidermal	Viral infection	Infection
	Acute dermatitis	Immunologic mechanism
Suprabasal	Pemphigus vulgaris	Immunologic mechanism
	Benign familial pemphigus	Inherited
	Darier's disease	Inherited
Subepidermal	Bullous pemphigoid	Immunologic mechanism
	Dermatitis herpetiformis	Immunologic mechanism
	Epidermolysis bullosa	Inherited
	Erythema multiforme	?Immunologic mechanism
	Lichen planus	Uncertain

[1] Differential diagnosis of bullae is important because of differences in etiology, prognosis, and treatment.

A. Pemphigus vulgaris

Roof—present only in early lesion

Intraepidermal vesicle— plane of separation is suprabasal

Basal cell attached to basement membrane but separated from one another (like a "row of tombstones")

IgG on surface attachment sites of prickle cells

Rounded acantholytic prickle cell in vesicle

Normal dermis

B. Bullous pemphigoid

Normal (thin, stretched) epidermis forms the roof

IgG deposited on basement membrane

Subepidermal fluid-filled vesicle

Eosinophil is dominant cell in vesicle

C. Dermatitis herpetiformis

IgA—patchy deposition on basement membrane

Subepidermal vesicle formed by coalescence of many papillary tip vesicles

Papillary microabscess with neutrophils in dermal papilla

Early vesicle formation at tip of papilla

Neutrophil is dominant cell in vesicle

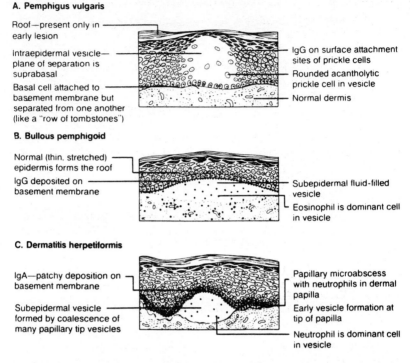

Figure 61–3. Differential histologic features of the 3 common immunologically mediated bullous diseases of the skin. **A:** Pemphigus vulgaris, characterized by a suprabasal vesicle caused by an IgG antibody directed at the intercellular attachments of the cells of the stratum spinosum. **B and C:** Bullous pemphigoid and dermatitis herpetiformis, in both of which there is subepidermal vesicle formation due to deposition of IgG and IgA, respectively, in the region of the basement membrane.

- Systemic symptoms such as fever and loss of weight are prominent.
- Without treatment, most patients die within 1 year.
- Treatment with steroids is effective in most cases.

Bullous Pemphigoid

This occurs mainly in the elderly (aged 60–80).

- It is associated with an IgG antibody that is deposited in linear fashion along the basement membrane of the skin.
- Separation of the basal cells from the dermis results in a subepidermal vesicle (Fig 61–3B) that contains eosinophils.

- Clinically, the vesicles are large and widespread. When they break, they produce denuded areas that show a tendency to heal.
- The condition is relatively benign. ·

Dermatitis Herpetiformis

This is a chronic disease that occurs in adults aged 20–40. It is associated with granular deposits of IgA at the dermoepidermal junction, especially at the tips of dermal papillae (Fig 61–3C).

- It is associated with gluten-induced enteropathy (celiac disease). The dermatitis does not improve with a gluten-free diet.
- Clinically, it is characterized by multiple erythematous vesicles and severe itching.
- Histologically, there are subepidermal vesicles containing neutrophils, and micro-abscesses at the tips of dermal papillae.
- It has a chronic course with spontaneous remissions and relapses.

Lupus Erythematosus

This is an autoimmune disorder that affects multiple systems and commonly shows skin involvement (see Chapter 68).

- Skin lesions may occur as:
  - Isolated involvement (discoid lupus erythematosus).
  - Part of systemic lupus erythematosus.
- Systemic and discoid lupus erythematosus are identical histologically, characterized by:
  - Epidermal atrophy and hyperkeratosis with follicular keratin plugs.
  - Liquefactive degeneration of the basal layers of the epidermis.
  - Lymphocytic vasculitis in the dermis.
  - Deposition of IgG and complement in the basement membrane.
- Systemic lupus shows IgG deposition in uninvolved skin, whereas discoid lupus shows it only in the lesions.

INHERITED DISEASES OF THE SKIN

Epidermolysis Bullosa

This includes several inherited variants characterized by onset in infancy and the formation of vesicles as a result of minor trauma.

- Epidermolysis bullosa simplex is dominantly inherited. It is usually a mild disease, healing without scarring.
- The recessive-dystrophic form:
  - Has extensive ulceration and scarring.
  - Has involvement of the oral mucosa.
- Histologically, vesicle formation occurs at various levels in the epidermis, probably as a result of defective intercellular attachments.

Darier's Disease (Keratosis Follicularis)

This is inherited as an autosomal dominant trait. It presents as a slowly progressive skin eruption consisting of hyperkeratotic crusted papules. Vesicles are rare.

- Histologic features consist of:
  - Acanthosis, hyperkeratosis, and dyskeratosis.
  - Suprabasal acantholysis, leading to the formation of clefts in the epidermis.

Benign Familial Pemphigus (Hailey-Hailey Disease)
This is inherited as an autosomal dominant trait. It is characterized by localized eruption of vesicles, commonly in the skin of the axillas and groins. Histologically, there is acantholysis and vesicle formation, but no immunoglobulin deposition.

Pseudoxanthoma Elasticum
This is a rare, recessively inherited disorder of elastic fibers.

- It produces soft yellowish plaques in the skin. The sides of the neck, the axillas, and the groins are most commonly affected.
- Histologically, there is accumulation of abnormal elastic fibers in the dermis.
- Other sites where elastic tissue is found may also show involvement:
  - The ocular fundi, showing diagnostic changes.
  - The arteries, leading to myocardial ischemia, gastrointestinal hemorrhage, and abnormal peripheral pulses.

Ichthyosis
Several forms of ichthyosis exist, having different inheritance patterns (dominant, recessive, X-linked) and varying degrees of severity. All are associated with hyperkeratosis, which may produce fishlike scales. Severe congenital forms may lead to early death.

IDIOPATHIC SKIN DISEASES

Psoriasis Vulgaris
This is common, affecting 1% of the population. It is a chronic disease of unknown etiology characterized by remissions and exacerbations.

- The lesions of psoriasis are sharply defined papules and red plaques covered by silvery scales.
- The nails are affected in 50% of cases.
- The basic defect in the epidermis is an increase in the rate of maturation (Fig 61–4).
- Microscopic examination shows:
  - Regular acanthosis, with clubbing and fusion of rete pegs.
  - Hyperkeratosis, with parakeratosis and an absent granular layer.
  - The presence of neutrophils in the epidermis, with abscesses in the stratum corneum (Munro microabscesses) and subcorneal layer (Kojog spongiform pustules).
- It is, rarely, associated with a destructive joint disease resembling rheumatoid arthritis.

Lichen Planus
This is a chronic disorder of unknown etiology characterized by the appearance of violaceous, itching papules and plaques on the skin, oral mucosa, and external genitalia.

- Women are affected more frequently than men, and the maximal age incidence is 30–60.

- The basic defect is a decrease in the rate of cellular proliferation (Fig 61–4).
- Microscopic examination shows:
  - Irregular acanthosis, hyperkeratosis, a prominent granular cell layer.
  - Vacuolar degeneration of basal cells.
  - A bandlike infiltrate in the upper dermis.

Erythema Multiforme

This is a common skin disorder that may affect patients of any age. The cause and pathogenesis are unknown, though an immunologic mechanism is suspected.

- It is associated with a large variety of diseases, including many infections, drugs, cancers, and autoimmune diseases.
- Clinically, it is characterized by diverse lesions, including macules, papules, vesicles, and target lesions.
- Microscopically, it is characterized by:
  - Epidermal changes, including spongiosis, dyskeratosis, and epidermal cell necrosis.
  - Dermal changes including vasculitis and edema.
- Minor forms are self-limited. The major form of the disease (**Stevens-Johnson syndrome**) is characterized by high fever, extensive bulla formation and necrosis, ulceration of skin and orogenital mucosa, and a high mortality rate.

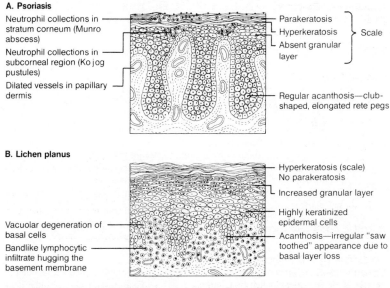

A. Psoriasis

Neutrophil collections in stratum corneum (Munro abscess)

Neutrophil collections in subcorneal region (Kojog pustules)

Dilated vessels in papillary dermis

Parakeratosis
Hyperkeratosis
Absent granular layer } Scale

Regular acanthosis—club-shaped, elongated rete pegs

B. Lichen planus

Vacuolar degeneration of basal cells

Bandlike lymphocytic infiltrate hugging the basement membrane

Hyperkeratosis (scale)
No parakeratosis
Increased granular layer

Highly keratinized epidermal cells

Acanthosis—irregular "saw toothed" appearance due to basal layer loss

Figure 61–4. Contrasting features of psoriasis (**A**) and lichen planus (**B**), both of which are characterized clinically by the formation of papular skin lesions with silvery hyperkeratotic scales. Psoriasis is the result of an increased rate of epidermal cell turnover; lichen planus is the result of decreased epidermal cell turnover.

Erythema Nodosum

This is the most common form of panniculitis (inflammation of subcutaneous fat).

- It is associated with:
  - Infections with β-hemolytic streptococci, tuberculosis, fungal infections, leprosy.
  - Drugs such as sulfonamides, iodides.
  - Sarcoidosis.
  - Acute rheumatic fever.
  - Inflammatory bowel disease.
  - Malignant neoplasms.
- Most cases of erythema nodosum have no associated disease.
- Clinically, there are multiple tender red nodules, commonly in the anterior tibial region. The disease remits spontaneously in 3 or 4 weeks without scarring.
- Histologically, there is a panniculitis and vasculitis.

Pityriasis Rosea

This is a common, self-limited condition occurring in adults aged 20–30.

- It is suspected of having a viral origin, though no agent has yet been isolated.
- The onset is typically with a sharply defined scaling plaque (herald patch), followed by an eruption of oval salmon-pink papules covered by thin scales.
- Histologically, the features are those of nonspecific subacute dermatitis.

Acanthosis Nigricans

This is characterized by velvety, dark patches that involve especially the skin of the groin area in middle-aged patients.

- Fifty percent of cases are associated with visceral carcinoma.
- Histologically, there is hyperkeratosis and papillomatosis, with increased melanin production.

Melanocyte Disorders

- Vitiligo is a relatively common disorder manifested by loss of pigmentation of the skin due to destruction of melanocytes.
- Albinism is a congenital failure of melanin production by melanocytes.
- Lentigo consists of small pigmented lesions in the young (lentigo simplex) or elderly (lentigo senilis or liver spots) due to hyperplasia of melanocytes.
- Ephelides (freckles) are pigmented spots resulting from increased melanin production by normal numbers of melanocytes.

CYSTS OF THE SKIN

Epidermal Cyst & Pilar Cyst

Epidermal cysts are lined by keratinizing squamous epithelium and filled with laminated keratin. Pilar cysts (also called trichilemmal cysts) are similar, but lack a granular layer and contain amorphous rather than laminated keratin. Clinically, these common cysts are filled with thick yellow material and are often incorrectly called "sebaceous cysts."

Dermoid Cyst

These are congenital cysts that occur at lines of embryonic skin closure and fusion, most commonly around the eyes (external angular dermoid). They are lined by an epithelium that shows various epidermal appendages, including hair follicles and sebaceous glands.

NEOPLASMS OF THE SKIN (Table 61–4)

BENIGN NEOPLASMS OF KERATINOCYTES

Verruca Vulgaris (Common Wart)

This is caused by a papillomavirus and is transmitted by direct contact.

- It may occur anywhere in the skin, with the fingers the most common single site.
- Histologically, the wart is a squamous papilloma with conspicuous keratohyaline granules.
- Large vacuolated cells in the proliferating squamous epithelium stain positively for papilloma virus by the immunoperoxidase technique.

Condyloma Acuminatum

These are similar to large warts, and are caused by a different serotype of papillomavirus. They occur in genital skin and mucosa and are sexually transmitted.

TABLE 61–4. NEOPLASMS OF THE SKIN

Cell of Origin	Benign	Malignant
Keratinocyte	Verruca vulgaris Condyloma acuminatum Molluscum contagiosum Keratoacanthoma	Carcinoma in situ (Bowen's disease) Squamous carcinoma Basal cell carcinoma
Skin adnexal cells	See Table 61–5	
Melanocyte	Nevocellular nevus Blue nevus	Lentigo maligna Superficial spreading malignant melanoma Nodular malignant melanoma
Merkel cell	. . .	Merkel cell carcinoma
Dermal mesenchymal cells	Dermatofibroma Fibroxanthoma Hemangioma Neurofibroma	Dermatofibrosarcoma protuberans Angiosarcoma Malignant schwannoma
Lymphocyte	. . .	Mycosis fungoides Sézary's syndrome
Mast cell	Urticaria pigmentosa Solitary mastocytoma	Systemic mastocytosis

Molluscum Contagiosum

This is caused by a virus of the poxvirus group.

- Lesions consist of small and discrete dome-shaped papules having an umbilicated center.
- They usually heal spontaneously.
- Histologically, the epidermis bulges downward into the dermis and the epidermal cells contain intracytoplasmic inclusion bodies known as molluscum bodies.

Seborrheic Keratosis

This is a very common lesion (probably not a true neoplasm), occurring on the trunk, extremities, and face, usually in elderly persons.

- The lesions are flat, raised, soft, sharply demarcated, and brown.
- Histologically, it is a flat, often pigmented squamous epithelial proliferation with many keratin-filled cysts.

Keratoacanthoma

This usually occurs in middle age, most commonly on the face or upper extremities. It is characterized by a rapid early growth phase, reaching maximum size in a few weeks, followed by a static phase (up to 1 year), after which the lesion spontaneously involutes with scarring.

- Histologically, keratoacanthoma appears as a cup-shaped lesion with an irregular keratin-filled crater in the center. There is no invasion at the base.
- Histologic distinction from squamous carcinoma may be difficult.

PREMALIGNANT LESIONS OF KERATINOCYTES

Actinic Keratosis

Actinic keratosis represents the effect of ultraviolet radiation of sunlight on skin. It occurs predominantly in fair-skinned individuals with a history of sunlight exposure.

- It appears as rough erythematous or brownish papules.
- Histologically, there is dysplasia of the epidermis and degeneration of dermal collagen.
- Actinic keratosis is a premalignant lesion with an increased risk of squamous and basal cell carcinomas.

MALIGNANT NEOPLASMS OF KERATINOCYTES

Bowen's Disease (Carcinoma in Situ)

Carcinoma in situ of the squamous epithelium may occur:

- On sun-exposed skin.
- On the vulva, oral mucosa, and glans penis.
- It is associated with visceral malignant disease.
- Rarely, it is caused by chronic arsenic exposure.
- It presents clinically as a slowly enlarging erythematous patch that on histologic

examination shows carcinoma in situ. There is no invasion of the basement membrane.

Basal Cell Carcinoma

Basal cell carcinoma is a common skin neoplasm, occurring in sun-exposed areas of light-skinned individuals over age 40.

- The face is the most common site.
- Rarely, multiple basal cell carcinomas arise in early life as part of an autosomal dominant inherited disorder in which abnormalities of bone, nervous system, and eyes are present (nevoid basal cell epithelioma syndrome).
- Clinically, early lesions appear as a waxy papule with small telangiectatic vessels on its surface. Late lesions are punched-out ulcers with pearly edges.
- Histologically, basal cell carcinoma arises from the basal layer of the epidermis and invades the dermis as nests resembling basal cells.
- Basal cell carcinoma is locally aggressive. It may invade deeply to involve bone and muscle.
- It almost never metastasizes.
- Complete surgical excision is curative.

Squamous Carcinoma

Squamous carcinoma of the skin is also very common, especially in sun-exposed skin of elderly, fair-skinned individuals.

- It is a locally aggressive neoplasm that rarely metastasizes (1% of cases).
- Squamous carcinoma may also occur in relation to chronic ulcers, burn scars, and infected sinuses. These have a much higher (20–30%) incidence of metastases.
- Clinically, squamous carcinoma presents as a shallow ulcer with a raised, everted, firm border.
- Histologically, the tumor is composed of large polygonal cells with abundant keratinized cytoplasm and cytologic features of malignancy. Invasion is present.
- Wide surgical excision of squamous carcinomas arising in sun-exposed skin is usually curative.

NEOPLASMS OF SKIN APPENDAGES

Neoplasms arising in skin appendages are usually benign. They are classified according to their differentiation (Table 61–5). All present clinically as painless skin nodules and are cured by simple surgical removal. Very rarely, adnexal skin tumors are malignant, with both locally infiltrative and metastasizing capability.

MELANOCYTIC NEOPLASMS (Fig 61–5)

Nevi develop from clusters of menalocyte precursor cells (nevus cells) that are arrested during migration from the neural crest to the epidermis. Nevi usually develop in childhood and are benign. Malignant melanomas develop by neoplastic transformation of melanocytes in the epidermis. They usually occur in adults.

Nevocellular Nevus (Melanocytic Nevus)

Melanocytic nevi are usually not present at birth but appear in childhood and stop growing soon after puberty.

TABLE 61–5. CLASSIFICATION OF SKIN ADNEXAL NEOPLASMS[1]

Neoplasm	Differentiation	Common Sites
Trichofolliculoma	Hair	Face, solitary
Trichoepithelioma	Hair	Face; may be multiple
Pilomatrixoma	Hair	All over body, mainly in children
Syringoma	Eccrine (sweat gland)	Lower eyelids, frequently multiple
Syringocystadenoma papilliferum	Eccrine	Face, scalp
Clear-cell hidradenoma	Eccrine	All over body
Eccrine poroma	Eccrine	Feet, hands; mainly in elderly
Eccrine spiradenoma	Eccrine	All over body
Hidradenoma papilliferum	Apocrine	Vulva in females
Cylindroma	Apocrine	Scalp; may be multiple
Nevus sebaceus	Sebaceous	Scalp, face; from birth
Sebaceous adenoma	Sebaceous	Rare

[1]These are all benign neoplasms. Their malignant counterparts occur very rarely, with sebaceous carcinoma being the most common.

- They are extremely common and are better regarded as hamartomatous growths than as true neoplasms.
- Clinically, they present as flat papular, papillomatous, or pedunculated pigmented (black or brown) lesions.
- Histologically, they are composed of nests of nevus (melanocytic) cells, which may be found:
  - In the dermis (intradermal nevus).
  - In the junctional zone of the epidermis (junctional nevus).
  - In both epidermis and dermis (compound nevus).
- They have low risk of malignant melanoma.

Congenital Melanocytic Nevus
This is an uncommon lesion that is present at birth but is not inherited.

- It presents as a pigmented, often hairy, lesion occurring anywhere on the body. It may be large and multiple.
- Histologically, congenital melanocytic nevus is a compound nevus with a tendency to neural differentiation.
- It carries a slight risk of developing malignant melanoma.

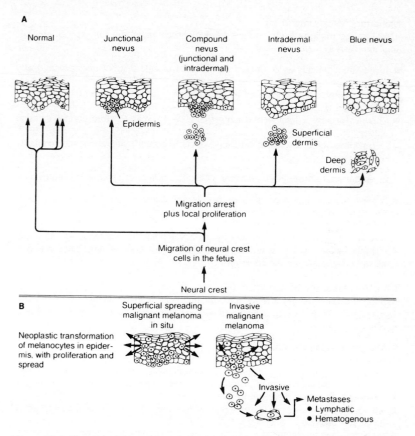

Figure 61–5. Melanocytic lesions. A: Melanocytic nevi result from the arrest of melanocytic cells during embryonic migration from the neural crest, followed by proliferation, usually during childhood. These are hamartomatous rather than neoplastic lesions. **B:** Malignant melanoma, which arises from the neoplastic transformation of normally located melanocytes in the epidermis, followed by proliferation. Intraepidermal (in situ) and invasive phases of proliferation are recognized. Malignant melanomas commonly arise in older patients.

Blue Nevus

These are common skin lesions presenting as small, well-circumscribed, bluish-black nodules.

- Histologically, they are composed of a poorly circumscribed collection of heavily pigmented dendritic melanocytes deep in the dermis.
- Except in very rare instances, blue nevi are benign.

Malignant Melanoma in Situ

A. Lentigo maligna (Hutchinson's freckle) occurs mainly in sun-exposed areas of skin in elderly persons.

- It presents clinically as an unevenly pigmented macule that becomes progressively larger.
- Histologically, it is characterized by a marked increase in the number of melanocytes in the basal layer.
- There is usually a long period (sometimes 10–15 years) before dermal invasion occurs.
- Dermal invasion is associated clinically with enlargement, induration, and nodularity of the macule.

B. Superficial spreading melanoma occurs regardless of exposure to sunlight.

- It presents as a pigmented and slightly elevated lesion.
- The in-situ phase is much shorter than in lentigo maligna, and invasion frequently occurs within months after onset.
- Invasion is characterized clinically by the development of ulceration and bleeding.
- Histologically, it is characterized by the presence of nests of large, atypical, neoplastic melanocytes in the epidermis.

Invasive Malignant Melanoma

Malignant melanoma may arise de novo, in a previous lentigo maligna, in a superficial spreading melanoma in situ, in a congenital giant pigmented nevus, or in a nevocellular nevus.

- Malignant melanoma occurs:
  - Most often in skin.
  - In extracutaneous sites, including the choroid layer of the eyes (common), the oral cavity, nasal mucosa, and pharynx (rare), the esophagus, bronchus, vaginal and anorectal mucosa (very rare).
- Clinically, it appears as an elevated pigmented nodule that grows rapidly and tends to bleed and ulcerate.
- Metastasis via the lymphatics and bloodstream tends to occur early.
- Histologically, it is characterized by:
  - Proliferation of cytologically abnormal melanocytes.
  - Invasion laterally and upward in the epidermis, and downward into the dermis from its origin in the basal epidermis.
- Diagnosis is established by:
  - The presence of melanin pigment in the neoplastic cells.
  - Electron microscopy, which shows premelanosomes and melanosomes.
  - Immunohistochemical demonstration of S100 protein or melanoma-related antigens (eg, HMB 45).
- Prognosis depends on several factors (Fig 61–6):
  - The depth of invasion, determined by measurement of vertical extent of tumor below the stratum granulosum.
  - Clark's level of invasion.
  - The clinical stage. The presence of lymph node metastases worsens the prognosis.

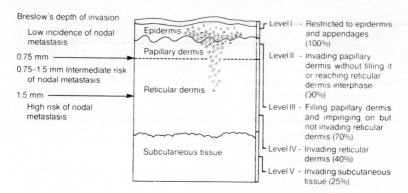

Figure 61–6. Two common methods of estimating the prognosis of malignant melanoma based on the degree of vertical invasion. On the left is Breslow's thickness, which is an actual measurement of the deepest invasion from the granular layer. On the right is Clark's level, which relates to involvement of different anatomic regions of the skin. The figures in parentheses given after individual Clark levels indicate disease-free 5-year survival rates. Note that metastasis, either lymph node or hematogenous, decreases survival drastically.

- When distant hematogenous metastases are present, the 5-year survival rate is less than 10%.

MERKEL CELL (NEUROENDOCRINE) CARCINOMA

This arises from Merkel cells, which are neuroendocrine cells situated in the basal epidermis.

- It presents as a nodular skin lesion, and usually occurs in patients over age 40.
- Histologically, it is composed of small cells with scanty cytoplasm and hyperchromatic nuclei arranged in nests and trabeculae.
- Diagnosis is made by:
  - Demonstrating neurosecretory granules on electron microscopy.
  - Positive staining by immunoperoxidase techniques for neuroendocrine markers such as neuron-specific enolase and chromogranin.
- A few tumors have been reported to secrete serotonin and calcitonin.
- Lymph node and distant metastases occur early in the course in about 25% of cases. In the remainder, wide local excision results in cure.

NEOPLASMS OF DERMAL MESENCHYMAL CELLS

Dermatofibroma (Cutaneous Fibrous Histiocytoma)

This is a common benign neoplasm that presents as a firm, slowly growing, nodular dermal lesion. Histologically, the dermal mass is composed of fibroblasts, histiocytes, and collagen in varying amounts.

Atypical Fibroxanthoma

This is a nodular lesion that commonly occurs in a sun-exposed area, usually the head or neck, of an elderly patient.

- It is usually solitary and small.
- Histologically, it is characterized by proliferation of fibroblasts and histiocytes, with marked atypia, pleomorphism, bizarre multinucleated giant cells, and numerous mitoses.
- Despite its malignant appearance, the lesion does not metastasize. It recurs locally if inadequately excised.

Dermatofibrosarcoma Protuberans

This is a slowly growing nodular skin lesion that may reach large size and result in ulceration of the overlying epidermis.

- It is locally invasive, frequently infiltrating subcutaneous fat.
- Histologically, it is a highly cellular spindle cell proliferation with cytologic atypia and increased mitotic activity.
- Wide surgical excision is necessary to prevent local recurrence.
- Metastases are rare, but may occur after many years, especially in lesions that have recurred several times.

MALIGNANT LYMPHOMAS

Cutaneous malignant lymphoma occurs primarily in the skin, and secondarily in the course of disseminated lymphoma (5–10% of patients with Hodgkin's lymphoma and 15–20% of patients with non-Hodgkin's lymphoma).

Mycosis Fungoides (Cutaneous T Cell Lymphoma)

Mycosis fungoides is a T cell lymphoma that affects the skin primarily.

- It is characterized by large malignant T lymphocytes (mycosis cells) with hyperchromatic, irregularly lobulated, cerebriform nuclei.
- The cells have a helper T cell phenotype.
- Clinically, the disease can be divided into three stages:
  - Erythematous stage, characterized by erythematous, scaling patches that itch severely. Histologically, the mycosis cells are around dermal blood vessels with migration into the epidermis.
  - Plaque stage, characterized by well-demarcated, indurated erythematous plaques. Histology shows a bandlike upper dermal infiltrate of mycosis cells.
  - Tumor stage, which is characterized by reddish-brown ulcerating nodules.
- Lymph node and visceral involvement occurs in up to 70% of cases and signifies a poor prognosis.
- The overall 5-year survival rate is less than 10%.

Sézary's Syndrome

This is a leukemic variant of mycosis fungoides.

- Clinically, it presents with generalized erythroderma with intense itching.

■ The histologic features are identical to those of the erythematous stage of mycosis fungoides.

■ Sézary cells (indistinguishable from mycosis cells) are present in the peripheral blood.

MAST CELL NEOPLASMS

This is characterized by proliferation of mast cells in the dermis.

◘ Mast cells contain basophilic cytoplasmic granules with Giemsa's stain.

■ Release of histamine, serotonin, and other vasoactive substances from proliferating mast cells in the skin causes urticaria and flushing.

■ Three variants are recognized:

● Urticaria pigmentosa is a benign condition occurring in infancy, characterized by multiple red-brown macules and papules all over the body.

● Solitary mastocytoma is an uncommon benign lesion usually occurring at or soon after birth and presenting as a nodule.

● Systemic mastocytosis is an uncommon malignant disease that resembles malignant lymphoma with mast cell infiltrates in skin, bone marrow, liver, spleen, and lymph nodes.

Section XV. The Nervous System

The Central Nervous System: I. Hydrocephalus; Congenital Diseases

62

THE CEREBROSPINAL FLUID

The cerebrospinal fluid (CSF) fills the ventricular system of the brain, the central canal of the spinal cord, and the subarachnoid space.

- It is secreted by the choroid plexuses and is absorbed into the venous system by the arachnoid villi in the superior sagittal sinus.
- It can be removed for examination by lumbar puncture.
- Abnormalities in the composition of CSF (Table 62–1) are important in diagnosis of diseases of the nervous system.

HYDROCEPHALUS

Hydrocephalus is defined as abnormal dilatation of the ventricles. It is readily diagnosed by computerized tomography.

- Hydrocephalus may result from (Table 62–2):
  - Increased secretion of CSF, as occurs very rarely with neoplasms of the choroid plexus.
  - Obstruction to the flow of CSF, either in the ventricular system or in the subarachnoid space.
  - Failure of absorption of CSF.

Classification
A. Anatomic classification:

- Noncommunicating (obstructive) hydrocephalus occurs when an obstruction in the ventricular system prevents CSF from passing into the subarachnoid space.
- Communicating hydrocephalus occurs when CSF passes normally out of the ventricular system, but flow is obstructed in the subarachnoid space or reabsorption is reduced.

B. Functional classification:

- High-pressure hydrocephalus is due to obstruction of CSF flow.

689

TABLE 62–1. CEREBROSPINAL FLUID ABNORMALITIES[1]

	Normal	Abnormalities
Color	Clear, colorless	Yellow (xanthochromic): indicates old hemorrhage, high protein, complete subarachnoid obstruction. Red: subarachnoid hemorrhage (if traumatic puncture is excluded). Turbid (purulent): bacterial meningitis. Clear with clot on standing: high protein, common in tuberculous meningitis.
Protein	20–50 mg/dL	Marked increase: infection, hemorrhage, tumor causing subarachnoid block. Moderate increase: many causes.
Oligoclonal protein bands[2]	. . .	Multiple sclerosis, syphilis.
Serology	. . .	VDRL positive in neurosyphilis.
Glucose	50–80 mg/dL (~75% of blood glucose)	Marked decrease in bacterial meningitis; increased in hyperglycemic states.
Cells	0–5 (mostly lymphocytes); no neutrophils are present	↑ Neutrophils: bacterial infection. ↑ Lymphocytes: viral, fungal, tuberculous meningitis, syphilis, cysticercosis, degenerative diseases. Malignant cells: cancer (various types).
Gram stain of sediment	Negative	Useful test in meningitis; positive finding may provide immediate diagnosis.
Culture	Negative	Positive bacterial, mycobacterial, fungal, and viral cultures.

[1]Always check for evidence of raised intracranial pressure prior to lumbar puncture. If pressure is normal in a recumbent patient, remove 3-mL samples in 3 separate sterile containers (1) for chemistry/serology, (2) for culture, (3) for cell count and cytology.
[2]Oligoclonal protein bands: 2–4 immunoglobulin bands seen on electrophoresis of cerebrospinal fluid.

- If obstruction occurs after fusion of skull sutures, it causes an increase in intracranial pressure (see following).
- When it occurs in the fetus or infant before fusion of the sutures, it causes the skull to expand.
■ Low-pressure (or normal pressure) hydrocephalus is associated with slow dilatation of the ventricles, free flow of CSF, cerebral atrophy, and dementia. The cause is unknown in most cases.

TABLE 62–2. CAUSES OF HYDROCEPHALUS

Noncommunicating hydrocephalus
Congenital
    Aqueductal stenosis and atresia
    Dandy-Walker syndrome

Acquired
    Neoplasms and cysts obstructing cerebral aqueduct
        and the third ventricle
    Gliosis and chronic inflammation involving aqueduct
    Obstruction of fourth ventricle openings
    Organized subarachnoid hemorrhage, obstructing
        flow at base of brain
    Organized meningitis involving base of brain

Communicating hydrocephalus Choroid plexus papilloma (increased secretion)
Arnold-Chiari malformation

Deficient absorption of cerebrospinal fluid
    Dural sinus thrombosis
    Organized subarachnoid hemorrhage
    Organized meningitis
    ?Deficiency of arachnoid villi

INCREASED INTRACRANIAL PRESSURE

Increased pressure is defined as elevation of the mean CSF pressure above 200 mm water (15 mm Hg) when measured with the patient in the lateral decubitus position.

Etiology (Table 62–3)

- Obstructive hydrocephalus.
- The presence of a space-occupying mass lesion in the cranial cavity. Rapidly expanding lesions produce greater rise in intracranial pressure than slowly expanding masses.
- Cerebral edema, which includes:
  - Intracellular cytotoxic cerebral edema, which is an early manifestation of cell injury most commonly seen in ischemic states.
  - Extracellular vasogenic edema is responsible for most cases of cerebral edema, occurring in infections, trauma, neoplasms, and metabolic disorders.

Pathology

The raised pressure within the fixed volume of the bony cranial cavity causes displacement of the brain (Fig 62–1).

- Supratentorial lesions cause caudal displacement of the entire brain stem, which may:
  - Stretch and paralyze the sixth cranial nerve.

TABLE 62–3. CAUSES OF INCREASED INTRACRANIAL PRESSURE

Hydrocephalus	(See Table 62–2)
Space-occupying lesions Hemorrhage or hematoma	Extradural, subdural, sub- arachnoid, or intra- cerebral
Infarction	With local edema or hem- orrhage
Neoplasm	Primary or secondary (mass effect and local edema)
Infection	Abscess (mass effect and local edema)
Cerebral edema Cytotoxic	Anoxia of any cause; hypo- glycemia
Vasogenic	Hypertensive encephalo- pathy; associated with altered capillaries of tu- mors, abscesses; toxins (eg, lead poisoning); uremia
Infection	Meningitis, encephalitis
Trauma	
Hypercapnia in chronic obstructive lung dis- ease	

- Cause rupture of perforating vessels passing from the basilar artery to the brain stem, resulting in brain stem hemorrhages (Duret's hemorrhages).
- Herniation of the uncinate gyrus of the temporal lobe through the tentorial opening (tentorial herniation):
  - Stretches and paralyzes the third nerve.
  - Compresses the pyramidal tract in the crus cerebri.
- Posterior fossa lesions cause herniation of the cerebellar tonsils through the foramen magnum, leading to compression of the medulla, with cardiorespiratory failure and death.

Clinical Features
Raised intracranial pressure presents with:

- Headache, typically present on waking, and bursting in nature.

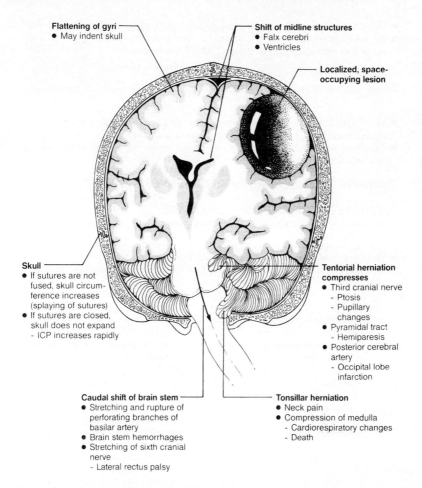

Figure 62–1. Possible consequences of raised intracranial pressure (ICP) resulting from a mass lesion in the right supratentorial compartment.

- ■ Vomiting, typically effortless and projectile.
- ■ Papilledema.
- ■ Raised intracranial pressure also produces false localizing signs, caused by displacement of the brain. These include:
  - ● Cranial nerve palsies, commonly the sixth and third nerves.
  - ● Pyramidal tract compression.
  - ● Brain stem hemorrhage, which may cause unconsciousness and death.

- Diagnosis of raised intracranial pressure is made by clinical examination.
- If raised intracranial pressure is suspected, lumbar puncture should not be performed because of the danger of precipitating tonsillar herniation.

Treatment
Raised intracranial pressure due to a mass lesion should be treated by removal of the mass.

- In hydrocephalus caused by a lesion that cannot be removed, decompression of the dilated ventricles may be achieved by a ventricular shunt.
- Raised intracranial pressure caused by cerebral edema may be treated with diuretics and high doses of corticosteroids.

CONGENITAL DISEASES OF THE NERVOUS SYSTEM

DEFECTIVE CLOSURE OF THE NEURAL TUBE
Defective closure of the neural tube may occur throughout its extent but is most common at either end.

- Defective closure of the caudal end (spina bifida) may result in:
  - **Spina bifida occulta,** which is the mildest form, and is characterized by failure of vertebral fusion only. The overlying skin often shows a dimple, a tuft of hair, or a fatty mass. In a few cases, a congenital dermal sinus passes from the epidermis through the vertebral defect into the spinal canal.
  - **Meningocele** is a more severe degree of spina bifida associated with protrusion of a meningeal sac filled with CSF through the vertebral defect.
  - **Myelomeningocele** is a still more serious defect characterized by the presence of parts of the spinal cord in the sac, and is often associated with severe neurologic defects in the lower extremities, bladder, and rectum.
  - **Spina bifida aperta,** the most severe form, results from complete failure of fusion of the caudal end of the neural plate.
- All types of spina bifida are associated with Arnold-Chiari malformation.
- Defective closure of the cranial end are less common, but may result in:
  - Anencephaly, which is a complete failure of development of the cranial end of the neural tube.
  - Occipital meningocele and encephalocele, which are similar to lumbar meningocele and meningomyelocele.

Clinical Features
Spina bifida occulta is a common abnormality that is usually asymptomatic. Rare patients with a dermal sinus present with recurrent meningitis in childhood.

- Meningocele, meningomyelocele, and spina bifida aperta present at birth with a detectable lesion in the lumbosacral region.
- Meningomyelocele is associated with lower limb weakness and with bladder and rectal dysfunction.
- Anencephaly and spina bifida aperta are almost always fatal in early life.
- Hydrocephalus often coexists due to the concomitant presence of the Arnold-Chiari malformation.

Antenatal Diagnosis

Raised levels of alpha-fetoprotein (AFP) in the amniotic fluid are present in over 95% of fetuses with neural tube defects. Ultrasound examination of the fetus is also an effective method of demonstrating the anatomic abnormality before birth.

Treatment

Meningocele, the commonest serious lesion, should be closed soon after birth before infection and ulceration occur. In many patients, surgical drainage of the associated hydrocephalus is required. Neurologic deficit in the legs in meningomyelocele presents a serious problem.

CEREBRAL PALSY

This is a common disorder characterized by a disturbance of motor function, usually nonprogressive, that is manifest at birth or comes on in early infancy. The following syndromes are recognized.

A. Spastic diplegia (Little's disease):

- Is characterized by spastic weakness of all four extremities.
- Is associated with prematurity, characterized by predominant involvement of the legs, associated with minimal mental retardation.
- Spastic diplegia associated with full-term delivery and difficult labor is believed to result from intrapartum asphyxia. The infant develops quadriplegia associated with mental retardation.

B. Infantile hemiplegia usually results from unilateral infection or thrombosis of cerebral vessels that occurs in utero or soon after birth. Mild mental retardation and convulsions are commonly associated.

TRISOMY 13 (Patau's Syndrome)

Trisomy 13 is characterized by failure of normal development of the forebrain, leading to:

- Formation of a brain with a single frontal lobe and a single ventricle (holoprosencephaly).
- Absence of the olfactory bulbs (arhinencephaly).
- A single median eye (cyclopia).
- Failure of formation of nasal structures.
- Patau's syndrome is usually fatal soon after birth.

CONGENITAL HYDROCEPHALUS

Hydrocephalus is a common abnormality, affecting about 0.1–0.5% of births. It is caused by several different congenital anomalies (Table 62–2).

1. AQUEDUCTAL STENOSIS & ATRESIA

Narrowing of the cerebral aqueduct is the commonest cause of congenital noncommunicating hydrocephalus. There is controversy about whether the narrowing is a developmental abnormality or whether it results from a fetal inflammatory process causing gliotic occlusion.

2. ARNOLD-CHIARI MALFORMATION

This is the commonest cause of congenital communicating hydrocephalus. It is characterized by:

- Elongation of the medulla oblongata, so that the fourth ventricular foramens open below the level of the foramen magnum.
- Obstruction of the subarachnoid space at the foramen magnum by protrusion of the cerebellum into the foramen magnum.
- Obstruction of cerebrospinal fluid passage at the foramen magnum.
- Arnold-Chiari malformation is commonly associated with:
  - Flattening of the base of the skull (platybasia).
  - Abnormalities in the cervical vertebrae.
  - Spina bifida and all its variants.
  - Syringomyelia.

3. DANDY-WALKER SYNDROME

This syndrome is a rare cause of congenital noncommunicating hydrocephalus, characterized by failure of development of the cerebellar vermis and obstruction of the fourth ventricular foramens of Luschka and Magendie.

SYRINGOMYELIA

This is an uncommon disease of adults, believed to result from abnormal development of the cervical spine and upper spinal cord.

- It is characterized by development of fluid-filled spaces in the spinal cord, mainly the cervical cord.
- Many cases are associated with Arnold-Chiari malformation.
- Pathologically, the cystic spaces occupy the central part of the cervical cord. The spaces are lined by reactive astrocytes.
- Clinical effects are characteristic, depending on the nerve fibers or tracts destroyed (Fig 62–2).

HEREDITARY HAMARTOMATOUS MALFORMATIONS

1. GENERALIZED NEUROFIBROMATOSIS (von Recklinghausen's Disease)

Neurofibromatosis is the commonest hereditary hamartomatous malformation, with an estimated prevalence of 1:3000 in the USA. It is inherited as an autosomal dominant trait with varying degrees of penetrance.

- The gene responsible is carried in chromosome number 17.
- Manifestations vary from asymptomatic disease characterized by a few skin lesions to severe disease that is fatal in early infancy.
- Clinically, it is characterized by café-au-lait skin patches—well-demarcated flat areas of brown pigmentation.
- Multiple neurofibromas may occur in the skin, intestine, autonomic nerve plexuses, and in relation to large peripheral nerve trunks.
- Diffuse proliferation of nerve elements (plexiform neurofibromatosis) may cause massive enlargement of tissues (elephantiasis neurofibromatosa).

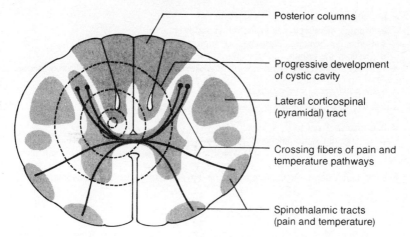

Posterior columns

Progressive development
of cystic cavity

Lateral corticospinal
(pyramidal) tract

Crossing fibers of pain and
temperature pathways

Spinothalamic tracts
(pain and temperature)

Figure 62–2. Syringomyelia. Transverse section of the cervical cord to illustrate the development of signs and symptoms. Dotted lines indicate the region where the cystic spaces develop, starting centrally and radiating outward. The initial symptoms are caused by involvement of the pain fibers crossing at the level of involvement from the dorsal nerve root to the spinothalamic tracts (shown). As the disease progresses, the more peripheral long tracts and the anterior horn are involved.

■ Malignant transformation of neurofibromas to form neurofibrosarcomas in 5–10% of patients.
■ Neoplasms of the nervous system (meningiomas, astrocytomas, optic nerve gliomas) and pheochromocytoma may be associated.

2. TUBEROUS SCLEROSIS (Bourneville's Disease)

This is a rare autosomal-dominant disease usually presenting in young adults. It is characterized by multiple hamartomas in the brain composed of giant astrocytes. Intraventricular tumors composed of these giant astrocytes (subependymal giant cell astrocytoma) are typical.

■ Mental retardation and epilepsy are usual.
■ Skin manifestations include:
  ● Nodules composed of fibroblastic and vascular proliferation (adenoma sebaceum) involve mainly the face.
  ● Larger confluent papular lesions called *shagreen patches* occur over the buttocks.
■ Visceral lesions include rhabdomyoma of the heart, pancreatic cysts, and, most commonly, angiomyolipomas of the kidney (Chapter 49).

3. VON HIPPEL-LINDAU DISEASE

This is a rare disease transmitted as an autosomal-dominant trait.

- It is characterized by:
    - Multiple hemangiomas in the retina and brain.
    - Cerebellar hemangioblastoma, a benign neoplasm.
    - Cysts in the kidneys and pancreas.
- There is an increased incidence of renal adenocarcinoma and pheochromocytoma.

STURGE-WEBER SYNDROME

Sturge-Weber syndrome is very rare.

- It is characterized by:
    - A large unilateral cutaneous angioma ("port wine stain") of the face.
    - A venous malformation involving the ipsilateral cerebral hemisphere and meninges.
- Patients develop cortical atrophy and epilepsy due to the cerebral angioma.

The Central Nervous System: II. Infections

63

MENINGEAL INFECTIONS

ACUTE LEPTOMENINGITIS

Acute leptomeningitis is an acute inflammation of the pia mater and arachnoid. Most cases are caused by infectious agents. Rarely, release of keratinoceous contents from an epidermoid cyst or teratoma causes a chemical meningitis. When the term *meningitis* is used without qualification, it means leptomeningitis.

Etiology & Classification
A. Acute pyogenic meningitis is caused mainly by bacteria.

- Neonatal meningitis:
  - Is acquired during passage of the fetus through the birth canal.
  - *Escherichia coli, Streptococcus agalactiae* and *Listeria monocytogenes* are the common agents.
- In children up to age 5, the most common pathogen causing meningitis is *Haemophilus influenzae.*
- In adolescents—in whom meningitis occurs most frequently—*Neisseira meningitidis* is the commonest cause.
- *Streptococcus pneumoniae* causes meningitis in all age groups, but most commonly at the extremes of life.
- The fungi *Cryptococcus neoformans, Histoplasma, Blastomyces,* and *Candida albicans* may cause meningitis in immunocompromised patients.
- Free-living amoebas belonging to the genera *Naegleria* and *Acanthamoeba* are rare causes of pyogenic meningitis.

B. Acute lymphocytic meningitis: A cellular response, consisting predominantly of lymphocytes, occurs in meningitis due to obligate intracellular organisms, usually viruses.

- Viruses commonly involved are enteroviruses, mumps virus, and lymphocytic choriomeningitis (LCM) virus.
- In about 30% of cases of acute lymphocytic meningitis, no virus can be isolated.

C. Tuberculous meningitis: Typically, this is a chronic meningitis. In the early stages there may be an exudative phase that resembles acute meningitis.

Routes of Infection of the Meninges

- Bloodstream spread accounts for the majority of cases.

- The primary entry site of the organism may be:
  - The respiratory tract (*N meningitidis, H influenzae, S pneumoniae, C neoformans,* and many viruses).
  - Skin (bacteria causing neonatal meningitis).
  - Intestine (enteroviruses).
- Meningitis may also result from:
  - Direct spread from an infected middle ear or paranasal sinus.
  - Skull fractures, especially those at the base of the skull.
  - Brain surgery and lumbar puncture.
- Rarely, organisms gain entry through the intact nasal cribriform plate (eg, free-living soil amoebas in stagnant swimming pools).
- Tuberculous meningitis may occur:
  - In severe tuberculous bacteremia (miliary tuberculosis).
  - By reactivation of a meningeal focus.

Pathology

- Grossly, the leptomeninges are congested and opaque and contain an exudate.
- Microscopically, there is hyperemia, fibrin formation, and inflammatory cells.
  - In pyogenic meningitis, neutrophils dominate.
  - In acute lymphocytic meningitis, neutrophils are rare and lymphocytes dominate.
  - In acute tuberculous meningitis, there is a mixture of neutrophils and lymphocytes.

Clinical Features

Acute meningitis presents with fever and symptoms of meningeal irritation, which include headache, neck pain, and vomiting.

- Physical examination reveals neck stiffness and a positive Kernig sign.
- Pyogenic meningitis is a serious disease with considerable risk of death.
- Viral meningitis is usually a mild self-limiting infection.
- Tuberculous meningitis has an insidious onset and a slow rate of progression, but frequently causes death if not treated.

Diagnosis

Diagnosis is made by examination of the CSF, a sample of which is obtained by lumbar puncture (Table 63–1).

Treatment

Antibiotic treatment is urgent in pyogenic and tuberculous meningitis.

- The initial choice of antibiotic should be based on a presumptive etiologic diagnosis as suggested by the clinical features and CSF findings, including Gram stain (Table 63–1).
- Viral meningitis requires only supportive treatment.

CHRONIC MENINGITIS

Chronic meningitis is caused by *Mycobacterium tuberculosi*, fungi, or *Treponema pallidum*.

TABLE 63–1. CEREBROSPINAL FLUID CHANGES IN INFECTIONS OF THE CENTRAL NERVOUS SYSTEM

	Encephalitis	Bacterial Meningitis[1]	Viral Meningitis	Tuberculous (Chronic) Meningitis	Brain Abscess
Pressure	Raised	Raised	Raised	Raised	May be very high
Gross appearance	Clear	Turbid	Clear	Clear; may clot	Clear
Protein	Slightly elevated	High	Slightly elevated	Very high	Elevated
Glucose	Normal	Very low	Normal	Low	Normal
Chloride	Normal	Low	Normal	Very low	Normal or low
Cells	Lymphocytes or normal	Neutrophils	Lymphocytes	Pleocytosis[2]	Pleocytosis
Gram stain	Negative	Positive in 90%	Negative	Negative	Occasionally positive
Acid-fast stain	Negative	Negative	Negative	Rarely positive	Negative
Bacterial culture	Negative	Positive in 90%	Negative	Negative	Occasionally positive
Mycobacterial culture	Negative	Negative	Negative	Positive	Negative
Viral culture	Positive in 30% or less	Negative	Positive in 70%	Negative	Negative

[1] Amebic and cryptococcal meningitis are diagnosed by the finding of these organisms in the smear.
[2] Pleocytosis is the presence of both neutrophils and lymphocytes in cerebrospinal fluid.

Pathology & Clinical Features

Chronic tuberculous or fungal meningitis is characterized by caseous granulomatous inflammation with fibrosis.

- Complications of chronic meningitis include:
  - Obliterative vasculitis, which may produce focal microinfarcts in the brain and brain stem.
  - Entrapment of cranial nerves in the fibrosis, resulting in cranial nerve palsies.
  - Fibrosis around the fourth ventricular foramens, causing obstructive hydrocephalus.
- Clinically, chronic meningitis is characterized by an insidious onset with low grade fever and focal neurologic symptoms.

Diagnosis & Treatment

Diagnosis is established by lumbar puncture (Table 63–1).

- Serologic tests for syphilis performed on both serum and CSF are positive in meningeal syphilis.
- Culture is commonly positive in cases caused by tuberculosis and fungal infection.
- Antibiotic therapy is indicated once the organism is identified.
- Treatment begun after extensive fibrosis has occurred does not produce complete recovery.

INFECTIONS OF THE BRAIN PARENCHYMA

CEREBRAL ABSCESS

Cerebral abscess is a localized area of suppurative inflammation in the brain substance.

Etiology

Cerebral abscesses are caused by a large variety of bacteria. Several organisms may occur in a single abscess, and anaerobic bacteria are common.

- Cerebral abscesses may occur as complications of:
  - Chronic suppurative infections of the middle ear and mastoid air spaces and of the paranasal sinuses.
  - Infective endocarditis with embolization to brain.
  - Right-to-left shunts (eg, in patients with congenital cyanotic heart disease).
  - Suppurative lung diseases such as chronic lung abscess and bronchiectasis.

Pathology

Grossly, a cerebral abscess appears as a mass lesion in the brain. It has a liquefied center filled with pus and a fibrogliotic wall whose thickness depends on the duration of the abscess. The surrounding brain frequently shows vasogenic edema.

Clinical Features & Diagnosis

Cerebral abscess presents with:

- Features of a space-occupying lesion, including evidence of raised intracranial pressure (headache, vomiting, papilledema) and focal neurologic signs, depending on the location of the abscess.

- Features relating to the source of infection, such as chronic otitis media, suppurative lung disease, and endocarditis.
- General evidence of infection, such as fever, rapid erythrocyte sedimentation rate, and weight loss in chronic cases.
- Diagnosis of cerebral abscess is made clinically and confirmed by CT scan or MRI.
- CSF may be normal or may show mild increases in protein, neutrophils, and lymphocytes (Table 63–1). Cultures may or may not be positive.

Treatment
Surgical evacuation of the abscess is followed by antibiotic therapy. The mortality rate is about 5–10%.

VIRAL ENCEPHALITIS
In the United States, about 1500 cases are reported every year. The etiologic virus is identified in only about 30% of cases.

- Epidemics of encephalitis are most commonly the result of arthropod-borne viruses (arboviruses) (Table 63–2).
- Sporadic cases of encephalitis may be caused by a large number of other viruses, most commonly herpes simplex.

TABLE 63–2. CAUSES OF VIRAL ENCEPHALITIS

Diffuse encephalitis
Epidemic (arbovirus) encephalitis
Eastern equine encephalitis
Western equine encephalitis
Venezuelan equine encephalitis
St. Louis encephalitis
California encephalitis
Japanese B encephalitis
Sporadic encephalitis
Herpes simplex
Enterovirus encephalitis
Measles
Varicella (chickenpox)
Encephalitis in the immunocompromised host
Herpes simplex
Progressive multifocal leukoencephalopathy
Cytomegalovirus
HIV (AIDS encephalitis)
Specific types of encephalitis
Poliomyelitis
Rabies
Subacute sclerosing panencephalitis
Slow virus infections

Pathology

The virus usually reaches the brain via the bloodstream. It infects brain cells, causing neuronal necrosis and cerebral edema, which in turn leads to acute cerebral dysfunction and increased intracranial pressure. Perivascular lymphocytic infiltration is characteristic.

Clinical Features

Viral encephalitis has an acute onset with fever, headache, and signs of brain dysfunction. In many cases, there is concomitant meningitis causing neck stiffness and CSF abnormalities. Lumbar puncture with examination and culture of CSF may provide an etiologic diagnosis.

Treatment

Control of cerebral edema with high doses of corticosteroids is useful to control raised intracranial pressure. The mortality rate is high, and patients who recover are frequently left with permanent neurologic deficits.

1. HERPES SIMPLEX ENCEPHALITIS

Incidence & Etiology

Herpes simplex encephalitis occurs in:

- Neonates, who are infected during delivery to a woman with active genital herpes. Herpes simplex type II is usually involved.
- Adults, who are infected through the bloodstream from a focus of viral replication, usually in the mouth. Herpes simplex type I is commonly involved.
- Immunocompromised hosts, particularly patients undergoing chemotherapy for cancer.

Pathology

This encephalitis affects the inferior frontal and temporal lobes. It causes a severe hemorrhagic necrotizing encephalitis. Patients who survive frequently have permanent neurologic damage.

Diagnosis & Treatment

Diagnosis may be made by:

- Brain biopsy, which shows Cowdry A intranuclear inclusions in infected cells. Immunohistochemical demonstration of viral antigens and electron microscopy are useful.
- Serologic studies show elevated Herpes simplex antibody levels.
- Treatment with antiviral drugs is effective in the acute phase.

2. POLIOMYELITIS

This is caused by the poliovirus, an enterovirus transmitted by the feco-oral route. It has become rare because of childhood immunization.

- The poliovirus selectively infects:
  - The meninges, causing an acute lymphocytic meningitis.
  - The lower motor neuron in the anterior horn of the spinal cord and medulla oblongata.

- Clinically, there is acute asymmetric flaccid paralysis of skeletal muscles. Muscle atrophy occurs rapidly.
- Death may occur in the acute phase from paralysis of respiratory muscles.
- Patients who recover commonly have permanent muscle paralysis.

3. RABIES

Rabies is rare in humans, but common in wild and domestic animals, particularly in underdeveloped countries.

- Humans are infected by the bite of an infected animal.
- The virus passes to the nervous system along the nerves. The incubation period is 1–3 months.
- Rabies virus causes a severe, necrotizing encephalitis that maximally affects the basal ganglia, hippocampus, and brain stem.
- Infected neurons show eosinophilic cytoplasmic inclusions (Negri bodies).
- Death is invariable. There is no treatment.

4. CYTOMEGALOVIRUS ENCEPHALITIS

This encephalitis occurs in neonates due to transplacental infection during the last trimester. It causes periventricular necrosis, leading to microcephaly and mental retardation. CMV encephalitis also occurs in immunocompromised hosts, particularly in AIDS.

5. PROGRESSIVE MULTIFOCAL LEUKOENCEPHALOPATHY (PML)

This is caused by papovavirus SV40. It occurs in immunocompromised hosts—commonly in AIDS and those undergoing chemotherapy for cancer. It is characterized by widespread focal demyelination of cerebral white matter with maximal involvement of occipital lobes.

- Giant astrocytes and intranuclear inclusions are present in biopsy specimens, and permit diagnosis.
- Clinically, PML presents as an acute illness characterized by severe cerebral dysfunction.
- The mortality rate is high.

6. SUBACUTE SCLEROSING PANENCEPHALITIS (SSPE)

This is an uncommon disease, usually affecting children. It is caused by the measles virus. The exact mechanism by which the measles virus causes SSPE is unknown.

- Pathologically, it is characterized by neuronal degeneration, mainly in the basal ganglia and gray matter.
- The white matter shows demyelination, edema, and lymphocytic infiltration.
- Clinically, presentation is with personality changes and myoclonic type seizures.
- SSPE is relentlessly progressive, leading to death 1–2 years from onset.

7. SLOW "VIRUS" INFECTIONS

These are characterized by a long latent period after infection. This is followed by an encephalitis of insidious onset and slow but relentless progression to a fatal outcome.

- Diseases included in this category are:

TABLE 63–3. NEUROSYPHILIS: PATHOLOGIC AND CLINICAL FEATURES

Type of Disease	Time Elapsed After Primary Infection	Principal Pathologic Features	CSF	Clinical Features
Asymptomatic	2–3 years	Mild lymphocytic meningeal infiltrate	Positive VDRL[1]	Very common; discovered by routine lumbar puncture in patients with secondary syphilis; penicillin is curative
Meningovascular syphilis Diffuse	3+ years	Chronic inflammation of meninges with fibrosis and endarteritis	Increased protein; mild lymphocytosis; positive VDRL	Meningeal symptoms; cranial nerve palsies; penicillin may be effective in early stage
Focal	3+ years	Gumma formation	Positive VDRL; increased protein, lymphocytosis	Very rare; acts as a space-occupying lesion
Parenchymatous syphilis General paresis	10+ years	Diffuse cerebral cortical neuronal loss; chronic encephalitis; spirochetes present	Positive VDRL; mild lymphocytosis	Progressive dementia and psychosis; cerebral atrophy with ventricle dilatation; penicillin not effective
Tabes dorsalis	10+ years	Demyelination of spinal cord (posterior columns) and sensory nerve root; spirochetes absent	Positive VDRL; mild lymphocytosis	Lightning pains, sensory loss, hypotonia, areflexia; penicillin not effective

[1]VDRL = Veneral Disease Research Laboratory serologic test for syphilis. This is positive in about 50% of all cases of neurosyphilis. The more sensitive FTA-ABS (fluorescent treponemal antibody test) is positive in 90%.

- Creutzfeldt-Jakob disease.
- Kuru, which occurs among cannibalistic tribes in Papua-New Guinea.
- Scrapie, an encephalitis of goats and sheep.
■ They are believed to be caused by prions.
■ Pathologically, it is characterized by progressive neuronal loss, demyelination, and edema.
■ Clinically, patients present with dementia followed by ataxia. There is no treatment.

NEUROSYPHILIS (Table 63–3)
Syphilis involves the nervous system in its late stage. Neurosyphilis has become rare, due to effective treatment of early syphilis.

■ The three different disease types are (Table 63–3):
- Meningovascular syphilis.
- Tabes dorsalis, which affects the spinal cord.
- General paresis which involves the cerebral cortex.
■ Manifestations of the different types may coexist in one patient.

GRANULOMAS OF THE BRAIN
Infectious granulomas of the brain are rare lesions caused by *M. tuberculosis* and fungi. They are characterized by an area of central caseous necrosis surrounded by epithelioid cells and fibrosis. They present clinically as mass lesions of the brain resembling neoplasms. Diagnosis is made by biopsy.

PARASITIC INFECTIONS

Toxoplasmosis
Toxoplasma gondii infection of humans occurs through contact with infected cats.

■ Congenital toxoplasmosis:
- Is by transplacental infection in the third trimester.
- Causes extensive necrosis of brain and retina.
- Many fetuses are stillborn. Those that survive may show microcephaly, calcification of the brain, mental retardation and visual disturbances.
■ Acquired toxoplasmosis:
- Causes cerebral infection in immunocompromised hosts, particularly AIDS patients.
- Is characterized by multiple necrotic mass lesions.
- Clinically, it presents with fever and symptoms of acute cerebral dysfunction. CT scan shows ring-enhancing lesions.
- Diagnosis is by identifying the protozoan in biopsy specimens.

Other Parasitic Infections
■ Cerebral malaria is caused by infection with *Plasmodium falciparum*.
■ African trypanosomiasis (sleeping sickness) is caused by *Trypanosoma rhodesiense* and *T gambiense*. It is transmitted by the tsetse fly.
■ Cysticercosis, hydatid cysts, trichinosis, schistosomiasis and amoebiasis infect the central nervous system rarely and only in endemic areas.

The Central Nervous System: III. Traumatic, Vascular, Degenerative, & Metabolic Diseases

64

TRAUMATIC NERVOUS SYSTEM LESIONS

CEREBRAL INJURIES

1. PENETRATING (OPEN) INJURIES
These injuries are caused by gunshots and severe blunt trauma. They are associated with severe brain damage and a high incidence of infection.

2. NONPENETRATING (CLOSED) INJURIES
These injuries are usually caused by blunt trauma.

A. Cerebral concussion is the transient loss of cerebral function, including loss of consciousness, that immediately follows head injury.

■ The brain shows no gross or histologic abnormality.
■ In severe cases coma may be prolonged, and in rare cases death may be the outcome.

B. Cerebral contusion is caused by rupture of small blood vessels and extravasation of blood into the brain substance.

■ Most commonly, it is caused by movement of the brain relative to the skull, causing it to strike bony prominences.
■ It may also occur:
   ● Subjacent to the point of impact, particularly if there is a depressed skull fracture.
   ● On the side opposite the point of impact (contrecoup injuries).
■ It may appear as an area of subpial hemorrhage. The lesion undergoes color change from red to brown.
■ Cerebral contusions may serve as a focus for epileptic activity.

C. Cerebral laceration is characterized by tearing of cerebral tissue, resulting in acute hemorrhage in the subarachnoid or subdural space.

■ It is often associated with profound neurologic dysfunction.
■ There is a high mortality rate.

SPINAL CORD INJURIES
These injuries result from forced movements (such as the "whiplash" injury of the cervical cord) or vertebral fractures and subluxations.

- Road traffic accidents, diving into shallow water, and sports injuries are common causes.
- These injuries in the spinal cord are similar to those in the brain: concussion, contusion, and laceration.
- With high cervical cord injury, quadriplegia occurs.
- Thoracic cord injuries may lead to paraplegia and dysfunction of the bladder and rectum.

MENINGEAL TEARS
Meningeal tears may occur with fractures of the base of the skull. They are manifested clinically as a leak of cerebrospinal fluid through the nose (CSF rhinorrhea) or ears (CSF otorrhea). The main risk is infection.

TRAUMATIC INTRACRANIAL HEMORRHAGE

1. ACUTE EXTRADURAL HEMATOMA
This is one of the commonest complications of nonpenetrating head injuries. It is an accumulation of blood between the skull and the dura (Fig 64–1). In 90% of cases, bleeding is from a branch of the middle meningeal artery. In the remainder, the bleeding is of venous origin.

- Laceration of the middle meningeal artery is often associated with fracture of the temporal region of the skull.
- With arterial bleeding, symptoms appear within hours after injury; with venous bleeding, progression is less rapid.
- The clinical history is characteristic:
  - It follows a head injury, often associated with concussion.
  - There is a lucid interval, during which the patient appears normal.
  - There is evidence of raised intracranial pressure with headache, vomiting, altered consciousness, and papilledema.
- Tentorial herniation rapidly follows (pupillary abnormalities and pyramidal tract compression).
- Coma and death rapidly ensue in untreated cases.
- It requires urgent diagnosis and treatment by surgical evacuation of the blood clot.

2. CHRONIC SUBDURAL HEMATOMA
This is a common lesion characterized by accumulation of blood in the subdural space (Fig 64–1). It occurs mainly in elderly patients with some degree of cerebral atrophy.

- The amount of trauma required is minimal, and many patients give no history of head injury.
- Bleeding is the result of rupture of veins passing from the cerebral cortex to the superior sagittal sinus.
- Chronic subdural hematomas are frequently bilateral.
- Bleeding is slow. The blood clot in the subdural space breaks down and exerts an osmotic effect that draws in fluid from the adjacent subarachnoid space.
- Clinically, patients present with slowly increasing intracranial pressure, causing headache, vomiting, papilledema, and fluctuating levels of consciousness.
- Treatment is by surgical evacuation of the fluid collection.

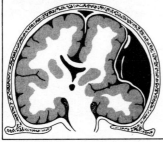

Extradural hematoma
- Trauma usually severe, associated with concussion and skull fracture
- Source: usually middle meningeal artery
- Course: acute (hours)

Subdural hematoma
- Trauma usually mild
- Source: usually communicating veins
- Course: slow (days to months)

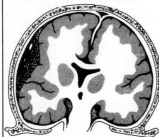

Subarachnoid hemorrhage
- Source: circle of Willis or cerebral arteries; usually berry aneurysm
- Course: acute (instantaneous or minutes)

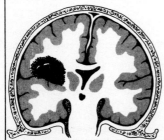

Intracerebral hemorrhage
- Source: small intracerebral arteries (especially lenticulostriate)
  - Microaneurysms
  - Hypertension
- Course: instantaneous

Figure 64–1. Common types of intracranial hemorrhage. Extradural and subdural hematomas are commonly caused by trauma, whereas subarachnoid and intracerebral hemorrhage are commonly the result of diseases involving the blood vessels.

CEREBROVASCULAR ACCIDENTS (Strokes)

The terms *CVA* and *stroke* denote a wide variety of nontraumatic cerebrovascular accidents of abrupt onset. Strokes have many causes (Table 64–1; Fig 64–2).

- Cerebral thrombosis with infarction is responsible for about 90% of cases.
- Stroke is one of the leading causes of death in developed countries, accounting for approximately 200,000 deaths per year in the USA.

ISCHEMIC STROKES

1. CEREBRAL INFARCTION

Etiology
A. Atherosclerosis:

- Atherosclerosis and thrombosis are responsible for most cases of cerebral infarction.
- Atherosclerosis tends to involve the large arteries—especially sites of arterial branching (such as the carotid bifurcation) and curvature (the carotid siphon).
- Occlusions promixal to the circle of Willis are usually compensated for by the collaterals in the circle.
- Arteries distal to the circle are functional end arteries, and their occlusion usually results in cerebral infarction.

B. Emboli may be responsible for many cases of "nonocclusive" infarction.

- Cerebral emboli occur:
  - After myocardial infarction, due to detachment of mural thrombi.
  - With infective endocarditis, due to detachment of valvular vegetations.

TABLE 64–1. CLASSIFICATION AND ETIOLOGY OF CEREBROVASCULAR ACCIDENTS (CVA; "STROKES")

Ischemic	Hemorrhagic
Cerebral infarction	Intracerebral hemorrhage:
Nonocclusive	hypertensive
Cerebral arterial	Subarachnoid hemor-
thrombosis	rhage: berry aneurysms
Cerebral embolism	Associated with vascular
Transient ischemic attack	malformations and
Hypertensive encephalopa-	neoplasms
thy with vasospasm	Associated with bleeding
Venous occlusion: in hy-	diathesis such as coag-
percoagulable states,	ulation disorders,
infection	thrombocytopenia; anti-
Arteritis: polyarteritis	coagulant therapy
nodosa, giant cell	
arteritis	
Dissecting aneurysm of the	
aorta	
Carotid injury	

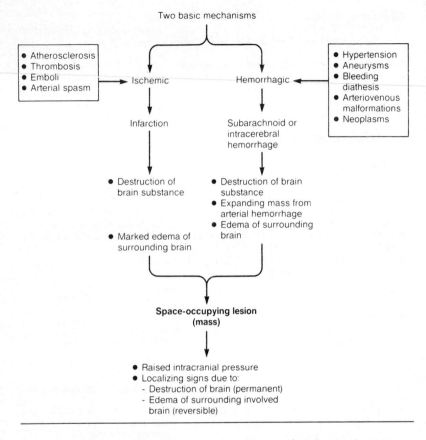

Figure 64–2. Etiology and pathogenesis of the 2 major types of cerebrovascular accident.

- With prosthetic cardiac valves.
- With mitral stenosis and atrial fibrillation.
- With atherosclerotic disease in the aortic arch, carotids, or circle of Willis.

C. Other Causes:

■ Rarely, cerebral ischemia is the result of vasculitides such as polyarteritis nodosa and giant cell arteritis (Table 64–1).
■ Cerebral venous occlusion is a rare cause. It occurs in hypercoagulable states.

Pathology

The earliest gross change after infarction occurs at about 6 hours and is a softening of the brain with loss of demarcation between gray and white matter.

- Microscopically, the neurons show nuclear pyknosis, cytoplasmic eosinophilia, and liquefaction.
- At 48–72 hours the cerebral infarct appears as a pale, soft area composed of liquefied necrotic cells. Foamy macrophages (gitter cells) are present in the wall.
- Ten to twenty percent of cerebral infarcts are hemorrhagic.
- After about three weeks, the debris has been cleared, producing a cystic fluid-filled cavity surrounded by a zone of reactive gliosis.

Clinical Features

Characterized by a sudden loss of neurologic function corresponding to the area involved (Table 64–2).

- The onset may be acute, but it is usually not as explosive as in cerebral hemorrhage. In many cases the neurologic deficit progresses over several hours to days.
- Infarction secondary to thrombosis has a slower onset than that caused by embolism.

TABLE 64–2. LOCALIZING SIGNS ASSOCIATED WITH OCCLUSION OF MAJOR CEREBRAL ARTERIES

Artery Occluded	Area Infarcted	Clinical Effect
Anterior cerebral artery	Frontal lobe	Confusion, disorientation
	Motor and sensory cortex (leg area)	Contralateral weakness maximal in leg; cortical-type sensory loss, maximal in leg
Middle cerebral artery	Lateral surface of hemisphere	Contralateral hemiparesis, face > leg; contralateral cortical-type sensory loss
	Speech area (if dominant hemisphere)	Expressive aphasia
	Optic radiation	Hemianopia
Posterior cerebral artery	Occipital lobe	Cortical-type visual loss
Vertebrobasilar arteries	Cerebellum	Intention tremor, incoordination, hypotonia
	Brain stem	Contralateral hemiparesis and sensory loss; ipsilateral cranial nerve palsies

■ Most patients show evidence of raised intracranial pressure due to the presence of edema.

Treatment & Prognosis
In the acute phase, corticosteroids and diuretics such as furosemide and mannitol are used to decrease cerebral edema and intracranial pressure. The overall prognosis for recovery of neurologic function after cerebral infarction is reasonably good.

2. TRANSIENT ISCHEMIC ATTACKS
TIAs are caused by platelet or cholesterol emboli originating in ulcerative atherosclerotic plaques in the carotid arteries or the aorta. They are characterized by sudden neurologic deficits lasting a few seconds to a few minutes. Full recovery (within 24 hours) is the rule.

■ The frequency of attacks varies from several times a day to once in several months.
■ The embolic fragments may sometimes be seen in the vessels of the optic fundus.
■ Thirty percent of patients having transient ischemic attacks suffer cerebral infarction within 5 years. Thirty percent of patients with cerebral infarction give a history of transient ischemic attacks.
■ Vascular surgery, anticoagulant therapy, and aspirin therapy may be used.

3. HYPERTENSIVE ENCEPHALOPATHY
This results from cerebral ischemia due to arterial spasm precipitated by extremely high blood pressure.

■ Spasm is temporary and results in cerebral edema, usually without necrosis.
■ Patients develop acute transient neurologic dysfunction, convulsions, and raised intracranial pressure.
■ It requires immediate treatment to reduce blood pressure and decrease cerebral edema. Recovery is the rule.

HEMORRHAGIC STROKES (Table 64–1)

1. SPONTANEOUS INTRACEREBRAL HEMORRHAGE
Cerebral hemorrhage is responsible for about 10% of strokes. Over 80% of intracerebral hemorrhages are secondary to hypertension. Most occur after age 40.

Pathology
The site of rupture is frequently a microaneurysm (Charcot-Bouchard aneurysm) in the lenticulostriate arteries.

■ Multiple microaneurysms occur at this location in 70% of hypertensive patients.
■ Rupture is commonly precipitated by a sudden increase in blood pressure.
■ The hematoma involves the basal ganglia and deep white matter, including the internal capsule.
■ The rapidly expanding blood clot dissects and destroys brain tissue and may rupture into the ventricular system or subarachnoid space.
■ The hematoma causes rapid and marked increase in intracranial pressure.

Clinical Features

This is characterized by an abrupt onset of headache, dense neurologic deficit, papilledema, and loss of consciousness ("cerebral apoplexy"). Hemiplegia from pyramidal tract involvement in the internal capsule is the commonest neurologic deficit. Cerebral hemorrhage has a high mortality rate.

2. SPONTANEOUS SUBARACHNOID HEMORRHAGE

This is less common than spontaneous intracerebral hemorrhage. In 95% of cases, it results from rupture of a berry aneurysm (saccular aneurysm) of the cerebral arteries. Berry aneurysms are generally located in the circle of Willis. The common sites are:

- The anterior communicating artery (30%).
- The junction of the posterior communicating and internal carotid arteries (30%).
- The middle cerebral artery (10%).
- The basilar artery (10%).
- In 10–20% of cases, multiple berry aneurysms are present.

Pathology

Rupture of a berry aneurysm may occur at any time, but is rare in childhood. The frequency of rupture increases with age.

- Rupture of an aneurysm may be precipitated by hypertension, exercise, or sexual intercourse.
- Many aneurysms never rupture and are found incidentally at autopsy.
- When aneurysms rupture, they usually cause rapid bleeding into the subarachnoid space. Rarely, they cause intracerebral hemorrhage.
- Intact berry aneurysms may become large enough to cause focal symptoms, eg, third nerve paralysis due to compression by a large posterior communicating artery aneurysm.

Clinical Features

- Subarachnoid hemorrhage presents with sudden onset of severe "bursting" headache associated with vomiting, pain in the neck, and rapid loss of consciousness.
- Marked neck stiffness is present.
- Raised intracranial pressure with papilledema is common. The retina may show an area of hemorrhage below the optic disk.
- Lumbar puncture shows blood in cerebrospinal fluid.
- Death may occur rapidly. In patients who recover, there is a high risk of recurrence, and surgical correction is urgent.

VENOUS OCCLUSION

Occlusion of cerebral veins and venous sinuses is an uncommon cause of cerebrovascular accident.

- Superior sagittal sinus thrombosis may occur in severely malnourished or chronically sick individuals. It is characterized by edema, hemorrhage, and infarction of both cerebral hemispheres.

- Thrombophlebitis of the cortical cerebral veins rarely occurs in women after childbirth or abortion. When extensive, it causes fever, convulsions, and infarction of the cerebral hemisphere.
- Thrombosis of the vein of Galen (internal cerebral vein) leads to hemorrhagic infarction of the thalamic region and deep white matter.
- Cavernous sinus thrombophlebitis may result from spread of infection from the face and orbit, and is associated with high fever, leukocytosis, orbital edema, congestion, and hemorrhage.
- Lateral sinus thrombophlebitis may occur as a complication of suppurative otitis media. It is accompanied by severe bacteremia and associated with high fever and pain in the back of the head.

DEMYELINATING DISEASES (Table 64–3)

MULTIPLE SCLEROSIS
Multiple sclerosis is the most common demyelinating disease. Its incidence varies greatly in different parts of the world:

- It is most common in the Scandinavian countries, with a prevalence of 80:100,000 in Norway.
- It is progressively rarer as one moves south (10:100,000 in southern Europe).
- In the United States, Massachusetts has a higher incidence than Florida.
- It is rare in the tropics (1:100,000) and in Asia, even in the northern latitudes of Japan.
- Individuals who migrate in early childhood from a low-risk to a high-risk area have the same risk of developing multiple sclerosis as those in the country to which they move. If the same move is made after adolescence, the risk remains low.
- Infection by an unidentified slow virus in childhood is thought to be responsible.
- The onset of multiple sclerosis is usually between ages 20 and 40.
- Both sexes are affected, and there is no racial predominance within geographic areas.
- There is an increased family incidence plus an increased frequency of HLA-A3, -B7, and -DR2.

Etiology
The etiology is uncertain.

- Patients with multiple sclerosis commonly have high measles antibody titers.
- Measles virus and canine distemper virus, a paramyxovirus that cross-reacts with measles antibody, have been suggested as possible causes.
- Immunologic hypersensitivity may play a role.

Pathology
It is characterized by the presence in the white matter of plaques of demyelination. These are irregular, well-demarcated, gray or translucent lesions.

- Multiple plaques, widely disseminated throughout the central nervous system, are common.
- Any area of the brain can be affected. Sites of predilection are:
  - The optic nerves.

TABLE 64–3. DEMYELINATING DISEASES

Disease	Comments
Multiple sclerosis (MS)	Possible viral or immune mediated
Neuromyelitis optica (Devic's disease)	Variant of MS with lesions focused in optic nerves, brain stem, and spinal cord
Experimental allergic encephalomyelitis (EAE)	Demyelination induced in animals by immunization against brain tissue
Acute disseminated encephalomyelitis	Apparent human analogue of EAE; occurs postinfection with or post-immunization for smallpox, rabies, or pertussis
Guillain-Barré syndrome	Resembles EAE but demyelination involves nerve roots and peripheral nerves; typically follows virus infection
Progressive multifocal leukoencephalopathy	Papilloma virus infection (see Chapter 63)
Subacute sclerosing panencephalitis	Delayed injury caused by measles virus (see Chapter 63)
Diffuse sclerosis (Schilder's disease)	Several variants, familial and sporadic; present early in life; may include several different entities
Dysmyelinative disorders	Disorders of myelin metabolism; metachromatic leukodystrophy, lipidoses, phenylketonuria
Demyelination secondary to systemic disease	Anoxia, toxic agents, nutritional disorders (eg, vitamin B_{12} deficiency)

- Paraventricular region and deep cerebrum.
- Brain stem.
- Cerebellum.
- Spinal cord.
■ Microscopically, the plaques show demyelination and tangled masses of preserved axons. Lymphocytic infiltration is present in areas of active demyelination.

Clinical Features
Multiple sclerosis is a chronic disease with an extremely variable clinical course, characterized by episodic relapses and remissions over several years.

■ The clinical manifestations depend on the area of brain affected. Common manifestations are:
- Abnormalities in vision.
- Cerebellar dysfunction.
- Paresthesias, weakness, and spinal cord dysfunction.

- The randomly disseminated nature of the lesions gives a characteristic clinical picture.
- The cerebrospinal fluid shows a mild increase in the number of lymphocytes, elevated protein, and oligoclonal immunoglobulin bands on immunoelectrophoresis.
- Treatment is limited to the management of complications. The course of the disease is not altered by treatment.

DEMYELINATION IN IMMUNOLOGIC INJURIES

1. EXPERIMENTAL ALLERGIC ENCEPHALOMYELITIS
Acute demyelination of nerve fibers in the central nervous system can be produced in many animals by injection of a brain emulsion in Freund's adjuvant. It is thought to be due to the action of sensitized T lymphocytes against myelin protein.

2. ACUTE DISSEMINATED ENCEPHALOMYELITIS
This is a group of diseases believed to have a pathogenesis similar to that of experimental allergic encephalomyelitis.

- It occurs:
  - After viral infections (postinfectious encephalomyelitis).
  - After immunization against smallpox, rabies, or pertussis.
- Lymphocytes from these patients exhibit cell-mediated immunologic reactivity against myelin protein in vitro.
- Pathologically, there is extensive acute demyelination of the white matter of the brain and spinal cord.
- The mortality rate is high.

3. GUILLAIN-BARRÉ SYNDROME
This is an uncommon disease believed to be the peripheral nervous system equivalent of experimental allergic encephalomyelitis. It follows viral infection in a majority of cases.

- Pathologically, Guillain-Barré syndrome is characterized by acute demyelination of multiple cranial and spinal nerve roots (polyradiculopathy).
- The cerebrospinal fluid shows cell-protein dissociation. The cell count is normal but the protein is markedly elevated.
- Clinically, there is a subacute onset with motor neuron weakness, mainly in the lower extremities. Sensory impairment is minimal.
- Paralysis progresses for 1–4 weeks and then slowly improves over several months.
- Ninety percent of patients recover completely.
- Treatment is supportive. Plasma exchange is helpful in severe cases or when respiratory muscle paralysis occurs.

DEGENERATIVE DISEASES

CEREBROCORTICAL DEGENERATIONS

1. ALZHEIMER'S DISEASE
Alzheimer's disease is very common. It is responsible for more than 50% of all cases of dementia (Table 64–4).

TABLE 64–4. PRINCIPAL CAUSES OF DEMENTIA

Alzheimer's disease: over 50% of cases
Chronic alcoholism
Tertiary syphilis (now rare)
Multiple cerebral infarcts
Creutzfeldt-Jakob disease
Huntington's chorea
Pick's disease
Chronic subdural hematoma
Aluminum toxicity, in chronic renal failure
Drugs
Deficiency of vitamins B_{12}, B_6, B_1
Hypothyroidism ("myxedema madness")
Chronic meningitis
Hydrocephalus, low pressure

Etiology

The cause is unknown. In some families, there is evidence of transmission as an autosomal dominant age-dependent trait.

- An abnormality of the chromosome 21 gene encoding the β-amyloid protein of Alzheimer's disease has been demonstrated.
- Deficient synthesis of acetylcholine has been demonstrated in some patients.
- High levels of aluminum have been detected in some lesions, and some patients have increased serum aluminum levels.

Pathology

- Grossly, there is atrophy of the cerebral cortex with thinning of the gyri and widening of the sulci. The frontal cortex is maximally affected.
- Microscopically, it is characterized by:
  - Neuronal loss and disorganization of the cerebrocortical layers.
  - Neurofibrillary tangles in the cytoplasm of affected neurons.
  - Argyrophilic plaques, which are large (150 μm) extracellular collections of degenerated cellular processes disposed around a central mass of β-amyloid protein.

Clinical Features

Usually it occurs in patients over age 50. It presents with slow onset of dementia, which progresses inexorably over 10–20 years. There is no effective treatment.

2. PICK'S DISEASE

This is an extremely uncommon cause of presenile dementia, occurring in the age group from 40 to 65 years. The cause is unknown.

- Clinically, the course is indistinguishable from that of Alzheimer's disease.
- Pathologically, neurofibrillary tangles and argyrophilic plaques are not present. Affected neurons contain round, eosinophilic cytoplasmic inclusions (Pick bodies).

BASAL GANGLIA DEGENERATIONS

1. IDIOPATHIC PARKINSON'S DISEASE (Paralysis Agitans)

This is a common disease, affecting 5% of persons over age 70. The exact cause is unknown. There is degeneration of the pigmented nuclei of the brain stem, particularly the substantia nigra, producing dysfunction of the extrapyramidal system. Failure of normal dopamine synthesis is postulated as the mechanism for the dysfunction.

Pathology

- Grossly, there is depigmentation of the substantia nigra.
- Microscopically, loss of pigmented neurons is accompanied by gliosis in the substantia nigra and other basal ganglia.
- Lewy bodies—rounded eosinophilic cytoplasmic inclusions—may be present in the remaining neurons; they are characteristic of Parkinson's disease.

Clinical Features

Onset is usually after age 50, and the disease is slowly progressive. It is characterized by increased rigidity of muscles, resting tremors, and slowness of movements (bradykinesia).

- Patients have a typical gait, walking stooped forward with short, quick, shuffling steps (festinating gait).
- Treatment with levodopa produces a good clinical response in most cases. As the disease progresses, control becomes difficult.
- Recently, transplantation of autologous adrenal medulla into the region of the basal ganglia has produced clinical improvement.

2. OTHER CAUSES OF PARKINSON'S SYNDROME

Clinical features identical to idiopathic Parkinson's disease may be caused by:

- Postencephalitic parkinsonism, which occurred in association with the influenza epidemic of 1914–1918, and tended to arise in younger individuals.
- Ischemic damage to the basal ganglia associated with atherosclerosis.
- Wilson's disease, due to deposition of copper in the basal ganglia (see Chapter 43).
- Damage to the basal ganglia from exposure to carbon monoxide and manganese.
- Drugs, notably the phenothiazines and reserpine.
- Shy-Drager syndrome, which consists of intractable hypotension with various autonomic defects and Parkinson's syndrome.

3. HUNTINGTON'S CHOREA

This is a rare disease that is inherited as an autosomal dominant trait with complete penetrance but delayed appearance. It is characterized by atrophy and loss of neurons of the caudate nucleus and putamen, associated with variable cerebrocortical atrophy, particularly in the frontal lobe.

- The disease has its onset in adult life, usually between ages 20 and 50.
- It is characterized by depression, dementia, and choreiform involuntary movements.
- The disease is slowly but inexorably progressive, leading to death in 10–20 years.

SPINOCEREBELLAR DEGENERATIONS

These rare diseases are usually inherited as autosomal recessive traits. They include:

- Friedreich's ataxia, in which there is degeneration of spinocerebellar tracts, posterior columns, the pyramidal tract, and the peripheral nerves (Fig 64–3).
- Olivopontocerebellar degeneration, in which there is degeneration of neurons in the cerebellar cortex, cerebellar nuclei, olivary nuclei, and pons.

MOTOR NEURON DISEASE

This disease is characterized by degeneration of both upper and lower motor neurons. The cause is unknown.

- Most cases occur in a sporadic manner. A high incidence of familial occurrence has been reported in Guam, the Marianas, and the Caroline Islands.
- Typically, it affects individuals over age 50.
- The neurologic deficit is purely motor (Fig 64–3).
- Depending on the distribution of lesions, four clinical variants of the disease are recognized:
  - Amyotrophic lateral sclerosis is characterized by degeneration of the corticospinal tracts in the spinal cord, causing upper motor neurone paralysis in the extremities.
  - Progressive muscular atrophy shows degeneration of anterior horn motor nuclei, causing lower motor neuron paralysis in the extremities.
  - Progressive bulbar palsy affects medullary motor nuclei, causing lower motor paralysis of the jaw, tongue, and pharyngeal muscles.
  - Pseudobulbar palsy is a disorder in which bilateral upper motor neuron paralysis of the jaw, tongue, and pharyngeal muscles occurs.
- The disease is slowly progressive. Death usually occurs 1–6 years from onset. There is no specific treatment.

NUTRITIONAL DISEASES

SUBACUTE COMBINED DEGENERATION OF THE CORD

This degeneration is caused by deficiency of vitamin B_{12} (see Chapter 24). It is characterized by demyelination involving (Fig 64–3):

- The posterior columns, leading to loss of position and vibration sense and loss of reflexes.
- The lateral columns, resulting in upper motor neuron paralysis.
- The peripheral nerves.
- Peripheral neuropathy or optic neuropathy may also occur as isolated lesions in patients with vitamin B_{12} deficiency.

WERNICKE'S ENCEPHALOPATHY

This is caused by thiamine deficiency (see Chapter 10), which is commonly seen in malnourished individuals and chronic alcoholics. It involves the floor of the third

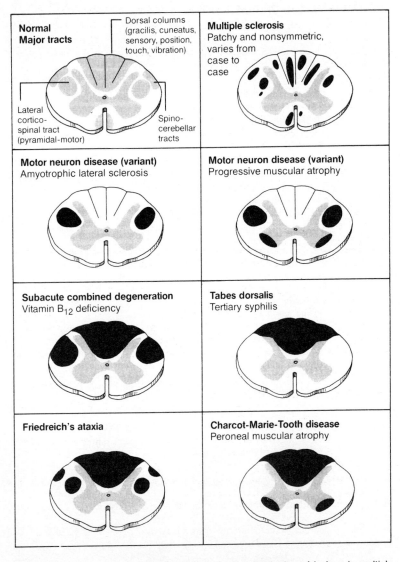

Figure 64–3. Sections of spinal cord, showing typical distribution of lesions in multiple sclerosis, motor neuron disease, Friedreich's ataxia, subacute combined degeneration, tabes dorsalis, and peroneal muscular atrophy.

ventricle and the periaqueductal region of the midbrain. The mammillary bodies are maximally involved.

- The early lesion is characterized by petechial hemorrhages and capillary proliferation. This is followed by atrophy and degeneration of neurons.
- The atrophic areas show brownish discoloration because of hemosiderin pigment deposition.
- Clinically, it is manifested by:
  - Ocular muscle paralysis and nystagmus.
  - Confusion and a psychotic state (Korsakoff's psychosis).

PELLAGRA ENCEPHALOPATHY

This is caused by nicotinamide deficiency. It is characterized by neuronal degeneration affecting the cerebral cortex, pontine nuclei, cranial nerve nuclei, and anterior horn cells in the spinal cord. Dementia is the most common clinical manifestation.

METABOLIC DISEASES

KERNICTERUS

Kernicterus (see Chapter 1) is a rare disease of neonates resulting from deposition of bilirubin in the brain, particularly in the basal ganglia.

- The disease occurs in premature infants who develop unconjugated hyperbilirubinemia due to hemolysis of red cells.
- Rh compatibility (hemolytic disease of the newborn) is the commonest cause.
- Severe kernicterus has a high mortality rate.
- Patients who survive show extrapyramidal dysfunction.

TABLE 64–5. CONGENITAL METABOLIC DISEASES (INBORN ERRORS OF METABOLISM) ASSOCIATED WITH MENTAL RETARDATION

Defects of amino acid metabolism
  Phenylketonuria (phenylalanine)
  Maple syrup urine disease (valine, leucine,
    isoleucine)
  Others (very rare)

Lipid storage diseases   Tay-Sachs disease

Mucopolysaccharidoses
  Hunter-Hurler syndrome
  Morquio's syndrome

Disorders of carbohydrate metabolism
  Galactosemia
  Glycogen storage diseases

WILSON'S DISEASE

Wilson's disease (see Chapter 43) is an inherited disorder characterized by deposition of copper in the liver and the basal ganglia, especially the lenticular nuclei. Extrapyramidal symptoms due to lenticular nucleus degeneration occur in early life, and include rigidity and involuntary movements.

INBORN ERRORS OF METABOLISM

Numerous inherited enzyme deficiencies are associated with diffuse cortical neuronal loss and mental retardation (Table 64–5).

The Central Nervous System: IV. Neoplasms

65

INTRODUCTION

Intracranial and spinal neoplasms may be primary or metastatic. Metastatic tumors are more common.

- Primary intracranial neoplasms number about 13,000 new cases a year in the USA and represent about 2% of deaths from malignant neoplasms.
- They are the second most common group of neoplasms in children, after leukemia/lymphoma.
- Sixty-five percent of primary intracranial neoplasms are gliomas, 10% meningiomas, 10% acoustic schwannomas, 5% medulloblastomas, and 10% others.
- Primary malignant lymphomas of the central nervous system are common in patients with AIDS.

Classification

A. Histogenetic classification is based on the cell of origin (Table 65–1).

B. Topographic classification: Intracranial neoplasms are classified as supratentorial or infratentorial.

- When the location of the neoplasm is combined with the patient's age, a clinically useful differential classification is arrived at (Table 65–2).
- Seventy percent of primary neoplasms in children are infratentorial. Seventy percent of primary tumors in adults are supratentorial.

C. Classification according to biologic potential:

- Even highly malignant intracranial neoplasms generally do not metastasize outside the craniospinal axis.
- Metastasis within the craniospinal axis via the cerebrospinal fluid does occur, most commonly with medulloblastoma, pineoblastoma, malignant ependymoma, and glioblastoma multiforme.
- Destructive infiltration of the brain is the major criterion of malignancy for intracranial neoplasms.
- The rate of growth of neoplasms also correlates well with malignant behavior. Rapidly growing neoplasms such as glioblastoma multiforme and medulloblastoma are highly malignant.
- Recurrence after treatment is almost invariable with malignant intracranial neoplasms. Recurrence also occurs with many benign neoplasms such as meningioma and craniopharyngioma, and recurrence of itself is not a criterion of malignancy.

TABLE 65-1. CLASSIFICATION OF NEOPLASMS OF THE NERVOUS SYSTEM ON THE BASIS OF HISTOGENESIS

Cell Type	Neoplasm
Cellular derivatives of the neural tube Glial cells	Glioma [1]
Astrocytes	Astrocytoma Glioblastoma multiforme
Oligodendroglia	Oligodendroglioma
Ependymal cells	Ependymoma Subependymoma Choroid plexus papilloma
Neurons	Medulloblastoma
Mixed glial and neuronal	Ganglioglioma
Pinealocyte	Pineocytoma Pineoblastoma
Cells derived from the neural crest Schwann cell	Schwannoma Neurofibroma
Arachnoid cell	Meningioma
Other cells Connective tissue cells	Sarcomas
Lymphoid cells	Malignant lymphoma
Vascular cells	Hemangioblastoma
Pituicytes	Pituitary adenoma
Embryonic remnants Ectodermal derivatives	Craniopharyngioma Epidermoid cysts Dermoid cysts
Notochordal remnants	Chordoma
Germ cells	Teratoma Germinoma
Melanocytes	Melanoma
Adipocytes	Lipoma
Metastatic neoplasms	
Tumors of bone (skull and vertebrae)	

[1] The term glioma has different applications. In its narrowest usage it is synonymous with astrocytomas; in its broadest usage it includes oligodendroglioma and ependymal neoplasms.

TABLE 65-2. COMMON INTRACRANIAL NEOPLASMS CLASSIFIED ACCORDING TO LOCATION AND AGE

Location	Children	Adults
Supratentorial Cerebral hemisphere	30%[1] Rare	70%[1] Glial neoplasms Meningiomas Metastases
Suprasellar	Craniopharyngioma Juvenile astrocytoma	Pituitary adenoma Craniopharyngioma Glial neoplasms
Pineal	Pineoblastoma Germ cell tumor (teratoma)	Pineocytoma Germ cell tumor (germinoma)
Infratentorial (posterior fossa) Midline	70%[1] Medulloblastoma Ependymoma	30%[1] Brain stem glioma
Cerebellar hemisphere	Juvenile astrocytoma	Metastases Hemangioblastoma
Cerebellopontine angle	Epidermoid cyst	Schwannoma (acoustic neuroma) Meningioma
Spinal cord Epidural	Rare Bone tumors	Common Metastases Bone tumors
Intradural but extramedullary	Rare	Neurofibroma Schwannoma Meningioma
Intramedullary	Ependymoma	Ependymoma Astrocytoma

[1] Percentages refer to frequency of intracranial neoplasms within each category; ie, in children, 70% of neoplasms are infratentorial and 30% are supratentorial, while in adults 70% of neoplasms are supratentorial and 30% are infratentorial.

Pathology & Clinical Features (Fig 65-1)

Intracranial neoplasms cause the following clinical and pathologic changes:

- Compression of adjacent neural tissues occurs with all expanding neoplasms. In general, relief of compression is followed by significant recovery of function.
- Destruction of neural tissues by direct infiltration with a malignant neoplasm produces an irreversible deficit.
- Cerebral edema is commonly present around infiltrative neoplasms and may be severe. Cerebral edema tends to be most marked in highly malignant neoplasms. It causes elevation of intracranial pressure.

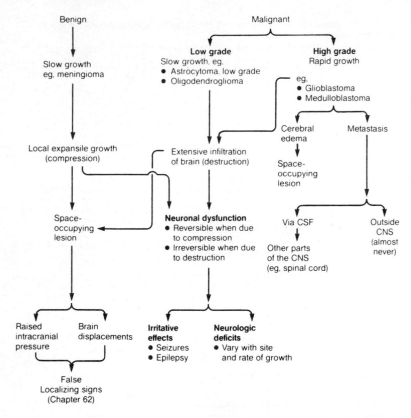

Figure 65–1. Clinical effects related to the biologic behavior of intracranial neoplasm.

- Irritation of neural tissues may occur, commonly resulting in focal epilepsy.
- Hydrocephalus due to obstruction of the ventricular system is especially common with tumors in the posterior fossa.
- Intracranial neoplasms cause increased intracranial pressure due to:
  - The mass effect of the neoplasm itself.
  - Cerebral edema.
  - Hydrocephalus.
- Many patients with intracranial neoplasms present with the effects of raised intracranial pressure—headache, vomiting, and papilledema.

ASTROCYTOMAS

1. CEREBRAL HEMISPHERE ASTROCYTOMA

The commonest primary neoplasm of the brain and occurs chiefly in adults (Table 65–

2). Astrocytomas originate from cerebral white matter astrocytes. They are graded by histologic criteria into the following.

A. Well-differentiated astrocytomas are infiltrative, slowly growing neoplasms that form firm, white ill-defined masses.

- Microscopically, they show slightly increased cellularity and astrocytes with mild cytologic atypia and absent mitotic activity, necrosis or proliferation of endothelial cells.
- Low-grade malignant neoplasms that progress slowly to cause death after 5–10 years.

B. Anaplastic astrocytomas are more rapidly growing neoplasm that forms a white infiltrative mass in the cerebral hemisphere.

- Microscopically, they are composed of astrocytes that show greater cellularity, more pleomorphism, neovascularization with proliferation of endothelial cells, and an increased mitotic rate.
- They cause death after 1–5 years.

C. Glioblastoma multiforme is the most common type of astrocytoma.

- It is one of the most malignant and rapidly growing neoplasms of the brain.
- Grossly, glioblastomas appear as large infiltrative masses that typically extend across the midline as the so-called "butterfly" tumor.
- Microscopically, they are composed of highly pleomorphic astrocytic cells with frequent mitotic figures. Necrosis and endothelial proliferation are important diagnostic criteria.
- Glioblastoma multiforme is highly malignant, with a median survival of 1 year after diagnosis.

2. JUVENILE PILOCYTIC ASTROCYTOMA

This is a neoplasm of children and adolescents found most commonly in the cerebellar hemispheres, but also in the hypothalamic region.

- It accounts for 25% of intracranial neoplasms in children under age 10.
- Grossly, it is well circumscribed and often cystic.
- Microscopically, it shows hypercellularity and is composed of cytologically uniform fibrillary astrocytes. Microcystic changes and the presence of enlarged astrocytic fibers (Rosenthal fibers) are characteristic features.
- A very slow-growing tumor that is almost benign in its biologic behavior.
- Surgical removal results in permanent cure in most cases.

OLIGODENDROGLIOMA

This occurs in the cerebral hemisphere in adults aged 30–50.

- Grossly, oligodendrogliomas are well-circumscribed solid neoplasms. Seventy-five percent of oligodendrogliomas have speckled calcification that is visible on X-ray.
- Microscopically, the neoplasm is composed of numerous small uniform oligodendroglial cells. Mitotic activity is scarce.
- Clinically, oligodendroglioma is a slowly growing neoplasm. The prognosis after surgical removal is good, though recurrence is common.

EPENDYMAL NEOPLASMS

1. EPENDYMOMA

Ependymoma is an uncommon neoplasm that occurs at all ages, but is relatively more common in children.

- It accounts for 60% of intramedullary spinal cord neoplasms. In the brain, 60% occur in the fourth ventricle.
- Grossly, ependymomas form well-circumscribed, reddish-brown nodular masses that occur in relation to the ventricular system.
- They grow slowly but have the ability to spread via the cerebrospinal fluid and should be considered as malignant neoplasms.
- Microscopically, ependymomas are highly cellular, with small polygonal cells that form ependymal tubules and perivascular pseudorosettes.
- Ependymomas tend to grow slowly and may be cured by complete surgical removal.
- Less well differentiated ependymomas infiltrate, grow rapidly, and have a bad prognosis.
- A specific type of ependymoma called myxopapillary ependymoma occurs in the filum terminale and presents as a cauda equina tumor in young adults.

2. CHOROID PLEXUS PAPILLOMA

This is a rare neoplasm that tends to occur in the ventricles of young children.

- Pathologically, it is characterized by a highly vascular papillary mass of benign cuboidal epithelial cells.
- Rarely, it may invade the brain (choroid plexus carcinoma).
- It may secrete increased amounts of cerebrospinal fluid and give rise to communicating hydrocephalus.

3. COLLOID CYST OF THE THIRD VENTRICLE

These are cysts occurring in the anterior third ventricle. They are unilocular cysts lined by cuboidal epithelium and containing thick gelatinous fluid. As they enlarge, colloid cysts block the foramen of Monro, producing obstructive hydrocephalus.

MEDULLOBLASTOMA

This is a neoplasm of primitive neuroectodermal cells. It occurs mainly in children, accounting for 25% of all intracranial neoplasms in children under age 10.

- Its most common location is the midline cerebellar vermis in the posterior fossa.
- Grossly, it appears as a grayish-white fleshy mass which extensively infiltrates the brain.
- Microscopically, it is highly cellular and composed of sheets of small primitive cells with hyperchromatic nuclei and scant cytoplasm.
- Medulloblastoma is highly malignant and frequently seeds the cerebrospinal fluid to produce metastases around the spinal cord.
- Chemotherapy and radiation are somewhat effective. The prognosis is poor.

PINEAL NEOPLASMS

Pineal neoplasms include both pinealocyte and germ cell neoplasms.

- Pinealocyte neoplasms include:

- Pineocytoma, which is a benign or low-grade malignant neoplasm that occurs in adults.
- Pineoblastoma resembles medulloblastoma. It occurs in childhood and is highly malignant.
■ The most common germ cell neoplasm is germinoma, which is identical to the testicular seminoma, and teratoma. Germinomas compress the dorsal aspect of the midbrain, causing abnormalities in ocular movement and hydrocephalus.

MENINGIOMA

These occur most frequently in middle-aged women, a sex distribution that may be related to the presence of estrogen receptors on the tumor cells.

■ They arise from the dura and grow as firm, encapsulated masses that compress adjacent structures and the brain.
■ They are frequently associated with hypertrophy of the overlying bone.
■ Rarely, they infiltrate the underlying brain and are then called malignant meningiomas.
■ Microscopically, they are composed of sheets and whorls of meningothelial cells, which are uniform and appear cytologically benign. Rarely, cytologic atypia is present. Psammoma bodies (round, laminated calcifications) are common.
■ Meningioma is a benign neoplasm. However, because of infiltration of dura and bone, they tend to recur after removal.
■ The clinical features depend on their location:
  - Parasagittal and falx meningiomas compress the leg area of the motor cortices causing paraplegia.
  - Meningiomas on the surface of the hemisphere cause focal epilepsy and cortical dysfunction.
  - Olfactory bulb tumors compress the optic nerve, producing blindness.
  - Sphenoidal ridge tumors compress the cranial nerves passing into the orbit, causing ophthalmoplegias.
  - Posterior fossa tumors cause features of a cerebellopontine angle tumor.
  - Spinal cord meningiomas cause spinal compression.

NERVE SHEATH NEOPLASMS

The commonest intracranial example is the eighth nerve (acoustic) schwannoma. It presents as a cerebellopontine angle mass, compressing adjacent cranial nerves and cerebellum. Neurofibromas and schwannomas also commonly arise from the spinal nerve roots, causing spinal compression.

CEREBELLAR HEMANGIOBLASTOMA

This is a benign neoplasm that occurs either sporadically or as part of von Hippel-Lindau disease (Chapter 62).

■ It appears as a well-circumscribed mass with cystic and solid components.
■ Microscopically, numerous endothelium-lined vascular spaces are separated by trabeculae of cells with lipid-laden cytoplasm.
■ Clinically, presentation is in adult life with cerebellar dysfunction and hydrocephalus.
■ It may secrete erythropoietin and cause polycythemia.
■ Surgical removal is usually curative.

MALIGNANT LYMPHOMA OF THE BRAIN

Primary malignant lymphoma of the brain is very uncommon in otherwise healthy individuals. Its incidence is greatly increased in immunocompromised patients, as in those with AIDS, or after renal transplantation.

■ Most commonly it occurs in the deep cerebral hemispheres and is frequently multifocal.
■ They are usually high-grade B cell lymphomas, most commonly B-immunoblastic lymphoma.
■ Treatment with chemotherapy is of limited efficacy, and the prognosis is poor.

NEOPLASMS DERIVED FROM EMBRYONAL REMNANTS

1. CRANIOPHARYNGIOMA

This is derived from Rathke's pouch, the epithelial remnant of the foregut that contributes to the origin of the pituitary gland. It occurs mainly in childhood in the suprasellar region.

■ Pathologically, they are composed of cystic and solid components, with local infiltration that makes complete surgical removal difficult.
■ Microscopically, the cystic spaces are lined by stratified squamous epithelium and contain an oily fluid containing cholesterol crystals. Calcification is usually present.
■ Craniopharyngiomas present with compression of:
  ● The pituitary, causing hypopituitarism. In children, growth retardation is common.
  ● The optic chiasm, causing visual field defects, commonly bitemporal hemianopia.
  ● The third ventricle, causing hydrocephalus.
■ Treatment is surgical, often followed by radiation therapy. The recurrence rate is high.

2. EPIDERMOID CYST

This cyst is derived from rare embryonic epidermal remnants.

■ The commonest locations are the cerebellopontine angle, the suprasellar region, and the lumbar region of the spinal cord.
■ They are benign cystic structures lined by stratified squamous epithelium and filled with keratin.
■ Surgical removal is curative.

3. CHORDOMA

Chordoma is derived from notochordal remnants in the skull and vertebral bodies.

■ Common locations are:
  ● The sacrococcygeal region, compressing the cauda equina.
  ● The clivus, from which it extends into the posterior fossa.
  ● The suprasellar region, where it compresses the pituitary stalk and third ventricle.
■ Grossly, appears as a lobulated mass that has a gelatinous appearance on cut section.
■ Microscopically, it is composed of large cells with abundant bubbly cytoplasm (physaliphorous cells).
■ Chordomas are malignant neoplasms that grow slowly but inexorably.

■ Complete surgical removal is rarely possible. Most patients die of their tumor, usually after several years.

METASTATIC NEOPLASMS

Metastatic neoplasms are the most common brain tumors. They are commonly derived from carcinomas of the lung, breast, kidney, stomach, and colon, and melanomas.

■ Meningeal involvement by metastatic neoplasms occurs frequently in acute leukemia.
■ Diagnosis is by biopsy or cytologic examination of the cerebrospinal fluid.

The Peripheral Nerves & Skeletal Muscle

66

DISORDERS OF PERIPHERAL NERVES

PERIPHERAL NEUROPATHY
Peripheral neuropathy is a clinical term that denotes nontraumatic disease of the nerves.

- Most peripheral neuropathies tend to affect the longest fibers first, producing a typical symmetric "glove and stocking" distribution of sensory loss and involvement of the muscles of the hands and feet.
- Sensory and mixed neuropathies are more common than pure motor neuropathy.
- Neuropathy affecting autonomic nerves results in autonomic dysfunction.
- Two basic pathologic lesions cause peripheral neuropathy: segmental demyelination and axonal degeneration.
- There are many causes of peripheral neuropathy (Table 66–1).

TRAUMATIC NERVE INJURIES
Peripheral nerve injuries resulting in transection of the nerve are common.

- Recovery from a nerve injury depends mainly on whether the continuity of the nerve sheath of the damaged axon is maintained.
- Where the nerve sheath is not disrupted, complete recovery is the rule. Axonal regeneration occurs at the rate of 1–2 cm per week.
- When the nerve sheath is disrupted, as in complete nerve transection, functional recovery is poor.
- Complications of nerve transection include:
  - Failure of return of function.
  - Return of abnormal function, due to establishment of incorrect innervation.
  - Development of traumatic neuromas at the severed nerve end composed of proliferating Schwann cells.

NEOPLASMS OF PERIPHERAL NERVES
Neoplasms of peripheral nerves are common. They are classified anatomically into:

- Neoplasms within the skull or spinal canal.
- Neoplasms that involve both the spinal canal and the paraspinal soft tissue ("dumbbell" tumors).
- Neoplasms arising in large peripheral nerves.
- Neoplasms in small peripheral nerve filaments that appear as soft tissue masses without obvious connections to nerves.

TABLE 66–1. CAUSES OF PERIPHERAL NEUROPATHY

Hereditary neuropathies
  Refsum's hypertrophic polyneuritis
  Peroneal muscular atrophy (Charcot-Marie-Tooth disease):
    X-linked dominant inheritance; distal leg muscles
    involved
  Neuropathies associated with heredofamilial amyloidosis

Ischemic neuropathies
  Diabetic neuropathy[1]
  Giant cell arteritis (high incidence of optic nerve
    involvement)
  Systemic lupus erythematosus
  Atherosclerosis

Toxic neuropathies
  Drugs (isoniazid, nitrofurantoin)
  Alcoholic polyneuropathy
  Heavy metals: arsenic, lead, gold, mercury
  Industrial substances: insecticides, solvents

Metabolic neuropathies
  Deficiency of vitamins B_1, B_6, B_{12}
  Diabetic neuropathy[1]
  Porphyria
  Amyloidosis
Infections and postinfection syndromes
  Leprosy
  Diphtheria toxin
  Guillain-Barré syndrome

**Carcinomatous neuropathy (noncompressive, nonmeta-
  static)**

---

[1] Diabetic polyneuropathy may result from either axonal degeneration caused by the osmotic effect of sorbitol accumulating in the nerve or diabetic microangiopathy involving the vasa nervorum.

- In a few patients, multiple neurofibromas occurs as an inherited disease (von Recklinghausen's disease, see Chapter 62).
- Pathologically, nerve sheath tumors are divided into the following.

A. Schwannoma (neurilemmoma) is a slowly growing benign neoplasm that commonly occurs in relation to large nerve trunks.

- Sensory cranial nerves (eighth and fifth nerves), the sensory root of spinal nerves, and the posterior mediastinum are common locations.
- Clinically, it presents as a mass lesion, often associated with pain and nerve paralysis.
- Grossly, schwannomas are encapsulated masses that compress the nerve of origin. Hemorrhage and cystic change may occur.

- Histologically, they are composed of spindle-shaped Schwann cells arranged in a compact (Antoni A) and loose (Antoni B) pattern.
- Immunohistochemical studies show the presence of S-100 protein in the Schwann cells.
- The malignant potential of schwannomas is very low.

B. Neurofibroma is a slowly growing benign neoplasm that occurs:

- In relation to large nerve trunks.
- In peripheral tissues such as skin, where it arises from very small nerves.
- Clinically, neurofibroma presents as a soft tissue mass, commonly associated with pain.
- Grossly, neurofibromas of large nerves appear as a firm, rubbery mass that expands the affected nerve and cannot be demarcated from it.
- Histologic examination shows a varied spindle cell population composed of Schwann cells and fibroblasts. The stroma shows myxomatous change.
- Neurofibroma carries a low but significant risk of malignant transformation.

C. Malignant peripheral nerve sheath tumor is synonymous with malignant schwannoma and neurofibrosarcoma.

- Most such tumors occur de novo. A few complicate preexisting neurofibroma, particularly in patients with von Recklinghausen's disease.
- Malignant peripheral nerve sheath tumors appear clinically as soft tissue neoplasms.
- The rate of growth varies, being slow in low-grade neoplasms and rapid in high-grade ones.
- Grossly, they are fleshy, frequently large, and show extensive infiltration. Areas of necrosis and hemorrhage are common.
- Microscopically, most are highly cellular spindle cell sarcomas with marked cytologic atypia and pleomorphism and a high mitotic rate.
- Diagnosis of malignant peripheral nerve sheath tumor may be made:
  - When an origin from a large peripheral nerve is apparent.
  - When a sarcoma of appropriate histologic type occurs in a patient with von Recklinghausen's disease.
  - When S-100 protein is demonstrated in the tumor cells.
  - When electron microscopy demonstrates features typical of Schwann cells.

DISORDERS OF SKELETAL MUSCLE

CLINICAL FEATURES OF MUSCLE DISEASE

Muscle Weakness
The causes of muscle weakness include:

- Neurologic diseases involving the lower motor neuron, which also causes muscle atrophy and loss of deep tendon reflexes.
- Upper motor neuron paralysis, which causes spasticity and brisk reflexes without significant muscle atrophy, at least initially.
- Failure of neuromuscular transmission.

■ Diseases involving skeletal muscle per se, including myositis, muscular dystrophies, and myopathies.

Muscle Pain
Inflammatory lesions of muscle (myositis) are commonly associated with pain and tenderness in the involved muscles.

DIAGNOSIS OF MUSCLE DISEASES

Clinical Examination
The diagnosis of many muscle diseases is based on the distribution of involvement, family studies, and other clinical features.

Electromyography
This measures action potentials generated in muscles by means of an electrode inserted into the muscle belly, and provides useful information.

Serum Enzyme Levels
Serum levels of creatine kinase, aldolase, transaminases, and lactate dehydrogenase become elevated in many muscle diseases, especially the dystrophies and myositis. Elevations of these enzymes, however, are not specific for muscle diseases.

Muscle Biopsy
Skeletal muscle biopsy is a highly specialized procedure. Routine light microscopy permits separation of denervation atrophy from primary muscle disease, and identification of inflammation. Special histochemical methods—to assess their enzyme content— and electron microscopy are used in diagnosis of specific primary muscle diseases.

PRIMARY MUSCLE DISEASES

1. MUSCULAR DYSTROPHIES
This is a group of rare inherited primary muscle diseases characterized by:

■ Onset in childhood.
■ Distinctive distribution of involved muscles.
■ Nonspecific histologic changes in muscle, consisting of random atrophy and hypertrophy of muscle fibers.
■ Several different clinical types are recognized (Table 66–2).

   A. Duchenne type muscular dystrophy is also called pseudohypertrophic muscular dystrophy. It is the most common type of muscular dystrophy.

■ It is inherited as an X-linked recessive trait, with females carrying the abnormal gene and transmitting it to 50% of their male offspring, who manifest the disease.
■ Affected individuals are normal at birth and manifest the disease in early childhood.
■ The disease progresses rapidly, with most children being disabled within a few years. Death commonly occurs by the end of the second decade.
■ Muscle weakness is symmetric and first affects the muscles of the pelvic girdle.

TABLE 66–2. MUSCULAR DYSTROPHIES

Type	Frequency	Inheritance[1]	Severity	Age at Onset	Distribution of First Involved Muscles
Duchenne (pseudohypertrophic)	Common	XR	Severe, fatal	0–12 years	Pelvis, legs
Becker	Rare	XR	Mild	10–70 years	Pelvis, legs
Facioscapulohumeral	Relatively common	AD	Mild	10–20 years	Face, shoulders
Limb girdle	Rare	AR	Moderate	Variable	Pelvis, shoulders
Distal	Very rare	AD	Variable	Adult	Hands, feet
Myotonic	Relatively common	AD	Variable, slow progression	Usually adult	Face, tongue, extremities

[1]X = X-linked; A = autosomal; R = recessive; D = dominant.

- The affected muscles appear larger than normal in the early stages. This is most easily seen in the calf muscles. Enlargement of muscles is caused by increased fat content (pseudohypertrophy).
- A few patients show evidence of myocardial dysfunction.

B. Myotonic dystrophy is characterized, not by muscle weakness, but by failure of relaxation of muscle after voluntary contraction.

- Onset is usually in adult life, and progression is very slow.
- Patients with myotonic dystrophy may have cataracts, gonadal atrophy, mental retardation, abnormal insulin metabolism, and cardiac arrhythmias.

2. CONGENITAL MYOPATHIES

This is a group of very rare primary muscle diseases characterized by:

- Onset at birth or in early infancy, with muscle weakness and decreased muscle tone ("floppy infant syndrome").
- A very slowly progressive or nonprogressive course, with long survival being the rule.
- Specific histologic changes on muscle biopsy that characterize individual entities within the group (Table 66–3).

3. ACQUIRED MYOPATHIES

This is characterized by muscle weakness without histologic changes in the involved muscle. Common causes of acquired myopathies are:

TABLE 66-3. CONGENITAL AND ACQUIRED MYOPATHIES (MORE COMMON TYPES ONLY)

Disease	Histologic Characteristic
Central core disease	Amorphous central core in myofibrils with absence of myofilaments.
Nemaline myopathy	Elongated crystalline rods composed of tropomyosin present beneath sarcolemma; show periodicity on electron microscope.
Centronuclear myopathy	Nuclei occupy the central part of the myofibril, which lacks myofilaments.
Secondary congenital myopathies	Myopathy is a feature of some forms of glycogen storage disease and certain disorders of lipid metabolism (eg, carnitine deficiency).
Acquired myopathies	Endocrine diseases: thyrotoxicosis, corticosteroid excess (Cushing's syndrome, exogenous steroid administration), acromegaly; osteomalacia (hypocalcemia); familial periodic paralysis (potassium deficiency or excess); malignant neoplasms (paraneoplastic syndrome).

- Endocrine diseases such as thyrotoxicosis, Cushing's syndrome, and acromegaly.
- Malignant neoplasms.
- Electrolyte abnormalities such as hypocalcemia and abnormal potassium metabolism.

INFLAMMATION OF MUSCLE (Myositis)
The causes of myositis are (Table 66–4):

- Infectious diseases.
- Autoimmune diseases. In polymyositis, inflammation of muscles is the dominant clinical manifestation (see Chapter 68).
- High-dosage radiation (most commonly in treatment of cancer).
- Myositis ossificans:
  - Is a rare disease of unknown etiology.
  - Characterized by bone formation in the involved muscle.
  - Presents as a hard mass in the muscle that may be mistaken for a neoplasm.

DISORDERS OF NEUROMUSCULAR TRANSMISSION

1. MYASTHENIA GRAVIS
Myasthenia gravis is one of the commoner muscle diseases, affecting 1:40,000 persons in the USA. The commonest age at onset is 20–40 years. There is a female preponderance when the disease occurs under the age of 40.

Etiology
Myasthenia gravis results from failure of neuromuscular transmission due to blockage of acetylcholine receptors by autoantibody (Fig 66–1).

TABLE 66-4. CAUSES OF MYOSITIS[1]

Infectious diseases
Bacterial
Local infection with pyogenic bacteria, usually
secondary to trauma, intramuscular injection
Bacteremic myositis, eg, in infective endocarditis,
typhoid fever, leptospirosis
Gas gangrene (clostridial infection)
Viral
Coxsackievirus (Bornholm disease); affects mainly
chest wall muscles
Influenza
Many other viruses
Parasitic
Trichinella spiralis (trichinosis)
Toxoplasma gondii
Cysticercosis (*Taenia solium*)
Trypanosoma cruzi (Chagas' disease)
Exotoxic
Diphtheria
Immune diseases
Polymyositis-dermatomyositis
Other autoimmune diseases: systemic lupus
erythematosus, progressive systemic sclerosis
Sarcoidosis
Myasthenia gravis: associated with anti-striated
muscle antibody in serum
Radiation
Ischemia
Myositis ossificans

[1]Myositis is characterized by the presence of inflammation on histologic examination.

- Acetylcholine receptor antibody is present in the serum of almost all patients. It is an IgG antibody and may cross the placenta in pregnancy, causing neonatal myasthenia in the newborn.
- Thymectomy often improves the condition, and it is believed that the thymus plays a role in the etiology of myasthenia gravis.
- The thymus is not the source of antibody, which is produced by the peripheral lymphoid tissue.

Pathology
Specific morphologic abnormalities are not seen on gross examination or light microscopy. Focal collections of lymphocytes (lymphorrhages) may be seen in affected muscle.

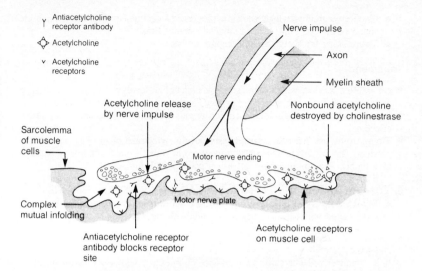

Figure 66–1. Pathogenesis of myasthenia gravis. Acetylcholine released at the nerve ending by the nerve impulse normally binds with acetylcholine receptors. This evokes the action potential in the muscle. In myasthenia gravis, antiacetylcholine receptor antibody binds to the acetylcholine receptor and inhibits the action of acetylcholine.

- Immunohistochemistry demonstrates the presence of IgG and complement components on the motor end plate.
- Electron microscopy shows damage to the motor end plate with loss of the normally complex folds.
- Thymic abnormalities are seen in many patients:
  - Thymic follicular hyperplasia in 70%.
  - Thymomas in 15%.

Clinical Features & Diagnosis

- It is characterized by muscle weakness that is typically aggravated by repeated contraction.
- The typical clinical presentation is weakness of ocular muscles (causing bilateral ptosis and diplopia).
- The disease slowly progresses to include facial muscles, limb girdle muscles, and respiratory muscles.
- Untreated, 40% of patients with myasthenia gravis will die of their disease within 10 years.
- The clinical diagnosis may be confirmed by:
  - The Edrophonium (Tensilon) test, which is positive.

- Electromyography, which shows a progressive decline in amplitude of muscle action potentials with repeated voluntary contraction.
- Serum assay for acetylcholine receptor antibody.

Treatment

■ Anticholinesterases, which increase the acetylcholine levels at the motor end plate and compensate for the receptor blockage, represent the mainstay of treatment.
■ In crisis situations, high-dosage corticosteroids and plasma exchange may prove effective.
■ Thymectomy produces variable remission of the symptoms of myasthenia in many patients. The improvement is most pronounced in young women with recent onset of myasthenia. The improvement is least in patients with thymoma.

2. OTHER CAUSES OF NEUROMUSCULAR TRANSMISSION FAILURE

A. Myasthenic syndrome (Eaton-Lambert syndrome) is a paraneoplastic syndrome associated with cancer, particularly small-cell carcinoma of the lung.

■ It is caused by an abnormality of acetylcholine release by nerve endings at the motor end plate.
■ It is characterized clinically by weakness of muscles, with early involvement of ocular muscles.
■ The muscle weakness is not aggravated by effort, and electromyography shows progressive increase of amplitude of action potentials upon repeated contraction.

B. Botulism The exotoxin of *Clostridium botulinum* in minute doses blocks release of acetylcholine at the motor end plate. Generalized muscle weakness rapidly leads to respiratory paralysis and death.

C. Tick Paralysis: Ticks of the species *Dermacentor andersoni*, the Rocky Mountain wood tick, and *Dermacentor variabilis*, the American dog tick, secrete a toxin that inhibits acetylcholine release. Removal of the tick is curative.

D. Aminoglycoside drugs in high dosage, especially in the presence of renal dysfunction, inhibit acetylcholine release and cause muscle weakness. These antimicrobial drugs should be avoided in patients with myasthenia gravis.

NEOPLASMS OF SKELETAL MUSCLE

1. BENIGN NEOPLASMS (Rhabdomyoma)

Benign neoplasms are extremely uncommon. Cardiac rhabdomyoma occurs rarely in patients with tuberous sclerosis (see Chapter 62).

2. MALIGNANT NEOPLASMS (Rhabdomyosarcoma)

Rhabdomyosarcoma is an uncommon soft tissue sarcoma. Three subtypes are recognized.

A. Embryonal rhabdomyosarcoma is the most common type, occurring especially in children under age 10.

■ It presents as a rapidly growing neoplasm involving the soft tissues of the extremities, retroperitoneum, orbit, nasal cavity, and a variety of organs.

- It is extremely infiltrative, and tends to metastasize via the bloodstream at an early stage.
- Histologically, embryonal rhabdomyosarcoma is highly cellular, being composed of small round and oval cells with primitive hyperchromatic nuclei and a high mitotic rate.
- Diagnosis is made by demonstrating skeletal muscle differentiation by:
  - The presence of scattered cells with abundant pink cytoplasm (strap cells) that show cross-striations.
  - The presence of irregular Z bands on electron microscopy.
  - The presence of muscle proteins such as myoglobin, myosin, actin, and desmin as shown by immunohistochemical studies.
- Treatment with chemotherapy is effective and has improved survival greatly.

B. Alveolar rhabdomyosarcoma is less common and occurs in the age group from 10 to 30 years.

- It presents as a soft tissue mass, commonly around the shoulder and pelvis.
- It is characterized by an alveolar arrangement of small primitive neoplastic skeletal muscle cells.
- It is rapid-growing and highly malignant.

C. Pleomorphic rhabdomyosarcoma is an uncommon neoplasm of soft tissue that mainly affects the extremities and retroperitoneum in elderly patients.

- Histologically, it is highly pleomorphic with numerous giant cells.
- It is highly malignant. Treatment is rarely effective.

Section XVI. Bones, Joints, & Connective Tissue

Diseases of Bones

67

CONGENITAL DISEASES OF BONE

ACHONDROPLASIA

Achondroplasia is a common disease, inherited as an autosomal dominant trait.

- It is characterized by failure of cartilage cell proliferation at the epiphyseal plates of the long bones, resulting in failure of longitudinal bone growth.
- Membranous ossification is not affected.
- Achondroplastic dwarfs have short limbs and normally developed skull, facial bones, and axial skeleton.
- General health and intelligence are not affected, and life expectancy is normal.

OSTEOGENESIS IMPERFECTA (Brittle Bone Disease)

Usually it has an autosomal dominant inheritance pattern with variable penetrance.

- It is characterized by defective synthesis of collagen by fibroblasts and osteoid by the osteoblasts.
- Abnormal collagen synthesis leads to loose-jointedness, blue scleras, thin skin, and development of hernias.
- Abnormal synthesis of osteoid leads to thin, poorly formed bones that tend to fracture easily.
- Fractures usually begin to appear a few years after birth and often require internal fixation because they do not heal well.
- Survival into adult life is common.

OSTEOPETROSIS (Marble Bone Disease; Albers-Schönberg Disease)

Osteopetrosis is very rare. There is a relatively mild autosomal dominant form and a lethal autosomal recessive form.

- It is characterized by bones that are greatly thickened, due to overgrowth of cortical bone.
- The marrow cavity is reduced and sometimes obliterated.
- The vertebrae, pelvis, and ribs are more affected than extremities.
- Though thickened, affected bones are brittle and susceptible to fracture.

■ Patients present with recurrent fractures or anemia due to decreased hematopoiesis.
■ The radiologic appearance of dense bones is diagnostic.

INFECTIONS OF BONE

ACUTE PYOGENIC OSTEOMYELITIS

Etiology
Most cases of pyogenic osteomyelitis occur in previously healthy, active individuals.

■ It is usually caused by *Staphylococcus aureus,* which reaches the bone via the bloodstream.
■ In a few cases, bone infection is a complication of compound fracture, or has spread to bone from a neighboring focus of infection.
■ Patients with sickle cell anemia have a special tendency to develop osteomyelitis caused by Salmonella species.

Pathology
The metaphyseal region of long bones of the extremities are most commonly involved. Acute inflammation leads to suppuration and bone necrosis, with intrametaphyseal abscess formation.

■ If not treated, the abscess extends:
  ● To the surface (subperiosteal abscess).
  ● Into an adjacent joint (pyogenic arthritis).
  ● Into the medullary cavity, leading to dissemination of the infection throughout the bone.

Clinical Features
The onset is rapid, with high fever and severe throbbing pain in the affected area. There is tenderness, swelling, and warmth over the inflamed bone.

■ There is almost invariably a neutrophil leukocytosis in the peripheral blood, and blood cultures are positive in 70% of patients.
■ Radiographs may be normal early. Later, when bone necrosis occurs, areas of lucency appear.

Treatment & Prognosis
Early treatment by surgical drainage of pus plus antibiotics is essential. With effective treatment, less than 10% of cases are complicated by chronic osteomyelitis.

Complications
Untreated acute osteomyelitis frequently progresses to chronic suppurative osteomyelitis, characterized by extensive bone necrosis and multiple abscesses which drain into the skin through sinuses. Complications of chronic osteomyelitis include secondary amyloidosis and squamous carcinoma of the overlying affected skin.

TUBERCULOSIS OF BONE

This has become rare in areas of the world where good control of tuberculosis has been achieved. It is still common in many developing countries.

- The vertebral column is the commonest site of disease (Pott's disease of the spine).
- Tuberculous osteomyelitis has an insidious onset, with low-grade fever and weight loss.
- Radiologic changes due to bone destruction are present.

METABOLIC BONE DISEASE

OSTEOPOROSIS

Osteoporosis is a decrease in the total mass of bone without other structural or chemical abnormalities in the bone. It is a form of bone atrophy.

Etiology & Pathogenesis

Senile osteoporosis:

- Is present to some degree in most individuals over the age of 50 years.
- Is generally more severe in women after menopause (postmenopausal osteoporosis), probably a consequence of declining levels of estrogen.
- Decreased physical activity and nutritional protein or vitamin deficiency may play a role.
- Prolonged immobilization of any bone causes disuse atrophy.
- Osteoporosis occurs in endocrine diseases such as Cushing's syndrome, hyperthyroidism, and acromegaly.
- Many patients are in negative calcium balance. Calcium supplements slow, but do not reverse, the process.

Pathology & Clinical Features

Osteoporosis most commonly produces symptoms in the major weight-bearing and stress areas (vertebral bodies and femoral neck).

- The vertebral bodies show changes in shape, decreased height, and compression fractures. Kyphosis is common.
- Osteoporosis of the femoral neck predisposes to pathologic fractures.
- Affected bones show thinning of the bony cortex and trabeculae (Fig 67–1).
- Diagnosis is possible both radiologically and histologically when severe osteoporosis is present.
- The structure of bone, as determined by chemical analysis of bone ash, shows no abnormality.
- Patients with osteoporosis have normal serum levels of calcium, phosphate, and alkaline phosphatase (Table 67–1).

OSTEOMALACIA

Osteomalacia is a structural abnormality of bone caused by defective mineralization of osteoid, which is produced in normal or increased amounts. Because it is not calcified

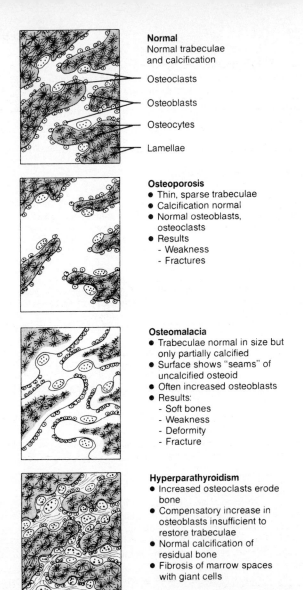

Normal
Normal trabeculae
and calcification

Osteoclasts

Osteoblasts

Osteocytes

Lamellae

Osteoporosis
- Thin, sparse trabeculae
- Calcification normal
- Normal osteoblasts,
  osteoclasts
- Results
  - Weakness
  - Fractures

Osteomalacia
- Trabeculae normal in size but
  only partially calcified
- Surface shows "seams" of
  uncalcified osteoid
- Often increased osteoblasts
- Results:
  - Soft bones
  - Weakness
  - Deformity
  - Fracture

Hyperparathyroidism
- Increased osteoclasts erode
  bone
- Compensatory increase in
  osteoblasts insufficient to
  restore trabeculae
- Normal calcification of
  residual bone
- Fibrosis of marrow spaces
  with giant cells

Figure 67–1. Pathologic changes in bone in metabolic bone diseases. In osteoporosis, the bone is qualitatively normal but decreased in amount; in osteomalacia and rickets, calcification does not occur normally in the osteoid produced by osteoblasts, resulting in wide uncalcified osteoid seams; in hyperparathyroidism, there is increased resorption of bone with proliferation of osteoclasts and fibrosis.

TABLE 67–1. LABORATORY FINDINGS IN METABOLIC BONE DISEASE

	Serum Calcium	Serum Phosphorus	Alkaline Phosphatase	Parathyroid Hormone (PTH)
Osteoporosis	N	N	N	N
Osteomalacia (rickets)	↓	↓(↑)[1]	↑	N(↑)
Primary hyperparathyroid bone disease	↑	↓	N↑	↑
Bone disease in renal failure—with secondary hyperparathyroidism	N↓	↑	↑	↑
Lytic bone neoplasms	N↑	N↑	N↑	N
Paget's disease of bone	N	N	↑	N

[1]Secondary increase in PTH production may elevate the serum phosphate level.

normally, affected bones are soft. The causes of osteomalacia have been discussed in Chapter 10 with reference to vitamin D.

Pathology & Clinical Features

Microscopic examination of undecalcified bone shows the presence of uncalcified osteoid, usually in the form of wide seams on the outer aspect of bony trabeculae (Fig 67–1).

- Serum calcium levels are usually low in patients with vitamin D deficiency (Table 67–1).
- Softening of bone leads to bone pain, and deformity.
- In the vertebral column, the vertebral bodies often become biconcave as a consequence of inward protrusion of the intervertebral disks.
- X-ray examination of long bones show deformities, decreased density, and the presence of radiolucent bands (pseudofractures, or Looser's zones).
- The changes of osteomalacia are reversible.

HYPERPARATHYROIDISM (Osteitis Fibrosa Cystica)

Etiology

Bone changes are caused by elevated parathyroid hormone (PTH) levels and occur in both primary and secondary hyperparathyroidism (see Chapter 59).

Pathology

Increased PTH levels stimulate osteoclastic and fibroblastic activity in bone. The bone becomes thinned with fibrosis and cyst formation (osteitis fibrosa cystica). Microscopically, there is marked proliferation of osteoclastic giant cells and fibroblasts (Fig

67–1). When this is focal, nodular masses called brown tumors may occur in the bone. These resemble giant cell tumor of bone.

Clinical Features

Bone changes of hyperparathyroidism are usually asymptomatic. Rarely, bone pain, fractures, cysts, and mass lesions occur. The bone changes regress when hyperparathyroidism is treated.

MISCELLANEOUS BONE DISEASES OF UNCERTAIN CAUSE

PAGET'S DISEASE OF BONE (Osteitis Deformans)

Paget's disease is very common. About 3% of the population over age 50 in the United States and Western Europe show radiologic evidence of Paget's disease.

- It is rare in blacks and in natives of Asia.
- Most cases are asymptomatic.
- Men are affected somewhat more commonly than women.

Etiology & Pathology

The cause is unknown. The finding of viruslike particles in affected bones has led to the suggestion that Paget's disease may represent a slow virus infection of bone.

- Paget's disease may involve one bone (monostotic) or many (polyostotic).
- The bones most commonly involved are the pelvis, skull, spine, scapula, femur, tibia, humerus, and mandible.
- The disease progresses through three stages:
  - Irregular osteoclastic resorption of bone.
  - Osteoblastic compensation, in which the new bone balances the osteolysis, but is disorganized.
  - Sclerotic phase, in which osteoblastic activity is greatly in excess of osteoclastic resorption, leading to marked thickening of bone.
- Histologically, affected bone shows thickened trabeculae with irregularly arranged cement lines (mosaic pattern).

Clinical Features

Early Paget's disease is asymptomatic. Pain in affected bone in the later stages is the most common symptom.

- Thickening of bone may cause deformities such as:
  - Enlargement of the head.
  - Abnormal vertebral curvatures.
  - Bowing of the tibias and femurs.
- Thickening of the bone may impinge on nerves that leave bony foramens, causing symptoms of nerve compression and radicular pain.
- Serum calcium, phosphorus, and parathyroid hormone levels are normal. Serum alkaline phosphatase levels are greatly elevated (Table 67–1).

Complications

The arteriovenous fistula effect resulting from extreme hypervascularity in involved bones may be sufficient to cause high-output heart failure. Paget's disease is associated with an increased risk (2–5%) of developing malignant neoplasms in the involved bones. Osteosarcoma is the most common.

FIBROUS DYSPLASIA

Fibrous dysplasia is a focal slowly expanding lesion in which the bone is replaced by a mass of fibroblasts, collagen, and irregular bony trabeculae.

A. Monostotic fibrous dysplasia:

- Fibrous dysplasia affecting a single bone is common and may occur at any age.
- Any bone may be involved, most often the lower extremities, skull, mandible, or ribs.
- Pathologically, there is replacement of the affected area by proliferating fibroblasts in which are scattered trabeculae of irregular bone.
- The lesion appears on X-ray as a well-defined circumscribed radiolucent area.
- Clinically, there is pain, deformity, or pathologic fracture.

B. Polyostotic Fibrous Dysplasia:

- Rarely, fibrous dysplasia affects many bones, causing deformities and fractures.
- Albright's syndrome is a form of polyostotic fibrous dysplasia in which there are multiple unilateral bone lesions associated with precocious puberty and unilateral pigmented skin lesions.

FIBROUS CORTICAL DEFECT

This is also called **nonossifying fibroma** or **fibroxanthoma**.

- It is a common lesion that is believed to be of developmental origin. It is not a true neoplasm.
- It occurs in children, most commonly affecting the tibia, fibula, and femur.
- Pathologically, it appears as a small, well-demarcated lesion in the cortex. It is soft, yellowish-gray and composed of fibroblasts, foamy histiocytes, and giant cells.
- Clinically, it is characterized by nocturnal pain in the legs.
- Radiologic examination shows a circular, punched-out area of lucency surrounded by normal bone.
- No treatment is necessary. The lesion disappears spontaneously after a variable interval.

BONE CYSTS

1. UNICAMERAL BONE CYST (Solitary Bone Cyst)

This is an uncommon lesion affecting long bones in children and young adults. It usually involves the metaphysis.

- It is thought to result from a developmental defect.
- The cyst contains clear or yellowish fluid and is lined by connective tissue.
- Commonly presents with pain, as a mass, or as a pathologic fracture.

2. ANEURYSMAL BONE CYST

This is an uncommon lesion that occurs most often in the age group from 10 to 20. It affects vertebrae and flat bones more commonly than long bones.

- Pathologically, it appears as a large destructive lesion causing expansion of bone.
- Microscopic examination shows large, endothelium-lined hemorrhagic spaces surrounded by proliferating cells closely resembling giant cell tumor of bone.
- Clinically, it presents with pain or a mass. The radiologic appearance is characteristic.

NEOPLASMS OF BONE (Table 67–2)

By far the commonest neoplasms of bone are leukemic involvement of bone marrow, and metastatic carcinoma.

- The most frequent tumors that metastasize to bone in adults are carcinomas of the lung, prostate, breast, thyroid, kidney, and colon.
- In children, neuroblastoma is the commonest skeletal metastasis.
- Eosinophilic granuloma and Hand-Schüller-Christian disease, part of the spectrum of histiocytosis X (see Chapter 29) also produce lytic lesions of bone.

BENIGN NEOPLASMS OF BONE

1. OSTEOCHONDROMA

This is called **osteocartilaginous exostosis.** It is the commonest benign bone neoplasm. Most occur in children and young adults.

- The common sites of involvement are the lower femur, upper tibia, humerus, and pelvis.
- The great majority are solitary. Rarely, multiple osteochondromatosis is inherited (called diaphyseal aclasis, multiple exostoses) with an autosomal dominant inheritance.
- Osteochondromas project outward from the cortex of the bone on a short stalk. Histologically, the stalk is composed of mature bone upon which there is a cap of hyaline cartilage.
- Malignant transformation of solitary osteochondromas is very rare. Chondrosarcoma occurs commonly (in 10%) in familial multiple osteochondromatosis.

2. CHONDROMA

Chondroma is a common benign neoplasm occurring most often in the diaphyseal medulla (enchondroma). The small bones of the hands and feet are the commonest sites, with ribs and long bones affected less frequently.

- About 30% of patients have more than one lesion.
- Multiple enchondromas may occur as an inherited, autosomal dominant disease (Ollier's disease).
- Enchondroma appears as a firm, well-circumscribed, glistening white mass that expands the bone from the center and causes thinning of the cortex.
- Microscopically, it is composed of lobules of hyaline cartilage of low cellularity.
- Malignant transformation does not occur in solitary enchondromas. There is an increased risk of chondrosarcoma in patients with Ollier's disease.

3. CHONDROBLASTOMA

Chondroblastoma is an uncommon benign neoplasm of bone, occurring mainly under age 20. There is a 2:1 male:female preponderance.

- Sites commonly affected are the distal femur, the proximal tibia, and the proximal humerus.
- Chondroblastoma occurs in the epiphyseal region.
- Radiologically, it appears as a well-demarcated lucent lesion that may show calcification.
- Microscopically, it appears as a cellular lesion composed of small uniform round cells and giant cells. Areas of cartilage formation are usually present.

4. GIANT CELL TUMOR OF BONE

Giant cell tumor is a relatively common bone neoplasm that usually occurs in patients in the age group from 20 to 40 years.

- Sites commonly affected are the distal femur, proximal tibia, distal radius, and proximal humerus.
- It is usually located in the epiphyseal region, with expansion of involved bone and thinning of the cortex.
- Radiologically, they appear as a lytic mass traversed by thin sclerotic lines ("soap-bubble" appearance).
- Grossly, composed of soft grayish tissue with hemorrhage and cystic degeneration.
- Microscopically, it shows proliferation of small spindle cells of unknown origin. Numerous osteoclastlike multinucleated giant cells are present.
- Most giant cell tumors are benign, but they have a high (50%) recurrence rate after surgical excision.
- Metastases occur in 10% of giant cell tumors, which must be regarded as being malignant.

5. OSTEOMA

This is an uncommon solitary benign neoplasm, almost totally confined to the skull and facial bones. It occurs commonly in patients with Gardner's syndrome (familial colonic adenomatous polyposis). Pathologically, it is composed of a circumscribed mass of dense sclerotic bone.

6. OSTEOID OSTEOMA

This is an uncommon benign neoplasm of bone, occurring mainly in the 10- to 30-year age group.

- Favored sites include the cortices of the femur, tibia, and humerus.
- Patients typically present with severe pain. X-rays show a well-demarcated lucent area (up to 1.5 cm in diameter) in the cortex with a circumscribed rim of sclerotic reactive bone.
- Microscopic examination shows the central nidus to be highly vascular, with numerous proliferating osteoblasts. The nidus is surrounded by a rim of sclerotic bone.
- Surgical removal is curative.

Metaphysis - Osteoid Osteoma (dt?)
Osteoblastoma (med)
Osteosarcoma (med)
Osteochondroma (ett?)
* Chondrosarcoma (?ues)
* Giant Cell (2 sites)

Epiphysis - Chondroblastoma
* Giant Cell

Diaphysis - Chondroma
Ewing's
* Chondrosarcoma

Other - Periosteal osteosarcoma
Osteoma

TABLE 67-2. BONE NEOPLASMS

Neoplasm	Behavior	Age	Bones Commonly Involved	Location	Histologic Features
Neoplasms of osteoblasts					
Osteoma	Benign	40–50	Skull, facial bones	Flat bones	Dense, mature lamellar bone.
Osteoid osteoma	Benign	10–30	Femur, tibia, humerus, hands and feet, vertebrae	Cortex of metaphysis	Sharply demarcated with a nidus composed of highly vascular osteoblastic connective tissue and osteoid. Surrounded by sclerotic bone; smaller than 2 cm.
Osteoblastoma	Benign; rarely aggressive	10–30	Vertebrae, tibia, femur, humerus, pelvis, ribs	Medulla of metaphysis	Resembles the nidus of osteoid osteoma; larger than 2 cm.
Osteosarcoma	Malignant; 20% 5-year survival rate	10–25	Femur, tibia, humerus, pelvis, jaw	Medulla of metaphysis	Highly cellular, pleomorphic, abnormal osteoblasts with high mitotic rate; osteoid present, invasive.
Parosteal osteosarcoma	Malignant; 80% 5-year survival rate	30–60	Femur, tibia, humerus	Periosteal surface	Spindle cells alternating with bone-forming osteoblasts; well-differentiated.

	Behavior	Age	Bones	Site	Histology
Neoplasms of chondroblasts					
Chondroma	Benign	10–40	Hands and feet, ribs	Diaphysis	Well-differentiated hyaline cartilage.
Osteochondroma (exostosis)	Benign	10–30	Femur, tibia, humerus, pelvis	Cortex of metaphysis	Projecting mass composed of bony stalk and cap of hyaline cartilage.
Chondroblastoma	Benign	10–25	Femur, humerus, tibia, pelvis, scapula, feet	Epiphysis	Uniform small round cells and giant cells; very cellular; chondroid areas.
Chondrosarcoma	Malignant; 30% (grade III) to 90% (grade I) 5-year survival rate	30–60	Pelvis, ribs, femur, vertebrae, humerus	Diaphysis and metaphysis	Malignant chondrocytes with variable anaplasia (grades I–III); chondroid stroma.
Unknown cell of origin					
Giant cell tumor	Benign; 50% recur locally	20–40	Femur, tibia, radius	Metaphysis and epiphysis	Very cellular, small spindle cells with numerous osteoclast-like giant cells.
Ewing's sarcoma	Malignant; 25% 5-year survival rate	5–20	Femur, pelvis, tibia, humerus, ribs, fibula	Diaphysis	Anaplastic small round cells with high mitotic rate.

7. OSTEOBLASTOMA

This is an uncommon bone neoplasm that occurs mainly in the age group from 10 to 30 years.

- They most commonly occur in the vertebrae.
- Patients usually present with pain and radiologically show an irregular lytic lesion.
- Microscopically, osteoblastoma is composed of a highly vascular proliferation of osteoblasts.
- Osteoblastomas are benign. Rarely, they behave in a locally aggressive manner, recurring after surgical removal.

MALIGNANT NEOPLASMS OF BONE

1. OSTEOSARCOMA

This is the commonest malignant neoplasm of bone. It affects mainly individuals in the age group from 10 to 25 years.

- There is a second peak in age incidence in the sixth decade, when osteosarcoma may develop in Paget's disease of bone.
- Osteosarcoma arises most commonly in the medullary cavity of the metaphyseal region of long bones. The lower end of the femur, the upper tibia, and the upper humerus are the commonest locations.
- Grossly, it presents as a fleshy destructive mass with areas of necrosis and hemorrhage. Bone and cartilage formation may be present.
- The tumor may infiltrate the medullary cavity and the soft tissue outside the bone.
- Radiologically, osteosarcomas present as irregular destructive lesions.
- Hematogenous metastasis, most commonly to the lungs, occurs early. Lymphatic metastasis and tumor involvement of lymph nodes is rare.
- Microscopically, osteosarcoma is composed of malignant osteoblasts with anaplasia and a high mitotic rate. Osteoid and bone are present in most cases.
- Based on the degree of anaplasia, osteosarcomas are classified grades I–III. Patients with grade I tumors have longer survival.
- In some tumors, vascular spaces dominate the histologic picture (telangiectatic osteosarcoma).
- Clinically, it presents with a rapidly growing bony mass, with or without pain.
- It is not uncommon for patients to have evidence of pulmonary metastases at the time of presentation.
- Osteosarcoma is sensitive to both radiation and modern chemotherapeutic agents. Surgery is the preferred treatment for early limb lesions.
- The 5-year survival rate is 25–30%.

2. CHONDROSARCOMA

Chondrosarcoma accounts for about 20% of primary malignant neoplasms of bone.

- It is most often seen in persons in the age group from 30 to 60 years.
- Males are affected twice as frequently as females.
- A few cases occur in patients with familial multiple osteochondromatosis and familial enchondromatosis (Ollier's disease).

- The pelvic girdle, ribs, shoulder girdle, long bones, vertebrae, and sternum are the common sites.
- Grossly, chondrosarcoma appears as a large destructive whitish translucent mass.
- Microscopically, they consist of malignant chondrocytes in a chondroid matrix. Three grades are recognized by differences in cellularity and cytologic atypia.
- Clinically, present as a bony mass or fracture.
- Metastasis occurs relatively late and usually through the bloodstream.
- Chondrosarcomas tend to be more radioresistant than osteosarcomas and do not respond to chemotherapy. Surgery is the principal means of treatment.
- The prognosis depends on the grade. The 5-year survival rate is 90% for Grade I and 30–40% for grade III lesions.

3. EWING'S SARCOMA

Ewing's sarcoma is uncommon. It occurs in children and young adults (5–30 years).

- Males are affected twice as frequently as females.
- It is believed to be derived from primitive neuroectodermal cells.
- The tumor cells show the consistent presence of a t (11–22) translocation, and C-*MYC* expression is frequently detectable.
- Ewing's sarcoma arises in the long bones, ribs, pelvic bones, and vertebrae, and expands rapidly to destroy the medullary cavity, bony cortex, and surrounding soft tissues.
- Radiologically, it appears as a destructive radiolucent lesion in the diaphysis, infiltrating the cortex from within.
- Grossly, the neoplasm is soft and friable, with areas of necrosis and hemorrhage.
- Microscopically, it is characterized by sheets of proliferating small round to oval cells with a hyperchromatic nucleus and scant cytoplasm. Mitotic figures are numerous.
- Positive reaction for glycogen with periodic acid-Schiff reagent, and neuron-specific enolase by immunohistochemistry are helpful diagnostic features.
- Ewing's sarcoma is a rapidly growing, highly malignant neoplasm that tends to spread via the bloodstream at an early stage.
- Response to chemotherapy has recently shown improvement.
- The prognosis is poor. The 5-year survival rate is about 10%.

4. LYMPHOID NEOPLASMS

The leukemias, multiple myeloma, and neoplasms of bone marrow are described in Chapters 26, 29, and 30.

Diseases of Joints & Connective Tissue

68

I. DISORDERS OF JOINTS

CONGENITAL DISORDERS OF JOINTS

CONGENITAL DISLOCATION OF THE HIP
This is caused by deficient development of the acetabulum, which allows the femoral head to ride upward out of the joint socket (subluxation) when weight-bearing begins.

- It is much more common in females and shows a familial tendency.
- Unless it is corrected soon after birth, abnormal stresses cause malformation of the developing femoral neck, with a characteristic limp (if unilateral) or waddling gait (if bilateral).
- Treatment consists of splinting of the hips in abduction during the first few months of life to allow development of the acetabulum.

TALIPES EQUINOVARUS & CALCANEOVALGUS (CLUBFOOT)
The two forms of clubfoot represent abnormal articulation of the small bones of the foot. They are caused by abnormal intrauterine forces, abnormal fetal muscle action, or defective ligament insertion.

INFECTIOUS DISEASES OF JOINTS

PYOGENIC ARTHRITIS
This is usually caused by *Staphylococcus aureus*. Less frequently, *Streptococcus pyogenes*, *Streptococcus pneumoniae*, *Neisseria gonorrhoeae*, and *Haemophilus influenzae* are responsible.

- The route of infection is hematogenous.
- In a few patients, pyogenic arthritis complicates acute osteomyelitis.

Pathology & Clinical Features
This is an acute inflammation that commonly involves a single large joint such as the knee or hip.

- It is characterized by severe pain, tenderness, redness, swelling, local warmth, and marked restriction of movement.

- The joint space becomes filled with a purulent exudate.
- High fever, often with chills and a neutrophil leukocytosis, is present in most cases.

Diagnosis & Treatment

Diagnosis of pyogenic arthritis is made by clinical examination.

- Drainage of the joint forms part of the treatment and provides fluid for culture (Table 68–1).
- Antibiotic therapy is usually effective.
- In untreated cases, infection spreads to the articular cartilage and adjacent bone, causing destruction and permanent disability.

TUBERCULOUS ARTHRITIS

Tuberculous arthritis has become rare in developed countries.

- It occurs in adults by reactivation of a dormant tuberculous focus in the joint and is often the only manifestation of tuberculosis in the body.
- It is characterized by involvement of a single large joint, most commonly the knee, hip, or wrist.
- The affected joint is swollen and painful.
- Diagnosis depends on examination of joint fluid (Table 68–1) or examination of a synovial biopsy specimen, which shows caseous granulomas and acid fast bacilli.

LYME DISEASE

Lyme disease is an infection caused by *Borrelia burgdorferi*. It is prevalent in northeastern USA, but cases have been reported elsewhere in the USA and in Europe.

TABLE 68–1. CHANGES IN SYNOVIAL FLUID IN DISEASE OF JOINTS

Disease	Findings
Pyogenic arthritis	Purulent fluid exudate; large numbers of neutrophils; culture positive for bacteria
Tuberculosus arthritis	Fluid exudate (high protein and specific gravity); neutrophils and mononuclear cells; culture positive for *Mycobacterium tuberculosis*
Rheumatoid arthritis	Clear fluid, high protein content; inflammatory cells: neutrophils and mononuclear cells; increased immunoglobulins and complement; rheumatoid factor present in many cases
Osteoarthrosis	Clear fluid, high protein content; no inflammatory cells
Gout	Urate crystals
Chondrocalcinosis	Calcium pyrophosphate crystals

■ The disease is transmitted by ixodid ticks, which become infected by biting deer and mice, the common reservoirs of infection.

■ Lyme disease is characterized by:
  ● A distinctive papular skin rash (erythema migrans) at the site of inoculation 1–4 weeks after the tick bite.
  ● Migratory acute arthritis, followed by chronic arthritis.
  ● Myocarditis and neurologic abnormalities.

■ Diagnosis of Lyme disease is confirmed by serologic tests. Demonstration of the spirochete in blood or infected tissues is rarely successful.

■ Treatment with penicillin is successful if started early.

IMMUNOLOGIC DISEASES OF JOINTS

RHEUMATOID ARTHRITIS

Incidence

Rheumatoid arthritis is common in the United States and Western Europe, affecting 1–3% of the population.

■ Females are affected 2–3 times more frequently than males.
■ The highest age incidence is between 30 and 50 years.
■ Rheumatoid arthritis is uncommon in tropical countries.

Etiology

The cause of rheumatoid arthritis is unknown, but evidence suggests an immunologic basis.

■ Rheumatoid factor—an autoantibody (usually IgM) reactive against the patient's own IgG—is present in the plasma of about 90% of patients.
■ Immune complexes composed of rheumatoid factor and IgG have been found in synovial fluid of some patients.
■ Complement levels are frequently decreased in active disease.

Pathology

The synovial membrane of affected joints becomes swollen, congested, and thickened, with granulation tissue containing numerous lymphocytes and plasma cells (pannus).

■ The pannus erodes articular cartilage, subchondral bone, and periarticular ligaments and tendons.
■ Progressive destruction of the joint follows, with fibrosis, increasing deformity, and restriction of movement.

Clinical Features

Typically, it presents with symmetric involvement of the small joints of the hands and feet—classically, the proximal interphalangeal joints.

■ Involved joints are swollen, painful, and stiff.
■ Swelling of the proximal interphalangeal joints produces a typical spindled appearance of the fingers.

- Many patients have systemic symptoms such as low-grade fever, weakness, and malaise.
- Joint deformity occurs early in severe cases.

Extra-articular Manifestations

In a minority of patients, tissues other than joints show significant pathologic change (Table 68–2).

TABLE 68–2. RHEUMATOID ARTHRITIS: SYSTEMIC MANIFESTATIONS AND LABORATORY FINDINGS

Systemic Manifestations	Description
Pyrexia, malaise	Mechanism unknown; ?lymphokines
Rheumatoid nodules	Subcutaneous granulomas with a central area of fibrinoid necrosis of connective tissue; tender 1- to 2-cm nodules at elbow and wrist particularly
Vasculitis	Particularly endarteritis; may lead to skin ulcers (ischemia), Raynaud's phenomenon, and peripheral neuropathy
Cardiac lesions	The myocardium is rarely involved (arrhythmias); pericarditis occurs in 10%
Lung lesions	Pleuritis, pleural effusions; large necrotizing rheumatoid nodules in lung; diffuse pulmonary fibrosis; nodular fibrosis of lung (in miners exposed to coal dust: Caplan's syndrome)
Neurologic lesions	Peripheral neuropathy (due to arteritis); mononeuropathy due to spinal nerve compression; carpal tunnel syndrome (median nerve compression); cervical cord compression (atlantoaxial joint involvement)
Ocular lesions	Keratitis, scleritis, granulomas, uveitis (iris inflamed)
Amyloidosis	Primary pattern of distribution (see Chapter 2)
Lymphadenopathy, splenomegaly	In up to 25% of cases, especially in juvenile form (Still's disease) and Felty's syndrome

Laboratory findings
Positive rheumatoid factor (90% of classic adult cases but < 20% of childhood cases)
Leukocytosis common (leukopenia in Felty's syndrome)
Raised erythrocyte sedimentation rate
Polyclonal hypergammaglobulinemia (in 50%)
Positive ANA (antinuclear antibody), usually in low titer (10–40%)

Course & Prognosis

Rheumatoid arthritis is usually slowly progressive.

■ In 10–20% of patients, the disease remits completely after the first attack.
■ Most other patients go on to develop a chronic disease characterized by relapses and remissions, with slowly progressive disability from joint destruction.
■ After 10 years of disease, about 10% of patients are severely disabled while about 50% are still fully employed.
■ Poor prognostic factors include:
  ● A classic pattern of disease with high levels of rheumatoid factor in the serum.
  ● The presence of rheumatoid nodules.
  ● Onset of disease before age 30 years.

VARIANTS OF RHEUMATOID ARTHRITIS

1. FELTY'S SYNDROME

This occurs in older individuals with long-standing rheumatoid arthritis and high titers of rheumatoid factor. It is characterized by splenic enlargement and evidence of hypersplenism, resulting in granulocytopenia, anemia, and thrombocytopenia.

2. SJÖGREN'S SYNDROME

Sjögren's syndrome is commonly associated with rheumatoid arthritis (see Chapter 31).

3. JUVENILE RHEUMATOID ARTHRITIS (Still's Disease)

Still's disease is rheumatoid arthritis in a patient under 16 years of age. It is characterized by acute onset with high fever, leukocytosis, splenomegaly, arthritis, and skin rash.

■ Pericarditis and uveitis may also occur.
■ Rheumatoid factor is usually not present.
■ Patients commonly have monarticular involvement, frequently of a large joint.
■ Fifty percent of patients undergo complete remission. Others progress to severe joint disease with extra-articular manifestations.

DEGENERATIVE JOINT DISEASES

ANKYLOSING SPONDYLITIS

Ankylosing spondylitis is a common disease affecting 0.5% of the population in the United States.

■ Predominantly it affects young men (males:females = 8:1), the maximum age incidence being between 15 and 30 years.
■ It has a very strong association with HLA-B27, which is present in the cells of 95% of patients with ankylosing spondylitis, compared with 3–7% of the general population.
■ The cause is unknown.

Pathology & Clinical Features

■ It maximally affects the sacroiliac joints.

- Chronic inflammation is associated with fibrosis and calcification, leading to bony fusion (ankylosis) of the joints.
- Low back pain and stiffness are the common presenting symptoms.
- Calcification of the vertebral joints and paravertebral ligaments produces a characteristic radiologic appearance ("bamboo spine"), and marked immobility of the lower back.
- Ankylosing spondylitis progresses slowly up the vertebral column.
- Involvement of the costovertebral joints and thoracic spine may result in restriction of chest expansion and rarely produces respiratory failure.

Extra-Articular Manifestations
Patients with ankylosing spondylitis may show degeneration of the media of the aorta, causing aortic valve incompetence, aortic dissection and aortic rupture. Twenty-five percent of patients have eye changes, most commonly iridocyclitis. Pulmonary fibrosis occurs in a few patients.

Course & Prognosis
Ankylosing spondylitis is a slowly progressive disease that causes increasing disability from pain and stiffness of the low back. Respiratory dysfunction and aortic disease represent life-threatening complications.

OSTEOARTHROSIS (Osteoarthritis)
Osteoarthrosis is a common degenerative joint disease characterized by primary abnormalities in the articular cartilage.

- Changes of osteoarthrosis are present in over 90% of individuals over age 50.
- Though only a few of these patients are symptomatic, osteoarthritis is the commonest cause of joint disability.

Etiology
Osteoarthrosis is caused by degeneration of articular cartilage of joints (Fig 68–1).

- The cause of articular cartilage degeneration is not known.
- Abnormalities in the ground substance, collagen, lysosomal enzyme activity, and changes in water content have been demonstrated in the articular cartilage in patients with osteoarthrosis.
- A few cases of osteoarthrosis occur secondary to articular cartilage diseases (eg, alkaptonuria) and severe trauma (eg, in football players).

Pathology (Fig 68–1)
The large weight-bearing joints of the vertebral column, hips, and knees are most affected, along with the distal interphalangeal joints of the fingers.

- The primary abnormality is thinning and fragmentation of the articular cartilage. The normally smooth, white articular surface becomes irregular and yellow.
- Continued loss of articular cartilage leads to exposure of subchondral bone, which appears as shiny foci on the articular surface (eburnation).
- Fibrosis, increased bone formation, and cystic change frequently occur in the underlying bone.

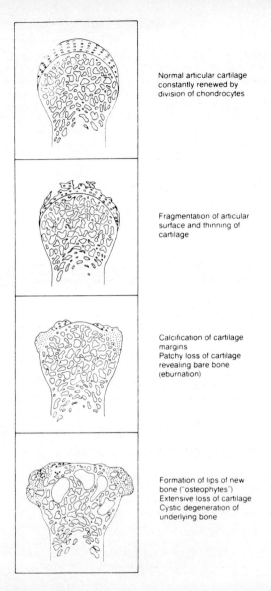

Normal articular cartilage constantly renewed by division of chondrocytes

Fragmentation of articular surface and thinning of cartilage

Calcification of cartilage margins
Patchy loss of cartilage revealing bare bone (eburnation)

Formation of lips of new bone ("osteophytes")
Extensive loss of cartilage
Cystic degeneration of underlying bone

Figure 68–1. Pathologic features of osteoarthrosis. Degeneration of the articular cartilage may result in fragments of cartilage breaking free into the joint space as loose bodies ("joint mice").

■ The loss of articular cartilage stimulates new bone formation, usually in the form of nodules (osteophytes) at the bone edges.
■ Inflammation is absent.

Clinical Features
There is pain, stiffness, and swelling of affected joints, with no evidence of acute inflammation.

■ Crepitus, a grating sound produced by friction between adjacent areas of exposed subchondral bone, is common.
■ Osteophytes may:
  ● Be visible clinically as bony masses, eg, Heberden's nodes over affected distal interphalangeal joints.
  ● Cause compressive symptoms, most notably in spinal osteoarthrosis, in which nerve and spinal cord compression may occur.

Course & Prognosis
Osteoarthrosis is a slowly progressive, chronic joint disability. Recent advancements in the technique of joint replacement with prostheses have improved the outlook of these patients considerably.

NEUROPATHIC JOINT (Charcot's Joint)
This results from loss of sensory innervation to the joint, as occurs in peripheral neuropathy, tabes dorsalis, diabetic neuropathy, and syringomyelia.

■ The lack of pain and protective reflexes result in progressive destruction of the joint with trauma.
■ Large joints such as the knees are usually involved.
■ The affected joint is swollen, unstable, and frequently shows an abnormally increased range of motion resulting from destruction of intra-articular ligaments.
■ The joint involvement is painless.

METABOLIC DISEASES OF JOINTS

ALKAPTONURIA (Ochronosis)
Alkaptonuria is a rare autosomal recessive disease in which there is a deficiency of homogentisic acid oxidase.

■ It is characterized by deposition of homogentisic acid in:
  ● Collagen (dermis, ligaments, tendons, endocardium, the intimal surfaces of blood vessels).
  ● Cartilage (nose, ear, larynx, tracheobronchial tree, intervertebral disks, and joint spaces).
■ All of these areas become black and radiopaque.
■ Diagnosis is made by detecting homogentisic acid in the urine. This is done at routine neonatal screening.
■ The major clinical effect of alkaptonuria is degeneration of affected cartilages, resulting in juvenile osteoarthrosis.

GOUT (Gouty Arthritis)

Etiology
Gout is the result of deposition of urate crystals in connective tissues, associated with elevated plasma uric acid levels.

A. Primary gout occurs mainly in elderly men and has a strong familial tendency. The basic abnormality in urate metabolism is not known, but it results in hyperuricemia.

B. Secondary gout occurs in diseases in which excess breakdown of purines leads to increased uric acid synthesis. It is most commonly seen in patients with leukemia, particularly at the start of treatment, when there is marked cell necrosis.

Pathologic and Clinical Features
A. Acute gouty arthritis is caused by deposition of microcrystals of sodium urate in the synovial membranes of joints.

- The first metatarsophalangeal joint (big toe) is affected in 85% of cases.
- Urate microcrystals produce an intense acute inflammation.
- The urate microcrystals can be recognized in joint fluid as birefringent needle-shaped crystals under polarized light.

B. Chronic tophaceous gout is the result of deposition of sodium urate as large amorphous masses known as *tophi*.

- Tophi occur commonly in the cartilage of the ear and around joints.
- Chronic inflammation and marked deformity result.
- Microscopically, tophi appear as pale pink amorphous masses surrounded by a foreign body type granulomatous reaction.
- Urate crystals can be identified by polarized light in tissue sections.

CALCIUM PYROPHOSPHATE DEPOSITION DISEASE (Chondrocalcinosis; Pseudogout)
This is a degenerative joint disease characterized by deposition of calcium pyrophosphate in the joints. Most cases involve the knee joints after trauma or surgery.

- Clinically, it is characterized by an acute arthritis involving one or many joints, most commonly the large joints of the lower extremity.
- The arthritis is self-limited, lasting 1–4 weeks.
- The synovial fluid contains numerous leukocytes and calcium pyrophosphate crystals, which are short and rhomboid and can be distinguished from urate crystals by their polarization characteristics.

TUMORS OF JOINTS

PIGMENTED VILLONODULAR SYNOVITIS
This is an uncommon disease characterized by proliferation of the synovial membrane of joints. It occurs in adults and most commonly involves the knee joint.

- Clinically, there is pain, swelling, and progressively increasing joint disability.
- The cause is unknown. It is believed that the lesion is a reactive and not neoplastic process.

- Grossly, the synovial membrane is thickened and shows orange-brown villous outgrowths.
- Microscopically, the villi consist of proliferating synovial epithelial cells, lymphocytes, plasma cells, and histiocytes, many of which contain hemosiderin. Multinucleated giant cells are frequently present.
- Surgical or arthroscopic removal of the abnormal synovium is effective, but local recurrence may occur.

SYNOVIAL CHONDROMATOSIS

This is an uncommon condition of unknown cause characterized by the occurrence of multiple foci of cartilaginous metaplasia in the synovial membrane.

- The cartilage appears as nodules that may undergo ossification and may become detached into the joint cavity as "loose bodies."
- The knee is commonly affected, with symptoms of pain, swelling, limitation of movement, and intermittent locking.
- Osteoarthrosis may result.

GANGLION

This is a common cystic lesion arising in the connective tissue of the joint capsule or in a tendon sheath. It most commonly occurs around the wrist.

- Microscopically, it is a cystic structure filled with myxomatous tissue and lined by collagen.
- Except for producing a lump, ganglions are of no significance clinically.

GIANT CELL TUMOR OF TENDON SHEATH

Giant cell tumor of tendon sheath is the only common benign neoplasm that involves the synovium.

- It occurs either inside the joint—usually the knee—or in relation to the tendon sheaths in the hands and feet.
- It presents as a mass that may become large and cause erosion of adjacent bone.
- Histologically, there is an admixture of foamy macrophages, multinucleated giant cells, and fibroblasts (**benign fibrous histiocytoma** is an alternative name).
- Treatment is surgical removal, which is curative.

SYNOVIAL SARCOMA

Synovial sarcoma is a rare malignant neoplasm arising from synovial epithelial cells.

- They occur much more commonly in relation to bursae and tendon sheaths than within joints.
- They tend to present as extra-articular soft tissue masses, most commonly near a joint in the extremities.
- Microscopically, they are highly cellular neoplasms with a biphasic pattern, being composed of spindle cells and epithelium-lined slit-like spaces.
- The cells contain keratin intermediate filaments in addition to vimentin.
- Synovial sarcomas are high-grade malignant neoplasms with a high rate of local recurrence and metastasis.
- They have a 5-year survival rate of about 50%.

II. DISEASES OF EXTRASKELETAL CONNECTIVE TISSUE

AUTOIMMUNE CONNECTIVE TISSUE DISEASES (Collagen Diseases)
This is a group of diseases characterized by:

- Involvement of multiple tissues.
- Evidence for an autoimmune basis.
- The presence of antinuclear antibodies in the serum.
- Inflammation of small blood vessels (vasculitis), frequently with fibrinoid necrosis of the wall.
- Polyarteritis nodosa (see Chapter 20), rheumatoid arthritis, and rheumatic fever (Chapter 22) are sometimes included within this category.

LUPUS ERYTHEMATOSUS
Lupus erythematosus exists in two clinical forms:

- Systemic lupus erythematosus (SLE), which is a progressive and often severe condition involving multiple systems.
- Discoid lupus erythematosus, in which skin involvement dominates the clinical picture (see Chapter 61).

Incidence
SLE is common in the United States, more so in blacks than whites. The disease is also common in Western Europe but less so in Asia. Women are affected 10 times more frequently than men. The usual age at onset of disease is 20–40 years.

Etiology
It is mediated by an abnormal immune response associated with the presence of antinuclear antibodies and immune complexes in the plasma (Fig 68–2). The cause of this response is widely believed to be autoimmune, though there is evidence for viral and genetic influences.

- A variety of antinuclear antibodies are present in the serum of all patients with systemic lupus erythematosus. Antibody against double-stranded DNA is highly specific for lupus erythematosus.
- Autoantibodies other than antinuclear antibodies found in SLE include:
  - Rheumatoid factor (20–30%).
  - Antibodies that give a false-positive reaction in serologic tests for syphilis.
  - Antibodies against plasma coagulation proteins, most commonly factor VIII, producing a bleeding diathesis.
  - Antibodies against antigens on erythrocytes, leukocytes, and platelets, which may lead to immune destruction of these cells.
- SLE is precipitated by drugs such as hydralazine and procainamide. Drug-induced SLE is similar to idiopathic SLE, including the presence of antinuclear antibodies. Withdrawal of the drug causes reversal of the disease.
- SLE is associated with the histocompatibility antigen HLA-DR2.

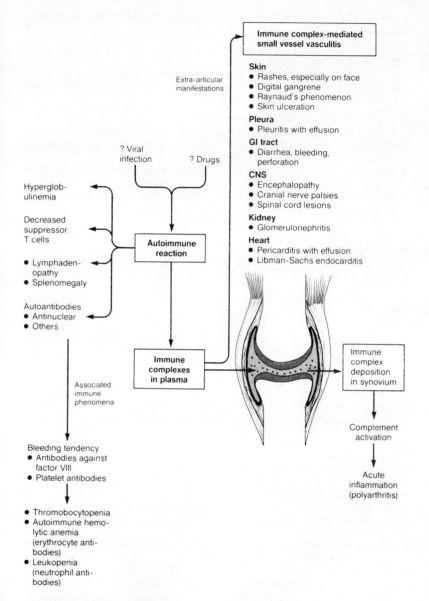

Figure 68–2. Etiologic factors and pathogenesis of systemic lupus erythematosus.

■ Patients with inherited deficiency of early complement factors (C1, C2, and C4) have an increased incidence of SLE.

Pathology & Clinical Features

Sites of immune complex deposition show evidence of tissue necrosis and acute inflammation. The pattern of disease in an individual patient depends on where immune complex injury takes place.

■ Acute small vessel vasculitis with ischemia:
  ● Is characterized by fibrinoid necrosis and inflammation of the media and thrombosis.
  ● Commonly affects the skin (digital gangrene and ulceration) and the gastrointestinal tract (diarrhea, bleeding, and perforation).
■ Hyperplasia of the lymphoid system causing enlargement of lymph nodes or spleen occurs in 50% of patients.
■ Skin involvement is present in 70% of patients and is characterized by:
  ● Immune complex deposition in the basement membrane.
  ● Erythematous rash, typically over the malar regions of the face ("butterfly rash").

■ Arthritis or arthralgia occurs in 90% of patients with SLE. Both large and small joints may be involved. Joint involvement in SLE is usually mild without deformity.
■ Cardiac lesions include pericarditis with effusion, myocarditis, and Libman-Sachs endocarditis (see Chapter 22).
■ Central nervous system involvement occurs in 25% of patients. Clinical manifestations include convulsions, psychosis, cranial nerve palsies, and spinal cord dysfunction.
■ Renal involvement occurs in approximately two-thirds of patients and represents the most common mode of death in SLE (see Chapter 48).

Diagnosis

The diagnosis of lupus erythematosus is confirmed by demonstration of serum antinuclear antibodies (ANA), particularly anti-double-stranded DNA. Less than 5% of patients with SLE are ANA-negative. Histologic examination of tissues such as the skin and kidney is often of diagnostic value.

Course & Prognosis

The course of SLE is variable.

■ Rarely, patients have a severe acute illness.
■ Most patients pursue a chronic course, with repeated exacerbations and remissions.
■ Corticosteroid therapy is usually effective in controlling exacerbations.
■ The survival rate is approximately 90% at 10 years.
■ Patients with discoid lupus erythematosus have a chronic skin disorder. About 10% of patients develop SLE.

PROGRESSIVE SYSTEMIC SCLEROSIS (Scleroderma)

This is an uncommon connective tissue disease characterized by vasculitis affecting small vessels and widespread deposition of collagen. It occurs more commonly in females and has its onset most frequently in the ages from 20 to 50 years.

Etiology

This is an autoimmune disorder closely related to SLE.

- Antinuclear antibodies are usually present in the serum.
- The most characteristic antinuclear antibody for progressive systemic sclerosis has specificity against nucleolar RNA.
- Deposition of immune complexes in tissues has been demonstrated in renal and vascular lesions.
- The mechanism underlying the excessive fibrosis is unknown.

Pathology

Pathologic changes in affected tissue include small vessel vasculitis, which is identical histologically with that seen in SLE.

- The disease tends to be chronic and marked fibrosis dominates the histologic appearance.
- Skin involvement is characterized by:
  - Initial edema, with vasculitis and often petechial hemorrhages.
  - Progressive fibrosis, involving the entire dermis and extending to the subcutaneous tissue.
  - Thinning of the epidermis, and atrophy of all adnexal structures (hair, sweat glands, etc).
  - Enlargement of vessels visible as telangiectases.
  - Trophic ulceration and dystrophic calcification.

Clinical Features

Progressive systemic sclerosis usually has an insidious onset. Systemic symptoms are uncommon.

- In many patients, the disease is restricted to the skin for many years before visceral involvement occurs.
- The skin is affected in 90% of cases, with involvement of fingers (claw-like hands) and face (restricted movements) being most common. Raynaud's phenomenon may occur.
- Gastrointestinal manifestation occur in 60% of patients, and include:
  - Esophageal fibrosis, causing dysphagia.
  - Small intestine fibrosis, which causes deficient peristalsis and malabsorption.
- Sixty percent of cases have evidence of glomerular and vascular changes due to immune complex deposition (see Chapter 48).
- Twenty percent of patients develop a diffuse pneumonitis and fibrosis (see Chapter 35). The end stage is a honeycomb lung with respiratory failure.

Course

The clinical course is usually chronic. The occurrence of symptomatic visceral disease (especially renal disease) is an ominous sign. Treatment with immunosuppressive drugs is of limited value.

POLYMYOSITIS-DERMATOMYOSITIS

This is an uncommon connective tissue disease affecting women twice as frequently as men.

■ Onset of disease is maximal between the ages of 40 and 60 years.
■ Antinuclear antibodies occur in the serum of most patients, and immune complex deposition can be demonstrated in many cases of dermatomyositis.
■ Patients with polymyositis-dermatomyositis have an increased risk for malignant neoplasms, mainly carcinoma of the lung.

Pathology & Clinical Features

It is a chronic disease that affects skeletal muscle in all cases and skin in 50% of cases. Visceral involvement is uncommon.

■ Myositis commonly affects the proximal muscles of the limb girdles.
■ In the acute phase, affected muscles slow edema, lymphocytic infiltration, and necrosis.
■ Chronic disease is characterized by muscle atrophy and fibrosis.
■ Clinically, there is muscle weakness associated with pain and tenderness.
■ In the acute phase, serum creatine kinase and aldolase levels are greatly elevated, and creatinuria may accompany muscle necrosis.
■ Muscle biopsy is useful to differentiate polymyositis from muscular dystrophy.
■ Skin changes:
  ● Result from a vasculitis.
  ● Typically consists of a violaceous edematous rash (heliotrope rash) involving the upper eyelids.
  ● Rayneud's phenomenon occurs in 30% of patients.
  ● Dermal atrophy and calcification occur in the later stages.

Course

Polymyositis-dermatomyositis has a chronic course characterized by increasing disability from muscle wasting. The main danger of the disease is from the associated malignant neoplasms.

MIXED CONNECTIVE TISSUE DISEASE

This is an uncommon disease with clinical features that overlap with systemic lupus erythematosus, progressive systemic sclerosis, and polymyositis ("overlap syndrome").

■ It is characterized by the presence in the serum of a high titer of antibodies against ribonucleoprotein.
■ Mixed connective tissue disease tends to run a more benign course than SLE, mainly due to a lesser frequency of renal involvement.

SOFT TISSUE NEOPLASMS

Soft tissue neoplasms may arise from any mesenchymal cell in extraskeletal connective tissue (Table 68–3).

■ Neoplasms of blood vessels (see Chapter 20), nerves (Chapter 66), and skeletal muscle (Chapter 66) have been considered elsewhere.
■ Benign soft tissue neoplasms are very common. Lipomas and hemangiomas are among the commonest neoplasms occurring in humans.
■ Malignant soft tissue neoplasms are rare.
■ Soft tissue neoplasms occur in almost any tissue of the body. They are most commonly found in the extremities and retroperitoneum.

TABLE 68–3. NEOPLASMS OF CONNECTIVE TISSUE ("SOFT TISSUE" NEOPLASMS)

Cell of Origin	Benign[1]	Low-Grade Malignant,[1] Locally Aggressive	Malignant[1]
Fibroblast	Fibroma	Fibromatosis, fibrosarcoma (low-grade)	Fibrosarcoma (high-grade)
Adipocyte	Lipoma, hibernoma	Liposarcoma (well-differentiated and myxoid)	Liposarcoma (pleomorphic and round cell)
Nerve sheath	Neurofibroma, schwannoma, granular cell tumor		Malignant peripheral nerve sheath tumor
Fibrohistiocyte	Fibroxanthoma, dermatofibroma	Atypical fibroxanthoma, dermatofibrosarcoma protuberans	Malignant fibrous histiocytoma
Smooth muscle	Leiomyoma	Leiomyosarcoma (low-grade)	Leiomyosarcoma (high-grade)
Skeletal muscle	Rhabdomyoma		Rhabdomyosarcoma
Vascular	Hemangioma	Hemangiopericytoma, hemangioendothelioma (low-grade)	Angiosarcoma, Kaposi's sarcoma
Synovial	Giant cell tumor of tendon sheath		Synovial sarcoma
Unknown			Ewing's sarcoma (extra-skeletal), alveolar soft part sarcoma, clear cell sarcoma,[2] epithelioid sarcoma

[1] Benign neoplasms are cured by surgical removal. Low-grade malignant soft tissue neoplasms are locally infiltrative and tend to recur locally after surgical removal. Their metastatic potential is low. Malignant neoplasms have a high metastatic potential as well as local infiltrative properties.
[2] Cells comprising clear cell sarcoma have been shown to contain melanosomes, and this neoplasm is now also called malignant melanoma of soft tissue.

BENIGN SOFT TISSUE NEOPLASMS

These are well-circumscribed encapsulated nodular masses that closely resemble the tissue of origin.

■ Local excision is curative.
■ Rarely, neurofibromas and lipomas occur in families, being inherited as an autosomal dominant trait—generalized neurofibromatosis (von Recklinghausen's disease), and generalized lipomatosis (Dercum's disease).

LOCALLY AGGRESSIVE SOFT TISSUE NEOPLASMS

This group of soft tissue neoplasms are locally infiltrative and tend to recur after surgical excision. They rarely metastasize.

- The best examples of this group are the fibromatoses (desmoid tumors), which:
  - Occur in skeletal muscle, most common in the rectus abdominis muscle.
  - Are slow-growing neoplasms that form large masses with extensive local infiltration along fascial planes, often with extensive tissue destruction.
- Unless excised with an adequately wide margin, the tumor recurs locally, often after several years.
- Despite their locally aggressive behavior which may result in death, desmoid tumors do not metastasize.

MALIGNANT SOFT TISSUE NEOPLASMS (Sarcomas)

Sarcomas are classified according to the cell of origin. They are generally much less common than carcinomas. The most common type of sarcomas are malignant fibrous hystiocytoma and liposarcoma.

- Sarcomas usually present as a soft tissue mass, often of large size. The extremities and retroperitoneum are the most common sites.
- The biologic behavior of sarcomas is extremely variable.

High-Grade Sarcomas

These are highly cellular neoplasms, being composed of poorly differentiated mesenchymal cells.

- They show necrosis and have a high mitotic rate.
- Because of their anaplasia, high-grade sarcomas are sometimes difficult to classify.
- Recognition of the cell of origin is sometimes possible by:
  - Immunohistologic techniques, demonstrating factor VIII antigen (angiosarcoma), myoglobin, desmin, and actin (myosarcomas), or keratin (synovial sarcoma).
  - Electron microscopic identification of differentiation towards striated muscle, lipoblasts, or Schwann cells.
- High-grade sarcomas grow rapidly, show extensive local invasion, and tend to metastasize early through the bloodstream.
- They are usually fatal, treatment being rarely successful.

Low-Grade Sarcomas

These are better-differentiated, less cellular, and tend to resemble the tissue of origin to some extent.

- They are characterized by a slower growth rate, a high risk of local recurrence after surgical removal, and a relatively low risk of metastasis.
- Patients typically survive a long time, with repeated local recurrences after surgery.
- Treatment of soft tissue sarcomas include:
  - Surgical removal of the tumor with a wide margin of normal surrounding tissue.
  - Radiotherapy is of limited value, mainly for local control of recurrences.
  - Chemotherapy, particularly preoperative intra-arterial chemotherapy, has proved to be of some benefit.

Index